THE PSYCHIATRIC THERAPIES

APA COMMISSION ON PSYCHIATRIC THERAPIES

THE PSYCHIATRIC THERAPIES

**The American Psychiatric Association
Commission on Psychiatric Therapies**

Chaired by Toksoz B. Karasu, M.D.

Published by the
American Psychiatric Association
1400 K Street, NW
Washington, DC 20005

NOTE: The contributors have worked to ensure that all information in this book concerning drug dosages, schedules, and routes of administration is accurate at the time of publication and consistent with standards set by the U.S. Food and Drug Administration and the general medical community. As medical research and practice advance, however, therapeutic standards may change. For this reason and because human and mechanical errors sometimes occur, we recommend that readers follow the advice of a physician directly involved in their care or the care of a member of their family.

Cover design: Tom Jones/Jane Kearns, Inc.
Text design: Richard E. Farkas
Typesetting: Unicorn Graphics
Printing: Port City Press

Library of Congress Cataloging in Publication Data
Main entry under title:

The Psychiatric therapies.

Editor: Toksoz B. Karasu.
Each pt. also issued separately.
Includes bibliographies and index.
Contents: pt. 1. The somatic therapies — pt. 2.
The psychosocial therapies.
    1. Psychotherapy. I. Karasu, Toksoz B. II. American
Psychiatric Association. Commission on Psychiatric
Therapies. [DNLM: 1. Mental disorders—Therapy. WM 400
P9734]
RC480.P78   1984   616.89′.1   84-3053
ISBN 0-89042-102-1

0-89042-102-1	The Psychiatric Therapies	(Part I and Part II casebound edition)
0-89042-104-8	The Somatic Therapies	(Part I paperback edition)
0-89042-103-X	The Psychosocial Therapies	(Part II paperback edition)

Printed in the U.S.A.

ACKNOWLEDGMENTS

I would like to express my thanks to the many people without whom this volume would not have been possible. My gratitude is extended to Jules H. Masserman, M.D., Donald G. Langsley, M.D., Daniel X. Freedman, M.D., H. Keith H. Brodie, M.D., and George Tarjan, M.D., who have served as Presidents of the American Psychiatric Association during the lifetime of the APA Commission on Psychiatric Therapies. They have given us unfailing support. My special thanks to Melvin Sabshin, M.D., Medical Director of the APA, for his loyal support, personal encouragement, and extraordinary commitment to this project. A special word of thanks to Judy Baker, APA Staff Liaison, for her dedication, steadfastness, and organizational ability.

I am most grateful to the members of the APA Commission on Psychiatric Therapies, the consultants, and the cooperative, altruistic authors who allowed their original work to be modified through the consultation process.

My sincere appreciation to Ronald McMillen, General Manager of the American Psychiatric Press, Inc., for his invaluable guidance, and to Richard E. Farkas, Production Manager, for his many suggestions. My gratitude is also extended to Margaret McDonald, who has faithfully edited and re-edited every chapter through the review process.

Also, I want to express my special gratitude to Louise Notarangelo, Philomena Lee, Rita Segarra, and Shirley Kreitman, who have typed and corrected the final drafts with great patience, diligence and exuberance.

Toksoz Byram Karasu

Contents

INTRODUCTION

By asking the impossible,
obtain the best possible.
—Italian Proverb

In 1977 Jules Masserman, M.D., as President of the American Psychiatric Association, appointed a Commission on Psychiatric Therapies and, with the approval of the Board of Trustees, charged the Commission to: (a) assay as many as possible of the somatic, dyadic, group, familial, and social therapies in current use by a thorough and critical examination of the literature as to techniques, duration, results, costs, and other characteristics; (b) gather other data from previous APA committee and task force reports by consultation with advocates of differing modalities, by direct observation of various treatments where practicable, by the viewing of video tapes, by supplementary questionnaires and by other means; and (c) analyze the findings as to the common vectors that are therapeutically effective, as distinguished from procedures that may be extraneous or counterproductive.

After considerable discussion and review of the current literature, the Commission decided to pursue two major goals. The first was the development of a volume that delineated the methodological problems of research in psychotherapy and that also examined in detail the literature regarding the efficacy of the various psychotherapies. This task has been completed; and the volume entitled "Psychotherapy Research: Methodological & Efficacy Issues," was published by APA in 1982.

The second goal of the Commission was to provide an overview of all psychiatric therapies currently practiced in the United States. We hope this volume fulfills that goal. In order to facilitate the presentation of this material and to maintain the integrity of each modality, the book includes chapters divided into two parts: Part I deals with "Somatic Therapies" and Part II with "Psychosocial Therapies." However, neither the division between Part I and Part II nor the divisions between the chapters imply their mutual exclusiveness in clinical application. Rather, didactic presentation necessitates the arbitrary drawing of some lines. In actual practice, there has been a trend toward theoretical and technical integration of multiple psychosocial and somatic approaches.

For the most part, we have limited ourselves to well established and widely practiced therapies. However, in Chapter 6, under the title "Other Somatic Therapies," we have reviewed relatively outdated, relatively new, or less common practices to give the most comprehensive presentation possible. And in Chapter 11 under the title "Experiential, Inspirational, Cognitive/Emotive and Other Therapies," we have reviewed some of the less traditional therapies. Strictly speaking, some of these may not be considered as therapies; nevertheless, they are often used by individuals who may be in psychological distress. Finally, some of the therapies that may fall between the somatic and psychosocial spheres appear in either Part I or II. There are some therapies that we did not cover (i.e., transcultural therapy, etc.) but the field does not lend itself to being exhaustive.

Because of the complex and sometimes overlapping boundaries of the treatments under discussion, readers may find some repetition in certain areas. In fact, a great deal of discussion went into making what may appear to be minor distinctions. Moreover, the length of the chapters varies, and not necessarily in proportion to the breadth or importance of the treatment modalities under discussion.

There is no single source available which systematically and comprehensively deals with all psychiatric treatments. Although there are publications that describe some of the therapies, many reflect the views of one or a few individuals. In contrast, the aim of the Commission was to establish a consultative process involving many individuals and viewpoints. We have held a relatively open attitude toward the different therapies, however, and have made no attempt to formulate a common language with which to describe them. Each therapeutic approach has been presented in its own terms.

The contributors and consultants to the present project were chosen by the Commission from many well qualified individuals on the basis of their national reputation, past accomplishments, and broad perspectives. This method of selecting contributors and consultants and the desire for integration and synthesis of divergent views led to multiple responses and challenges. We believe this approach has had a salutary effect on the outcome of the chapters.

In order to achieve some degree of uniformity in the presentation of the material, the contributors were requested to follow a standard format which included sections devoted to the historical background of the mode of therapy under consideration; the basic theoretical issues implicit or explicit in its formulation; and a description of its strategies and techniques, indications and limitations and developmental and age-related issues. In some therapies the latter issues were large enough to justify separate chapters. Other areas contributors were to address included the nature of the training required of the therapist and financial, legal, and ethical aspects of the therapies. Some contributors deviated from these guidelines in order to present the unique aspects of each therapy in the most effective way.

Once a draft was prepared by the contributor or contributors selected by the Commission, it was then sent to three to five consultants, chosen by the contributor(s) for comments. Draft II was then prepared by the contributors(s) on the basis of the consultants' suggestions. The Commission then sent Draft II without the names of the author(s) to five to ten consultants considered experts in that field. A special effort was made to consult individuals with various views. The comments and critiques of these individuals were then sent to the original contributor(s) for preparation of Draft III. Draft III was then reviewed and finalized by the Commisssion. This complex process of consultation and review produced chapters that reflect the input and ideas not only of the contributors but of the members of the Commission and its consultants.

A few other points should be made about the content and structure of the chapters. For the most part, the chapters do not deal with diagnostic issues except as related specifically to a given form of treatment, e.g., sexual dysfunctions.

With two exceptions, (interpersonal therapy and cognitive/behavior therapy), wherein practice and research have been inextricably linked, questions of efficacy, evaluation, and research for all psychosocial therapies were dealt with collectively in one chapter, rather than individually, because of common methodological issues. Likewise, issues related to treatment planning for all therapies have been incorporated into the first two chapters.

* * * * * * * * * *

Future directions will entail increasing refinement of significant variables toward a greater understanding of individual differences in response to somatotherapies and psychotherapies. Such refinement will depend on further research, which must take into account specific interventions. Future work must also consider specific disorders or patient subgroups of responders and nonresponders, specific doses, durations, and combinations and sequences of treatment - in short, the ultimate establishment of carefully delineated criteria for selecting and timing psychiatric therapies.

T. B. K.

Contributors to Part I

Ross J. Baldessarini, M.D.
Professor of Psychiatry and Neuroscience
Harvard Medical School
Interim Director, Laboratories for Psychiatric Research
Mailman Research Center, McLean Hospital
Belmont, MA

John Donnelly, M.D., Sc.D.
Senior Consultant, The Institute of Living
Professor of Psychiatry, University of Connecticut Medical School
Hartford, CT

Todd Wilk Estroff, M.D.
Associate Director, Neuropsychiatric Evaluation, Unit II
Research Facilities
Fair Oaks Hospital
Summit, NJ

Irl Extein, M.D.
Medical Director
Falkirk Hospital
Central Valley, NY

Fred H. Frankel, M.B. Ch.B., D.P.M.
Director, Clinical Psychiatry, Beth Israel Hospital
Professor of Psychiatry, Harvard Medical School
Boston, MA

Mark Glenn, M.D.
Clinical Associate, Department of Psychiatry
Duke University Medical Center
Staff Psychiatrist, Lumberton Psychiatry Associates
Lumberton, NC

Mark S. Gold, M.D.
Director of Research
Fair Oaks Hospital
Summit, NJ

Robert N. Golden, M.D.
Laboratory of Clinical Science
National Institute of Mental Health
Bethesda, MD

Seymour L. Halleck, M.D.
Professor of Psychiatry
University of North Carolina Medical School
Chapel Hill, NC

Malcolm Lader, D.Sc., Ph.D., M.D.
Institute of Psychiatry
London, England

Stanley Lesse, M.D., Med.Sc.D.
Faculty of Neurology, College of Physicians and Surgeons
Columbia University
New York, NY

Morris A. Lipton, Ph.D., M.D.
Professor of Psychiatry & Biochemistry
Director, Biological Sciences Research Center
University of North Carolina Medical School
Chapel Hill, NC

A.L.C. Pottash, M.D.
Medical Director, Regent Hospital, New York City
Medical Director, Psychiatric Associates of New Jersey
Fair Oaks Hospital
Summit, NJ

Ronald J. Taska, M.D.
Assistant Professor of Psychiatry
Department of Psychiatry
Duke University Medical Center
Durham, NC

Contributors to Part II

Charles S. Adler, M.D.
Chief, Division of Psychiatry
Rose Medical Center
Denver, CO

Sheila Morrissey Adler, Ph.D.
Clinical & Developmental Psychology
Denver, CO

Arthur M. Bodin, Ph.D.
Mental Research Institute, Palo Alto
Associate Clinical Professor of Medical Psychology
UCSF School of Medicine
San Francisco, CA

Cynthia M. Briggs, M.M. CMT/RMT
Assistant Professor and Director
Music Therapy Education
Hahnemann University
Philadelphia, PA

Dale Richard Buchanan
Chief, Psychodrama
St. Elizabeth's Hospital
Washington, DC

Stanley H. Cath, M.D.
Associate Clinical Professor of Psychiatry
Tufts University School of Medicine
Medical Director, Family Advisory Service & Treatment Center
Belmont, MA

Eve S. Chevron, M.S.
Clinical Psychologist
Yale University School of Medicine
New Haven, CT

Hope R. Conte, Ph.D.
Associate Professor of Psychology
Albert Einstein College of Medicine/Montefiore Medical Center
Bronx Municipal Hospital Center
Bronx, NY

Dianne Dulicai, M.A., ADTR
Assistant Professor & Director
Movement Therapy Education
Hahnemann University
Philadelphia, PA

Aaron H. Esman, M.D.
Professor of Clinical Psychiatry
Cornell University Medical College
Director of Adolescent Services
Payne Whitney Clinic
New York, NY

Allen Fay, M.D.
Assistant Clinical Professor of Psychiatry
Mount Sinai School of Medicine
City University of New York
New York, NY

Susan B. Fine, M.A., OTR, FAOTA
Director of Therapeutic Activities
Payne Whitney Clinic, New York Hospital
Faculty, Department of Psychiatry
Cornell University Medical College
New York, NY

Paul J. Fink, M.D.
Chairman, Department of Psychiatry
Albert Einstein Medical Center - Northern Division
Medical Director, Philadelphia Psychiatric Center
Professor & Deputy Chairman, Department of Psychiatry
Temple University Health Services Center
Philadelphia, PA

Ronnie M. Fuchs, M.D.
Assistant Clinical Professor, University of California at San Francisco
Medical Director, Psychiatric Emergency Service
Mt. Zion Hospital
San Francisco, CA

Marc Galanter, M.D.
Professor & Director
Division of Alcohol
Department of Psychiatry
Albert Einstein College of Medicine
Bronx, NY

Fred Gottlieb, M.D.
Associate Professor of Psychiatry, UCLA
Director of the Family Therapy Programs in Child Psychiatry
& Mental Retardation
Neuropsychiatric Institute of Los Angeles
Los Angeles, CA

Saul I. Harrison, M.D.
Professor of Psychiatry and Director of Child Psychiatry
Harbor/UCLA Medical Center
Torrance, CA

Ronald Hays, M.S., ATR
Assistant Professor & Director
Art Therapy Education
Hahnemann University
Philadelphia, PA

David Read Johnson, Ph.D., RDT
Assistant Clinical Professor
Yale University School of Medicine
Psychology Service, VA Medical Center
West Haven, CT

Helen S. Kaplan, M.D., Ph.D.
Clinical Professor of Psychiatry and
Director of Human Sexuality Program
New York Hospital - Cornell University Medical Center
New York, NY

Toksoz Byram Karasu, M.D.
Professor of Psychiatry and Deputy Chairman
Department of Psychiatry, Albert Einstein College of Medicine
Montefiore Medical Center
Director of Psychiatry, Bronx Municipal Hospital Center
New York, NY

Martha J. Kirkpatrick, M.D.
Associate Clinical Professor of Psychiatry
University of California at Los Angeles
Los Angeles, CA

Gerald L. Klerman, M.D.
George Harrington Professor
Harvard University Medical School
Director, Stanley Cobb Research Laboratories
Psychiatry Service, Massachusetts General Hospital
Boston, MA

Lawrence C. Kolb, M.D.
Distinguished Physician
Veterans Administration
Professor of Psychiatry, Albany Medical College
Albany, NY

Arnold A. Lazarus, Ph.D.
Distinguished Professor of Psychology
Graduate School of Applied and Professional Psychology
Rutgers - The State University of New Jersey
New Brunswick, NJ

Lawrence W. Lazarus, M.D.
Assistant Professor of Psychiatry
Rush Medical College, Chicago
Director, Geropsychiatric Program
Illinois State Psychiatric Institute
Chicago, IL

Myra F. Levick, Ph.D., ATR
Director, Creative Arts Therapy
Hahnemann Medical College & Hospital
Philadelphia, PA

Judd Marmor, M.D.
Adjunct Professor of Psychiatry
UCLA School of Medicine
Franz Alexander Professor Emeritus
University Southern California School of Medicine
Los Angeles, CA

Jules Masserman, M.D.
Professor Emeritus, Psychiatry & Neurology
Northwestern University
Director, Psychiatric Training,
Illinois Psychiatric Institute
Chicago, IL

James Lawrence Moodie, M.D.
Psychiatry Service
Kaiser Permanente Health Service
San Diego, CA

John C. Nemiah, M.D.
Professor of Psychiatry, Harvard Medical School
Psychiatrist-in-Chief, Beth Israel Hospital
Boston, MA

Nancy A. Newton, Ph.D.
Associate, Department of Psychiatry
Northwestern University Medical School
Staff Psychologist, Older Adult Program
Northwestern Memorial Hospital
Chicago, IL

Joseph D. Noshpitz, M.D.
Professor of Psychiatry & Behavioral Sciences
George Washington University Medical School
Sr. Attending Staff Psychiatrist
Children's Hospital
National Medical Center
Washington, DC

John M. Oldham, M.D.
Associate Clinical Professor of Psychiatry
Cornell University Medical College &
Director, Division of Acute Treatment Service
New York Hospital, Westchester Division
White Plains, NY

Robert Plutchik, Ph.D.
Professor of Psychiatry
Albert Einstein College of Medicine/Montefiore Medical Center
Bronx Municipal Hospital Center
Bronx, NY

Douglas Robbins, M.D.
Assistant Professor of Psychiatry &
Director of Adolescent Psychiatry Service
University of Michigan
Ann Arbor, MI

Bruce J. Rounsaville, M.D.
Assistant Professor of Psychiatry
Yale University School of Medicine
New Haven, CT

A. John Rush, M.D.
Betty Jo Hay Professor
Director, Affective Disorders Unit
Department of Psychiatry
Southwestern Medical School
Dallas, TX

Theodore Shapiro, M.D.
Professor of Psychiatry and Professor of Psychiatry in Pediatrics
Director of Child and Adolescent Psychiatry
Cornell University Medical Center
Payne Whitney Clinic
New York, NY

Miriam Sherman, M.D.
Associate Professor of Clinical Psychiatry in Psychiatry & Pediatrics
Cornell University Medical College
Director of Pediatric Mental Health
New York Hospital, Cornell Medical Center
New York, NY

David Spiegel, M.D.
Associate Professor, Psychiatry & Behavioral Sciences
Stanford University School of Medicine
Palo Alto, CA

Herbert Spiegel, M.D.
Lecturer, Columbia University College of Physicians and Surgeons
New York, NY

Myrna M. Weissman, Ph.D.
Professor of Psychiatry & Epidemiology and
Director of Depression Research Unit
Yale University School of Medicine
New Haven, CT

Consultants

Paul L. Adams, M.D.
W. Stewart Agras, M.D.
Erma Dosamantes-Alperson, Ph.D., DTR
Elwyn James Anthony, M.D.
Roberta J. Apfel, M.D.
Stephen Appelbaum, Ph.D.
Frank J. Ayd, Jr., M.D.
Jeanette Bair, MBA, OTR
James T. Barter, M.D.
John Basamajian, M.D.
Robert Beavers, M.D.
Aaron T. Beck, M.D.
Leopold Bellak, M.D.
Elissa P. Benedek, M.D.
John Benjamin, M.D.
Norman R. Bernstein, M.D.
C. Lee Birk, M.D.
H. Waldo Bird, M.D.
Harvey Bluestone, M.D.
Sheila B. Blume, M.D.
John Paul Brady, M.D.
Saul L. Brown, M.D.
James Bugental, Ph.D.
Robert J. Campbell, III, M.D.
Robert Cancro, M.D.
Gerald Caplan, M.D.
Patrick F. Carone, M.D.
Pietro Castelnuovo-Tedesco, M.D.
Paul Chodoff, M.D.
Bruce M. Cohen, M.D., Ph.D.
Sheldon B. Cohen, M.D.
Lee Combrinck-Graham, M.D.
Ann Conway, OTR
Arnold M. Cooper, M.D.
Raymond J. Corsini, Ph.D.
Daniel D. Cowell, M.D.
Harold B. Crasilneck, Ph.D.
John M. Davis, M.D.
Herman C.B. Denber, M.D., Ph.D.
Paul A. Dewald, M.D.
Robert R. Dies, Ph.D.
Paul D. Ellsworth, MPH, OTR, FAOTA
Parkash G. Ettigi, M.D.
James Fadiman, Ph.D.
Thomas A. Falci, M.D.
Gail S. Fidler, OTR, FAOTA
Jay W. Fidler, M.D.
Stephen Fleck, M.D.
T. Corwin Fleming, M.D.
Jerome D. Frank, M.D., Ph.D.
Cyril M. Franks, Ph.D.
Shervert H. Frazier, M.D.
Alfred M. Freedman, M.D.
Daniel X. Freedman, M.D.

Erika Fromm, Ph.D.
Donald S. Gair, M.D.
Linda Gantt, M.A., ATR
Alan Jay Gelenberg, M.D.
Robert W. Gibson, Jr., M.D.
Merton M. Gill, M.D.
Meg Givinsh, M.A., Cert., TEP
Ira D. Glick, M.D.
Myron L. Glucksman, M.D.
John S. Golden, M.D.
Joshua S. Golden, M.D.
Marvin R. Goldfried, Ph.D.
Naomi Goldstein, M.D.
Jerome Goldsmith, M.D.
Warren H. Goodman, M.D.
Mark S. Gould, M.D.
Robert L. Goulding, M.D.
George S. Greenberg, D.S.W.
Lillian Gross, M.D.
Doris Gruenewald, Ph.D.
Donald W. Hammersley, M.D.
Leston L. Havens, M.D.
Peter B. Henderson, M.D.
Marijan Herjanic, M.D.
Josephine R. Hilgard, M.D., Ph.D.
Mardi J. Horowitz, M.D.
Frederic W. Ilfeld, Jr., M.D.
Eleanor C. Irwin, Ph.D.
Kristine Jensch, M.A., ATR
Virginia T. Jorgensen, M.D.
Leslie B. Kadis, M.D.
Lothar B. Kalinowsky, M.D.
Francis J. Kane, Jr., M.D.
Stanley S. Kanter, M.D.
Eugene H. Kaplan, M.D.
Robert A. Karlin, Ph.D.
Edward Karmiol, Ph.D.
Sylvia R. Karasu, M.D.
Alfred H. Katz, D.S.W.
David R. Kessler, M.D.
Howard D. Kibel, M.D.
Donald F. Klein, M.D.
Irvin A. Kraft, M.D.
David J. Kupfer, M.D.
Deborah R. Labovitz, Ph.D., OTR
Donald G. Langsley, M.D.
Zigmond M. Lebensohn, M.D.
Jary M. Lesser, M.D.
Alexander N. LeVay, M.D.
Jerome Levine, M.D.
Jerry M. Lewis, M.D.
Robert P. Liberman, M.D.
E. James Lieberman, M.D.
Harold I. Lief, M.D.

Joel Lubar, Ph.D.
R. Bruce Lydiard, M.D., Ph.D.
Isaac M. Marks, M.D., D.P.M.
Judah M. Maze, M.D.
Myrene McAninch, Ph.D.
John F. McDermott, Jr., M.D.
John J. McGrath, M.D.
Robert Michels, M.D.
Robert Millman, M.D.
Salvador Minuchin, M.D.
Steven Mirin, M.D.
Ronald Moline, M.D.
Connie Moore, M.D.
Zerka T. Moreno
Thurman Mott, Jr., M.D.
O. H. Mowrer, Ph.D.
Richard L. Munich, M.D.
Thomas Munson, M.D.
Melvin Muroff, Ph.D.
Neville Murray, M.D.
Edgar P. Nace, M.D.
Carol C. Nadelson, M.D.
Geoffrey J. Newstadt, M.D.
Frank John Ninivaggi, M.D.
William C. Offenkrantz, M.D.
Martin T. Orne, M.D.
Herbert Pardes, M.D.
Irving Philips, M.D.
George H. Pollock, M.D.
Samuel Rabison, M.D.
Frank T. Rafferty, M.D.
Judith H. L. Rapoport, M.D.
Morton F. Reiser, M.D.
William H. Rickles, M.D.
Leigh M. Roberts, M.D.
Carolyn B. Robinowitz, M.D.
Terry C. Rodgers, M.D.
Judith A. Rubin, Ph.D., ATR
Virginia A. Sadock, M.D.
Kenneth M. Sakauye, M.D.
Clifford J. Sager, M.D.
Lindbergh Sata, M.D.
Saul Scheidlinger, M.D.
Jerome M. Schneck, M.D.
Henry E. Schniewind, Jr., M.D.
Nancy J. Schoebel, M.D., ATR
Mark S. Schwartz, Ph.D.
Melvin L. Selzer, M.D.

Richard I. Shader, M.D.
Diane S. Shapiro, M.S., OTR
Steven S. Sharfstein, M.D.
Peter E. Sifneos, M.D.
Henry K. Silberman, M.D.
George M. Simpson, M.D.
Paul Slawson, M.D.
William C. Sorum, M.D.
Wilford W. Spradlin, M.D.
Henry I. Spitz, M.D.
Jeanne Spurlock, M.D.
Frederick J. Stare, M.D.
Aaron Stein, M.D.
Marvin Stein, M.D.
Solomon Steiner, Ph.D.
Harvy Sternbach, M.D.
Alan A. Stone, M.D.
Lawrence A. Stone, M.D.
Scott D. Stoner, M.S., ATR
Manuel Straker, M.D.
Nicholas E. Stratas, M.D.
Charles F. Stroebel, III, M.D., Ph.D.
Albert J. Stunkard, M.D.
Arthur A. Sugarman, M.D.
John A. Talbott, M.D.
George Tarjan, M.D.
Daniel Tarsey, M.D.
Elizabeth G. Tiffany, M.Ed., OTR, FAOTA
George A. Ulett, M.D.
Gene L. Usdin, M.D.
Hugo Van Dooren, M.D.
Harold M. Visotsky, M.D.
Lawrence A. Vitulano, M.D.
Robert S. Wallerstein, M.D.
George J. Wayne, M.D., Ph.D.
Richard D. Weiner, M.D., Ph.D.
Walter H. Wellborn, Jr., M.D.
Carl A. Whitaker, M.D.
Robert W. Whitener, M.D.
G. Terence Wilson, Ph.D.
Laurie J. Wilson, Ph.D., ATR
Lewis R. Wolberg, M.D.
Joseph Wolpe, M.D.
Henry H. Work, M.D.
Richard J. Wurtman, M.D.
Irvin R. Yalom, M.D.
Charlotte M. Zitrin, M.D.

THE PSYCHIATRIC THERAPIES

THE SOMATIC THERAPIES

**Part I of
The Psychiatric Therapies**

1
Treatment Planning

1

Treatment Planning

INTRODUCTION

Any effort to address treatment planning must begin by acknowledging the difficulties of the task and the vast and complex mass of data involved. So many variables must be considered in each treatment decision that the task of defining them all and describing their relationships may seem insurmountable. There is also considerable disagreement as to how the critical variables should be defined and measured. No studies are available which address the relative merits of various comprehensive treatment plans, each of which may consist of several elements.

Lewis and Usdin (1982) have edited a treatment planning book in which five treatment modalities—psychodynamic, group, marital and family, behavior, and biological therapies—were put into some perspective based on their theoretical orientations. Few other efforts have been made to provide theoretical models of treatment planning. The complexity of this task is certainly one factor that may have discouraged such conceptualization. To the extent that treatment planning is not adequately conceptualized, patients with mental disorders are unlikely to receive the best possible treatment because care givers may tend to use only a single type of treatment, that which they know best, or a haphazard blending of treatments. The exclusive use of pharmacotherapy, psychotherapy, behavior modification, and family or group therapy with a particular patient may not be sufficient. The number of treatments used and their timing and duration should be based on a rational system of planning.

Insurors are putting new pressures on the field to produce research evidence justifying the use of given interventions, but these demands often raise critical moral problems for researchers and practitioners. Until now, treatment outcome studies have not dealt sufficiently with such dimensions of outcome as the quality of life a patient achieves or the level of his usefulness to society. It has been easier to address relatively simpler outcome variables such as symptom removal or staying out of the hospital, for which the cost-effectiveness is easier to calculate. When treatment practices are designed to produce outcomes that do not include subjective feelings and greater personal effectiveness, however, serious moral questions must be raised. The patient whose symptoms have improved to the extent that hospitalization is unnecessary may still be intensely miserable, incapable of working, or a burden to society.

The development of a framework—or treatment planning—should produce models that will guide the clinician in day-to-day practice and facilitate the development and assimilation of new knowledge. Such models may be based on the following premises:

A. Treatment planning needs to be comprehensive. It may be based on a structured approach to the integration of a wide group of variables, including those related to the patient, to treatment modalities, to outcome goals, and to ethical and legal considerations.

B. Patients with different diagnoses and different personal characteristics are likely to respond to different treatments. Some treatments are better for some patients than for others.

C. The therapist must be aware of the available interventions. This implies some knowledge of the empirical evidence for the usefulness of the various treatments, a measure of understanding of the manner in which they work, and an acceptable degree of skill in their use. Finally, the therapist must have extensive knowledge of the possible adverse side effects of each intervention. The patient should receive as many different types of intervention as are needed but certainly no more than necessary.

The planning process is facilitated by obtaining a rich mix of data, indeed, as much as possible, about the patient and the patient's environment. These data arise from the traditional medical and psychiatric examinations, which include:

A. History,
B. Mental status examination,
C. Physical examination,
D. Appropriate laboratory tests,
E. Psychological testing when indicated,
F. Interviews with others (members of the family, friends, social agencies, etc.) when indicated.

This chapter will not deal with routine diagnostic issues and will assume that treatment planning was preceded by a thorough diagnostic work-up.

PROCESS OF FORMING TREATMENT DECISIONS

Once the diagnosis has been made, the first component of treatment planning is to relate this diagnosis to one's scientific knowledge of what has been proven effective in treating other patients with the same diagnosis. The outlook is empirical. The second component is to consider possible causes of the disorder and to relate treatment to hypotheses of etiology. The third is to consider decisions made on the basis of the first two components in terms of appropriate patient-related factors.

A. Empiricism

Certain interventions are known to have various degrees of proven efficacy in treating certain disorders. For example, if the patient fits the criteria for bipolar disorder, good evidence suggests that lithium therapy is useful.

The empirical clues to the treatment of most psychiatric disorders, however, are more equivocal. In many, if not most, situations, clinical wisdom and experience will supplement experimental data in dictating the day-to-day treatment of disturbed patients. It is well known, for example, that highly psychotic individuals benefit by being protected from an environment containing too many stimuli, that depressed patients may do a little better if they can involve themselves in tasks at which they can succeed, that some patients benefit at times from having someone provide them with nurturance and support, and that certain patients sometimes benefit from being left alone. When it is unclear what type of treatment may be best, the sophisticated clinician reaches back into experience, tries to find similarities between the patient being treated and other patients he has known, and proceeds to use interventions that were successful in comparable circumstances.

B. Etiology

While many treatments are still discovered by trial and error or by accident, medicine does not advance by empiricism alone. As causes of various disorders are discovered, treatments become more specific and refined. It is the doctor's understanding of the processes that cause disease which has facilitated so many advances in modern medicine. In this area, psychiatry must do some catching up with the rest of the field.

The good clinician will routinely hypothesize a potential physical cause for all the behavioral disorders he treats. This practice includes careful physical and laboratory examinations to determine the nature of any physical process that may be contributing to the disorder. (A thorough discussion of the laboratory evaluation in the treatment planning begins on page 31). Lack of concern with theories of etiology would also handicap efforts to attain preventive goals. When the clinician hypothesizes that sources of psychological stress in the patient's environment play a role in causing the disorder, he can seek to identify these stresses; try to test the degree of their etiologic force; and, if appropriate, do something to minimize them. Failure to consider etiology, from both internal and external sources, could lead to treatments that produce adverse consequences.

In dealing with a highly complex set of hypotheses, the clinician must develop a systematic and comprehensive approach. Some or all of many etiological hypotheses may be relevant to the treatment of a particular patient at a particular time. In planning treatment, the clinician must review all reasonable hypotheses of etiology and relate them to potential interventions.

A great deal of theoretical and empirical knowledge about etiology is available and is probably used regularly in treatment planning. However, it is not ordinarily systematized. The approach recommended here requires that the clinician routinely consider five classes of hypotheses: biological, learning, cognitive or apperceptive, psychodynamic, and environmental. Systematic evaluation of each of these hypotheses complements empiricism as a guide to one or more therapies.

1. Biological Hypotheses. A variety of anatomical and physiological dysfunctions cause organic brain syndromes. Hence, in dealing with this type of disorder, finding the right causative factor or factors may often suggest definitive treatment.

One also assumes that there is a significant biological dysfunction at the heart of the more serious psychoses and the more severe depressions. Every time the patient is given a major psychotropic agent such as a neuroleptic, lithium, or a tricyclic antidepressant, the practitioner bases this intervention, in part, on the speculation that he is modifying a pathophysiological process. As knowledge of brain chemistry and physiology improves, one can reasonably expect that some of these hypotheses will become facts.

2. Learning Hypotheses. In putting together a case history and trying to understand how the patient's symptoms have developed, clinicians always try to relate current dysfunction to past learning. Here, two types of questions are critical. First, what has the patient learned in the past which is influencing his maladaptive behavior now? Are there specific behaviors we would have him unlearn? Second, what has the patient failed to learn which might have helped him adapt more effectively to his current situation? Learning hypotheses are essential to developing plans for intervention based on behavior modification. They are also an inherent part of the psychodynamic approach.

3. Cognitive or Apperceptive Hypotheses. Because much maladaptive behavior can, in theory, be traced to deficient assimilation of knowledge or inaccurate knowledge, consideration of these processes is also critical. The following types of cognitive or apperceptive hypotheses may be considered:

A. The patient lacks awareness of how he influences others.

B. The patient lacks awareness of how others influence him.

C. The patient lacks awareness of how past experiences influence present conduct.

D. The patient lacks awareness of current environmental expectations.

E. The patient possesses erroneous information about himself, others, or the environment.

The terms "knowledge" or "awareness" used here describe a subtype of learning which includes awareness of affective states. These terms are also more or less synonymous with the commonly used term "insight." By approaching the problem of insight in terms of inaccuracies or deficits of knowledge or awareness, the terminology used becomes subject to operational definition. More specific hypotheses concerning cognitive or apperceptive deficits have been generated by psychodynamically-oriented clinicians, who are especially concerned with the emotional states associated with learning.

4. Psychodynamic Hypotheses. The basic propositions of the psychodynamic point of view are:

A. All psychological behavior can be understood in terms of psychological causes—the concept of psychic determinism.

B. All behavior is designed to fulfill human needs that originate at various levels of development and range from basic biologically determined needs (e.g., attachment to the parent) to those that represent complex goals and values (e.g., the willingness to die for a cause). Thus, behavior can be understood as motivated and generally tending toward the avoidance of pain and the maintenance of pleasure and security—the pleasure-unpleasure principle.

C. These needs and wishes often conflict with each other or with inner values and prohibitions. Because this state of intrapsychic conflict, although inevitable and ubiquitous, can be painful and frightening, a variety of defense mechanisms develop for removing these conflicts from conscious awareness. These mechanisms involve an active process, repression, and result in important aspects of thinking, feeling, and decision making becoming psychodynamically unconscious, i.e., not available to awareness by an act of will.

D. Early life experiences, the vicissitudes of maturation and development, have a lasting effect on behavior; the adaptations made during each developmental stage affect the succeeding stages. This genetic point of view dictates that an understanding of the antecedents of any behavior is necessary for a full understanding of current behaviors. Significant failures to develop the appropriate phase-specific capacities at each stage of development can result in life-long arrest of these capacities.

E. The individual is always engaged in making the best adaptation possible out of the mix of inner needs, values, and fears and the requirements of outer reality. These adaptive efforts often require unconscious compromises among opposing needs, and these compromises may present as symptoms (Lewis and Usdin, 1982).

F. The individual's repertoire of available behaviors is limited and repetitive. Therefore, a detailed examination of these behaviors in a relatively neutral setting, e.g., the psychodynamic treatment situation, can yield evidence concerning the person's behavior in other settings. The perceptions, needs, and quality of interactions which the individual creates in relationship to the therapist tend to reflect past experiences and ongoing needs imposed upon current relationships and are often markedly discrepant with the realities of the relationship.

G. It is useful to view many functions of mental life as coalescing into a group of structures, i.e., stable ways in which groups of experiences are organized. In psychoanalytic theory, such comprehensive structural systems of mental life are organized around the major functions of wishing (id), restraining (superego), mediation of conflict and recognition of reality (ego), and maintenance of a cohesive inner organization (self). Psychopathology may occur either as a result of failure of adequate structure formation due to developmental vicissitudes or as a result of conflict between or within structures.

5. Environmental Hypotheses. These complicated hypotheses have been developed largely by family theorists, learning theorists, and social psychologists. In general, clinicians look for two elements of environmental causation. First, they are concerned with the manner in which stresses generated by the environment have influenced the patient. (The classes of hypotheses are often interrelated. An obvious stress generated by a vital part of the environmental sector such as the family might be the withholding of accurate information. Such withholding might be viewed as part of a cognitive or apperceptive hypothesis.) Second, they are concerned with how reinforcements provided by the environment perpetuate symptomatology.

In general, the family is a critical part of the patient's environment, and the clinician will routinely try to discern the manner in which the family system stresses the patient and reinforces symptoms. Sometimes the critical environmental variables are the patient's friends, the school environment, the community, or even the culture as a whole. In considering the environment as an etiological agent, it is necessary to examine environmental factors at different times in the patient's life. In particular, attention must be focused on the time frame directly preceding and following the illness. In the pre-symptomatic environment, the emphasis is usually on stress as a causative factor. Sometimes stress is created by events outside of the patient's control, such as an accident, illness, or economic conditions. Sometimes it is related to developmental needs such as entrance into school, puberty, marriage, the birth of a child, or retirement. Very often, however, patients create their own stressful environment as a result of repetitive and maladaptive behavior patterns. Cognitive and affective processes that are heavily influenced by earlier learning patterns may play a significant role in causing patients to make maladaptive responses.

The post-symptomatic environment is of interest insofar as behavior associated with the patient's illness may create aversive environmental responses (the environment becomes more stressful) or elicit responses that reinforce symptoms. Thus, the patient who becomes paranoid may alienate others; they, in turn, respond in a way that adds new stresses to the patient's life. The patient who receives more attention from family members when symptomatic than when well will have powerful encouragement toward maintaining symptomatology. Another important consideration relates to the kinds of interventions the patient has received after the appearance of symptoms but before the current evaluation. Doctors and others may have done a variety of things to help the patient; some of them, however, may have complicated the illness. These effects have to be defined and hypotheses formulated regarding their etiological significance.

In the above cited method the clinician is encouraged to compartmentalize hypotheses temporarily for the sake of systematic inquiry; at the same time it must be emphasized that all classes of hypotheses are interrelated. Biological deficits influence learning and the acquisition of information. So do environmental variables. Reciprocally, learning, cognitive, and environmental factors will also influence biological states. The clinician must try to synthesize these various etiological approaches.

C. Modifications Suggested by Patient Variables

Three important patient variables are part of Axes III, IV, and V of *DSM-III* (APA, 1980). These are:

Coexisting Physical Illnesses or Complications (Axis III). Certainly the patient's physical status will influence the variety and the extent of biological intervention. Patients with other illnesses may be using medications that exert a direct effect on their mental status or interact with psychotropic medications in ways that require modifications of conventional psychopharmacologic practice. Sometimes the treatment of the nonpsychiatric disorder must be modified. If a patient is severely depressed, the clinician may have to recommend changes in the use of drugs or procedures that increase depression. (See Chapter Two of this volume for an elaboration of the interface between physical/medical and psychological conditions.)

Other physical disabilities may influence treatment choice by creating urgent situations. The psychiatrist will be more concerned with the anorexia of the depressed patient who is also diabetic than with that of the depressed person who does not have diabetes.

The Degree of Stress That Preceded the Onset of Symptomatology, Which May Be Regarded as a Major Precipitating Factor in the Illness (Axis IV). As a rule, when pre-symptomatic stress has been high, therapy or crisis intervention is more practicable. The goal is rapid restoration of the prior level of functioning. High levels of pre-symptomatic stress tend to be associated with a better prognosis, but not always. If the patient does not respond quickly, the clinician must be prepared to initiate alternative interventions.

The Patient's Highest Level of Adaptive Functioning in the Past Year (Axis V). As a rule, patients who have attained high levels of functioning prior to their illness will have a better prognosis. The former level of adaptive functioning also influences the choice of which type of psychotherapy to use. It is generally agreed that psychotherapies that are directed only toward growth or character change should be reserved for those who have adequate psychological resources.

The clinician may consider a number of other factors in treatment planning. Most of these we will simply name or categorize; a few will be discussed. Following the listing of these variables, we will consider how the clinician should use his or her awareness of them in formulating treatment plans.

Ability to communicate verbally
Acceptance or rejection of treatment
Age and developmental phase
Attributive styles
Compliance with treatment
Cultural factors
Current family status
   a. Role in family
   b. Sibling pattern
   c. Family structure, immediate and extended
   d. Marital status
Danger to self or others
Degree and quality of motivation
Early developmental history
Education
Financial status
Genetic/family history
Geographic factors
History of antisocial tendencies
Insurance coverage
Intelligence
Interests and activities
Legal status
Occupation or school status
Past treatment experience

Presence and nature of any learning disabilities
Previous occurrence of the disorder
Psychological mindedness
Psychological strengths and weaknesses
Psychosocial supports available
Quality of object relationships
Race and ethnicity
Religious factors
Severity of pre-symptomatic stress
Sexual development—sex role and gender identity
Stage of illness

Treatment Goals. In planning the treatment of any patient the clinician should have specific goals in mind. The patient also has some share in determining goals. Sometimes the goals of patient and clinician are identical, but not always. At the beginning of treatment of suicidal, psychotic, or delinquent behavior, for example, the goals of the clinician will be quite different from the stated goals of the patient.

One goal may be symptom removal or behavioral change, which implies alleviating the patient's suffering. Usually, the patient and clinician agree that this goal is desirable; occasionally, however, they do not. Disagreements arise when the patient does not perceive the therapist as helpful or even benign, when the patient is too alienated to perceive the therapist as other than an enemy, or when he is too pleasure oriented to see his own behavior as anything other than desirable. When the patient's symptoms or behavior are more painful to others than to himself, the therapist may have difficulty enlisting the patient's help in seeking symptom removal. Another source of patient-therapist discord can arise when the treatment itself is risky. When major somatic interventions are used to alleviate symptoms, both clinician and patient must evaluate the benefits and risks of each intervention.

The goal may be to bring the patient back to the pre-morbid state, which requires that symptoms be removed without the treatment's handicapping the patient in any way. Except under unusual circumstances, patients and therapists will agree that this goal is desirable. The goal of restoration implies that the patient has sufficient coping skills to deal with potential future stress. Often restoration is viewed as a process that simply modifies extremely stressful situations or developmental crises. To be sure, it must do so in a manner that protects the patient and preserves his opportunity to re-enter the normal process of development.

The goal may also be emotional growth or character change. Psychiatry is committed to a treatment goal of bringing the patient to a state where he is better off than he was before he showed symptoms of illness. Clinicians will often try to change long-standing maladaptive behavior patterns that were part of the patient's life even before symptoms appeared. This goal is frequently viewed as essential to the prevention of recurrences. Not surprisingly, the patient may be unaware of the relationship between maladaptive character traits and certain symptomatology. He has usually entered treatment merely to obtain relief from his symptoms, only to learn that healing may be contingent on emotional growth or character change. In such a case the conflict between the goals of the clinician and those of the patient must be resolved through clarification, interpretation, or negotiation.

By seeking to change aspects of the patient which were never experienced as troublesome or as related to symptoms, the therapist asserts an unusual definition of the healing role and thus enters into an area of ethical vagueness. In recent years, some schools of psychotherapy have elevated the goal of growth above all others and have argued that it is, in itself, a sufficient indication for treatment. Indeed, the growth-promoting techniques have been used extensively with people who were never symptomatic in the first place.

Finally, it is important to consider that when one works with adults, the values that pertain to growth are themselves only beginning to be defined. Some of them may vary at any given time and place with the transient political and economic climate or the views of a given subculture. A therapeutic approach, for example, which defines sexual freedom as growth is likely to be condoned only by certain segments of the population. Within the realm of child practice, there is greater uniformity—although still no unanimity—of accepted criteria for development.

The goal of treatment may be primarily managerial and prophylactic—to get the patient into a psychiatric hospital; to keep the patient out of such a hospital; or, if he must be admitted, to help him achieve good hospital adjustment. The goal may be not only to keep the patient out of the hospital but also to have him continue in school, work, or as a competent self-sustaining member of the community. In a parallel sense, the goal may be to keep the patient out of jail or other institutions, or to avoid unnecessary surgery, an outbreak of delinquency, addiction to drugs or alcohol, or any other unhealthy situation.

Defining Who Is the Patient

Ordinarily the person who comes or is sent for help is seen as the patient. Sometimes, however, the social system of which that person is a member is viewed as "the patient." In the latter case, the focus of treatment is often on marital or family disharmony. In the case of a child, the parents may be in great need, other siblings in the family may also be troubled, or the entire family may be an obvious target of intervention.

Clinicians may also evaluate individuals for agencies such as employers, schools, insurors, or courts. Here the clinician is concerned with the agency as well as the individual, and treatment may not be the major consideration.

Treatment planning may become an issue only if the patient should seek help during the course of the evaluation; under such circumstances treatment should be undertaken only with special precautions and with the patient's full awareness of the clinician's mixed allegiances. It may be better to refer the patient to another clinician for treatment.

In most medical practice an agreement or implied contract places the person seeking help in the status of patient. In psychiatry some people are placed under medical care involuntarily and do not consent to the patient role. Psychiatrists have the duty to treat these patients with the same concern and dedication they give voluntary patients.

The Age and Developmental Phase of the Patient. The patient's age and stage of development are likely to be major factors in every treatment decision. The very young and the very old may be unusually sensitive to certain pharmacological agents, for example. As a rule, the dosage of a drug will vary with age. Some clinicians may be reluctant to use more powerful modalities such as neuroleptic medication or ECT with younger people because of concern about long-term adverse consequences. Issues such as separation, intimacy, autonomy, and loss are likely to be critical in all forms of psychotherapy. The manner in which they are presented and dealt with will depend on both the age related conflicts of the patient and the therapist's view of the outcome of conflict resolution.

Decisions as to the best milieu for the particular patient's treatment will likewise be influenced by developmental level. Children are particularly vulnerable to destructive home environments, and the effective treatment of youngsters exposed to such environments may require a drastic change of milieu (Marsden et al., 1977). The elderly may require transfer to a setting that gives them an optimal amount of sensory input (Pieroni, 1981).

Indications for conjoint family therapy or for other therapies that alter the patient's environment are also age related. As a rule, children cannot be treated effectively without paying considerable attention to the environment. Either the family members and important care givers (such as school teachers) must be worked with separately, or there must be conjoint therapy. Adult patients can usually be treated without involving the family of origin and frequently can be helped by marital therapy or conjoint therapy with their own children. The aged, too, will often need treatment that involves their children or principal care givers.

The patient's age and developmental level will also influence goals. Many clinicians believe that the natural growth processes will overcome most of the difficulties young people face if the problems that are temporarily blocking growth can be resolved. There is a tendency to provide adolescents and youth with briefer treatment, in the hope that such patients will avoid identification with the "ill role" and will come to rely on real-life events as their prime means for gratification. On the other hand, for the sicker youngsters, patient care tends to last longer than with adults.

With the elderly, growth potential is often seen as limited. Accordingly, when life expectancy is anticipated to be brief, there may be reluctance to invest energy in expensive long-term interventions. On the whole, in dealing with the elderly, goals tend to be less ambitious.

Early Developmental History. In assessing developmental history, the clinician will be concerned with temperament and constitution. These factors, plus any complications of pregnancy or delivery, set the stage for future vulnerabilities.

The infant may encounter numerous forms of trauma. Of special importance are losses of significant figures in early life. A history of multiple losses is usually associated with a greater potential for all types of depression (Cytryn and McKnew, 1980). A history of emotional deprivation in early life may also influence treatment decisions. Maternal depression, multiple foster home placements, child abuse and neglect, major patterns of rejection, and other such states will contribute to this outcome. Patients who received little nurturance as children may, as adults, lack the capacity to relate well to other people or to deal with stress (Ainsworth, 1973). Any disorder they bring to treatment is likely to require prolonged intervention. A history of severe deprivation may also make the clinician hesitate to recommend the growth-oriented psychotherapies that tend to induce stress.

Finally, the clinician may discover that specific events occurred during critical phases of development (such as sexual seduction by a mature adult during the prepubescent period). A history of such trauma may, in adult patients, be related to patterns of unsatisfactory object relationships. An awareness of such untreated experiences may influence the clinician's assessment of the potential for modifying the adult pattern. Affectively loaded learning experiences, that is, those occurring at critical phases of development, may need immediate attention (Ewing, 1978).

Sex. The patient's gender will often influence the nature of biological intervention. The side effects of psychotropic medication may vary with the sex of the patient, a factor that may influence the choice of drug treatment.

Men and women also differ in their susceptibility to nonpsychiatric medical disabilities. A higher incidence of coronary artery disease in men may necessitate using psychotherapies that emphasize serenity rather than achievement. Women requiring surgery for breast cancer may need special types of supportive psychotherapy in dealing with changes in body image following mastectomy.

Given the learning of sexual roles in our society, boys and girls, and later, men and women will differ in their responses to developmental crises. Girls are more resistant to behavior disorder in childhood and enter puberty much earlier than boys. Precocious menarche sometimes predisposes girls to major emotional and identity crises. Likewise, women responding to the hormonal changes associated with menopause may have periods of emotional instability. Men, although they may have similar responses to changes associated with aging, are more vulnerable in the face of the realities of waning physical strength and eventual retirement (Ewing, 1978).

In considering any psychotherapeutic intervention, the issue of sex stereotyping must be weighed. Therapists must be aware of the values they impose upon patients. Currently, many female patients are uncomfortable with therapists who are insensitive to issues related to feminism. Some of those patients prefer a therapist of the same sex; when this preference is present it should be considered. Some clinicians believe that the sex of the therapist is a critical variable in the outcome of psychotherapy (Landfield, 1977). They argue that some patients will do better with a therapist of the same and others with a therapist of the opposite sex. The data in this area, however, are not conclusive.

Race and Ethnicity. Different races and ethnic groups show some differences in susceptibility to various physical illnesses; when these illnesses and psychiatric disorders coexist, standard treatment may have to be modified. Blacks, for example, are highly susceptible to hypertension, the medication for which may increase their vulnerability to depression. The issues involved in genetic counseling and adjustment to physical illness will also vary with race and ethnicity.

In the course of psychotherapy with members of any minority group, their prior experience with oppression based on prejudice must be considered. Minority group members tend to suspect prejudice on the part of care givers who belong to majority races or other ethnic groups. Fear or prejudice may influence their willingness or capacity to cooperate in psychotherapy. The therapist's prejudice, particularly if it is beyond his awareness, will diminish the likelihood of a successful therapeutic outcome.

Therapists and patients of different races and ethnicity may have difficulty understanding one another. Sometimes these problems are complicated by ethnic language mannerisms or different connotations that impede communication. Therapy is obviously facilitated when patients and doctors understand one another's idiom. As a rule, patients will do better with therapists of similar background (Strupp et al., 1977).

With black patients, family therapy may also be a problem. For a variety of reasons, mainly socioeconomic, the typical nuclear family consisting of father, mother, and children is less common in the black culture. The therapist who wishes to use family psychotherapy with black patients may have to develop a broad concept of the family unit and include members of the extended family as part of the therapeutic system.

Intelligence. As a rule, intelligence facilitates the use of most interventions. Patients with normal I.Q.'s can assist the process of drug therapy by monitoring side effects and taking part in the determination of appropriate dosages. Such patients are also likely to be highly motivated and cooperative participants in psychotherapy and are capable of carrying out homework assignments in the behavioral therapies. (There are, however, exceptions. Sometimes patients with high intellectual endowment use these abilities to resist therapeutic change.) To the extent that the patient has greater capacity to understand the nature of the disorder, its prognosis, and its treatment, he is more likely to become a full partner in making treatment decisions.

Limited intelligence creates problems in regard to consent. If a patient does not have sufficient intelligence to understand an explanation concerning the side effects or risks of various treatments or the availability of alternative treatments, the clinician should advise family members or others that the patient may be adjudicated incompetent in order to obtain substitute consent.

Some individuals with limited intelligence who have had a hard time in their lives will have had many maladaptive learning experiences; they are likely to develop symptoms that resist modification. These considerations will influence the choice of the type of psychotherapy. Limited intelligence may also be a factor in favoring forms of treatment which do not require high levels of communication between therapist and patient. The patient's intelligence may also be a factor in determining the treatment milieu. More intelligent patients may be allowed to take care of some of the details of their treatment, such as regulating medication outside of the hospital. Patients with limited intellectual resources may benefit from day hospitals and sheltered workshops.

Education. The patient's educational level will have implications for treatment planning similar to those of intelligence but with minor differences. The clinician will encounter many individuals who are innately intelligent but who have had poor educational experiences. Here, the clinician may become a type of educator or may actively arrange for necessary educational exposure; the educative process can then be considered a form of psychotherapy. Patients with limited education may benefit from repeated and comprehensive explanations of diagnosis, prognosis, and treatment, an aspect of care that may require more time and effort on the part of the clinician.

Religious Factors. Occasionally, persons of certain religious denominations such as Christian Science will refuse to take medication on religious grounds. Such attitudes may have to be honored. Other patients may adhere to religious principles that make them wary of drug treatment although not *unalterably* opposed to it. Such patients may be educated about the use of appropriate biological interventions.

Religious beliefs may influence the choice of psychotherapeutic intervention as well. Some religious groups view the tenets of certain schools of psychotherapy as offensive. Members of denominations that oppose masturbation, contraception, divorce, abortion, or nonmarital sex may be conflicted if they are treated by therapists who have different sexual and marital values. When the patient feels ideologically alien to a particular form of psychotherapy, the clinician may try to match the patient with a therapist of the same or similar religion who is in a better position to deal with the patient's ideological concerns.

Religions also differ in their emphasis on self-realization. Some religions view emotional growth as a fundamental spiritual value. Others are more concerned with advancing such qualities as loyalty, faithfulness, compliance, and "doing right."

Some adolescents pose special problems because of their intense adherence to religious sects that advocate a variety of stands with respect to physical and mental health. Sometimes the views of the adolescent patient and his family may be radically at odds, and the therapist's neutrality or capacity to form a therapeutic alliance will be sorely tested.

Finally, the nature of family therapy may be influenced by religious beliefs. Some religions stress family interaction. Others stress individual autonomy and may reinforce the attitude that sharing burdens with family members is undesirable.

Sociocultural Factors. Sociocultural factors are important in determining the patient's willingness to participate in certain treatments and in assessing responsivity to those treatments. In subcultures of poverty, many people view the doctor as someone who intervenes actively in treatment. Members of such groups tend to favor biological intervention and may be puzzled by "talking therapy" (Clausen and Huffine, 1975). The members of some cultures perceive the degree of promptness, self-disclosure, and regularity required by many psychotherapeutic interventions as strange and unnecessary. These individuals may try to cooperate; but unless the therapist is extremely persistent and successful in reinforcing motivation, treatment is unlikely to work. Cultural factors may also exert influences similar to religious factors. Ideological inconsistencies may occur between patient and doctor which create conflict in the therapy situation.

Sociocultural issues are relevant to advantaged as well as disadvantaged groups. Highly educated individuals from urban environments tend to view certain forms of psychotherapy as more sophisticated and desirable than others. They may be less cooperative with therapies they feel lack this cachet.

Geographic Factors. The patient who is geographically isolated may require hospitalization to receive standard treatment. Beginning lithium therapy, for example, requires close monitoring and the availability of a laboratory where blood levels can be checked. Patients who live in rural areas may have difficulty finding therapists who can provide intensive psychotherapy, and the cost of commuting to therapy may be prohibitive.

The patient's geographical closeness to various family members will also influence the use of family therapy. If the patient is living hundreds of miles away from close family members, the use of family therapy obviously will be unlikely.

History of Antisocial Tendencies. In dealing with individuals who are known to have antisocial tendencies, the clinician must be wary of the sincerity of the patient's motivation from the beginning of treatment planning. Often these patients' initial enthusiasm is not sustained. The clinician must keep particularly careful records as antisocial patients are more likely than some others to become involved in litigation, a situation in which documentation of therapeutic events is important. If the patient tends to be violent, the situation is especially complicated. Here, the clinician will at times have to consider committing the patient or violating his confidentiality to inform the police or others if he believes the patient is likely to be violent.

The techniques of individual psychotherapy have not met with great success in treating antisocial patients. Most clinicians who work with these people recommend group or family therapy as preferable. Often the antisocial patient cannot be treated in an outpatient setting and must be managed in a more controlled milieu.

Quality of Interpersonal Relationships. The quality of the patient's interpersonal relationships is usually given a good deal of weight in determining prognosis and is a useful predictor of how the patient will respond to psychotherapeutic intervention. The patient who has formed close relationships with family members and friends is likely to trust the clinician and to welcome the closeness associated with long-term psychotherapy.

The clinician may note specific areas of strength and weakness in the quality of the patient's relationships. A given individual, for example, may have difficulty with authority figures or with persons of the opposite sex, may be anxious when faced with the threat of closeness, or may tend to eroticize relationships. Children may show either unusual fear or a too ready affinity for strangers. Often psychotherapeutic intervention, particularly group psychotherapy, can be tailored to deal with these deficiencies. Sometimes techniques associated with behavior modification such as assertiveness training may be used in a similar manner.

Genetics—Family History. In making treatment decisions, consideration of how other family members responded to previous psychiatric intervention is especially useful. Often patients with similar genetic patterns will have similar disorders and responses to the drugs used to treat them. If the patient is depressed and if his parent or sibling has been depressed and has responded favorably to a drug such as imipramine, there is a high probability that the patient will also respond to that drug (Ayd, 1975). Such predictability probably extends to other treatment modalities.

Genetic issues may also lead to modifications in the process of psychotherapy and counseling. People with a family history of heavy genetic "loading" for certain types of illness (such as affective disorders) worry a great deal about their susceptibility to these conditions. They need reassurance about the realities of their situation. Sometimes patients who have serious mental disorders need genetic counseling as to the advisability of having children. In dealing with families, the clinician may also wish to counsel family members who are not identified patients. If the two oldest of four siblings, for example, have had manic episodes, the younger siblings will need some type of counseling.

Current Family Status. A primary planning question involves whom in the family to include and whether to do so separately or conjointly (in the same room at the same time) or in a combination of the two. Four issues must be considered. First is age. Many questions arise about including younger children, or any children, where parental intimacies are among the central issues. Second is the patient's role in the family. If the patient is consistently in a position of family "scapegoat," "arbitrator," or the "responsible one," the psychotherapeutic effort may have to be directed specifically toward modifying that situation. Where the patient is a child, the marital relationship may be maintained by displacing all tensions onto the child's symptomatic behavior. The clinician must also be aware that the patient who assumes an authoritarian or responsible role in the family might be reluctant to participate in family therapy and expose his frailties. Third is family structure, a factor that is having a growing influence on who should be involved in treatment. With divorce and remarriage so commonplace, the clinician may have to decide whether the individuals to be included in treatment should be biologically related or be members of the new or "amalgamated family." Fourth is the individual's marital status. Marital therapy implies a marriage but may be considered broadly for any couple involved in an intimate relationship. Even people in the process of separation or divorce may benefit from an approach designed to ease the process.

Current family status may also be relevant to the issue of placement in a new milieu. On the one hand, children may have to be removed from a highly pathogenic family. On the other, hospitalization of seriously ill individuals can sometimes be avoided where family interest and responsibility are high.

Occupation or School Status. The level of success an individual has attained at work or in school may give the clinician important clues as to prognosis and the presence or absence of the psychological strength required for some psychotherapeutic interventions. The patient's occupation may, likewise, be critical in determining the use of specific biological approaches. Patients who rely on visual acuity in their work have to be warned, for example, that neuroleptic medications may temporarily blur their vision, necessitating interruptions at work. People who rely on muscular dexterity may have more serious problems and may be severely troubled by the extrapyramidal side effects of neuroleptic medications. These considerations will influence the clinician's aggressiveness in pursuing the use of anti-parkinsonism treatment. Sometimes, more esoteric occupational issues must be considered. For example, one would probably not want to give monoamine oxidase inhibitors to a wine or cheese taster.

Occupation and school status are important in creating therapeutic hospital milieus. Some patients who have been severely disabled may do better if they take on occupational tasks with which they are familiar. Other patients may profit from working at new and different tasks. For example, a person whose occupation requires primarily intellectual skills may enjoy some kind of manual activity in the course of his recovery. During hospital treatment, continuation of education activities may be desirable. Younger children and adolescents who need hospitalization of any duration will also need continued education tailored to their capacities and current impairments.

Past Treatment Experience. In general, the patient's past responsiveness to treatment will predict future responsiveness. If the patient has done well with a particular biological intervention, the clinician will want to think of using that same pattern of treatment if symptoms reappear. If previous treatment was unsuccessful, the clinician knows what interventions should not be used.

Prior treatment experiences also have a more subtle influence on treatment planning. The previous treatment may have resulted in the reinforcement of certain symptomatology. Some patients respond to quite appropriate treatment by becoming chronic seekers of medical attention. When the clinician encounters such patients, he must try to undo the effects of this previous reinforcement.

Past treatment experiences may become an issue related to demoralization. If previous prolonged treatment or a variety of treatments were not successful, the clinician may have to help the patient adjust to the possibility of chronic illness or seek to maintain the patient's morale while pursuing a new avenue of intervention.

Acceptance or Rejection of Treatment. A patient's consent to treatment is not meaningful unless it is voluntary, competent, and based on adequate information. Most patients need to be informed fully in as tactful but honest a manner as possible of the potential outcome of no treatment, of all risks and side effects of any given treatment, and of the existence of alternative treatments. Armed with this information, voluntary and competent patients have an absolute right to refuse any treatment recommended by the clinician. They may ask for an alternative treatment or they may elect no treatment. If they request an alternative treatment, the physician may not wish to provide it himself, in which case he is obliged to recommend someone who will (Halleck, 1980).

If the clinician feels that the patient who rejects treatment is making an incompetent decision, he has the ethical responsibility either to initiate or to assist the family in initiating legal procedures to allow involuntary treatment. There is considerable disagreement as to whether civil commitment alone, which must usually be based on the patient's dangerousness to himself or others, accomplishes this task (Roth, 1982). In many situations incompetency proceedings will also be needed.

Degree and Quality of Motivation. One way to evaluate motivation is to ask the patient what sacrifices he is willing to make to achieve the goals of treatment. These sacrifices might include money, time, or inconvenience; or they might entail enduring the pain relating to the embarrassment, loss of privacy, and anxiety engendered by certain interventions. Patients who are unwilling to commit much time to their treatment are not good candidates for long-term psychotherapy. Patients who are unwilling to abdicate their privacy to some extent are not good candidates for group psychotherapy. (Patients who have highly sensitive jobs in government or industry can have an unusual need for confidentiality that, at times, may militate against their receiving group psychotherapy.)

Motivation is, in part, an interactional process. An assessment of the degree and quality of the patient's motivation depends on the clinician's enthusiasm for using a particular form of treatment. Careful analysis of the clinician's own rationale makes for a more accurate appraisal of the patient's motivations.

In the case of children and adolescents, the clinician often finds himself working with unwilling patients or, at best, with patients who did not initiate the wish to come for help, even though they may accept its presence. It is often part of the nature of the discipline to work under these conditions.

Compliance with Treatment. The issue of likely compliance is important in considering any form of treatment. Where extremely disturbed patients are noncompliant, hospitalization may be necessary. On the other hand, highly cooperative patients, even when severely incapacitated, may be able to stay out of the hospital. The degree of patient compliance may influence choice of medication. Certain neuroleptics can be administered at widely spaced intervals and are, therefore, used for unreliable patients. The use of a depo form of antipsychotic drug is not necessary in patients known to have a high degree of compliance. It is obvious that any intervention that involves some risk is more safely used with the patient who follows the doctor's directions explicitly.

Excessive compliance can also create problems. Some patients remain in long-term psychotherapy, not out of a strong motivation for growth, but because of dependency, passivity, and/or a wish to please the doctor. The clinician should be wary of prescribing long-term and expensive interventions for patients who are too compliant.

Danger to Self or Others. The patient's potential dangerousness to self or others will influence the aggressiveness of treatment as well as decisions involving hospitalization. As a rule, mentally ill patients who are dangerous to self or others will be hospitalized. Such intervention, however, may not be necessary. Sometimes, even in the outpatient setting, sufficient surveillance to provide protection can be made available. Thus, the patient can be observed carefully by family members, can be seen more frequently by the clinician, and can have drug therapy monitored on a day-to-day basis. Once the patient is hospitalized, treatment decisions with regard to milieu structuring will be influenced by the degree of dangerousness to self and others. Some patients will require such careful observation that they cannot participate in all ward activities. Powerful suicidal tendencies may also be an indication for electroconvulsive therapy (ECT).

Psychosocial Supports Available. The psychosocial supports available to the patient will influence the planning for the best setting in which to provide care. When psychosocial support systems are strong, hospitalization can often be avoided. The clinician may also want to include individuals who play a significant role in the patient's life in some form of family therapy, sometimes even if these people are not part of the patient's nuclear or extended family.

Psychological Mindedness. Evaluation of psychological mindedness helps the clinician decide whether psychotherapeutic intervention should be favored in his planning. Patients who have a high capacity for insight, a readiness for self-exploration, and are interested in psychological concepts are more accepting of dynamic psychotherapy. When qualities of psychological mindedness are uncorrectable, the clinician may give more consideration to behavioral or biological interventions.

Attributive Styles. Patients have different ways of explaining their illness to themselves and others. Some will attribute their difficulties to forces they cannot control such as fate or the malevolence of others. Others tend to view their difficulties as problems of will. Another way of conceptualizing this issue is in terms of how people take responsibility for their own lives.

An analysis of attributive styles gives the clinician some hints as to the kinds of intervention which are most likely to be effective—and the kinds to avoid. Where individuals view their problems as having been inflicted upon them, they will not respond comfortably to growth psychotherapies that require them to assume responsibility for their own behavior.

The clinician must consider the possibility that the patient's view of responsibility could be erroneous. Some patients blame fate or others for their difficulties when relatively slight modifications of their own behavior might ameliorate the problem. Other patients insist that they are entirely responsible for having created their illness even though they are afflicted with a disorder that clearly was not theirs to elect. The skilled clinician tries to learn something about each patient's limits and capacities. He then tries to shape optimal behavior by holding patients responsible for behaviors within their control and by never demanding that they perform beyond their capacities.

Psychological Strengths and Weaknesses. The patient's psychological make-up encompasses a variety of subfactors which can be described in terms of capacities and defenses. The clinician should evaluate the patient's capacity to accept substitute gratification. High capacity favors a good therapeutic outcome for long-term psychotherapy, and it may also suggest the use of certain environmental interruptions that provide substitute gratification in times of stress. The patient's capacity to compromise may be important. Patients who are willing to accept partial solutions to their problems are generally more cooperative partners in any therapeutic venture and tend to be good candidates for psychotherapy.

Some patients are very much in tune with their environment and regulate their activities in accordance with environmental stimuli. Others rely more on inner cues. This variable may suggest modifications in types of individual, group, or family psychotherapy. The field dependent individual may be taught to become more aware of and responsive to inner cues. The field independent person may need to learn to be more responsive to the environment.

The patient's characteristic psychological defense mechanisms may be considerably relevant to treatment planning. Some people are resistant to experiencing regression and are obviously poor choices for treatment with psychoanalytically-oriented psychotherapy. Patients who regularly use denial mechanisms tend to have a high degree of emotional disturbance and are usually not good candidates for intensive psychotherapy. Patients who tend to project their difficulties onto others will not, as a rule, benefit from psychotherapies that put them under stress or require insight. These individuals, too, are more likely to benefit from a supportive approach. Patients who respond to conflict by impulsive action may require considerable modification of treatment plans and may need to be seen more frequently. Impulsive patients also cannot be given prescriptions for large amounts of potentially lethal drugs.

Some people try to resolve conflicts by turning inward and seeking to change some aspects of themselves. Their adaptational styles are called *autoplastic*. Others try to change the environment. Their styles are called *alloplastic*. As a rule, successful adaptation depends on a proper mix of both adaptational modes. When one or the other mode of adaptation is used exclusively, the clinician may need to be concerned with balance. Patients who rely heavily on autoplastic defenses may sometimes be more responsive to group or family therapies. By the same token, patients who resort primarily to alloplastic defenses are, as a rule, not good candidates for growth-oriented psychotherapy unless they can be treated in a controlled setting.

Financial Status. In the best of all possible worlds, the patient's financial status should not be an important variable in planning treatment. The realities are otherwise. Many patients cannot afford long-term treatment, and sometimes treatment is tailored to meet the patient's financial capacities. To the extent that insurance coverage is adequate, the clinician may consider a variety of treatments according to the patient's needs. One of the peculiarities of many insurance policies is that inpatient treatment may be covered but similar interventions provided in an outpatient setting are not.

In this situation, hospitalization may be considered. There is a risk-benefit evaluation involved here, however. The benefits of providing the patient with a wide variety of interventions without bankrupting him must be weighed against the risks of hospitalization, which include inconvenience, stigmatization, and an increased likelihood that the patient may learn new dependency and illness behaviors. These judgments must, of course, be made under the constraints imposed by utilization review committees. When strict criteria for hospitalization prevail, the range of choices is narrowed.

ETHICAL AND LEGAL ISSUES

Certain ethical values regularly dominate the practitioner's consciousness as he goes through the process of selecting treatment and will influence his goals and choice of intervention. The most obvious values are efficiency and economy. One is always seeking the most successful treatment at the least expense. But other values, while not as apparent, may be equally important. They are:

A. **Respecting the Patient's Autonomy.** In effect, this means that one assigns major importance to the patient's goal and, to the extent feasible, allows the patient's preference to have considerable weight in determining the choice of treatment. It seems evident that early in the process of evaluation, many patients are unable to articulate their treatment goals clearly. Nor do they know much about which modes of treatment are most likely to be efficacious. Indeed, the information patients do possess regarding either somatic or psychotherapeutic interventions may well be erroneous. There is no satisfactory way to consider the patient's wishes seriously unless one is sure the patient has received a great deal of information about various treatments, their risks, and their side effects, and, more importantly, has assimilated this information. To arrive at this point, the patient needs instruction and guidance.

The issue of informed consent is quite relevant to treatment planning. In determining what to do with patients, the more committed practitioners become to providing them with full information, the more they find themselves sacrificing some of their own freedom to decide and to act. At the same time, however, once treatment begins, they may reap some advantages from this new state of affairs for they may well find themselves dealing with patients who are more active and cooperative partners in the therapeutic process.

B. **Not Compromising the Patient's Future Potentialities.** In the long run, the treatment that has been most economic and efficient over the short term may nonetheless turn out not to be the most helpful approach. This issue has been discussed at length by social psychiatrists and family therapists (Haley, 1963; Halleck, 1971). Conscientious therapists must ponder these alternatives in making treatment decisions.

C. Compassion. Sometimes the severity of the patient's illness is such that even though his long-term interests might be compromised by some form of rapid intervention, the need for providing immediate relief supersedes all other values. In emergency situations, concern for the patient's autonomy may be eclipsed by overriding safety issues. Given such circumstances, the practitioner will also worry less about how treatment might compromise the patient's social position.

These days the clinician must be cognizant of legal issues from the outset of treatment planning. In the case of nonconsenting competent patients, the critical intervention of hospitalization is frequently not available. Even with committed patients, if they are competent and refuse consent, the use of pharmacotherapy may be severely restrained. Even where the patient has consented, some states have attempted to limit the administration of certain so-called intrusive treatments. Under specific circumstances, the timing of such an intervention may have to be delayed until issues of competency and consent are litigated. It is also likely that fears of malpractice suits influence how one plans for treatment. When a psychiatrist encounters a clinical situation that is ripe for litigation or when he considers a given patient to be exceptionally litigious, the natural tendency is to opt for the most conservative treatment. Often this is not the modality he thinks is best, but it is the one likely to be viewed as least controversial. This situation is lamentable, but it is a reality of modern day treatment planning.

The patient himself may be embroiled in or on the point of involvement in legal actions. Sometimes, the patient may be facing criminal charges. Here, the clinician must be aware that treatment may be sought primarily to avoid punishment.

Another possibility is that the clinician may be dealing with a patient who is not competent. If a need for consent arises, it cannot be obtained by the usual method. The patient may have to be adjudicated incompetent and substitute consent obtained from a family member or guardian.

A common problem arises when a patient seeks compensation for a disability or injury. Such a patient may put inordinate pressure on the physician to overestimate the extent of his incapacity. In this situation, psychotherapy must be modified to some extent. Efforts should be made to keep the patient from using psychiatric treatment primarily to gain monetary rewards. This is not only an ethical issue; there is the added danger that such a patient will learn to depend on the reinforcement he receives as a result of being sick and will not get better.

A final legal consideration involves patients struggling with marital conflicts; if divorced, they may want the psychiatrist to assist them in obtaining custody of their children. This issue is especially important in marital therapy. It may be necessary to warn patients involved in marital therapy that material generated during therapeutic hours is not always privileged and may end up being revealed in court. Following such a warning some patients will prefer individual psychotherapy where the patient's disclosures are more likely to be privileged.

Other treatment planning issues do not fit neatly into the format thus far proposed and can best be phrased as questions:

How much evaluation does the patient need for the clinician to establish a competent treatment plan? The answer depends on a number of variables, including the clinician's skills and the urgency of the patient's problem. In terms of time, there is unlikely to be much agreement among clinicians as to what constitutes a minimally acceptable work-up. Even in the hands of the most competent clinician, several hours of examination will often be essential. With a child, the necessity for interviewing parents and perhaps conducting a family interview and/or a home or school visit would be essential parts of the process.

When should therapy be stopped? This question has received surprisingly little discussion in the literature. The naive answer is that therapy should be stopped when the patient is better. Since the word "better" is so elusive, this statement provides practically no guidance. The issue is partly one of economics. Ideally, treatment planning should include some consideration of when treatment will be terminated if it is effective and at which point to discontinue it if it is not. In the first instance, the problem is how much treatment is enough. In the second, the problem is when should the clinician frankly acknowledge that the patient is not improving and that nothing more can be done, a new form of intervention should be tried, or a new therapist may be desirable.

Under what circumstances should the patient be advised that no treatment is indicated? It is likely that many patients who are given a diagnosis are also told that they do not need treatment. There may be a variety of reasons for this response. The patient may not want treatment or be able to afford it, or the therapist may believe the patient can handle the problem without outside assistance. The therapist may also believe that no adequate treatment for the patient's condition is available or that treatment will make the patient worse. It is axiomatic that in the process of evaluation a certain amount of therapy takes place; indeed, it is possible that the diagnostic evaluation is all the treatment the patient will need (Bloom, 1981). Many factors that make for change such as hope, a renewal of faith in the powers of the healer, catharsis, identification, clarification, and new learning or insight can all take place in the course of a single hour. One option that must be considered in the process of treatment planning, then, is that treatment is not needed (Bloom, 1981).

REFERENCES

Ainsworth MDS: The development of infant-mother attachment, in Review of Child Development Research, vol 3. Edited by Caldwell BM, Ricuitti HN. Chicago, University of Chicago Press, 1973

Ayd FJ (ed): Rational Psychopharmacotherapy and the Right to Treatment. Baltimore, Ayd Medical Communications, 1975

Bloom BL: Focused single-session therapy: initial development and evaluation, in Forms of Brief Therapy. Edited by Budman SH. New York, Guilford Press, 1981

Clausen JA, Huffine CL: Sociocultural and social-psychological factors affecting social response to mental disorder. J Health Soc Behav 16:405-420, 1975

Cytryn L, McKnew DH: Affective disorders, in Comprehensive Textbook of Psychiatry, vol 3, 3rd ed. Edited by Kaplan HI, Freedman AM, Sadock GJ. Baltimore, Williams & Wilkins, 1980

Diagnostic and Statistical Manual of Mental Disorders, 3rd ed. Washington, DC, American Psychiatric Association, 1980

Ewing CP: Crisis Intervention as Psychotherapy. New York, Oxford University Press, 1978

Haley J: Strategies of Psychotherapy. New York, Grune & Stratton, 1963

Halleck SL: The Politics of Therapy. New York, Science House, 1971

Halleck SL: Law in the Practice of Psychiatry. New York, Plenum, 1980

Landfield AW: Personal Construct Systems in Psychotherapy. Chicago, Rand-McNally, 1977

Lewis J, Usdin G: Treatment Planning. Washington, DC, American Psychiatric Press, 1982

Marsden G, McDermott SF, Minor D: Selection of children for residential treatment. J Am Acad Child Psychiatry 16:437-438, 1977

Pieroni RE: Geriatrics Review. Lexington, Mass, The Collamore Press, 1981

Roth LH: Competency to consent to or refuse treatment, in Psychiatry 1982: The American Psychiatric Association Annual Review. Edited by Grinspoon L. Washington, DC, American Psychiatric Press, 1982

Strupp HH, Hadley SW, Gomes-Schwartz B: Psychotherapy for Better or Worse: The Problem of Negative Effects. New York, Jason Aronson, 1977

Laboratory Evaluation
in Treatment Planning

INTRODUCTION

The laboratory evaluation of the psychiatric patient has changed dramatically over the last decade. One of the many factors that has contributed to this change is *DSM-III* (APA, 1980). Logically enough, all of the Axis I conditions have as an inclusion criterion "not due to any organic mental disorder" since, as any experienced clinician knows, a number of organic disturbances may have associated behavioral, cognitive, mood, and personality disturbances. As psychiatrists have begun vigorously to rule out such competing medical diagnoses, the procedures available for laboratory evaluation and diagnosis have been expanded and, in some cases, rediscovered by clinicians.

Any procedure that can lead to more accurate diagnosis, safer use of medications, or speedier clinical decision making has critical benefits in terms of patient safety and humanitarian interest in decreasing the needless suffering of the misdiagnosed patient. However, the benefit can also be financial. A procedure that decreases hospital stay by even one day saves the patient money far in excess of the cost of most tests. When, for example, an antidepressant level comes back from the lab so low as to reveal clear noncompliance, and if the psychiatrist can get the patient to improve compliance, consequences ranging from wasted hospital days or outpatient treatment to nonresponse and relapse can be avoided. Thus, laboratory procedures can improve the quality of care. Psychiatrists, like their colleagues in other medical specialties, will increasingly be able to use lab tests as an adjunct to their obviously crucial clinical skills.

PHYSICAL-PSYCHOLOGICAL INTERFACE

Many patients are being treated for psychiatric disorders without full attention to physical illnesses or drug or alcohol abuse (Hall et al., 1978; Hall et al., 1981; Koranyi, 1979; Herridge, 1960). Psychiatric symptomatology can be and frequently is the first manifestation of a reversible physical illness. It has been repeatedly documented that physical illness needs to be excluded as part of making a psychiatric diagnosis (Hall et al., 1978; Hall et al., 1981; Koranyi, 1979; Herridge, 1960). For example, Hall et al. (1978) studied 658 consecutive psychiatric outpatients and found that 9.1 percent had medical disorders that produced psychiatric symptoms. In another study of outpatients Koranyi (1979) excluded all patients who were immediately hospitalized as well as those who failed to complete a comprehensive assessment. A final sample of 2,090 patients who had been evaluated was examined. Forty-three percent of these patients suffered from one or several major physical illnesses, 46 percent of which were undiagnosed at the time of referral; 7.74 percent of the total population had a physical illness that caused the psychiatric symptoms. Herridge (1960) studied 209 consecutive admissions to an inpatient unit and found that at least five percent had major physical illnesses that were causative and presented as a psychiatric disorder. Hall et al. (1981) conducted a prospective study of 100 patients admitted to a state hospital. Patients with known physical disorders along with sociopathic personality disorders and persons with significant histories of alcohol or drug abuse were excluded. An intensive search for causative physical illness revealed that 46 percent of the patients had a previously unrecognized and undiagnosed physical illness that was specifically related to their psychiatric symptoms and either caused these symptoms or substantially exacerbated them. Hall et al. (1981) note that "28 of 46 patients evidenced dramatic and rapid clearing of their psychiatric symptoms when medical treatment for the underlying physical disorder was instituted. Eighteen patients were substantially improved immediately following medical treatments." These studies clearly show that physical illness is often either a precipitant or an associated condition that needs to be considered in any diagnostic formulation. More recently, sophisticated and provocative testing techniques have been used to help diagnose thyroid disease (Gold et al., 1981a, 1981b) and identify low-dose drug and alcohol abuse in psychiatric patients (Pottash et al., 1982). These new tests may expand even further the percentage of medical illnesses found to include psychiatric symptoms.

Physical illness can cause or worsen psychiatric symptoms to a variable extent. Therefore, it is important to be as specific as possible when discussing the interaction of physical and psychiatric illnesses. The previously cited studies refer only to physical illnesses that presented as psychiatric disorders and caused the psychiatric symptoms in whole or in part. Other patients can present with physical and psychiatric diseases that are concomitant and are not related; when the physical disorder is treated, the psychiatric symptoms are not affected. Finally, some psychiatric illnesses present as and are mistaken for physical illness and are often treated incorrectly as such by nonpsychiatric practitioners. Hoffman (1982), in reporting on 215 patients referred to a specialized medical neuropsychiatric inpatient evaluation unit for further evaluation, found the referring diagnosis to be inaccurate in 41 percent of the cases; in 24 percent of the cases, diagnoses were reclassified from physical to psychiatric or from psychiatric to physical illness.

There also exists a group of diseases, reviewed elsewhere (Estroff, 1984), which may be called the "great imitators in psychiatry." These disorders are truly on the borderline of psychiatry and internal medicine and neurology. Most of them are not detectable by physical examination or by "routine" laboratory screening. The diagnosis may not be made unless the attending physician is aware of the existence of these diseases and the diagnosis is actively pursued through aggressive specialized testing.

From the previously described studies and many others, it becomes clear that no matter how closely the first presentation of a psychiatric patient may conform to classical *DSM-III* descriptive criteria, this does not guarantee that the patient is suffering from a psychiatric disorder. One of the best examples of this fact is the presenting symptom of catatonia. For many years it has been clear that catatonia is not specific for schizophrenia and may be caused by a variety of neurologic, metabolic, psychiatric, and other disorders (Sripada, 1982; Gelenberg, 1976; Abrams and Taylor, 1976). The differential diagnosis includes: arteriolosclerotic parkinsonism and lesions of the basal ganglia, viral encephalitis, akinetic mutism, vascular lesions of the temporal lobes, tumors of the septum pellucidum infringing on the fornix, tumors and traumatic hemorrhage in the region of the third ventricle, focal lesions of the thalamus, frontal lobe tumors and lesions, anterior cerebral arterial aneurysms, AV malformations of the posterior cerebral circulation, diffuse brain trauma, diffuse encephalomalacia following closed head injuries, petit-mal epilepsy, status epileptus, the postictal phase of epilepsy, Wernicke's encephalopathy, tuberous sclerosis, general paresis of syphilis, narcolepsy, the acute phase of encephalitis lethargica, and cerebral-macular degeneration. In addition, many metabolic conditions are associated with catatonia: diabetic ketoacidosis, hypercalcemia from parathyroid adenomas, pellagra, acute intermittent porphyria, homocystinuria, membranous glomerulonephritis, and hepatic encephalopathy. It has also been associated with poisoning with organic fluorides, metals, illuminating gas, mescaline, large quantities of ethyl alcohol, chronic intoxication with amphetamines or cocaine, and acute phencyclidine (PCP) intoxication. Finally, catatonia has been associated with medications such as aspirin overdoses, ACTH, and antipsychotic medications. This list is clearly long (Weddington et al., 1980). Yet, even if all of the previously mentioned disorders have been ruled out, and the diagnosis of a psychiatric disorder is fairly certain, there is still no guarantee that the catatonia is due to schizophrenia. Abrams and Taylor (1976) found that out of 55 patients who displayed one or more catatonic signs, only four met research criteria for the diagnosis of schizophrenia, while 39 had affective disorders, three had a reactive psychosis, and nine had organic brain disease.

This nonspecificity of specific behavioral syndromes applies to other disorders as well. The differential diagnosis of depression is long and involved. Giannini et al. (1978) list 91 possible disorders that can present as depression. Hall (1980) lists 24 medical illnesses that frequently induce depression and 77 medical conditions that can present as depression. Giannini lists 28 causes of auditory hallucinations, 26 causes of euphoria, eight causes of mania, 56 causes of delusions, 21 causes of depersonalization, and 12 causes of hyperventilation. Hall et al. (1978) found that visual hallucinations were present almost exclusively in medically induced psychiatric disorders. Thus, a variety of physical disorders can cause the same symptomatology.

Recently introduced diagnostic systems, such as *DSM-III* (APA, 1980), have put added emphasis on the need to diagnose major depression accurately and to rule out medical illnesses that may manifest symptoms similar to, or indistinguishable from, major depression. One illness that can mimic depression is hypothyroidism, which often presents with and includes major depressive symptomatology (Whybrow et al., 1969; Brown, 1980). In general, hypothyroidism is routinely considered in the differential diagnosis of depressive and anergic states and is screened for with thyroid function tests such as serum thyroxine (T_4), triiodothyronine (T_3)-uptake, and basal thyroid stimulating hormone (TSH) (Cohen and Swigar, 1979). In the past, this thyroid screening approach may not have enabled the clinician to identify the majority of depressed patients who have thyroid disease as the primary diagnosis or who have thyroid failure as a major precipitant to their depression. During the past decade, however, our understanding of clinical hypothyroidism has broadened, and with the aid of improved laboratory tests the diagnosis can now be made much earlier in the natural history of the illness (Evered et al., 1973).

The most useful laboratory tests for hypothyroidism are total T_4, T_3-uptake, free thyroxine index (FTI), free T_4, T_3RIA, baseline TSH, and TRH stimulation test. In patients with evidence of overt Grade 1 hypothyroidism, T_4 and TSH will both be abnormal and will confirm the clinical diagnosis. Patients with possible Grade 2 or 3 hypothyroidism may require a TRH stimulation test to establish the diagnosis. All patients with a ΔTSH of ≥ 20 need to be tested for anti-thyroid antibodies.

Independent of the utility of the blunted TRH test response in the evolving biochemical nosology of depression (Gold et al., 1980a; Gold et al., 1981c; Prange et al., 1972) is the protirelin test's use in psychiatric medicine (Snyder and Utiger, 1972) in the evaluation of the depressed, anxious, anergic patient with possible hyperthyroidism, hypothyroidism, or subclinical hypothyroidism.

Another diagnosis that can present as depression is substance abuse. Drug intoxication and most drug withdrawal diagnoses require identification of the drug in exhaled breath, blood, or urine. Routine "drug screens" may not have the sensitivity necessary to measure psychiatrically relevant quantities of these drugs; and more specific, antibody-based tests may need to be ordered. The psychiatrist can test specifically for additional abusable substances on the basis of the patient's signs, symptoms, history, and age and the family's description of the phenomenology and assessment of drug use/abuse. A negative history of drug use or abuse, however, is not sufficient to replace negative specific tests for drugs of abuse.

Newer urine drug abuse screens that use enzymatic assays are sensitive to concentrations of drugs in the abuse range, as opposed to the older thin-layer chromatographic assays, which are less sensitive. Gas chromatograph/mass spectroscopy (GC/MS) assays for all major drugs of abuse in blood are now available and can aid diagnosis when urine testing is inconclusive or is not capable of detecting psychoactive quantities of the drug(s) in question or when the drug in question has a known blood level-behavior relationship.

Many patients have been so intoxicated and sedated from the medications they are abusing that they do not remember all the drugs they have taken, even within the previous 24 hours. Quite often drug-abusing patients do not actually know what drugs they are taking. Many times they may be using what they think is cocaine or heroine but actually is an adulterated drug. Pills or other injectable drugs that are sold as one medication may actually be something else. PCP is commonly substituted for other drugs.

As soon as the patient has been interviewed and the physical examination has been performed, samples of blood and urine should be sent to the laboratory for identification and quantification of the drugs of abuse. One may use antibody-based urine assays for most drugs of abuse, including alcohol. Quantitative, capillary column/GC, or GC/MS analysis of blood for specific drugs not easily detectable in urine (e.g., glutethimide, PCP, cocaine, Δ9THC) are ordered when clinically indicated. When urine is used to detect drug abuse, a *supervised* first void morning urine is essential. Concurrent urine specific gravity is used to ensure that the sample is the concentrated first void morning urine.

NEUROENDOCRINE TESTING

The neuroendocrine testing strategy involves measuring changes in peripheral hormone concentrations, sometimes after provocation, as potential markers of major psychiatric disorders. Because the monoamine neurotransmitters, norepinephrine (NE), serotonin (5HT), and dopamine (DA) regulate the hypothalamic factors that control the pituitary and hence other glands (Martin et al., 1977), changes in neuroendocrine systems reflect changes in the monoamine systems thought to be involved in mood disorders. For this reason, the neuroendocrine strategy has been called the "window into the brain." It may not be coincidence that the neurotransmitter systems involved in mood regulation and endocrine regulation are similar. The vegetative symptoms of depression, including disturbances in sleep, appetite, weight, and libido—the hypothalamic symptoms of depression—have long suggested neuroendocrine abnormalities.

Patients with major depressive disorder have been reported to have a number of reproducible neuroendocrine abnormalities (Table 1). Patients

Table 1. Summary of Neuroendocrine Abnormalities in Patients with Major Depressive Disorders.

Hormone	Basal	Challenged
GH	—	insulin, L-Dopa amphetamine, and clonidine stimulation ↓ TRH stimulation ↑
PRL	↑	TRH stimulation ↓
LH	↓	LHRH stimulation ↑
TSH	—	TRH stimulation ↓ (unipolar)
ACTH/cortisol	↑	dexamethasone non-suppression; amphetamine stimulation ↓

with major depression have a decreased growth hormone (GH) response to a number of provocative stimuli, including insulin-induced hypoglycemia (Sachar et al., 1971), L-dopa (Sachar et al., 1975), clonidine (Matussek et al., 1980), and amphetamine (Langer et al., 1976), and an augmented GH response to thyrotropin-releasing hormone (TRH) (Gold et al., 1981a, 1981c). Other neuroendocrine abnormalities that have been reported in major depression include increased prolactin (PRL) secretion (Halbreich et al., 1979), decreased luteinizing hormone (LH) (Robins and Guze, 1970), decreased LH response to gonadotropin releasing hormone (LHRH) (Brambilla et al., 1978), increased cortisol secretion (Sachar et al., 1973), failure to suppress cortisol production on the dexamethasone suppression test (DST) (Carroll et al., 1981a), decreased cortisol secretion in response to dextroamphetamine (Sachar et al., 1981), and decreased thyroid-stimulating hormone (TSH) and PRL response to TRH (Prange et al., 1972; Kastin et al., 1972; Extein et al., 1981a; Loosen and Prange, 1982). Neuroendocrine tests may have multiple uses in the diagnosis and treatment of the depressed patient (Table 2).

Table 2. Clinical Uses of Neuroendocrine Tests in Depression

1. Diagnosis
2. Prediction of treatment response
3. Documentation of biological state change with treatment.
4. Prediction of relapse

The focus of the following discussion will be on two neuroendocrine challenge tests—the dexamethasone suppression test (DST) and the thyrotropin-releasing hormone (TRH) test—which may be useful state markers for major depression.

The DST (Dexamethasone Suppression Test)

It has been well documented that a significant proportion of patients with major depressions secrete abnormally high amounts of cortisol from the adrenal gland (Sachar et al., 1973). This has been shown by serum cortisol measurement at multiple time points throughout a 24-hour period as well as by more integrated measures such as 24-hour urinary-free cortisol secretion. Recent studies have suggested that measurement of serum cortisol over a three-hour period from one to four p.m. correlates well with 24-hour cortisol secretion and may be useful as an index of integrated cortisol secretion. In addition to hypersecretion of cortisol, many major depressives show loss of the normal diurnal variation in cortisol secretion. The normal

#1 Normal diurnality, no hypersecretion
#2 Cortisol hypersecretion (e.g., primary affective illness. Cushing's disease)
#3 Loss of Diurnality; Cortisol hypersecretion

Figure 1. Diurnal Cortisol Patterns

circadian rhythm of cortisol consists of secretory bursts that decrease from four p.m. to midnight and peak around nine a.m. (Figure 1) (Martin et al., 1977).

Secretion of cortisol by the adrenal is stimulated by the pituitary hormone adrenocorticotrophic hormone (ACTH). ACTH production is, in turn, controlled by corticotropin-releasing hormone (CRH). This hypothalamic-pituitary-adrenal (HPA) axis shows inhibitory feedback control, which is used in the DST, a test of HPA regulation (Martin et al., 1977).

When a patient is given the synthetic corticosteroid dexamethasone, the normal response is that this excess corticosteroid is "read" by the pituitary and hypothalamus as an excess of cortisol, and cortisol production is suppressed for at least 24 hours. Failure to suppress cortisol on such a challenge was first used as a diagnostic test for Cushing's syndrome. The finding of importance to psychiatry is that approximately 45 percent of patients with major depressive illness fail to suppress cortisol values below $5\mu g8\%$ at any time in the 24 hours after dexamethasone administration (Figure 2). Thus, while most patients with major depression do not have true Cushing's syndrome, about half of them have a Cushing's-like biochemical profile.

Figure 2. Dexamethasone Suppression Test

Carroll et al. (1981a), who have pioneered the use of the DST as a laboratory test in psychiatry, have reported a rate of nonsuppression as high as 67 percent in a melancholic subgroup of major depressives and have proposed the DST as a diagnostic test for this disorder. The DST does not seem to differentiate between unipolar and bipolar depression. However, DST nonsuppression seems clearly to differentiate major depressions from nonmajor depressions and primary from secondary depressions. Failure to suppress on the DST has been reported to be rare in psychiatric disorders other than major depression, with a false positive rate of less than five percent in appropriately pre-screened populations. However, some recent studies suggest higher levels of nonsuppression in certain subgroups of patients with psychiatric disorders other than major depression.

Carroll et al. (1981a) have reported the diagnostic confidence level of an abnormal DST in the diagnosis of major depression in a mixed population of psychiatric patients to be approximately 95 percent. This means that in such a population the failure to suppress on the DST identifies a patient with a major depression 95 percent of the time. One must keep in mind that the diagnostic confidence (or predictive value) of the DST, like any diagnostic test, will vary depending on the prevalence of the illness in question in the population tested (Galen and Gambino, 1975). In fact an APA Task Force on the Use of Laboratory Tests in Psychiatry has taken the cautious position that available scientific data do not yet support the use of the DST for general diagnostic purposes although it may be useful in specific cases.

The DST as typically performed begins with administration of 1 mg of dexamethasone orally at about 11 p.m. The patient will experience no subjective effects from this test. Small samples of blood are obtained by venipuncture at a number of time points in the 24 hours after dexamethasone administration for assay of serum cortisol. Competitive protein binding and radioimmunoassay (RIA) are the two most commonly used assays. The clinician using this test must be sure that the laboratory being used has a cortisol assay that is sensitive and reliable in the lower ranges of cortisol from 3 to 8 μg% which are crucial for the DST in psychiatry (Carroll et al., 1981a, 1981b).

Carroll et al. (1981a) and others have used two post-dexamethasone time points for determination of cortisol: four p.m. and 11 p.m. By increasing the number of time points in the 24 hours post-dexamethasone to six, the sensitivity of the test for major depression is increased by about 40 percent with only a small loss of specificity. Specificity has been reported to be increased and sensitivity decreased with an increase in dosage of dexamethasone from 1 mg to 2 mg. It has been suggested that a cut-off of 4 μg% or lower for nonsuppression may be optimal, depending on the assay. The optimal parameters for the DST in psychiatry need to be studied further.

Certain factors that can affect the validity of the DST must be taken into account in screening psychiatric patients for DST administration (Carroll et al., 1981a). For example, while usual therapeutic doses of benzodiazepines, neuroleptics, tricyclics, and lithium do not affect the DST, other medications can. Barbiturates, phenytoin, carbamazepine, and other medications that induce hepatic enzymes and, hence, speed the metabolism of dexamethasone can cause false positives. It is noteworthy, however, that a recent study showed that the DST can be useful three to four weeks after detoxification to identify those alcoholics with major depression (Dackis et al., in press).

Failure to suppress on the DST and hypercortisol secretion are dissociated in some patients (Gold et al., 1981a; Sternbach et al., 1982). In other words, some major depressives have elevated diurnal cortisol levels while showing normal suppression on the DST, and some do not suppress on the DST despite normal diurnal cortisols. More research is needed to explain this dissociation. However, a practical implication of the finding is that measurement of diurnal cortisol may complement the DST as a measure of HPA axis hyperactivity.

What are the mechanisms of HPA axis activation in major depression? Studies measuring ACTH levels before and during the DST, while not in complete agreement, suggest that DST nonsuppression is associated with increased ACTH levels. At the level of the brain, loss of noradrenergic inhibition and increased serotonergic stimulation of the HPA axis in some depressions may account for DST nonsuppression (Martin et al., 1977). The recent identification and synthesis of corticotropin releasing hormone (CRH) mark the beginning of a new generation of studies which may further elucidate the mechanism of HPA axis hyperactivity in major depression.

The TRH Test (Thyrotropin-Releasing Hormone Test)

A large number of independent investigators have confirmed the finding that patients with major depression have a blunted response of the pituitary hormone TSH to an infusion of the hypothalamic tripeptide TRH (Prange et al., 1972; Kastin et al., 1972; Extein et al., 1981a; Loosen et al., 1982). There is some controversy as to whether unipolar and bipolar depressives differ on the TRH test (Gold et al., 1979). The TRH test is a standard endocrinological procedure first used in the diagnosis of thyroid disease (Martin et al., 1977). It has been suggested that the TRH test has utility as a diagnostic test in psychiatry in euthyroid patients with affective disorders (Gold et al., 1979; Gold et al., 1981c; Extein et al., 1981a; Extein et al., 1980).

The TRH test consists of measurement of TSH response to infusion of TRH. An indwelling venous catheter is placed in patients who are at bedrest at eight a.m. after an overnight fast. At nine a.m. 500 μg of synthetic TRH is administered over 30 seconds through the catheter. The patient experiences only mild, transient autonomic symptoms such as the urge to urinate. Before and 15, 30, 60, and 90 minutes after TRH administration, small samples of blood are obtained via the catheter for measurement of serum TSH in duplicate by RIA. The maximum TSH response, or ΔTSH, is determined for each patient by subtracting the baseline TSH from the peak TSH level after TRH infusion. GH and PRL also may be measured after

TRH infusion since patients with major depression may have a positive GH response to TRH or a blunted PRL response not found in most other psychiatric patients or normal controls.

Several factors can decrease the TSH response to TRH, and they must be taken into account in interpreting TRH test results in depression (Martin et al., 1977). These include hyperthyroidism, corticosteroids, some drugs of abuse, alcoholism, and age over 60 in men. Factors that can augment the TSH response to TRH include hypothyroidism and lithium. Many commonly used psychotropics, including benzodiazepines, neuroleptics, and tricyclic antidepressants, do not significantly interfere with the TRH test (Kirkegaard et al., 1977).

Manic patients also tend to have a blunted TSH response to TRH, whereas patients with schizophrenic psychoses tend to have a normal response (Extein et al., 1982a). It is important to differentiate these two groups of patients, who can appear similar in the acute phase of their illness, because of the better prognosis and response to lithium of the manic patient. Finally, patients with abnormalities on both the DST and TRH test may represent a subgroup of more severely ill depressives with characteristic treatment responses.*

Special Diagnostic Uses of Neuroendocrine Tests

A number of areas of diagnosis present particular difficulties to the clinician. In these, a laboratory test may be useful.

Depressed mood is almost ubiquitous in the course of patients with borderline personality disorder. It is often difficult to know whether the dysphoria represents a true depressive illness requiring antidepressant medication or whether it is more accurately seen and treated as part of the character disorder. Several studies have shown a high rate of DST and TRH test abnormalities in borderline patients, suggesting that many borderline patients have depressions similar to major depressions in nonborderlines† (Carroll et al., 1981b).

The diagnosis of major depression and, hence, choice of antidepressant medication treatment can be more difficult in children and adolescents because of developmental changes that color the diagnostic picture. In a study of inpatient adolescents without drug or alcohol abuse, eight of 15 adolescents with major depression showed nonsuppression on the DST, whereas only one of 12 adolescent patient controls failed to suppress

---

*Kirstein L, Extein I, Gold MS, et al: Neuroendocrine tests and treatment in depression. Presented at 134th annual meeting of the American Psychiatric Association, New Orleans, La, May, 1981

†Extein I, Pottash ALC, Gold MS: Neuroendocrine tests in depressed borderlines. Presented at 134th annual meeting of the American Psychiatric Association, New Orleans, La, May, 1981

(p<.025) (Extein et al., 1982b). Thus, the DST appears to have the same utility in adolescents as in adults as a possible marker for major depression.

The DST has also been suggested as a test that can help differentiate patients with so-called "depressive pseudomentia," who may respond to antidepressant treatment, from patients with true dementia (Carroll et al., 1981b). There have been conflicting reports in this area, however (Spar and Gerner, 1982). DST nonsuppression has also been suggested as a marker for the subgroup of patients with catatonia and schizoaffective disorder who have an illness more like an affective illness and who may respond to medications such as tricyclic antidepressants and lithium.*

LABORATORY TESTS IN TREATMENT; NEUROENDOCRINE TESTS

Neuroendocrine tests bridge the gap between procedures used in diagnosis and those used in treatment. The possibility that neuroendocrine tests may aid the clinician in predicting responses to treatment is an exciting area of current research (Gwirtsman et al., 1982). Several groups have reported preliminary studies suggesting that suppressors on the DST are more likely to respond to the so-called "serotonergic" tricyclics such as amitriptyline and chlorimipramine while nonsuppressors are more likely to respond to "noradrenergic" tricyclics such as desipramine and imipramine (Brown and Shuey, 1980). Other groups have reported simply that depressed patients with neuroendocrine abnormalities are more likely to respond to, and hence are candidates for, somatic treatment, be it antidepressant medications or ECT (Carroll et al., 1981a). One study of patients with schizophrenic and schizoaffective disorders showed that DST nonsuppression was a better predictor of response to tricyclics and lithium than clinicians' judgment.* And preliminary data suggest that although TRH and DST abnormalities are not associated with response to tricyclics in major depressives, patients with abnormalities on *both* the DST and TRH test are more likely to need ECT.† This is an area for further research.

Failure to suppress on the DST and blunted TSH responses on the TRH test in major depressions tend to normalize with clinical and neurobiological improvement during the course of treatment (Kirkegaard et al., 1977; Extein et al., 1981b; Greden et al., 1980; Gold et al., 1980b). By repeating the DST and TRH tests during the course of treatment, the clinician can obtain

---

*Carman JS, Wyatt E, Hole KR, et al: DST and thymoleptic response in RDC schizophrenics. Presented at the 134th annual meeting of the American Psychiatric Association, New Orleans, La, May, 1981

†Kirstein L, Extein I, Gold MS, et al: Neuroendocrine tests and treatment in depression. Presented at 134th annual meeting of the American Psychiatric Association, New Orleans, La, May, 1981

prognostic information about when the neurobiological abnormalities of depression are in remission. This information may help determine when antidepressant medication or ECT is no longer needed and when continued or different treatment is needed.

Several studies have shown that patients whose DST or TRH test abnormalities persist after treatment have a higher probability of relapse, regardless of clinical appearance or outcome up to that time (Kirkegaard et al.,1977; Greden et al., 1980). Patients who have not normalized on the TRH test, despite apparent recovery, may need closer monitoring, prophylactic antidepressants for a longer time, and other appropriate measures in view of their higher likelihood of relapse. The prognostic value of the DST and TRH tests in depression has exciting and practical potential application to clinical practice.

LABORATORY TESTS IN TREATMENT: THERAPEUTIC DRUG MONITORING

Pharmacological treatment can be enhanced in some patients by the monitoring of blood levels of the medications given to the patient. This is particularly important for the poorly responsive patient. Monitoring blood levels can be of practical benefit to the treating physician and patient by ensuring compliance, identifying rapid or slow metabolism so dosage can be adjusted accordingly, and minimizing side effects without loss of efficacy.

With antidepressants, the use of standard dose regimens unrelated to plasma levels has been identified as a major source of nonresponse. The reasons for this fact are numerous but include pharmacokinetic, pharmacodynamic, and other factors (Amsterdam et al., 1981). The main factor determining variation in blood levels of tricyclics among patients given the same dose is rate of metabolism by the liver. Liver microsomal enzymes metabolizing antidepressants and converting tertiary tricyclics to secondary may show large intersubject variability. Antidepressant absorption from the gastrointestinal tract is highly variable among patients and in the same patient over time. Absorption may be markedly affected by antacids, sodium bicarbonate, and vitamin C, for example. Drug interactions may seriously affect blood levels of antidepressants. Antipsychotic medications often increase antidepressant levels, while smoking and prior or current drug abuse will often lower levels. Physicians sometimes forget that poor compliance is a major factor in drug nonresponse even in the most motivated patient. In the psychiatric patient, compliance should never be assumed and should always be confirmed. All of these factors explain why routine measurement of antidepressant levels is indicated for patients on these medications. This use of laboratory technology enables the physician to ensure compliance, individualize dosage, reduce side effects, and guarantee the integrity of the medication trial.

Laboratories vary greatly with regard to methodology and accuracy of test performance. Measurement of antidepressant levels, for example, is a complicated and sensitive procedure performed accurately by few laboratories. When a laboratory does not itself perform the test, it must send the sample to a reference laboratory, which in many cases increases test result turnaround time. Clearly, for antidepressant levels to be useful clinically, the clinician needs the results rapidly to enable him or her to use the test when making decisions about dosage. It should take a laboratory no more than 24 hours to perform the assay.

Antidepressant Levels

For any given dose of an antidepressant medication, interindividual variations in resultant steady-state antidepressant concentrations are marked. Some patients have 30 times the blood level of other patients given the identical dose. Increasing evidence, as recently reviewed by numerous authors, suggests that for many antidepressants critical thresholds or ranges of steady-state plasma concentrations of parent antidepressants and psychoactive metabolites must be achieved for optimal efficacy. These ranges may not be achieved in approximately 40 percent of patients given standard therapeutic dosages, (i.e., imipramine 200 mg/day or trazodone 150 mg/day). Furthermore, even when therapeutic plasma concentrations are attained, these antidepressant levels may be altered and clinical response reversed by exogenous factors such as weight change, dietary alterations, changes in smoking status, differences in bioequivalence among pharmaceutical preparations, and the addition or withdrawal of concurrent medications. Subsequently, toxicity or clinical relapse may occur. Even when therapeutic ranges are wide or when there is a linear relationship between plasma antidepressant concentration and clinical response, plasma level determinations may occasionally be useful to minimize toxicity or reduce adverse side effects by adjusting dosage to maintain therapeutic levels but at lower concentrations.

Individuals who are at increased risk for toxic effects from antidepressants, including children and the elderly, may benefit from frequent plasma level monitoring. While most antidepressants have adverse effects, knowing plasma level-response relationships and using plasma levels can reduce or even eliminate side effects. In certain patients with cardiovascular disease, prolonged atrioventricular conduction times may lead to ventricular arrhythmias and, potentially, death. Consequently, any patient particularly at risk for toxic effects of antidepressants (e.g., advanced age, cardiovascular disease, drug and/or alcohol abuse history, liver disease, family or personal history of side effects from low doses of antidepressants) may be medicated with nortriptyline using concurrent frequent plasma level monitoring to remain within the lower limits of the therapeutic range to minimize any potential toxicity.

Even some patients in clinical remission on maintenance antidepressants may benefit from plasma antidepressant concentration determinations. As noted above, a variety of exogenous factors may alter steady-state concentrations of antidepressant medications. For example, neuroleptics, methylphenidate, corticosteroids, disulfiram, dipropylacetamide, vitamins, and weight loss may all markedly increase plasma levels of antidepressants and potentiate toxicity or cause relapse when the patient is being treated with those antidepressant agents with "therapeutic windows." Conversely, barbiturates and tobacco smoking may markedly lower plasma tricyclic concentration and allow relapse in patients treated with all classes of antidepressants. There are likely to be numerous other drug-drug interactions affecting tricyclic plasma concentrations in the outpatient; when adding to or deleting a concurrent medication from a patient's pharmacological regimen, a plasma level determination may be appropriate.

Finally, differences in bioequivalence among pharmaceutical preparations of the same tricyclic agent have resulted in changes in plasma tricyclic concentrations and have caused clinical relapse or precipitated toxicity; the clinician must always be alert to this possibility if an outpatient changes pharmacies.

Neuroleptic Levels

Recent studies of the relationship of plasma levels of neuroleptic medications and clinical response in schizophrenic patients have suggested a therapeutic range or threshold for therapeutic effect for antipsychotics with few, if any, active metabolites. These relationships have been worked out most extensively for haloperidol (Magliozzi et al., 1981; Extein et al., 1981c; Seeman et al., 1976). Because dopamine inhibits prolactin secretion, elevation of serum prolactin by neuroleptics has been proposed as an index of neuroleptic dosage adequacy (Gruen et al., 1978). This measurement of prolactin has been of limited practical use due to a ceiling effect. The antipsychotic potencies of neuroleptics are directly related to their ability to block dopamine receptors (Seeman et al., 1976). Dopamine receptor binding assays of plasma are therefore being used to quantify the dopamine blocking activity achieved by a given dose of a neuroleptic in a given patient (Creese and Snyder, 1977). The dopamine receptor binding assays allow for monitoring of neuroleptics with numerous active metabolites. The use of laboratory monitoring of therapeutic drug levels does not eliminate the need for clinical judgment of multiple factors in treatment, but it does take some of the guesswork out of the assessment of neuroleptic medication trials. The identification of optimal plasma levels for neuroleptic response above which side effects increasingly occur with no increase in efficacy can allow clinicians to individualize dose and narrow the risk/benefit ratio. Neuroleptic levels or composite, additive serum neuroleptic activity by dopamine blockade may be particularly helpful in ensuring against unnecessarily high dosages of neuroleptics which cause unnecessarily high plasma levels and debilitating extrapyramidal side effects or increase the risk of tardive dyskinesia. These measures may also help monitor patient noncompliance, a major cause of relapse, as well as control for other pharmacokinetic factors and identify nonresponding patients who are being treated with ineffective medication dosages as determined by blood levels.

Monoamine Oxidase (MAO)

Platelet MAO activity has been measured and found decreased in schizophrenia, mania, alcoholism, and other disease states (Wise et al., 1980; Rosen et al., 1982). While the use of platelet MAO as a confirmatory diagnostic test is controversial, quantitative measurement of platelet MAO activity before and during MAO inhibition treatment is used in many medical centers.

CONCLUSION

It is important to remember that laboratory tests are not in themselves diagnostic nor do they decide treatment. They should not be used without regard for the entire clinical presentation or as a substitute for medical observation and judgment. For example, our knowledge of depressive illness is being clarified and operationally defined by the combination of systematic interviews and DST, TRH, and other reliable biological tests, which can help guide treatment and assess treatment response and prognosis (Gold and Pottash, 1981; Ettigi and Brown, 1977; Sachar et al., 1980; Kupfer, 1976). As additional tests are studied and proven to be sensitive and reliable, they, too, may be of use in psychiatry.

REFERENCES

Abrams R, Taylor MA: Catatonia, a prospective clinical study. Arch Gen Psychiatry 33:579-581, 1976

Amsterdam JD, Winokur A, Caroff S: Effect of tricyclic antidepressants on the dexamethasone suppression test. Am J Psychiatry 138:1245-1246, 1981

Brambilla F, Smeraldi E, Sacchetti E, et al: Deranged anterior pituitary responsiveness to hypothalamic hormones in depressed patients. Arch Gen Psychiatry 35:1231-1238, 1978

Brown WA, Shuey I: Response to dexamethasone and subtype of depression. Arch Gen Psychiatry 37:747-751, 1980

Carroll BJ, Feinberg M, Greden JF, et al: A specific laboratory test for the diagnosis of melancholia: standardization, validation, and clinical utility. Arch Gen Psychiatry 38:15-22, 1981a

Carroll BJ, Greden JF, Feinberg M, et al: Neuroendocrine evaluation of depression in borderline patients. Psychiatr Clin North Am 4:89-99, 1981b

Cohen KL, Swigar ME: Thyroid function screening in psychiatric patients. JAMA 242:254-257, 1979

Creese I, Snyder SH: A simple and sensitive, radioreceptor assay for antischizophrenic drugs in blood. Nature 270:180-182, 1977

Dackis CA, Bailey J, Gold MS, et al: Neuroendocrine tests in alcoholics with and without major depression, in Problems of Drug Dependence, 1982. Edited by Harris LS. Rockville, Md, NIDA Research Monograph Series 43:266-272, in press

Diagnostic and Statistical Manual of Mental Disorders, 3rd ed. Washington, DC, American Psychiatric Association, 1980

Estroff TW: Psychiatric misdiagnosis, in Advances in Psychopharmacology: Predicting and Improving Treatment Response. Edited by Gold MS. Boca Raton, Fla, CRC Press, 1984

Ettigi P, Brown GM: Psychoneuroendocrinology of affective disorder: an overview. Am J Psychiatry 134:493-501, 1977

Evered DE, Ormston BJ, Smith PA, et al: Grades of hypothyroidsim. Br Med J 1:657-662, 1973

Extein I, Pottash ALC, Gold MS, et al: Using the protirelin test to distinguish mania from schizophrenia. Arch Gen Psychiatry 39:77-81, 1982a

Extein I, Rosenberg G, Pottash ALC, et al: The dexamethasone suppression test in depressed adolescents. Am J Psychiatry 139:1617-1619, 1982b

Extein I, Pottash ALC, Gold MS: The thyrotropin-releasing hormone test in the diagnosis of unipolar depression. Psychiatry Res 5:311-316, 1981a

Extein I, Pottash ALC, Gold MS: Relationship of thyrotropin-releasing hormone test and dexamethasone suppression test abnormalities in unipolar depression. Psychiatry Res 4:49-53, 1981b

Extein I, Augusthy KA, Gold MS, et al: Plasma haloperidol levels and clinical response in acute schizophrenia. Abstracts, Annual Meeting of the American College of Neuropsychopharmacology 70, 1981c

Extein I, Pottash ALC, Gold MS: The TRH test in depression (ltr). N Engl J Med 302:923-924, 1980

Galen RS, Gambino SR: Beyond Normality: The Predictive Valve and Efficiency of Medical Diagnosis. New York, John Wiley & Sons, 1975

Gelenberg AJ: The catatonic syndrome. Lancet 1:1339-1341, 1976

Giannini, AJ, Black HR, Goettsche RL: Psychiatric, Psychogenic, and Somatopsychic Disorders Handbook. New York, Medical Examination Publishing, 1978

Gold MS, Pottash ALC, Extein I: Hypothyroidism and depression: evidence from complete thyroid function evaluation. JAMA 245:1919-1922, 1981a

48   PART I / SOMATIC THERAPIES

Gold MS, Pottash ALC, Mueller EA, et al.: Grades of thyroid failure in 100 depressed and anergic psychiatric inpatients. Am J Psychiatry 138:253-255, 1981b

Gold MS, Pottash ALC, Extein I: The TRH test in the diagnosis of major and minor depression. Psychoneuroendocrinology 6:159-169, 1981c

Gold MS, Pottash ALC, Extein I, et al.: Diagnosis of depression in the 1980s. JAMA 245:1562-1564, 1981d

Gold MS, Pottash ALC: Depression: diagnosis and treatment with tricyclic antidepressants. Postgrad Med 69:104-117, 1981

Gold MS, Pottash ALC, Ryan N, et al: TRH-induced TSH response in unipolar, bipolar, and secondary depressions: possible utility in clinical assessment and differential diagnosis. Psychoneuroendocrinology 5:147-155, 1980a

Gold MS, Pottash ALC, Extein I, et al: Dexamethasone suppression tests in depression and response to treatment (ltr). Lancet 1:1190, 1980b

Gold MS, Pottash ALC, Davies RK, et al: Distinguishing unipolar and bipolar depression by thyrotropin release test (ltr). Lancet 2:411-412, 1979

Greden JF, Albala AA, Haskett RF, et al: Normalization of dexamethasone suppression test: a laboratory index of recovery from endogenous depression. Biol Psychiatry 15:449-458, 1980

Gruen P, Sachar E, Altman N, et al: Relation of plasma prolactin to clinical response in schizophrenic patients. Arch Gen Psychiatry 35:1222-1227, 1978

Gwirtsman H, Gerner RH, Sternbach H: The overnight dexamethasone suppression test: clinical and theoretical review. J Clin Psychiatry 48:321-327, 1982

Halbreich U, Grunhaus L, Ben-David M: Twenty-four-hour rhythm of prolactin in depressive patients. Arch Gen Psychiatry 36:1183-1186, 1979

Hall RCW, Gardner ER, Popkin MK, et al: Unrecognized physical illness prompting psychiatric admission: a prospective study. Am J Psychiatry 138:629-635, 1981

Hall RCW, Psychiatric Presentations of Medical Illness. New York, SP Medical and Scientific Books, 1980

Hall RCW, Popkin MK, Devaul RA, et al: Physical illness presenting as psychiatric disease. Arch Gen Psychiatry 35:1315-1320, 1978

Herridge CF: Physical disorders in psychiatric illness: a study of 209 consecutive admissions. Lancet 2:949-951, 1960

Hoffman RS: Diagnostic errors in the evaluation of behavioral disorders. JAMA 248:964-967, 1982

Kastin AJ, Ehrensing DS, Schalch DS, et al: Improvement in mental depression with decreased thyrotropin response after administration of thyrotropin-releasing hormone. Lancet 2:740-742, 1972

Kirkegaard C, Bjorum N, Cohn D, et al: Studies on the influence of biogenic amines and psychoactive drugs on the prognostic value of the TRH stimulation test in endogenous depression Psychoneuroendocrinology 4:131-136, 1977

Koranyi EK: Morbidity and rate of undiagnosed physical illnesses in a psychiatric clinic population. Arch Gen Psychiatry 36:414-419, 1979

Kupfer DJ: REM latency: a psychobiologic marker for primary depressive disease. Biol Psychiatry 11:159-174, 1976

Langer G, Heinze G, Reim B, et al: Reduced growth hormone responses to amphetamine in endogenous depressive patients. Arch Gen Psychiatry 33:1471-1475, 1976

Loosen PT, Prange AJ: Serum thyrotropin response to thyrotropin-releasing hormone in psychiatric patients: a review. Am J Psychiatry 139:405-416, 1982

Magliozzi JR, Hollister LE, Arnold KV, et al: Relationship of serum haloperidol levels to clinical response in schizophrenic patients. Am J Psychiatry 138:365-367, 1981

Martin JP, Reichlin S, Brown GM: Clinical Neuroendocrinology. Philadelphia, Penn, Davis Co, 1977

Matussek N, Ackenheil M, Hippius H, et al: Effect of clonidine on growth hormone release in psychiatric patients and controls. Psychiatry Res 2:25-36, 1980

Pottash ALC, Gold MS, Extein I: The use of the clinical laboratory, in Inpatient Psychiatry Diagnosis and Treatment. Edited by Sederer LI. Baltimore, Williams & Wilkins Co, 1982

Prange AJ, Lara PP, Wilson IC, et al: Effects of thyrotropin-releasing hormone in depression, Lancet 2:999-1002, 1972

Robins E, Guze SB: Establishment of diagnostic validity in psychiatric illness: its application to schizophrenia. Am J Psychiatry 126:983-987, 1970

Rosen AJ, Wirtshafter D, Pandey GN, et al: Platelet monoamine oxidase activity and behavioral response to pharmacotherapy in psychiatric patients. Psychiatry Res 6:49-59, 1982

Sachar EJ, Altman N, Gruen PH, et al: Human growth hormone response to levodopa. Arch Gen Psychiatry, 32:502-503, 1975

Sachar EJ, Asnis G, Halbreich U, et al: Recent studies in the neuroendocrinology of major depressive disorders, Psychiatr Clin North Am 3:313-316, 1980

Sachar EJ, Finkelstein J, Hellman L: Growth hormone response in depressive illness; I: response to insulin tolerance test. Arch Gen Psychiatry, 25:263-269, 1971

Sachar EJ, Halbreich U, Asnis GM, et al: Paradoxical cortisol responses to dextroamphetamine in endogenous depression. Arch Gen Psychiatry 38:1113-1117, 1981

Sachar EJ, Hellman L, Roffwarg HP, et al: Disrupted 24-hour patterns of cortisol secretion in psychotic depression. Arch Gen Psychiatry 28:19-24, 1973

Seeman P, Lee T, Chau-Wong M, et al: Antipsychotic drug doses and neuroleptic/dopamine receptors. Nature 261:717-719, 1976

Snyder PJ, Utiger RD: Response to thyrotropin-releasing hormone (TRH) in normal man. J Clin Endocrinol Metab 34:380-385, 1972

Spar JE, Gerner R: Does the dexamethasone suppression test distinguish dementia from depression? Am J Psychiatry 139:238-240, 1982

Sripada P: Catatonia: a non-specific syndrome. Resident and Staff Physician 28:41-44, 1982

Sternbach H, Extein I, Gold MS: Diurnal cortisol: DST and TRH tests in depression, in Continuing Medical Education Syllabus and Scientific Proceedings in Summary Form. 135th annual meeting of the American Psychiatric Association, Toronto, May 15-21, 1982

Weddington WW, Marks RC, Verghese JP: Disulfiram encephalopathy as a cause of the catatonia syndrome. Am J Psychiatry 137:1217-1219, 1980

Whybrow PC, Prange AJ, Treadway CR: Mental changes accompanying thyroid gland function. Arch Gen Psychiatry 20:48-63, 1969

Wise CD, Potkin S, Bridge P, et al: Sources of error in the determination of platelet monoamine oxidase: a review of methods. Schizophr Bull 6:245-253, 1980

2
Pharmacotherapies

Antianxiety Drugs

INTRODUCTION

The antianxiety drugs are part of a spectrum of agents which extends from anesthetics at one end, through hypnotics and sedatives, to antianxiety drugs (tranquilizers) and then to muscle relaxants. The distinctions among these classes are often arbitrary, depending on dosage and mode of administration rather than on fundamental pharmacological differences. For example, diazepam, a typical antianxiety drug, is an effective hypnotic in a larger dose at night and can be given intravenously as premedication or as a light anesthestic during minor operative procedures. It is widely used in states of muscle spasm and also has anticonvulsant properties.

This group of drugs is among the most widely prescribed of all classes of drugs, and in many countries it is the single most frequently prescribed group of drugs on repeat prescription. Recently, prescriptions for antianxiety agents have decreased in several countries as both medical and lay commentators have expressed their concern regarding habitual use and potential abuse. Paradoxically, there are some indications that patients' long-term use of antianxiety drugs is actually increasing, although the benefits and risks of this practice are poorly documented. Thus, the prescriber must consider carefully the need for anxiolytic agents in each case and review patients regularly so that long-term use does not supervene insidiously.

The use of antianxiety agents is among the most controversial in psycho-pharmacology, psychiatry, and medical practice. For example, family physicians typically regard antidepressants as useful drugs, whereas anti-anxiety drugs are often relegated to the status of necessary but troublesome. Attitudes vary among prescribers. Psychiatrists often see anxious patients who have failed to respond well to these drugs in primary care, leaving the physicians unimpressed by the drugs' effects. In addition, they may subscribe to the view that antianxiety agents, at best, offer purely symptomatic relief and, at worst, may interfere with reparative processes in dealing with the "underlying neurosis." Various factors affect response to antianxiety agents and, again, the views of prescribers will be influenced by the types of patients who present to them.

Thus, there is a glaring discrepancy between the attitudes of specialist prescribers and the extent of usage in primary care. In general, the prescribing figures betoken a high level of patient satisfaction with the currently available antianxiety drugs.

Another problem with antianxiety medications concerns the lack of systematic evaluation of their use. With a few notable exceptions, most clinical trials have tried only to establish drug-placebo differences. Consequently, guidelines on the management of the anxious patient tend to reflect the personal experience of the psychiatrist rather than a distillate of an extensive and systematic review of the literature. The inchoate nature of the classification of anxiety disorders has not helped.

In dealing with antianxiety drugs, the emphasis must inevitably fall heavily on the benzodiazepines. The barbiturates and meprobamate are still used but are obsolescent if not obsolete. Other medications are available but play a limited role.

Usually, antianxiety drugs are an adjunct to other therapies, particularly those based on psychodynamic and behavioral theories. Nevertheless, the symptomatic relief obtained is often substantial and should not be gainsaid. A balance must be kept between the usefulness of antianxiety drugs and the drawbacks, particularly of long-term use, including dependence.

HISTORICAL BACKGROUND

The term "sedative" was originally defined as a substance that has the property of allaying, assuaging, or calming. More recently it has come to imply feelings of drowsiness or torpor, a state originally called "oversedation" and often attributed to the barbiturates and other older drugs such as chloral hydrate. In place of sedative, the term "tranquilizer" was introduced to attempt to distinguish in the practitioner's schema between the older sedatives and the newer drugs, particularly the benzodiazepines. But this distinction is mainly specious as, apart from safety in overdosage, the benzodiazepines sufficiently resemble the barbiturates to justify sharing the same class. Another term enjoying some popularity is "anxiolytic," a word of dubious etymology. Perhaps the most logical term is "antianxiety drugs," in line with "antidepressants" and "antipsychotics"; this term will be used in this chapter.

The use of anxiety-allaying drugs goes back thousands of years to the discovery that grape juice and grain mashes were fermentable and that the resulting alcoholic beverages possessed beguiling psychotropic properties. Opium derivatives were known in the historical Middle and Far East and in ancient Greece. Other herbal remedies were discovered, but opium and alcohol remained the mainstays of treatment until the last century, and were used to anesthetize, to subdue the mentally disturbed, to allay anxiety, and to induce sleep.

The nineteenth century saw the development of inorganic and, later, organic chemistry. Bromides were introduced as sedatives and became widely used. Their poor effectiveness, cumulative toxicity, and likelihood of abuse become apparent by the 1930's. Even so, 20 years ago some mental hospitals routinely screened all newly admitted patients for serum bromide to detect the occasional bromide-induced toxic psychosis.

Organic chemistry in the second half of the nineteenth century developed anesthetics such as ether and chloroform and sedatives such as chloral hydrate and paraldehyde. These compounds pharmacologically resemble ethanol. Chloral hydrate still has some therapeutic usefulness but paraldehyde is unpleasant to take, may result in psychological and physical dependence, and may induce toxic psychotic states. At the end of the nineteenth century the first barbiturates were introduced, with many members of this class being synthesized during the twentieth century. Many different compounds were introduced, divided into the ultrashort-acting (e.g., anesthetic induction agents such as thiopental), short-acting (e.g., amobarbital and secobarbital), medium-acting (e.g., butobarbital), and the long-acting (e.g., phenobarbital) anesthetics. In fact, it is now apparent that thiopental owes its short action after intravenous administration to its rapid redistribution from brain to the rest of the body; and, apart from a few long-acting compounds such as phenobarbital, the rest are of medium duration with elimination half-lives of 16 hours or so.

As with the bromides, more than 50 years elapsed before the disadvantages of the barbiturates were appreciated. Their side effects of drowsiness and torpor, tolerance to their effects, dangers of overdose and of physical and psychological dependence, with consequent dangerous withdrawal syndromes, led to a growing dissatisfaction with these drugs. The scene was set for the the phenomenal, albeit short-lived, popularity of meprobamate. This drug was developed from mephenesin, which was a muscle relaxant acting mainly on the spinal cord. Meprobamate was introduced as the first of the tranquilizers, but its advantages over the barbiturates proved negligible. Nevertheless, it is still used as a sedative and muscle relaxant (Greenblatt and Shader, 1971). Other nonbarbiturate sedatives and hypnotics were developed, including glutethimide, methyprylon, ethchlorvynol, and the ill-fated thalidomide. The eager acceptance of these newer drugs evinced the growing dissatisfaction with the barbiturates; but, in turn, disillusion with the nonbarbiturate substitutes set in as experience grew of oversedation, toxicity in overdose, and dependence liability. Although some of these drugs still have their advocates, in general they have little place in modern therapy. Intravenous amobarbital is used to facilitate abreactive interviews and occasionally to sedate the severely disturbed patient who has failed to respond to antipsychotic medication.

The discovery of the benzodiazepines provides yet another instance of serendipity with respect to psychotropic agents (Cohen, 1970). In the 1930's, Sternbach in Poland became interested in the heptoxdiazepines, compounds with seven-membered rings. Twenty years later, now working for Roche Laboratories, Sternbach decided to screen these compounds for biological activity. Forty derivatives were synthesized but were biologically inert. The last compound, a methylamine derivative, was not tested immediately but put aside. In 1957, this compound was finally evaluated after a clean-up at the laboratory and was found to have actions similar to those of meprobamate in cats but with several times the potency. Futher studies followed, but it was some time before the chemical structure of this compound, called chlordiazepoxide, was established. It turned out to have a seven-membered ring, the methylamine being incorporated into the quinazoline ring to form a 1:4 benzodiazepine (Figure 1). More than 1,000 benzodiazepines and related compounds have been synthesized, including diazepam, the most successful of all.

Because of the dominant position of the benzodiazepines, any account of antianxiety medication must inevitably concentrate on the properties and use of these compounds. However, other types of medication have also been advocated in the management of anxiety states, and they will be outlined later.

THE BENZODIAZEPINES

Pharmacokinetics

While many similarities exist among the benzodiazepines, certain pharmacokinetic differences are important (Shader and Greenblatt, 1977). For the rational prescriber, two aspects of the pharmacokinetics of the benzodiazepines are particularly relevant: the speed of onset and the duration of action. The speed of onset of action depends on the mode of administration, the dissolution of the drug formulation, the rapidity of absorption, and the rate of entry into the brain. Diazepam is rapidly absorbed when taken orally and enters the brain quickly. It can thus be used

Figure 1. Formulae of Some Benzodiazepines

Table 1. Elimination Half-Lives of Some Benzodiazepines and Major Active Metabolites in Healthy Adults

Drug	Half-life of parent drug (hr)	Active metabolite	Half-life of metabolite (hr)
Chlordiazepoxide	7-14	Demoxepam	
		Desmethyldiazepam	50-100
Diazepam	14-90	Desmethyldiazepam	50-100
Oxazepam	6-24	—	
Clorazepate	—	Desmethyldiazepam	50-100
Lorazepam	9-22	—	
Prazepam	—	Desmethyldiazepam	50-100
Halazepam	—	Desmethyldiazepam	50-100
Flurazepam	1-2	N-desalkylflurazepam	50-100
Temazepam	4-10	—	

to give prompt relief of acute panic states. Given intravenously, it is a prime treatment for stopping repeated epileptic seizures. By contrast, oxazepam is slowly absorbed and takes more time to reach the brain. Desmethyldiazepam takes a little longer than diazepam. Lorazepam is also relatively slow in its entry into the brain but can be used intravenously as a sedative for prolonged investigative or minor surgical procedures. Diazepam is slowly and erratically absorbed after intramuscular injection (Assaf et al., 1975). It can be given by suppository, the plasma concentrations attained generally surpassing those after intramuscular injection (Kanto, 1975). Suppositories should be considered in patients who are vomiting, and they also have been used successfully in the management of status epilepticus in children.

Plasma protein binding of the benzodiazepines is generally extensive (Boxenbaum et al., 1977; Van der Kleijn et al., 1971) but is of little direct clinical relevance.

Benzodiazepine metabolism can be divided into Phase I and Phase II. The former comprises mainly oxidation and dealkylation, the latter conjugation to form glucuronides, sulfates, and acetylated compounds. Benzodiazepines can be divided into those that undergo both Phase I and Phase II metabolism—examples are diazepam, chlordiazepoxide, and flurazepam—and those undergoing Phase II metabolism alone—including lorazepam, oxazepam, and temazepam. As a general rule, the liver has a much greater capacity for Phase II than for Phase I metabolism. Consequently, drugs metabolized by Phase II processes alone will be better tolerated than Phase I/Phase II drugs in patients with impairments of liver function such as alcoholics. Also, Phase I metabolism tends to become slower with advancing age so that the elderly are more likely to suffer toxic effects from Phase I/Phase II drugs than Phase II only drugs.

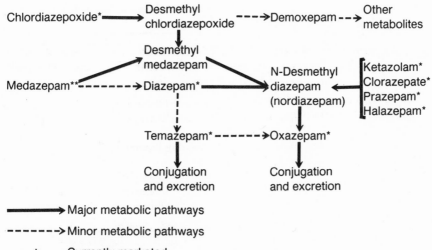

Lorazepam is a chlorinated derivative of oxazepam. Triazolam, flurazepam and clonazepam have separate metabolic pathways.

Figure 2. Metabolic Pathways of Some Benzodiazepines

The type of metabolism does not necessarily determine the rate of metabolism, and the elimination half-lives of the benzodiazepines vary greatly (Table 1). A key compound is N-desmethyldiazepam (nordiazepam), the major metabolite of diazepam (Figure 2), which has psychotropic activity as a tranquilizer. Its half-life is very long, typically over 100 hours (Mandelli et al., 1978). Consequently, it accumulates over the first month of treatment, reaching higher plasma and body concentrations than the parent compound, diazepam. N-desmethyldiazepam is also the major metabolite of clorazepate, prazepam, ketazolam, halazepam, medazepam, and to some extent chlordiazepoxide (Greenblatt et al., 1978a). Consequently, the clinical actions of these drugs are similar, as they share this common and major metabolite. Switching from one of these compounds to another during pharmacotherapy is almost always unproductive.

In contrast to these long-lasting N-desmethyldiazepam precursors, lorazepam, oxazepam, temazepam, and lormetazepam have half-lives of around six to 24 hours (Table 1), as the body eliminates much of each dose between each administration. These compounds are particularly suitable for acute, short-lived anxieties; fluctuating levels of anxiety; and for use as hypnotics. Triazolam is even shorter acting, its half-life being less than four hours. Flurazepam, long the most popular benzodiazepine hypnotic in the United States, has a similar short half-life; but it has an active metabolite with a prolonged action so residual effects may persist the next day. It is not an ideal hypnotic unless daytime sedation is also required, as in the case of an anxious insomniac.

Several studies have tried to relate clinical response to plasma concentrations of benzodiazepines. Most have failed to establish any significant relationships (Norman and Burrows, 1980), although, as is to be expected, side effects are more common at higher plasma concentrations. Further studies are needed and may be more fruitful, especially as radioreceptor assays are now available. These techniques are simple, inexpensive, and give some indication of the biological activity of both the parent drug and any active metabolites.

Basic Pharmacology

The mode of action of the benzodiazepines and other antianxiety drugs was obscure until recently. It is now probable that the benzodiazepines potentiate the inhibitory neurotransmitter, gamma amino butyric acid (GABA). It has been estimated that this transmitter is involved in 40 percent of all synapses, making it among the most ubiquitous of all neurotransmitters. Any drugs potentiating GABA would have widespread inhibitory actions. Benzodiazepines enhance transmission at all GABA-ergic synapses specifically investigated to date, both presynaptic and postsynaptic. However, this activity varies greatly from one part of the brain and spinal cord to another and even at different synapses within a given structure (Haefely, 1983). The molecular mechanism involved is a modification of the GABA receptor-chloride channel coupling so that these channels are opened more frequently, thereby increasing inhibition (Paul et al., 1981). Whether a natural transmitter acts on benzodiazepine binding sites or receptors has not been proven (Mohler, 1981). Barbiturates do not bind to these same sites but may also have some action on chloride transport mechanisms is neuronal membranes. A benzodiazepine antagonist has been developed (Mohler et al., 1982) and may be of use in overdose cases (Scollo-Lavizzari, 1983).

Because of their widespread inhibitory neuropharmacologic effects, benzodiazepines can alter the turnover of neurotransmitters such as norepinephrine and 5-hydroxytryptamine. The sites of action of the benzodiazepines include the spinal cord, where muscle relaxant effects are mediated; the brain stem, perhaps accounting for anticonvulsant properties; the cerebellum (perhaps causing ataxia); and limbic and cortical areas involved in the organization of emotional experience and behavior.

Clinical Pharmacology

Although the benzodiazepines have some effects on respiration and the cardiovascular system, these are slight; and virtually all the effects of these

Table 2. Psychological Measures Affected by Benzodiazepines

Much Effect	Little Effect
Critical Flicker Fusion	Complex visuo-motor coordination
Learning tasks	Visual spatial performance
Memory tasks	Auditory perception
Digit Symbol Substitution	Simulated driving
Cancellation task	
Card-sorting	
Tapping test	
Actual driving	

drugs result from other actions on the central nervous system. The most prominent of these are the allaying of anxiety, induction of sleep, muscle relaxation, and anticonvulsant effects. The benzodiazepines are normally regarded as devoid of analgesic or antidepressant effects, although alprazolam is reported to have some efficacy in elevating mood. Unlike the barbiturates, alcohol, and other sedative drugs, the benzodiazepines are not general neuronal depressants. Thus, with increasing dosage, sedation merges into sleep and stupor, but no true general anesthesia occurs. Despite sporadic claims by drug manufacturers, it is not clear whether the antianxiety properties of the benzodiazepines are separate from their sedative and hypnotic properties or are an intrinsic part of this action.

The psychological effects of single and repeated doses of benzodiazepines in normal subjects have been studied extensively (McNair, 1973). Marked variations are found in the extent to which various psychometric tests are affected (Table 2). In anxious patients, psychological impairment is much more difficult to detect. The reason is probably that anxiety itself impairs performance so that the benzodiazepine's side effect in further impairing performance is outweighed by its therapeutic effect in lessening anxiety and, thereby, improving performance.

Several reviews have surveyed clinical trials of benzodiazepines, and most concur in confirming the effectiveness of this class of compounds as antianxiety agents (Rickels et al., 1978; Rosenbaum, 1982). For example, in a coruscating review of the pharmacotherapy of anxiety with benzodiazepines, Greenblatt and Shader (1978b) state:

> Despite the elusive, evanescent and relatively nonspecific manifestations of clinical anxiety as well as the methodologic problems in reliable and relevant quantitation, most clinicians and investigators seem to agree that benzodiazepine derivatives are more consistently effective than placebo in well-controlled, short-term trials of anxiolytic drug therapy.

Despite extensive clinical use of the benzodiazepines, few studies have evaluated their long-term effects. It is not clear whether therapeutic effects are maintained for longer than a few weeks or months or whether any late, deleterious changes in neuropsychological functioning can be detected.

There are some minor differences among the benzodiazepines with respect to their pharmacodynamic profiles of action. For example, diazepam is more anticonvulsant than chlordiazepoxide, and lorazepam seems particularly sedative and is potent in producing amnesia after intravenous use or after large oral doses.

UNWANTED EFFECTS

Unwanted medication effects are due to interactions between the drug and the patient's pathophysical and psychological state. All antianxiety drugs are liable to have adverse effects on the central nervous system; the main problems are oversedation and impairment of higher cerebral functions. Relatively innocuous but frequent side effects occur during short-term treatment. In overdosage benzodiazepines are much safer than their predecessors. But comparatively little is known about potentially adverse, long-term effects, such as chronic psychological impairment. There is growing evidence that benzodiazepine dependence may be more widespread than previously assumed. These various aspects will be reviewed in turn (Edwards, 1981).

Acute Toxicity

Overdosage with the benzodiazepines occurs frequently; but, fortunately, deaths as a result of benzodiazepines *alone* are rare (Finkle et al., 1979). Although fatal overdose statistics contain deaths attributed to benzodiazepines alone, many such attributions are suspect. Often, other drugs, particularly alcohol, have been taken. Only in children and the physically frail, especially those with respiratory problems, are the benzodiazepines hazardous. Patients who have taken overdoses become drowsy or stuporous and fall into a deep sleep (Busto et al., 1980). A few develop rigidity or twitching of limbs or a skin eruption. Usually, blood pressure drops minimally, and respiration is hardly affected. Sleep lasts 24 to 48 hours but patients are generally rousable. Plasma benzodiazepine concentrations are understandably high on admission of such a patient to the hospital but are often still around the same levels when the patient wakes up and seems conscious and oriented. It may be that the brain can overcome the depressant effects of the drug, a form of acute tolerance (Greenblatt et al., 1978). In the case of barbiturates, however, drowsiness may progress to stupor or coma, with a life-threatening effect on the cardiovascular system and respiration.

Side Effects during Therapy

The most common unwanted side effects are tiredness, drowsiness, and torpor, these being most marked within the first two hours after large doses. Drowsiness is more frequently a complaint during the first week of treatment and then wanes and disappears, suggesting that tolerance outweighs any accumulation of long-acting compounds or metabolites. Accordingly, patients should be warned of the potential side effects of any prescribed benzodiazepine. The dosage should initially be cautious until the effects of the drug can be gauged. In particular, patients should be advised not to drive a vehicle during the initial adjustment of dosage. If driving is essential for their livelihood, very small doses should be used initially and increased under close supervision until symptom relief is obtained or adverse effects begin to occur. Once the dosage providing the optimal balance between symptom relief and side effects has been determined, interference with mechanical skills such as driving or operating dangerous machinery should not be a problem. Powers of judgment and memory are thought to be impaired in some patients during the first week or two of drug treatment, so important decisions should be deferred (Petersen and Ghoneim, 1980).

As with most CNS-depressant drugs, the effects of alcohol and benzodiazepines together can be greater than with either alone. It is not established whether this is a simple additive pharmacological effect or whether some potentiation (i.e., multiplication of effects) can occur (Linnoila et al., 1979). Also, pharmacokinetic interactions have been described: For example, the absorption of chlordiazepoxide, but not diazepam, was slowed by the simultaneous administration of alcohol (Linnoila et al., 1974). Patients must be warned not to drink alcohol when taking benzodiazepines, either chronically or intermittently. In particular, the combination of alcohol and a benzodiazepine may profoundly impair ability to drive, even when the patient has been taking the benzodiazepine for some time (or is an alcoholic). Generally speaking the benzodiazepines can be given safely in combination with other drugs. As with other tranquilizers, however, they may enhance the sedative effects of antipsychotic drugs, antidepressants, narcotic analgesics, and antihistamines. Unlike the barbiturates, the benzodiazepines are weak inducers of liver microsomal enzymes. Interactions with other drugs are generally minor. The only one of any real significance is between benzodiazepines metabolized by oxidation and desmethylation and cimetidine. Thus, diazepam and cimetidine compete for the same enzymes and the effects of diazepam can be enhanced, producing sedation. Cigarette smoking, a well known inducer of liver enzymes, may lessen diazepam's side effects (Boston Collaborative Drug Surveillance Program, 1973).

Other Adverse Reactions

Patients taking benzodiazepines may show so-called "paradoxical" behavioral responses (Hall and Disook, 1981). Such phenomena may include increased aggression and hostility, uncharacteristic criminal activities such as shop-lifting, sexual improprieties or offenses such as importuning or self-exposure, and excessive emotional responses such as uncontrollable giggling or weeping. This phenomenon is by no means confined to the benzodiazepines: Alcohol provides a cardinal example of a drug that may be associated with otherwise unexpected aggressive or criminal behavior. With the benzodiazepines, paradoxical reactions are most common during the first one or two weeks of treatment or following dosage increase. Often such reactions subside spontaneously but if they do not, dosage adjustment, usually downward, is generally successful. Hostile, aggressive, and irritable feelings often baffle the patient who fails to attribute them to the drug he is taking. It is wise to question patients routinely about any unexplained emotions that may be troubling them.

Administration of benzodiazepines can cause respiratory depression in patients with respiratory problems such as bronchitis and emphysema. The respiratory center in the brain becomes less sensitive to arterial carbon dioxide, which thus builds up. This is a particular problem after intravenous benzodiazepines.

Other side effects may include excessive weight gain, skin rash, impairment of sexual function, menstrual irregularities, and rarely, blood abnormalities. Benzodiazepines should be avoided during pregnancy, especially during the first three months; but claims that diazepam is associated with a higher than normal incidence of cleft lip with or without cleft palate in the fetus have not been sustained in large-scale retrospective surveys (Goldberg and DiMascio, 1978). Benzodiazepines readily cross the blood-placenta barrier (Kanto et al., 1973) and have been suspected of causing respiratory depression in the newborn. Benzodiazepines also pass into the mother's milk and can oversedate the baby (Cole and Hailey, 1975) so breast feeding may need to be discontinued if a benzodiazepine is required for the mother.

Tolerance and Dependence

Although benzodiazepines have a reputation for causing only a low rate of abuse and dependence, the possibility of this adverse effect of prolonged use is currently a subject of much concern. Tolerance certainly develops to some of the effects of antianxiety drugs, but the subsequent need for dosage escalation is much less than is the case with the opiates. Tolerance due to more rapid metabolism is probably of little clinical importance, but there is experimental evidence to show that pharmacological tolerance supervenes at the level of the receptor sites and is accompanied by physiological tolerance, i.e., of function. Tolerance to benzodiazepines confers cross-tolerance to methaqualone; barbiturates; and, to some extent, alcohol.

Although numerous reports describe human abuse and dependence, the number of case reports with convincing evidence of dependence is small in relation to the extensive and widespread use of benzodiazepines (Marks, 1978). Furthermore, relatively few patients escalate their dosage to levels so high that the prescriber suspects that dependence has supervened. When escalation does occur, each elevation of dosage seems to be related to a temporary increase in distress. Most patients can usefully increase their intake of antianxiety medication under distressing circumstances but reduce the dose once a crisis is past. A few patients maintain their increased dose and increase the dose still further when the next set of problems occurs. No definite features characterize such patients except that they may previously have abused alcohol or a barbiturate.

A withdrawal syndrome has been described in patients who have steadily increased their dose of benzodiazepine and have been above the maximum recommended dose for a few months or more. The mildest symptoms are anxiety, tension, apprehension, dizziness, insomnia, and anorexia. More severe physical dependence is manifested by withdrawal symptoms of nausea and vomiting, tremor, muscle weakness, and postural hypotension. This syndrome closely resembles that of withdrawal from barbiturates and has many features in common with the alcohol withdrawal syndrome. It is distinct from the narcotic withdrawal syndrome. Occasionally, hyperthermia, muscle twitches, convulsions, and confusional psychoses may occur. All benzodiazepines seem capable of producing this high-dose withdrawal syndrome.

Tolerance and dependence in patients who take therapeutic doses of benzodiazepines for long periods of time are less easy to establish. On withdrawal of medication, symptoms often appear which resemble those for which the benzodiazepine was originally prescribed, for example, anxiety, tension, insomnia, trembling, palpitations, and sweating. These are sometimes taken as evidence that the anxiety has continued, merely being kept under control by the drug, and that the symptoms have re-emerged when the drug was withdrawn, rather than being regarded as a true withdrawal syndrome (Rickels, 1981). Recent evidence suggests that some patients on standard therapeutic doses (i.e., up to 30 mg per day of diazepam or equivalent) who report difficulty in discontinuing their drugs develop a full-blown withdrawal syndrome if their drug is stopped suddenly (Petursson and Lader, 1981). On withdrawal, affective and perceptual changes occur, identical in nature, extent, and severity to those experienced in patients discontinuing supratherapeutic doses (see Table 3). Many patients may be reluctant to have their medication withdrawn because of previous unpleasant experiences when attempting to lower the dose them-

Table 3. Withdrawal Symptoms from Benzodiazepines

Symptom	Frequency
anxiety, tension	+ + + +
agitation, restlessness	+ + +
bodily symptoms of anxiety	+ +
irritability	+ +
lack of energy	+ +
impaired memory and concentration	+ +
depersonalization, derealization	+
sleep disturbance	+ + + +
tremor, shakiness	+ + +
headache	+ + +
muscle pains, aches, twitchings	+ +
loss of appetite	+ +
nausea, dry retching	+ +
depression	+
perspiration	+
metallic taste, hyperosmia	+ + + +
blurred vision, sore eyes, photophobia	+ + +
incoordination, vertigo	+ + +
hyperacusis	+ +
paresthesia	+ +
hypersensitivity to touch, pain	+ +
paranoid reaction	+

selves. This was apparent in one study in which only 40 out of 86 suitable patients consented to withdrawal (Tyrer et al., 1981).

The withdrawal reaction is most pronounced one to seven days after medication has been stopped. This delay depends on the half-life of the benzodiazepine or its active metabolites, being short with oxazepam, long with diazepam. Anxiety rises sharply during withdrawal, to incipient panic in many patients, but usually subsides to prewithdrawal levels over the next two to four weeks. Patients commonly experience bodily symptoms of anxiety, such as a choking feeling, dry mouth, hot and cold feelings, "legs like jelly," etc. (Table 3). Some become irritable, and a few complain of unpleasant feelings of depersonalization and derealization. All experience significant sleep disturbance, some experience hand tremor and profuse perspiration, and others have severe headaches and generalized muscular aches and pains. Many lose their appetite and suffer from nausea and vomiting in the mornings. Clinical depression is present in some patients but is usually neither severe nor prolonged. Many patients undergoing withdrawal experience mild to moderate perceptual disturbances. Some complain of intolerance to loud noises or bright lights, numbness or paresthesia, unsteadiness and a feeling of motion, or the sensing of strange smells and a metallic taste. Withdrawal epileptic seizures and psychotic episodes of a paranoid type may occasionally supervene.

The likelihood of a withdrawal reaction is lessened if the dose of benzodiazepine is gradually tapered off over the course of two to six weeks. Nevertheless, some patients, even those discontinuing from therapeutic doses, may still experience some withdrawal symptoms however gradual the cessation. The clinician may need to rely on help and support from the patient's family or friends to ease the patient over the worst of the withdrawal period, which is usually the first two weeks. Some patients experience prolonged withdrawal, with the perceptual symptoms and muscle tension persisting for up to several months. Substitution of an antipsychotic drug such as chlorpromazine is not advisable because the convulsive threshold is lowered. Propranolol, a beta-adrenoceptor antagonist, may help physical symptoms of withdrawal such as tremor. In patients experiencing many difficulties withdrawing from a medium-acting compound such as lorazepam, substitution of a long-acting drug such as clorazepate may facilitate withdrawal.

OTHER DRUGS AS ANTIANXIETY DRUGS

Antipsychotic Drugs

Antipsychotic drugs (neuroleptics) such as chlorpromazine, haloperidol, and thioridazine have been advocated to treat anxiety (Goldberg and Finnerty, 1979a; Finnerty et al., 1976). The suggested dose is quite low, typically half or less of the usual antipsychotic dose. Even at this low dosage, however, the antipsychotic drug may be poorly tolerated by the anxious patient because autonomic side effects such as dry mouth and dizziness too closely resemble his own symptoms. Even more upsetting are extrapyramidal symptoms such as restlessness (akathisia) and mild parkinsonism with paucity of voluntary movements and a coarse tremor. Such unwanted effects are relatively uncommon at low doses but can and are often overlooked. Of more concern, a few cases of tardive dyskinesia, even from low doses, have been recorded; and this possibility is a compelling reason against the routine use of low-dose antipsychotic medications for anxiety.

A theoretical advantage of antipsychotic drugs in the management of anxiety is that dependence on these drugs is virtually unknown. Accordingly, a common rationale for their use is as a short-term adjunct to nonpharmacological therapies in patients with a history of dependence on other CNS depressant drugs such as alcohol or a barbiturate. Dosage should be cautious and reviewed periodically, and careful observations should be made to establish whether any therapeutic benefit is accruing. Extrapyramidal signs should be carefully sought and, if observed, the dose should be lowered. Anticholinergic antiparkinsonism drugs should be avoided.

Sedative Antihistamines

Drugs such as diphenhydramine and hydroxyzine are sometimes used in anxious patients who have previously abused psychotropic drugs or alcohol. However, response is unpredictable especially in the young, who may be excited and stimulated rather than sedated. Also, when sedation is produced it can be peculiarly unpleasant with marked torpor.

Buspirone

Buspirone is a chemically novel compound probably acting on 5-HT mechanisms. Preliminary studies suggest antianxiety properties with low abuse potential (Goldberg and Finnerty, 1979b; Rickels et al., 1982; Cole et al., 1982).

Tricyclic Antidepressants

Several tricyclic antidepressants such as amitriptyline and doxepin have useful secondary sedative actions, perhaps reflecting their antihistaminic properties. They are often a good choice in depressed patients with anxiety or agitation. Clinical trials have established that the sedative properties of many tricyclic antidepressants are therapeutically useful in anxious patients. Nevertheless, they are not appropriate for patients with primary generalized anxiety disorders (nonphobic, nonpanic) because of their range of side effects, dangers in overdose, and interactions with other drugs. However, the distinction between primary depressive and primary anxious illnesses is not always obvious, especially in the milder cases frequently encountered in general practice. If a patient with anxiety fails to respond to simple antianxiety treatment, the possibility of an underlying depressive panic or phobic illness should seriously be considered. These sedative antidepressants can be used to treat insomnia in depressed patients by giving the bulk of the daily requirement as a night-time dose. Caution with such a regimen is necessary in the elderly and in the middle-aged with a history of cardiac disease because of the cardiotoxicity of some of these antidepressants in patients with pre-existing cardiac pathology.

Monoamine Oxidase Inhibitors

The monoamine oxidase inhibitors are used to treat so-called "atypical" depressive disorders. While some patients with phobic anxiety respond well to full doses of phenelzine or tranylcypromine, nonphobic anxiety is not usually helped.

Beta-Adrenoceptor Antagonists

Many different bodily symptoms in patients with anxiety states are mediated by the sympathetic nervous system. In particular, palpitations, tremor, and gastrointestinal upset are related to overactivity of beta-adrenergic sympathetic systems. Consequently, blockade of this activity by means of beta-adrenoceptor antagonists might be expected to help patients with anxiety, especially those with autonomic symptoms. Many trials have been carried out in the last 15 years using various beta-blockers. The results have consistently indicated that only those symptoms mediated by the beta division of the sympathetic nervous system are helped by administration of drugs such as propranolol or sotalol (Tyrer, 1980). Somatic symptoms such as headache, presumably otherwise mediated, and some aspects of psychological distress are not usefully improved. Whether a patient finds relief on a beta-blocker depends on his symptom profile. Patients with predominant complaints of palpitations, trembling, and gastrointestinal upset such as diarrhea are often much improved. Even so, the improvement may be limited to those symptoms alone, and other anxiety symptoms may be unchanged. A few patients may even worsen on beta-blockers. For example, somatic symptoms may signal to a phobic patient that he or she is entering a phobic situation. Loss of these symptoms may alarm a patient who thus fears loss of control. Beta-blockers may help some patients with panic disorders where awareness of palpitations or tremor exacerbates the condition.

Beta-blockers should not be used in patients with a history of asthma, and a cardiologist's advice should be sought for those with heart disease. A test dose, say 20 mg of propranolol, should be administered to detect undue sensitivity as shown by bradycardia below 60 beats/min at rest. If no sensitivity is found, the dose can be instituted at 20 mg three times a day and, if necessary, increased over the course of a week or two to 40 mg four times a day. The resting pulse rate should be monitored and used as the "end-point": Dosage should be maintained at that necessary to keep the pulse at normal levels. It is usually unhelpful to push the dose beyond 160 mg/day in total. At these dose levels, the drug predominantly acts peripherally on symptom mechanisms rather than centrally.

CLINICAL INDICATIONS AND LIMITATIONS

The fundamental problems faced by the therapist treating the anxious patient are whether the benefits of antianxiety medication outweigh the

Table 4. Symptoms of Anxiety and Differential Diagnosis

	Symptoms	Differential Diagnosis

Psychological	Anxiety
	Nervousness
	Fear
	Panic
	Mental disintegration
	Apprehension and
	  anticipation of the worst
		Early schizophrenia
		Drug abuse, especially
		  amphetamine and cocaine
		Excessive use of caffeine
		Temporal lobe epilepsy

Cardiovascular	Palpitations Rapid heart beat Tightness in chest Face flushing	Cardiac dysrhythmias Angina, hypertension Pheochromocytoma
Respiratory	Breathlessness Air hunger Paresthesiae	Asthma Respiratory failure Neurologic conditions
Gastrointestinal	Difficulty swallowing Nausea and vomiting Diarrhea	Esophageal pathology Gastric pathology Ulcerative colitis
Genitourinary	Frequency of micturition Impotence and premature ejaculation Frigidity	Bladder pathology Neurological conditions
Skin	Sweating	Thyrotoxicosis
Somatic	Aches and pains Headache Restlessness Fatigue Tremors	Rheumatology conditions Migraine Chronic infections, e.g. TB Neurologic conditions
Sleep	Insomnia Nightmares	Specific syndromes
General/metabolic	Dizziness Faintness	Hypoglycemia Adrenal insufficiency

risks of dependence (physical or psychological), whether problems that may be viewed as interpersonal or environmental should be "medicalized," and whether the physician should resort again to drugs in treating future episodes (Table 4). The main criterion for giving an antianxiety agent is generalized anxiety so severe that it hinders the patient's ability to cope with his symptoms and other responsibilities. Often, acute severe anxiety requires pharmacological treatment to tide the patient over a week or two of distress until he feels well enough to face up to his difficulties. For example, sedation after a particularly tragic bereavement may be appropriate, but the routine administration of tranquilizers after a long-expected death in the family usually is not. Control of symptoms by prompt and vigorous treatment enables the patient to regain mastery of his own symptoms and to approach his difficulties realistically when the symptoms subside. Also, although most acute anxiety states subside spontaneously, a few seem to become chronic if the symptoms are allowed to persist unabated for more than a week or two. When tranquilizers are intended to help combat a crisis, the patient must be warned to expect that the drugs will be given for a limited period only.

A more difficult decision concerns episodes of generalized anxiety of more than six months' duration. Drug administration will necessarily be long-term with the risk of dependence. Again the criteria should be the severity of the anxiety and the distress it causes the patient. If the anxiety interferes with everyday functioning, thus handicapping the patient, and the treatment helps the patient, then antianxiety drugs are indicated. Even so, such episodes do eventually resolve, and in the younger patient maturation is often accompanied by better coping responses and mastery of anxiety. The practitioner must reassess the patient from time to time to see whether reduction in dosage and eventual discontinuation are feasible.

Yet, the most complex decisions concern the patient with life-long anxiety. Here the anxiety constantly permeates the individual's existence. Every decision is an agony of doubt, every departure from routine a catalog of apprehensions, every encounter with a stranger a signal for a panic, and so on. Yet the individual functions after a fashion, may be married and have children, and may even be materially successful. To withhold anxiolytics or to insist on psychotherapy only can become a moral judgment. The essential fact to establish is whether the patient functions better on than off drugs with respect to interpersonal, social, occupational, and leisure activities and is relatively free from anxiety symptoms. If these facts can be established, then long-term or indefinite treatment may be in the patient's interests. The implications of such chronic treatment should be discussed frankly with the patient.

Choice of Drug

The choice of the most appropriate drug follows from the discussion of the pharmacokinetics of the benzodiazepines (Table 5). No consistent evidence indicates the superiority of one benzodiazepine over another in the reduction of anxiety. Clinicians have their preferences, and prescribing fashions do change. For example, diazepam has largely supplanted chlordiazepoxide in hospital practice although family doctors still use the latter quite widely. In general, though, the choice of drug is dictated by the type of anxiety,

Table 5. Antianxiety Drugs

	Adult daily dose (mg)	
Generic	Minor symptoms	Major symptoms
Benzodiazepines		
Chlordiazepoxide	20-40	40-100
Diazepam	6-15	15-30
Oxazepam	45-90	90-180
Clorazepate	15	15-30
Lorazepam	1-4	4-10
Prazepam	10-20	20-60
Flurazepam (hypnotic indication)	15	30
Temazepam (hypnotic indication)	10-20	20-40
Propanediols (obsolescent)		
Meprobamate	200-600	600-1800
Tybamate	250-500	500-2000
Barbiturates (obsolete)		
Amobarbital	30-90	90-200
Phenobarbital (anti-epileptic)	30-60	60-90
Antihistamines		
Diphenhydramine	50-100	100-300
Hydroxyzine	75-150	150-400
Tricyclic antidepressant		
Amitriptyline	50-75	75-150
β-adrenoceptor blocking agent		
Propranolol (N.B. not approved by F.D.A. for treating anxiety or panic disorder)	20-60	60-180

which should be matched to the pharmacokinetic properties of the various drugs, particularly the rate of absorption and duration of action.

In particular, the initial choice of benzodiazepine should take into account the temporal pattern of the anxiety state. A benzodiazepine with a long half-life, such as diazepam or clorazepate, is appropriate if the anxiety levels are high and sustained. Because of the long half-life, two daily or one nightly dosage is sufficient. Even so, some patients prefer more frequent dosage because they can detect the sedative effects following each dose and are reassured by them. For episodic anxiety, shorter-acting compounds such as lorazepam or alprazolam can be used, taken 30 minutes or so before entering an anxiety-provoking situation. If the episode has already started, diazepam should be given and will exert a fairly prompt action. However, full-blown panic attacks may not respond well to benzodiazepines. Some patients are reassured by carrying some alprazolam or similar compounds for just such an eventuality, which might be dubbed a "talismanic" use. Oxazepam is also short-acting, but its absorption rate is too slow for emergency use of this type.

Many patients report increases in anxiety on the background of an already raised anxiety level. Here, theoretically, the most appropriate drug, from the point of view of its pharmacokinetics, is diazepam. A proportion, perhaps half, of the daily dose can be given before the patient goes to bed. This amount acts as a hypnotic because of its rapid absorption and transient peak levels. During the day, the long half-life of diazepam and its major metabolite, N-desmethyldiazepam, provides a background antianxiety effect. Superimposed on this base, small doses of diazepam can be given during the day as required. Shorter-acting drugs can also be prescribed as regular doses, plus additions if required; however, divided doses are necessary to maintain the base levels.

Some patients take antianxiety medication regularly, but many take it only when feeling particularly anxious or when they feel they are about to encounter a particularly anxiety-provoking situation. Most such patients keep to a small dose of benzodiazepine, say diazepam, 5 mg, but supervision is necessary lest the dosage be insidiously increased.

Beta-adrenoceptor antagonists can be considered when the patient complains of somatic symptoms, especially palpitations. Therapeutic results can be gratifying when a symptom such as palpitations assumes overwhelming importance. Phobic patients may not respond so well. The combination of a beta-blocker and a benzodiazepine may be a reasonable therapy in patients with mixed somatic and psychological symptoms.

Doses

The keynote for treatment should be great flexibility within reasonable limits to accommodate the individual needs of the patient. If repeated daily doses of a short-acting drug are indicated, it is helpful if the patient keeps a daily log of his panic attacks and of drug usage. This practice facilitates the adjustment of the dosage which the patient undertakes and increases his sense of participation in a therapeutic process rather than his being a passive recipient. Many patients can be allowed substantial responsibility in the management of their drug use (Winstead et al., 1974).

The rules of establishing dosage are to obtain the best clinical response commensurate with the patient's ability to tolerate the side effects. The long-acting drugs are easier to stabilize in this respect although the rapid absorption of diazepam may give rise to a transient peak with concomitant drowsiness. On the other hand, such a rapid and detectable effect may be reassuring to the patient.

Despite the rationale of usage arising from the pharmacokinetics of the various benzodiazepines, too rigid adherence to dosage schedules can be self-defeating. Thus, one patient may manage well on one dose of clorazepate at night, another on minute doses of diazepam six or more times during the day, a third on eight-hourly oxazepam.

Duration of Therapy

Short courses of treatment are appropriate for the acutely anxious patient. As remission is likely to occur anyway, treatment should be planned in terms of one to two weeks rather than months. The patient must not be allowed to persist with marginally effective treatment—it must either be made effective by dosage manipulation or discontinued. Some patients with recurrent episodes of anxiety keep a store of antianxiety medicines and are adept at reverting to them for a short course of treatment during a crisis. It is best to encourage this form of self-medication but to ask the patient to inform the doctor when such an episode occurs. Disapproval of such a course only leads to the patient's taking antianxiety drugs clandestinely.

With chronic anxiety, courses of treatment are obviously prolonged; and with the abnormally anxious personality, treatment is indefinite. Nevertheless, the therapist should always be alert to any tendency to escalate the dosage and should seek to lower the dosage when the patient is stabilized in a quiescent period.

Drug Discontinuation

With the short-acting drugs given intermittently, no accumulation will have occurred so withdrawal can be abrupt. With the long-acting compounds, withdrawal is best carried out over a few weeks, especially when dosage has been above normal therapeutic levels or treatment prolonged beyond six months. The patient should be seen a week after final discontinuation as withdrawal effects may become apparent then.

Response to Treatment

Rickels and co-workers have carried out a large series of studies on response to treatment in anxious patients (Rickels et al., 1978). As might be expected, anxiety and somatic complaints are the symptoms most sensitive to antianxiety drug effects. Depressive symptoms respond occasionally, and obsessional symptoms rarely respond. Interpersonal sensitivity (i.e., feelings easily being hurt) is also unresponsive. Hostility, by contrast, is usually reduced by antianxiety treatment, although exceptional paradoxical increases may occur.

Rickels' group has also analyzed extensive data with respect to prognostic variables. Their replicated predictors are set out in Table 6. It should be added, however, that the establishment of rapport is important, and confidence in using drugs maximizes their effect.

Table 6. Predictors of Good Outcome (Rickels)

Patient:
   More educated
   Expects drug treatment
   Realizes problems are emotional
   Female without menopause or hysterectomy

Physician:
   Feels comfortable with patient
   Likes patient
   Considers drug therapy most appropriate

Illness and treatment related:
   Acute duration
   Diagnosis of anxiety
   No previous drugs
   Good response to previous drugs

Presenting psychopathology:
   Less severe obsessive-compulsive
   Less severe interpersonal sensitivity
   Less severe depression
   More severe anxiety

Panic Attacks and Antianxiety Drugs

The traditional treatment for severe panic attacks is sodium amobarbital, up to 500 mg, intravenously or intramuscularly. Intravenous diazepam (5-10 mg) is also effective (Kelly et al., 1973). Clonidine has also been advocated.

The prevention of panic attacks is more problematic. Constant antianxiety therapy may lessen their frequency and/or blunt their severity in some patients, but most complain that the panic attacks often persist despite amelioration of the background anxiety. Antidepressants, both tricyclics and MAOI's, are becoming established as antipanic agents; and many trials attest to their efficacy (Zitrin et al., 1983; Sheehan et al., 1980; Marks et al., 1983; Pohl et al., 1983).

Insomnia and Antianxiety Drugs

The largest use for short-acting benzodiazepines is in the management of insomnia, especially that related to stress and anxiety and the so-called "idiopathic" cases. The essential criterion for a hypnotic in patients not desiring an antianxiety effect during the daytime is that the drug should not accumulate on repeated dosage during the course of treatment (Nicholson, 1981). To this end, its half-life should not exceed eight to ten hours on the average. Triazolam has a very short half-life, but that of flurazepam (and metabolites) is too long to meet this criterion. For short-term insomnia temazepam is the drug of choice. In many patients with insomnia, a daytime antianxiety effect is important as the insomnia is but one symptom in a response to stress. Accordingly, diazepam or flurazepam may be given to act as both a night-time hypnotic and as a daytime sedative.

Other Indications

Benzodiazepines are in great vogue as skeletal muscle relaxants in the management of acute conditions such as tetanus, trauma, and chronic conditions such as the relief of spasticity and athetosis in patients with neurological illnesses. In this indication, diazepam acts on the spinal cord independently of any action in the brain (Cook and Nathan, 1966), although doses that reduce muscle tone are often sedative. The dosage is initially 6 mg per day but may be increased up to 30 mg a day if necessary; 15 mg is the average daily dose. As the effect on spasticity may last longer than its sedative action, unwanted effects are reduced if the daily dose is taken at bedtime. Diazepam reduces both clonus and pain, but baclofen more effectively reduces spasms and increases mobility (Burt and Currie, 1978). Clonazepam has also been evaluated and found effective (Cendrowski and Sobczyk, 1977). Benzodiazepines can be used as adjuncts to various types of relaxation therapy, especially if the patient is very tense, anxious, and unable to commence relaxation. Diazepam or lorazepam can be administered by mouth 30 to 60 minutes before the relaxation therapy session or, in the more severe cases, by careful and slow intravenous injection.

Other uses for which the short-acting benzodiazepines are appropriate are as pre-operative medication and as deep sedation for minor operative procedures. While diazepam is not a true anesthetic, only a sedative, sedation alone is sufficient for some procedures. The main problem with intravenous diazepam in its usual dose of 0.2 mg/kg is its variable and unpredictable effect; even large doses may prove ineffective (Brown and Dundee, 1968). A second problem is that dizziness may recur after initial recovery (Baird and Hailey, 1972), perhaps due to remobilization of the redistributed diazepam or to slow accumulation of the active metabolite, desmethyldiazepam. Other problems are the well known superficial venous thrombosis at the site of injection (Mikkelsen et al., 1980). Lorazepam injection seldom causes pain or venous thrombosis but is slow in its onset of action (Dundee et al., 1979).

Benzodiazepines are now the standard treatment in the management of alcohol withdrawal, due in part to the cross-tolerance between alcohol and benzodiazepines. A typical schedule is 50 mg of chlordiazepoxide or 10 mg of diazepam four to six times a day for a mild alcohol abstinence syndrome and up to three times this amount for major syndromes and delirium tremens. After the symptoms are controlled, the dose is reduced gradually over five to ten days. Oral medication is preferred to intramuscular injections, which are absorbed erratically. It must be remembered that the duration of action of some benzodiazepines, such as chlordiazepoxide, may be markedly prolonged in patients with cirrhosis of the liver (Roberts et al., 1977).

To summarize this section, the recommendations of the American Medical Association (1974) are still timely:

A. Reserve tranquilizers for the relief of severe symptoms, not for minor ephemeral complaints.

B. Diagnose and treat any underlying disorders before settling for merely symptomatic relief.

C. Avoid drugs when the patient has a history of drug or alcohol abuse.

D. Keep doses modest so that psychological impairment does not supervene.

E. Be familiar with the need for gradual withdrawal with much support and encouragement when abuse does occur or when discontinuing after long-term use.

F. Monitor the possibility of dependence when patients are on long courses of treatment. Four to six months' duration seems to be the crucial time when the risk of dependence becomes appreciable.

G. Limit the amount of drug prescribed to that appropriate to the interval between visits.

H. Warn patients that sedation may occur, especially early in treatment, and that interactions with alcohol and other depressants are frequent, major, and hazardous.

I. Warn patients to keep the drugs for themselves and not to offer them to other people or allow children access to them.

J. Emphasize that the drugs are only part of an overall strategy for management and treatment.

Sedative-Facilitated Interviewing

The drugs most commonly used to facilitate interviewing and to produce "abreactions" are the barbiturates. The most favored barbiturates are intravenous sodium amobarbital or methohexital. While a sedative-facilitated interview has been shown to be beneficial on occasion, other possible, if not well established, indications include use of sedatives:

A. For mobilizing stuporous, catatonic, withdrawn schizophrenic patients, although the underlying schizophrenic symptomatology is not altered.

B. For lessening negative affect associated with traumatic and stressful experiences (Post-traumatic Stress Disorder, Chronic or Delayed). In the latter, the patient may experience a "flash-back" and relive his experiences, often with extreme affective and behavioral disturbances, shouting, cringing in fear, screaming in anger, etc. Afterward, there may be little recall of the session but the catharsis is deemed quite successful in lessening anxiety, panics, and especially nightmares. Although formal trials are lacking for this indication, there have been several large series of such treatment in wartime.

Sedative-facilitated interviews have also been used in interviewing people suspected of criminal offenses, using the so-called "truth-drug." Courts vary in whether they will accept disclosures after the drug as evidence. Although material incriminating or absolving of guilt may be uncovered, fantasy material or lies may just as easily be released.

AGE RELATED FACTORS

The use of tranquilizers in children is a topic of much controversy and few data. Benzodiazepines and barbiturates often make children irritable and drowsy. In addition, there is little convincing evidence that tranquilizers are useful in children with minor neurotic disturbances marked by disturbed sleep and anxiety. However, a few severely anxious children benefit from benzodiazepines. In children with situational anxiety such as school phobia, the impairment of intellectual function by the high doses needed usually outweighs any modest therapeutic benefit.

A special use of diazepam is in the management of sleep disorders such as night terrors which are associated with deep slow-wave sleep. Diazepam reduces or abolishes deep sleep, and the pavor nocturnus is reduced accordingly. Ordinary nightmares are not helped.

Barbiturates and benzodiazepines are tolerated less well in the elderly than in younger adults. Confusional states and paradoxical agitation are common. Ataxia may result in disastrous falls. If a benzodiazepine is deemed appropriate in elderly patients for treatment of insomnia, dosage should be cautious. It is wise to start with between a third and a half of the young adult dose and to increase it slowly until symptomatic relief is obtained. Benzodiazepines such as lorazepam and temazepam with Phase II metabolic patterns involving only glucuronidation are usually better tolerated in the elderly than those such as the N-desmethyl precursors, diazepam, prazepam, etc., whose metabolic pathways are more complex.

ETHICAL, SOCIAL, AND POLITICAL ISSUES

The benzodiazepines have largely replaced their predecessors, the barbiturates, and are now among the most widely used of all prescribed drugs. By the 1970's diazepam was the most frequently prescribed drug in the United States. Its close analog, chlordiazepoxide, was the third most often prescribed (Blackwell, 1973). More than 70 million prescriptions were filled for these two agents at a cost of over $200 million dollars and comprised more than half of all the prescriptions for psychotropic drugs. In addition, the benzodiazepines are the commonest drugs on repeat prescriptions.

During the past 20 years, about 500 million people have taken a benzodiazepine. Several surveys in different countries have suggested that about one in ten adult men and one in five adult women take tranquilizers or hypnotics, mainly benzodiazepines, at some time during the course of each year (Balter et al., 1974). Of these people, between half and two-thirds take tranquilizers for at least a month at a time, and perhaps two percent of the adult population does so consistently throughout the year. Usage goes up with age in women but is not age-related in men. Usage is higher in the lower social classes and in women.

Most prescriptions for benzodiazepines are written by nonpsychiatrists, in particular by family physicians, general physicians, orthopedic specialists, gynecologists, and pediatricians (Lasagna, 1977). In such benzodiazepine usage in nonpsychiatric practice, tranquilization is the major desired action. Anxious patients referred for psychiatric consultation are typically the more severely or chronically ill or those with personality or social problems. The former two categories of patients are likely to benefit from benzodiazepines, but the latter group often derives little symptomatic relief.

RESEARCH CONSIDERATIONS

How much of the long-term use of tranquilizers is the legitimate prescription of powerful psychotropic drugs for a chronically distressing condition, and how much is the provision of tranquilizers to unfortunate patients who suffer withdrawal problems if they try to discontinue medication remains an open question. Properly conducted epidemiological surveys are needed.

Another unknown quantity is the extent of therapeutic benefit that accrues to patients taking benzodiazepines beyond six months of treatment or longer. This question needs to be balanced against the possibility of psychometric impairment on chronic administration of tranquilizers in setting up benefit/drawback balance sheets of tranquilizer use. Economic cost, however, is not usually a pressing concern, as benzodiazepines, particularly generic preparations, are not expensive compared to some other modern drugs. When the cost of the doctor's, nurse's, or psychotherapist's time is taken into account, it is not difficult to see why such facile resort is made to the use of drugs (Wheatley, 1973).

CONCLUSION

The exploitation of drugs and other substances to produce tranquility is as old as mankind, alcohol and opiates being the main indigenous agents. In the present century the pharmaceutical industry has developed other anxiolytic/sedative agents, the foremost being the barbiturates and the benzodiazepines. Unfortunately, problems of dependence and abuse have always accompanied the use of such medications. Hence, the introduction of new and supposedly safer drugs in this class has been eagerly welcomed. Typically, the antianxiety drug is introduced as a major innovation; and only much later do questions of efficacy and safety arise, followed finally, by a much belated recognition of its dependence potential. Attitudes to tranquilizer use have, therefore, often been less than rational, and have gone from one extreme to the other.

The benzodiazepines represent the latest and most effective class of tranquilizers. Introduced in 1961, they quickly became the most widely used of all psychotropic drugs and have all but ousted their main predecessors, the barbiturates. Although there is some evidence that phenomenal use of the benzodiazepines has begun to level off somewhat, and may actually have dropped in some countries, their extensive use is of considerable concern to health authorities, clinicians, and lay people. This class of drugs is now undergoing a critical re-evaluation; in particular, their dependence potential is now being thoroughly investigated. Recently, the World Health Organization recommended placing the benzodiazepines on Schedule 4 of the Psychotropic Drug Convention. However, as long as no real substitutes materialize, the benzodiazepines are unlikely to meet with the same fate as their predecessors. At present they are without serious rivals in the symptomatic treatment of anxiety and related conditions, and it would be hard to imagine modern medical practice without effective antianxiety agents. In the short term , tranquilizers are invaluable; in the long term, their risks and benefits are unclear. The wise physician will continue to use them judiciously and sparingly.

REFERENCES

AMA Committee on Alcoholism and Drug Dependence: Barbiturate-like drugs: considerations in their medical use. JAMA 230:1440-1441, 1974

Assaf RAE, Dundee JW, Gamble JAS: The influence of the route of administration on the clinical action of diazepam. Anaesthesia 30:152-158, 1975

Baird ES, Hailey DM: Delayed recovery from a sedative: correlation of the plasma levels of diazepam with clinical effects after oral and intravenous administration. Br J Anaesth 44:803-807, 1972

Balter MB, Levine J, Manheimer DI: Cross-national study of the extent of antianxiety/sedative drug use. N Engl J Med 290:769-774, 1974

Blackwell B: The role of diazepam in medical practice. JAMA 225:1637-1641, 1973

Boston Collaborative Drug Surveillance Program: Clinical depression of the central nervous system due to diazepam and chlordiazepoxide in relation to cigarette smoking and age. N Engl J Med 288:277-280, 1973

Boxenbaum HG, Geitner KA, Jack ML, et al: Pharmacokinetics and biopharmaceutic profile of chlordiazepoxide HCL in healthy subjects: multiple-dose oral administration. J Pharmacokinet Biopharm 5:25-39, 1977

Brown SS, Dundee JW: Clinical studies of induction agents, XXV: diazepam. Br J Anaesth 40:108-112, 1968

Burt AA, Currie SA: Baclofen spasticity and cerebral pathology, in Double-blind Controlled Trial of Baclofen and Diazepam in Spasticity due to Cerebral Vascular Lesions. Northampton, UK, Cambridge Medical Publication, 1978

Busto U, Kaplan HL, Sellers EM: Benzodiazepine-associated emergencies in Toronto. Am J Psychiatry 137:226-227, 1980

Cendrowski W, Sobczyk W: Clonazepam, baclofen and placebo in the treatment of spasticity. Eur Neurol 16:257-262, 1977

Cohen IM: The benzodiazepines, in Discoveries in Biological Psychiatry. Edited by Ayd FJ, Blackwell B. Philadelphia, JB Lippincott, 1970

Cole AP, Hailey DM: Diazepam and active metabolites in breast milk and their transfer to the neonate. Arch Dis Child 50:741-742, 1975

Cole JO, Orzack MH, Beake B, et al: Assessment of the abuse liability of buspirone in recreational sedative users. J Clin Psychiatry 43:69-74, 1982

Cook JB, Nathan PW: On the site of action of diazepam in spasticity in man. J Neurol Sci 5:33-37, 1966

Dundee JW, McGowan WAW, Lilburn JK, et al: Comparison of the actions of diazepam and lorazepam. Br J Anaesth 51:439-446, 1979

Edwards JG: Adverse effects of antianxiety drugs. Drugs 22:495-514, 1981

Finkle BS, McCloskey KL, Goodman LS: Diazepam and drug-associated deaths: a survey in the United States and Canada. JAMA 242:429-434, 1979

Finnerty RJ, Goldberg HL, Nathan L, et al: Haloperidol in neurotic outpatients. Dis Nerv Sys 37:621-624, 1976

Goldberg HL, DiMascio A: Psychotropic drugs in pregnancy, in Psychopharmacology: A Generation of Progress. Edited by Lipton MA, DiMascio A, Killam KF. New York, Raven Press, 1978

Goldberg HL, Finnerty RJ: A double blind study of prochlorperazine, chlordiazepoxide and placebo in psychoneurotic outpatients with dominant symptoms of anxiety. Int Pharmacopsychiatry 14:264-277, 1979

Goldberg H, Finnerty RJ: Comparative efficacy of buspirone and diazepam in the treatment of anxiety. Am J Psychiatry 136:1184-1187, 1979b

Greenblatt DJ, Shader RI, MacLeod SM, et al: Clinical pharmacokinetics of chlordiazepoxide. Clin Pharmacokinet 3:381-394, 1978

Greenblatt DJ, Woo E, Allen MD, et al: Rapid recovery from massive diazepam overdose. JAMA 240:1872-1874, 1978

Greenblatt DJ, Shader RI: Pharmacotherapy of anxiety with benzodiazepines and β-adrenergic blockers, in Psychopharmacology: A Generation of Progress. Edited by Lipton MA, DiMascio A, Killam KF. New York, Raven Press, 1978

Greenblatt DJ, Shader RI: Meprobamate: a study of irrational drug use. Am J Psychiatry 127:1297-1304, 1971

Haefely W: Benzodiazepine receptors: summary and commentary, in Pharmacology of Benzodiazepines. Edited by Usdin E, Skolnick P, Tallman JF, et al. London, MacMillan, 1983

Hall RCW, Disook S: Paradoxical reactions to benzodiazepines. Br J Clin Pharmacol 11 (Suppl 1):99S-104S, 1981

Kanto J, Erkkola R, Sellman R: Accumulation of diazepam and N-desmethyldiazepam in the fetal blood during labor. Ann Clin Res 5:375-379, 1973

Kanto J: Plasma concentrations of diazepam and its metabolites after peroral, intramuscular, and rectal administration. Int J Clin Pharmacol 12:427-432, 1975

Kelly D, Pik R, Chen CN: A psychological and physiological evaluation of the effects of intravenous diazepam. Br J Psychiatry 122:419-426, 1973

Lasagna L: The role of benzodiazepines in non-psychiatric medical practice. Am J Psychiatry 134:656-658, 1977

Linnoila M, Mattila MJ, Kitchell BS: Drug interactions with alcohol. Drugs 18:299-311, 1979

Linnoila M, Otterstrom S, Antilla M: Serum chlordiazepoxide, diazepam, and thioridazine concentrations after the simultaneous ingestion of alcohol or placebo drink. Ann Clin Res 6:4-6, 1974

Mandelli M, Tognoni G, Garattnini S: Clinical pharmacokinetics of diazepam. Clin Pharmacokinet 3:72-91, 1978

Marks IM, Gray S, Cohen D, et al: Imipramine and brief therapist-aided exposure in agoraphobics having self-exposure homework. Arch Gen Psychiatry 40:153-162, 1983

Marks J: The Benzodiazepines: Use, Overuse, Misuse, Abuse. Lancaster, UK, MTP Press, 1978

McNair DM: Antianxiety drugs and human performance. Arch Gen Psychiatry 29:609-617, 1973

Mikkelsen H, Hoel TM, Byrne H, et al: Local reactions after iv injections of diazepam, flunitrazepam and isotonic saline. Br J Anaesth 52:817-819, 1980

Mohler H: Benzodiazepine receptors: are there endogenous ligands in the brain? Trends Pharmacol Sci 2:116-118, 1981

Nicholson AN: The use of short and long-acting hypnotics in clinical medicine. Br J Clin Pharmacol 11:61S-69S, 1981

Norman TR, Burrows GD: Plasma levels of benzodiazepine anti-anxiety drugs and clinical response, in Handbook of Studies on Anxiety. Edited by Burrows GD, Davies B. Amsterdam, Elsevier, 1980

Paul SM, Marangos PJ, Skolnick P: The benzodiazepine-GABA-chloride ionophore receptor complex: common site of minor tranquilizer action. Biol Psychiatry 16:213-229, 1981

Petersen RC, Ghoneim MM: Diazepam and human memory: influence on acquisition, retrieval, and state-dependent learning. Prog Neuropsychopharmacol 4:81-89, 1980

Petursson H, Lader MH: Withdrawal from long-term benzodiazepine treatment. Br Med J 283:643-645, 1981

Pohl R, Berchou R, Rainey JM: Tricyclic antidepressants and monoamine oxidase inhibitors in the treatment of agoraphobia. J Clin Psychopharmacol 2:399-407, 1983

Rickels K, Downing RW, Winokur A: Antianxiety drugs: clinical use in psychiatry, in Handbook of Psychopharmacology, Vol 13: Biology of Mood and Antianxiety Drugs. Edited by Iversen LL, Iversen SD, Snyder SH. New York, Plenum, 1978

Rickels K, Weisman K, Norstad DO, et al: Buspirone and diazepam in anxiety: a controlled study. J Clin Psychiatry 43:81-86, 1982

Rickels K: Benzodiazepines: use and misuse, in Anxiety: New Research and Changing Concepts. Edited by Klein DF, Rablin JG. New York, Raven Press, 1981

Roberts RK, Wilkinson GR, Branch RA, et al: Effect of age and cirrhosis on the disposition and elimination of chlordiazepoxide (Librium). Gastroenterology 73:1243, 1977

Rosenbaum JF: The drug treatment of anxiety. N Engl J Med 306:401-404, 1982

Scollo-Lavizzari G: First clinical investigation of the benzodiazepine antagonist Ro 15-1788 in comatose patients. Eur Neurol 22:7-11, 1983

Shader RI, Greenblatt DJ: Clinical implications of benzodiazepine pharmacokinetics. Am J Psychiatry 134:652-656, 1977

Sheehan DV, Ballenger J, Jacobsen G: Treatment of endogenous anxiety with phobic, hysterical and hypochondriacal symptoms. Arch Gen Psychiatry 36:51-59, 1980

Tyrer P, Rutherford D, Huggett T: Benzodiazepine withdrawal symptoms and propranolol. Lancet 1:520-522, 1981

Tyrer PJ: Use of β-blocking drugs in psychiatry and neurology. Drugs 20:300-308, 1980

Van der Kleijn E, van Rossum JM, Muskens ETJM, et al: Pharmacokinetics of diazepam in dogs, mice and humans. Acta Pharmacol Toxicol Suppl 3:29, 109-127, 1971

Wheatley D: Psychopharmacology in Family Practice. London, William Heinemann Medical Books, 1973

Winstead DK, Anderson A, Eilsers MK, et al: Diazepam on demand: drug seeking behavior in psychiatric inpatients. Arch Gen Psychiatry 30:349-351, 1974

Zitrin CM, Klein DF, Woerner MG, et al: Treatment of phobias, I: comparison of imipramine hydrochloride and placebo. Arch Gen Psychiatry 40:125-138, 1983

Antidepressants and Lithium

INTRODUCTION

Specific pharmacologic agents for the treatment of affective disorders have been available for only three decades. However, since the introduction of antidepressants and lithium in the 1950's, major advances in the theory and clinical management of depression, bipolar disorder, and other allied disorders have been made. The brain amine hypotheses focused on the possibility that depressive symptoms could be related to changes in brain chemistry, and more recent neuroendocrine studies have associated hypothalamic-pituitary dysregulation with affective disorders. So-called "new generation" antidepressants have provided alternatives to standard tricyclic agents although unexpected complications have tempered some initial expectations of these agents. Monoamine oxidase inhibitors and lithium have remained extremely useful drugs for treating affective disorders. Future developments in the psychopharmacology of affective disorders no doubt will be enhanced by current research on neurotransmitter activity; receptor site function and specificity; and brain hormones, including endorphins.

Cade (1949) observed that a lithium salt induced sedation in guinea pigs and reasoned that lithium might calm manic patients. He administered the drug to ten manic patients and reported substantial improvement in all ten. Since Cade's original report, many controlled studies have established that lithium is effective in treating and preventing mania (Schou et al., 1954; Maggs, 1963; Bunney et al., 1965; Goodwin et al., 1969).

Until the late 1950's, there was no widely accepted pharmacological treatment for depression. Amphetamines had been tried for depressions characterized by psychomotor retardation while barbiturates had been tried for agitated depressions; however, minimal therapeutic benefit was generally noted. In 1951, isoniazid and its isopropyl derivative, iproniazid, were developed for the treatment of tuberculosis. Both compounds, but especially iproniazid, had mood-elevating effects in patients with tuberculosis. As a result, iproniazid was used to treat depressed patients, and its antidepressant properties were confirmed. Iproniazid was also discovered to be a potent and irreversible inhibitor of the amine-catabolizing enzyme, monoamine oxidase (MAO). Other MAO inhibitors were subsequently discovered to have antidepressant activity.

During the late 1950's the second major class of antidepressant drugs, the tricyclic antidepressants, was introduced into psychiatric practice. Iminodibenzyl, the parent compound of the tricyclic antidepressants, was synthesized in 1891 by Thiel and Holzinger. However, it was not until the mid-1950's that clinical trials with this agent were begun. Initially, iminodibenzyl was investigated as an antipsychotic drug because of its structural resemblance to chlorpromazine. Although schizophrenic psychoses showed little response to iminodibenzyl, later clinical trials confirmed the antidepressant property of this drug. Subsequently, imipramine was introduced in Europe in 1958 and to North America the following year. Amitriptyline, doxepin, and other tricyclics were introduced shortly thereafter.

The "new generation" antidepressants have been introduced more recently in an effort to improve specificity, efficacy, and safety. Amoxapine, trimipramine, maprotiline, and trazodone have been made available for clinical use in the United States in recent years; and other new antidepressants are also near to being marketed. Although these newer agents have been proposed to have advantages in terms of more rapid onset of action, less cardiotoxicity, and fewer anticholinergic side effects, more research and clinical experience are needed with these agents to evaluate their efficacy, safety, and side effects.

THEORETICAL ISSUES

While lithium's mechanism of action in affective disorders is unknown, several interesting aspects of its effects have been elucidated. Mandell and Knapp (1976) have found that administration of lithium to laboratory animals produces changes in serotonin synthesis. Administration of lithium for one to five days results in increased intracellular tryptophan in the forebrain and an associated increase in its conversion to serotonin. Such increased availability of serotonin has been associated with facilitation of the behavioral activation syndrome seen after loading with L-tryptophan, monoamine oxidase inhibition, or both (Grahame-Smith and Greene, 1974). Repeated treatment of animals with a lithium salt (ten to 21 days) results in persistent increase in tryptophan uptake, although a decrease in tryptophan hydroxylase activity soon returns conversion to serotonin to basal levels (Mandell and Knapp, 1976). These biochemical events in serotonergic neurons may alter neurotransmitter synthesis therapeutically by returning "receptor stimulation toward control levels" (Knapp and Mandell, 1975). This accords well with the hypothesis that, in mania, brain catecholamines may be functionally overactive.

With regard to biological predictors of lithium response, Sullivan et al. (1977) have reported a correlation between low platelet monoamine oxidase activity and poor response to lithium therapy in manic patients. Manic patients with normal platelet monoamine oxidase activity, however, may respond better to lithium therapy.

The "amine hypothesis" of affective disorders proposes that depression may be due to a functional deficiency of amine neurotransmitters in the brain, while mania may be due to overactivity of such amines. Monoamine oxidase inhibitors prevent inactivation of amines by the catabolic enzyme monoamine oxidase and thereby potentiate their actions. The intraneuronal storage of biogenic amines is blocked by reserpine, thus permitting increased destruction by monoamine oxidase; this effect may account for the depressive symptoms noted in many patients who have taken reserpine. Tricyclic antidepressants block uptake of amines into presynaptic nerve endings. Most research has suggested that norepinephrine and serotonin are the two main neurotransmitters depleted in depression.

MHPG (3-methoxy-4-hydroxyphenethyleneglycol) has been reported to be the major metabolite of brain norepinephrine in cats, rats, and dogs (Schanberg et al., 1968; Mannano, 1963; Maas and Landis, 1968). In humans, MHPG has been shown to be the major norepinephrine metabolite in the CSF (Post et al., 1973). Studies in animals indicate that at least 25 percent of the MHPG excreted in the urine comes from the metabolism of brain norepinephrine (Maas et al., 1973). Thus, the urinary MHPG level may reflect the state of catecholamine metabolism in the brain of the depressed patient. Several recent studies (Fawcett and Maas, 1972; Maas et al., 1973; Schildkraut, 1973; Beckman and Goodwin, 1975) have examined the relationship between pretreatment urinary MHPG excretion and clinical response to tricyclic antidepressants. A low pretreatment urinary MHPG level appears to be correlated with a favorable clinical response to imipramine and a poor response to amitriptyline. A normal or high pretreatment urinary MHPG level appears to be correlated with a favorable clinical response to amitriptyline but a poor response to imipramine. The effects of activity and anxiety on MHPG excretion remain unclear; however, urinary MHPG levels may be an epiphenomenon of depression greatly influenced by activity and anxiety (Taska, 1977).

The principal metabolite of serotonin is 5-HIAA (5-hydroxyindoleacetic acid). There have been several reports (Asberg et al., 1973; Maas, 1978) that patients with low CSF 5-HIAA tend to respond to drugs that work primarily in the serotonin reuptake system, such as amitriptyline. Hence, decreased levels of 5-HIAA in the CSF may reflect a brain serotonin deficit that needs to be treated by a drug inhibiting the serotonin reuptake system. One difficulty with this idea is that metabolites present in lumbar CSF may be derived from the spinal cord or capillaries rather than the brain.

The development of clinically effective antidepressants that neither inhibit MAO or the uptake of biogenic amines has challenged some aspects of the amine hypotheses. Antidepressant drugs may exert part of their action on mood by changing the receptor mediated aspects of neuronal information transfer. Studies of the norepinephrine receptor coupled adenylate cyclase system in the brain have shown that reserpine and propranolol increase, or up-regulate, the sensitivity of this system while antidepressant drug administration and electroconvulsive therapy decrease, or down-regulate, its sensitivity. Specifically, down-regulation refers to a decrease in the density of beta-adrenergic receptors available for transmission of a neuronal signal. A functional link between reduced sensitivity to norepinephrine and the reduction of beta-adrenergic receptors appears to exist. Thus, the classical amine hypotheses may prove to be oversimplified as receptor-mediated neuronal events become better understood.

In addition to urinary MHPG and CSF 5-HIAA assays, several other laboratory tests may be useful as biological markers of affective disorders or as predictors of treatment response. These include the dextroamphetamine challenge test, dexamethasone suppression test, EEG findings, and the thyroid releasing hormone (TRH) stimulation test.

In the dextroamphetamine challenge test (Fawcett and Simopoulos, 1971; Van Kammen and Murphy, 1978), a depressed patient is examined and then given 30 mg of dextroamphetamine orally. If, during subsequent evaluations (about two hours after the administration of the oral dextroamphetamine), the patient shows an improvement in mood or psychomotor activity, the test is said to be positive. Two groups of investigators (Fawcett and Simopoulos, 1971; Van Kammen and Murphy, 1978) have found that a positive dextroamphetamine challenge test is correlated with a therapeutic response to imipramine or desipramine.

Sachar et al. (1973) have reported that some depressed patients hypersecrete cortisol, particularly during the sleeping hours. In accordance with the catecholamine hypothesis of affective disorders, this hypersecretion might be caused by low brain norepinephrine levels. Since norepinephrine inhibits the production of corticotropin releasing factor (CRF), low brain norepinephrine levels lead to increased production of CRF from the hypothalamus, which, in turn, leads to increased adrenocorticotrophic hormone (ACTH) production by the pituitary and a subsequent increased production of cortisol by the adrenals. Hence, the subgroup of depressed patients who hypersecrete cortisol may be a subgroup with brain norepinephrine depletion illness.

Carroll et al. (1981) have reported an early loss of dexamethasone suppression of cortisol output in melancholic patients. This resistance to dexamethasone suppression could be secondary to the increased levels of cortisol in depressed patients or to the decreased levels of brain norepinephrine in depressed patients which may be important in mediating a feedback effect on the hypothalamus. According to Carroll et al. (1981), the failure of dexamethasone to suppress plasma cortisol levels serves as a potentially useful laboratory test for the diagnosis of melancholia. Using their standardized procedure, a patient receives 1 mg of dexamethasone at 11:30 p.m. Plasma cortisol samples are then drawn from the patient at 4:00 p.m. and 11:00 p.m. the following day. If either sample contains a plasma cortisol level greater than 5 μg/dl, the test is considered positive. Moreover, if certain diseases such as Cushing's disease and anorexia nervosa are excluded, and there is no concurrent use of certain medications that stimulate dexamethasone metabolism, such as barbiturates and anticonvulsants, then such an abnormal test may help confirm the diagnosis of melancholia. However, not all investigators have been able to replicate these findings; and false positives have been reported by several researchers, including Amsterdam et al. (1982) and Dewan et al. (1982). On the other hand, a normal dexamethasone suppression test (both plasma cortisol levels below 5 μg/dl) does not rule out depression since false negative results do occur. Interestingly, the abnormal dexamethasone test has been reported to return to normal in many depressed patients after recovery from depression. Since radioimmunoassays (RIA) of cortisol may be unreliable, research and clinical data using such assays should be interpreted with caution.

Several EEG findings may also be biological indications of depression. Shortened REM latency (the period of time between the onset of sleep and the onset of REM sleep) is one of the most frequently reported EEG markers (Kupfer et al., 1981). Moreover, prolongation of this shortened REM latency for one or two nights following the administration of tricyclics appears to be a good predictor of response to tricyclic antidepressant therapy (Kupfer et al., 1981).

In the TRH stimulation test, patients' blood levels of thyroid stimulating hormone (TSH) are measured before and after a dose of intravenous TRH, typically 150 μg, which should stimulate TSH production. A blunted TSH response of 7 μg/ml or less over baseline levels is often found in depressed patients (Gold et al., 1981). Using a more stringent definition of TSH blunting, which requires an increase of only 4 μg/ml or less, Loosen and Prange (1982) found that TSH blunting occurred in 13 of 50 (26 percent) patients with primary depression. With the stricter definition of TSH blunting, almost no false positives should occur. In another study of 73 normal men and women, Loosen and Prange (1982) found that the lowest maximum change in TSH in this entire group of patients was 5.6 μg/ml. Gold et al. (1981a) found that TSH blunting was frequently associated with unipolar, but not with bipolar or secondary, depression. The pathophysiological significance of a blunted TSH is not understood. The anterior pituitary is regulated by the hypophyseal portal venous system through hormones secreted by neurons in the hypothalamus. These neurons, in turn, are influenced by nerve cells from other areas of the brain which use substances such as acetylcholine, norepinephrine, dopamine, and serotonin (Martin et al., 1977; Reichlin, 1974; Frohman, 1975) as neurotransmitters. If the relevant neural connections were known in detail, conclusions about amine transmitters might be derivable from pituitary hormone measurements. Unfortunately, these associations are affected by complex interactions at multiple levels of the brain which make it extremely difficult to decode specific neuroendocrine/amine interrelationships.

BASIC SCIENCE ISSUES

Current chemotherapy of affective disorders involves a wide variety of psychotropic medications. Table 1 categorizes the agents in current use along with brand names and lists some experimental antidepressants that may be clinically available in the near future.

Lithium

Lithium has no metabolites and is excreted almost entirely by the kidney in unchanged form. It has a half-life of 24 ± 8 hours, depending on the individual and how long he or she has been taking the drug. Lithium excretion is influenced by sodium intake and sodium excretion. Patients on low sodium diets, for example, retain lithium. Patients using sodium depleting diuretics, patients perspiring heavily in hot weather, patients with sodium depleting diarrhea, and patients with high fevers may also retain lithium. Patients can be treated simultaneously with lithium and thiazide diuretics, but this usually necessitates about 30 percent reduction in the lithium dosage and close monitoring of serum lithium levels (Himmelhoch et al., 1977).

Before starting lithium therapy, kidney function should be evaluated. Since lithium is excreted primarily by the kidneys, patients with impaired renal function are susceptible to lithium toxicity. Baseline thyroid functions are also useful prior to starting treatment since lithium can produce goiter and other thyroid complications.

To begin inpatient treatment of an acute manic episode, lithium carbonate can usually be started at a dose of about 300 mg three times daily plus 500-600 mg at bedtime. Stokes et al. (1976) recommend using a dose in mg equal

LITHIUM COMPOUNDS
Lithium carbonate: Lithobid, Lithonate, Lithotabs, Eskalith
Lithium citrate: Cibalith-S

TRICYCLIC ANTIDEPRESSANTS
Amitriptyline hydrochloride: Elavil, Endep, Amitid
Imipramine hydrochloride: Tofranil
Doxepin: Adapin, Sinequan
Amoxapine: Ascendin
Desipramine hydrochloride: Norpramin, Pertofrane
Nortriptyline hydrochloride: Pamelor, Aventyl HCL
Trimipramine maleate: Surmontil
Protriptyline hydrochloride: Vivactil

BRIDGED TRICYCLICS
Maprotiline hydrochloride: Ludiomil
Oxaprotiline

TETRACYCLICS
Mianserin

MAO INHIBITORS
Isocarboxazid: Marplan
Phenelzine sulfate: Nardil
Tranylcypromine sulfate: Parnate

ATYPICAL ANTIDEPRESSANTS
Trazodone hydrochloride: Desyrel

EXPERIMENTAL ANTIDEPRESSANTS
Zimelidine
Fluoxetine
Fluvoxamine
Nomifensine
Alprazolam: Xanax
Bupropion
Carbamazepine: Tegretol

COMBINATION DRUGS CONTAINING ANTIDEPRESSANTS
Perphenazine and amitriptyline hydrochloride: Etrafon, Triavil
Chlordiazepoxide and amitriptyline hydrochloride: Limbitrol

Table 1. Psychotropic agents in current use

to ten times the body weight in pounds (e.g., a 150-pound person would receive 1,500 mg of lithium per day). Since clinical response to lithium usually takes seven to 14 days (Baldessarini and Lipinski, 1975), antipsychotic or sedative medication is often added during this period to help control manic symptoms. During an acute manic episode, the optimal serum lithium level should be between 1.0-1.5 mEq/L. Serum should be drawn in the morning before the morning dose of medication. Serum lithium levels above 1.5 mEq/L often produce toxicity, especially in elderly patients; and serum lithium levels above 5.0 mEq/L can be fatal. Following an acute manic episode, patients can usually be prophylactically maintained at a serum level of 0.5-1.2 mEq/L in order to prevent relapses of bipolar and unipolar illness.

Tricyclic Antidepressants

The tricyclic antidepressants are mainly metabolized by hydroxylation and desalkylation. Desipramine and nortriptyline are the demethylated metabolites of imipramine and amitriptyline, respectively. Hydroxylated metabolites may be pharmacologically active but are relatively water soluable and so are rapidly excreted. Compounds such as barbiturates (Burrows and Davis, 1971; Glassman and Perel, 1973) and cigarette smoking stimulate the enzymatic rate of hydroxylation, thus increasing the rate of excretion and decreasing plasma concentrations of the tricyclic antidepressants. Phenothiazines, methylphenidate, and amphetamine, on the other hand, inhibit the enzymatic rate of hydroxylation, thus decreasing metabolism of these antidepressants and increasing plasma concentrations. Elderly patients have slower enzymatic rates of hydroxylation and hence develop higher plasma concentrations than nonelderly adults (Nies et al., 1977). Thus, elderly patients should be treated with one-half to two-thirds of the tricyclic dose that nonelderly adults receive.

The tricyclic antidepressants usually take about two to three weeks to exert their antidepressant action, which is theorized to be caused by inhibition of the reuptake of norepinephrine and/or serotonin at brain neuronal receptor sites. This theory, however, may be an oversimplification since questions regarding whether amine receptors can become hypersensitive in depression and whether antidepressants down-regulate receptors remain unanswered.

It has been reported that amitriptyline works primarily in the serotonin system and imipramine in the norepinephrine system. The demethylated metabolites, nortriptyline and desipramine, have been reported to have a greater influence than their parent compounds in the norepinephrine system (Goodwin et al., 1978). Recent research, however, seems to indicate that most antidepressant drugs affect both norepinephrine and serotonin systems and that attempts to divide most antidepressants into serotonin or norepinephrine drugs is an oversimplification (Richelson, 1983).

Protriptyline is usually prescribed at a dose of 10 mg QID, and its dose may be increased to about 90 mg per day. It is more stimulating than the other tricyclics. Therapy with the other tricyclics is usually initiated at a dose of 50 mg. The dose can be increased about 50 mg every other day until a total dose of 150 to 200 mg is reached. Patients are usually maintained on this dose for two to three weeks in order to receive an adequate therapeutic trial. The dose of nortriptyline is appropriately started at a dose half that of imipramine because of its increased milligram potency and is usually not increased above 150 mg per day. The dose of imipramine, desipramine, amitriptyline, or doxepin can be increased to as much as 300 mg per day if the patient does not respond to lower doses. The tricyclics have half-lives of approximately 24 hours and a reasonable therapeutic index. Thus, much of the daily dose of these drugs (generally up to 150 mg) can be given at night. Such bedtime dosing often increases medication compliance by decreasing the complexity of the regimen. Doxepin has been reported to be less potent *in vivo* than the other tricyclics (Hollister, 1974) and hence may need to be used at higher doses in order to produce equivalent antidepressant activity.

L-triiodothyronine (T$_3$) in doses of 25-50 μg per day may be useful in improving the response to imipramine, especially in women during the first three weeks of imipramine therapy (Prange et al., 1969). According to Prange et al. (1969), T$_3$ acts mainly to accelerate the onset of the antidepressant action of imipramine. Other investigators have been unable to replicate the effectiveness of this T$_3$-imipramine combination (Steiner, 1980).

Goodwin et al. (1982) studied six women and six men who suffered from major affective disorder and who had not responded to imipramine or amitriptyline, 150-300 mg/day, during periods of 26 to 112 days. After the addition of 25 or 50 μg/day of L-triiodothyronine to their regimens, eight of these patients showed marked improvement.

If a patient responds to an antidepressant drug, he should be maintained on this medication for several months to a year in order to decrease the likelihood of relapse. If the patient has had multiple, frequent relapses, he may well need to be maintained on the antidepressant indefinitely. It has been shown that maintenance on an antidepressant significantly reduces the probability of relapse during the year after the patient has recovered from a depressive episode (Klerman, 1978; Davis, 1976). Quitkin et al. (1976) estimated this reduction in the risk of relapse during the first year after recovery at 20 to 50 percent. Seager and Bird (1962) reported that 69 percent of placebo-treated patients relapsed during the first six months after remission.

Several groups of investigators, as reviewed by Taska et al. (1979), have reported great variations in steady-state plasma concentrations in patients administered a standard dose of a tricyclic antidepressant and have tried to correlate clinical response with steady-state tricyclic antidepressant plasma concentrations (reached after about ten days of therapy with a constant dose). In 1971, Asberg (1971) reported that depressed patients treated with a fixed dose of nortriptyline showed less clinical improvement at very low (less than 50 ng/ml) or very high (greater than 140 ng/ml) steady-state plasma concentrations. The investigators referred to this relationship as a "therapeutic window" and in interpretating their data postulated that reduced clinical effect may occur at high plasma concentrations because the tricyclic antidepressants may block the monoaminergic receptors. This initial report of a therapeutic window for nortriptyline has been supported by three subsequent studies (Kragh-Sorenson et al., 1973, 1976; Ziegler et al., 1976a). Burrows et al. (1972, 1974), in contrast, found no correlation between plasma nortriptyline concentrations and clinical response. Their data have been criticized because their studies excluded patients with severe depressive illness who were treated with electroconvulsive therapy instead of nortriptyline and because the patients included in their study showed large fluctuations in their plasma nortriptyline concentrations from week to week and, therefore, did not reach steady-state kinetics. Whyte et al. (1976) have reported that a therapeutic window (166 to 237 ng/ml) may exist for protriptyline.

Several investigators have studied the relationship between clinical response and plasma concentrations in patients treated with imipramine. Glassman et al. (1977) reported poor clinical response to imipramine in patients whose plasma concentrations of imipramine plus desipramine (active metabolite) were below 150 ng/ml. The response rate, however, rose sharply between 150 and 200 ng/ml and appeared to plateau at about 250 ng/ml. These investigators found no evidence for an upper limit in imipramine plasma concentrations above which clinical response is reduced. Braithwaite et al. (1976) reported that in patients treated with amitriptyline, total plasma concentrations (amitriptyline plus its active metabolite, nortriptyline) of less than 120 ng/ml are correlated with poor response to amitriptyline therapy. Ziegler et al. (1976b) found that patients with total plasma concentrations (amitriptyline plus nortriptyline) above 95 ng/ml had better clinical response to amitriptyline. Available data concerning doxepin and desipramine plasma concentrations are limited, and therapeutic ranges of blood concentrations of these two drugs are not established.

Plasma concentrations are best evaluated after the drug has reached "steady-state," or a balance of intake and output, which typically requires about ten days of therapy at constant dose. A blood sample is usually drawn before the morning dose of medication. The plasma samples should be drawn in Venojet tubes or syringes since the rubber stoppers of Vacutainer tubes may contain a substance that causes tricyclics to shift from the plasma protein bound pool to red blood cells and other tissues, causing spuriously low plasma concentrations (Brunswick and Mendels, 1977).

Monoamine Oxidase Inhibitors

There are two major types of monoamine oxidase inhibitors (MAOI's), namely hydrazine and non-hydrazine compounds. Phenelzine and isocarboxazid are hydrazine compounds. Tranylcypromine is a nonhydrazine compound. Phenelzine and tranylcypromine are the most frequently used monoamine oxidase inhibitors. The usual daily dosage range is 15 to 90 mg for phenelzine and 20 to 30 mg for tranylcypromine. Other monoamine oxidase inhibitors currently available in the United States include pargyline and nialamide. Pargyline is marketed for hypertension rather than depression (Levy, 1966).

Hydrazine MAOI's undergo metabolism by acetylation. Rates of acetylation are genetically determined and show substantial interindividual variation (Evans et al., 1960; Evans and White, 1964). On the basis of studies that have categorized patients by their rate of acetylation of isoniazid or one of the sulfas, it has been suggested that the clinical effects of phenelzine treatment are different in so-called fast as compared to slow acetylators. Side effects of phenelzine, for example, have been reported to be more common among slow acetylators (Evans et al., 1965). Johnstone and Marsh (Johnstone and Marsh, 1973; Johnstone, 1976) have reported that slow acetylators also show greater clinical responsiveness to phenelzine than fast acetylators. Other investigators (Robinson et al., 1978a, 1978b), in contrast, have found no relationship between acetylator status and clinical response to phenelzine.

Platelet monamine oxidase inhibition correlates with inhibition of brain monoamine oxidase inhibition in laboratory animals and may be useful in monitoring the effect of some MAOI's in humans (Quitkin et al., 1979). Robinson et al. (1978a) studied the relationships of platelet monoamine oxidase inhibition and clinical improvement and found that 68 percent of patients achieving at least 80 percent inhibition of platelet monoamine oxidase had a favorable response to phenelzine. Of those who achieved 90 percent inhibition, 79 percent improved. This relationship between at least an 80 percent inhibition of platelet monoamine oxidase activity and clinical response has also been supported in a subsequent study by Robinson et al. (1978b).

Other Antidepressants

Several new antidepressants have been marketed recently, including maprotiline, amoxapine, trimipramine, and trazodone. Other antidepressants that are likely to be marketed in the United States soon are mianserin, zimelidine, and bupropion. Antidepressant agents for which further research is needed prior to marketing include oxaprotiline, fluoxetine, fluvoxamine, and nomifensine. Alprazolam (Xanax) is a marketed triazolo-benzodiazepine with many typical benzodiazepine-like characteristics at doses of 1-5 mg/day. There is also some evidence that it has antidepressant properties, especially at higher doses, in anxious dysthymic patients.

Maprotiline and oxaprotiline are bridged tricyclics, and mianserin is a tetracyclic compound. Maprotiline is a selective inhibitor of norepinephrine reuptake and has little or no serotonergic effect. Typical daily doses range from 50-300 mg and can be given on a divided schedule or as a single bedtime dose. Maprotiline has a 40- to 50-hour half-life and, hence, is particularly suitable for single dose maintenance therapy. Oxaprotiline is a hyroxy-analog of maprotiline and is an even more potent norepinephrine reuptake inhibitor than maprotiline (CIBA-Geigy, 1982). A dosage range of 50 to 150 mg is typical in research studies. Mianserin, likewise, has little effect on the serotonin reuptake system. It functions as a presynaptic blocker and increases the production and release of norepinephrine. The usual dosage range for mianserin is 30 to 150 mg per day.

Amoxapine, a dibenzoxazepine, is a metabolite of the antipsychotic drug loxapine. Amoxapine may have a more rapid onset of action than the other antidepressants—four to seven days rather than the usual 14 to 21 days. The clinical dosage range for amoxapine is usually between 200 and 400 mg, but inpatients may require up to 600 mg per day. The main active metabolite of amoxapine in humans is 8-hydroxyamoxapine, which, along with the parent agent, is a potent norepinephrine reuptake inhibitor but with a longer (30-hour) half-life. Amoxapine may, therefore, be given as a single bedtime dose if desired. A 7-hydroxymetabolite of amoxapine is a potent dopamine antagonist, and plasma samples from patients given amoxapine show significant levels of neuroleptic-like activity. As a result, patients may develop extrapyramidal system side effects (such as akathisia) while being treated with amoxapine, and the possibility of their developing tardive dyskinesia with prolonged use should be considered.

Trimipramine is an iminodibenzyl tricyclic antidepressant with serotonergic activity and has had many years of use in other countries. It has a relatively short half-life, ranging from three to eight hours, depending on which metabolites are examined. Although only recently marketed in the United States, its effectiveness has been shown in many clinical trials (Settle and Ayd, 1980).

Zimelidine, fluoxetine, and fluvoxamine are fairly selective inhibitors of serotonin reuptake, with minimal effects on dopamine or norepinephrine. The mechanism of action of trazodone is not understood. Trazodone has a usual dosage range of 50 to 800 mg and is usually given in divided doses because of its short half-life. Zimelidine is a bicyclic compound with a typical dosage range of 100 to 300 mg per day. Dosages of fluoxetine and fluvoxamine which usually result in antidepressant effects with minimal side effects range from 20 to 80 mg per day and 100 to 300 mg per day, respectively.

Nomifensine has actions as both a norepinephrine and a dopamine reuptake inhibitor (Brogdon et al., 1979). A tetrahydroisoquinoline compound, it is readily absorbed and is rapidly conjugated to the glucuronide metabolite and excreted mainly in the urine. Dosages range from 50 to 200 mg with a divided daytime schedule for administration.

Alprazolam is a triazolobenzodiazepine. It is a potent and effective anxiolytic but was noted to have significant antidepressant effects in clinical trials (Fabre and McLendon, 1976; Fabre, 1976). Although further study is indicated to support use of this agent clinically, antidepressant effects have been observed with dosages of 0.5 to 4.0 mg per day, given in divided doses, with the majority of the total daily dosage given at bedtime. Higher doses (greater than 5.0 mg/day) generally result in greater antidepressant effects.

Bupropion is chemically a chlorpropiophenone. It has no significant effect on norepinephrine or serotonin and only very mild, likely insignificant, dopaminergic or stimulant activity. It has no effect on monoamine oxidase. At this time its mechanism of action is unknown. Antidepressant responses have been achieved in outpatients on dosages from 300 to 450 mg per day, but inpatients have required dosages in the 450-700 mg per day range.

Folks et al. (1982) have reported on the treatment of inpatients with affective disorders using carbamazepine. Their experience with ten patients suggested both antimanic and antidepressant effects for carbamazepine. Lipinski and Pope (1982) have shown a possible synergy between carbamazepine and lithium carbonate in the treatment of mania. In three cases they noted that mania responded to treatment with simultaneous administration of these agents when trials of each individually were unsuccessful. Dosages of carbamazepine required range from 600 to 1,600 mg per day, with desired blood levels ranging from 8-12 μg/ml.

CLINICAL ISSUES: INDICATIONS, SIDE EFFECTS, LIMITATIONS

Lithium

Lithium appears to be the drug of choice in the treatment of mania (Prien et al., 1973), but since its clinical effect may require seven to 14 days, neuroleptic or sedative drugs, in addition to lithium therapy, are often used in the treatment of acute severe mania.

Cade (1949) originally reported that lithium was not effective in the acute treatment of depression. Many subsequent studies (Stokes et al., 1971; Gershon and Yuwiler, 1960; Hartigan, 1963; Gershon, 1974; Fieve et al., 1968) have likewise reported that lithium does not have short-term antidepressant activity. Other investigators, however, have reported that lithium may have an acute antidepressant effect, especially in bipolar patients (Goodwin et al., 1969, 1972; Mendels et al., 1972; Johnson, 1974; Noyes et al., 1974; Mendels, 1976).

The prophylactic use of lithium was first reported in 1963 by Hartigan (1963), who found that maintenance treatment with lithium carbonate prevented manic as well as depressive relapses in bipolar patients. Since then, several well controlled studies (Prien et al., 1973; Baastrup and Schou, 1967; Coppen et al., 1971; Hullin et al., 1972; Stallone et al., 1973) have proven the prophylactic effectiveness of lithium in preventing the recurrence of manic and depressive episodes in bipolar patients. Investigators have also reported that lithium is prophylactically effective in preventing recurrent depressions in patients without bipolar illness (Prien et al., 1973; Baastrup and Schou, 1967; Coppen et al., 1971).

There has been substantial debate concerning the effectiveness of lithium in treating schizophrenia. Several investigators have reported that lithium is ineffective in treating schizophrenia. (Fieve et al., 1968; Goodwin et al., 1972; Mendels et al., 1972; Johnson, 1974; Noyes et al., 1974; Mendels, 1976; Baastrup and Schou, 1967; Coppen et al., 1971; Hullin et al., 1972; Stallone et al., 1973; Hollister, 1972; Bailey et al., 1975; Hekimian et al., 1969; Shopsin et al., 1971; Johnson, 1970). Recently, in contrast, Alexander et al. (1979) have reported a controlled study suggesting that schizophrenic patients are responsive to lithium. In addition, Hirschowitz et al. (1980) have reported that lithium is effective in treating some cases of schizophrenia. Moreover, other research has indicated that lithium may be effective in treating some schizoaffective patients, especially when the lithium is used as an adjunct to antipsychotic therapy (Taylor and Abrams, 1973; Dinsmore and Ryback, 1972; Gleisinger, 1954; Biederman et al., 1979).

Other reported uses of lithium therapy include chronic alcoholism (Merry et al., 1976), morbid impulsive aggression (Schou, 1978), premenstrual tension (Sletten and Gershon, 1966), cluster headaches (Ekbon, 1977; Kudrow, 1977), and the prophylactic treatment of corticotropin-induced psychosis (Falk et al., 1979). A recent report by Price et al. (1982) described positive clinical response in five out of six patients with delusional depression when lithium was combined with neuroleptic and tricyclic agents. These patients had all been unresponsive to neuroleptic-tricyclic treatment regimens.

It should be emphasized that close monitoring of side effects, not serum lithium concentrations, is the ultimate criterion for lithium toxicity. Cases of severe lithium toxicity have been reported (Strayhorn and Nash, 1977) with serum lithium concentrations below 1.6 mEq/L. Elderly patients (Van Der Velde, 1971) and patients with brain damage (Shopsin et al., 1973) may be particularly susceptible to neurotoxicity at the usual therapeutic serum concentrations. If a patient develops signs and symptoms of lithium toxicity, then lithium dosage should be decreased regardless of the serum lithium concentration. Signs and symptoms of lithium toxicity or overdosage include tremor, weakness, ataxia, drowsiness, dysarthria, blurred vision, tinnitus, nausea, vomiting, hyperactive deep tendon reflexes, nystagmus, confusion, seizures, and coma. Some patients develop marked polyuria and polydipsia during prolonged lithium therapy. These side effects are reversible if the dose of lithium is decreased. Pretibial and pedal edema can also occur as lithium side effects. Lithium can produce hand tremor, which can often be alleviated by the addition of 15-60 mg per day of propranolol. Lithium salts may also result in gastric distress, including nausea, vomiting, and diarrhea; for this reason, it is usually prescribed in small divided doses during the day near mealtimes. Urinary retention might also be one of lithium's moderately common and somewhat troublesome side effects. Another possible complication of lithium intake is leukocytosis, with white blood cell count in the 10,000 to 14,000 range (Baldessarini and Lipinski, 1975). Cogwheel rigidity, which is unresponsive to anticholinergic agents, is another potential side effect of lithium therapy (Shopsin et al., 1973; Branchey et al., 1976; Kane et al., 1978; Asnis et al., 1979).

An increased incidence of cardiovascular abnormalities has been reported in the offspring of mothers treated with lithium during pregnancy (Goldberg and DiMascio, 1978). There have also been reports of lithium-induced teratogenicity in animal studies (Goldberg and DiMascio, 1978). Thus, lithium therapy should be avoided during pregnancy, especially during the first trimester. Lithium should also be avoided during nursing since it is excreted in breast milk (Goldberg and DiMascio, 1978).

Lithium has been reported to produce euthyroid goiter (four percent incidence), goiter plus hypothyroidism (6.5 percent incidence), and hypothyroidism without goiter (one percent incidence) (Gershon and Shopsin, 1978). About 90 percent of the patients developing thyroid symptoms in this study were women. Cho et al. (1979) have confirmed that the incidence of lithium-related thyroid side effects is much higher in women than men.

The possibility that lithium can produce renal damage remains controversial. In 1977 Hestbach et al. (1977) reported that 14 patients on prolonged lithium therapy had a considerable reduction in creatinine clearance associated with nonspecific chronic renal lesions, including tubular atrophy, interstitial fibrosis, and glomerulosclerosis. Scully et al. (1981) have reported a case of renal failure secondary to chronic interstitial nephritis in a patient who received lithium therapy. Gerner et al. (1980) did extensive testing of renal function in 43 patients who had been taking lithium from one to 120 months. Their only abnormal finding was that the urine concentrating ability of these patients was moderately but asymptomatically impaired. DePaulo et al. (1981) studied renal function in 99 lithium-treated patients and reported a relationship between chronic lithium therapy and declining glomerular filtration rate. Thus, it is possible that lithium may cause some bothersome changes in renal function tests, but the risk of clinically significant renal damage in patients treated with therapeutic serum concentrations of lithium appears to be small (Scully et al., 1981).

Lithium may also induce hyperparathyroidism with increased serum calcium concentration, decreased serum phosphate concentration, and decreased urinary calcium excretion (Tupin et al., 1968; Gerner et al., 1977; Mellerup et al., 1976; Christensson, 1976; Cervi-Skinner, 1977; Davis et al., 1981).

A question has been raised as to whether certain combinations of an antipsychotic agent with lithium may increase the risk of central nervous system toxicity. Cohen and Cohen (1974) reported on four patients who developed serious, irreversible neurotoxic symptoms on lithium and haloperidol within a short period of time. A careful review of these cases, however, raises the question of whether the patients were suffering from an encephalitis or some other illness not associated with lithium toxicity. Baastrup et al. (1976) subsequently retrospectively reviewed the records of 425 patients who had been treated with lithium plus haloperidol and found no cases of the type of neurotoxicity described by Cohen and Cohen. In 1979 Spring (1979a, 1979b) described six cases of combined neuroleptic and lithium toxicity, five with thioridazine and one with fluphenazine. More recently, Spring and Frankel (1981) have reported a case of combined lithium and haloperidol toxicity characterized by hyperpyrexia, severe rigidity, mutism, and the development of irreversible tardive dyskinesia. Weight gain can also occur as a side effect of lithium therapy. Vendsborg et al. (1976) reported that 45 of 70 patients treated with lithium incurred a mean weight gain of 10 kg.

Lithium generally should not be prescribed for patients with serious renal or cardiovascular disease, severe dehydration or sodium depletion, or for patients receiving potent diuretics. However, if the psychiatric indication is potentially life threatening, lithium can be administered in such situations with extreme caution, frequent monitoring of serum lithium levels, and the lowest possible doses required to achieve the desired effect. In such cases hospitalization is usually a necessity.

Tricyclic Antidepressants

Tricyclic antidepressants are usually the treatment of choice for major depression and for depressive episodes of bipolar disorder. In a review of 85 controlled studies comparing the efficacy of the tricyclic antidepressants and placebo, Morris and Beck (1974) reported that tricyclics were significantly more effective than placebo in 66 percent of the studies. Klein and Davis (1969) have reviewed a number of double-blind studies conducted with imipramine and reported that 70 percent of 734 depressed patients improved when treated with imipramine, in contrast to a 39 percent improvement rate in 606 patients treated with placebo.

Bielski and Friedel (1976) have reported that predictors of positive response to tricyclics include insidious onset, weight loss or anorexia, middle and late insomnia, and psychomotor disturbance. They found that predictors of poor response to tricyclics include hypochondriasis, hysterical traits, multiple prior episodes, and delusions.

In addition to being useful in treating depression, tricyclic antidepressants have also been used in treating childhood nocturnal enuresis (imipramine in doses of 25-50 mg per night), school phobias (similar doses of imipramine), migraine headaches, narcolepsy, and panic attacks. Imipramine at doses generally used for treating cases of depression has been useful in decreasing the frequency of panic attacks. However, a recent report by Nurnberg and Coccaro (1982) indicated that in two patients with panic disorder and major depression, their panic attacks responded while depressive symptoms remained prominent after six weeks' treatment with imipramine.

The tricyclic antidepressants have pronounced anticholinergic side effects including dry mouth, blurred vision, exacerbation of acute narrow angle glaucoma, urinary retention, constipation, palpitations, and tachycardia. As reviewed by Taska (1977), the incidence of these side effects shows little correlation with tricyclic antidepressant plasma levels. Hence, the presence of anticholinergic side effects cannot be used as a predictor of an adequate therapeutic plasma level. The urinary retention side effect can often be alleviated by treatment with bethanecol chloride, a peripherally acting cholinergic agonist that does not cross the blood-brain barrier (Everett, 1975).

Snyder and Yamamura (1977) have reported that amitriptyline is the tricyclic with the most anticholinergic activity and desipramine the tricyclic with the least. Hence, troublesome anticholinergic side effects may be handled by switching to a different tricyclic with less anticholinergic activity. The tricyclics may be listed in order of decreasing anticholinergic activity as follows: amitriptyline, doxepin, nortriptyline, imipramine, and desipramine.

Orthostatic hypotension is a common side effect of tricyclics. Glassman et al. (1979) reported that 14 percent of their patients on imipramine had either falls or ataxia. Another seven percent had treatment stopped or modified because of severe dizziness. With time, most patients develop some tolerance to the sedative and anticholinergic side effects of the tricyclics. In one study, however, orthostatic hypotension remained unchanged during four weeks of treatment with imipramine (Glassman et al., 1973).

Tricyclics can also lower the seizure threshold (Sovner and DiMascio, 1978) or produce sedation, with amitriptyline usually observed to be the most sedating. In addition, tricyclics can produce sexual difficulties such as slowness in achieving erection, delayed ejaculation, nonejaculation, and retrograde ejaculation (Comfort, 1979). Another possible complication of tricyclic therapy is precipitation of a manic episode (Van Scheyen and Van Kammen, 1979). Because of potentially serious incompatibility with sympathomimetic drugs, tricyclic antidepressants should be discontinued prior to surgery in which these drugs may be used.

Tricyclics can also precipitate an anticholinergic psychosis characterized by delirium, confusion, and disorientation. The risk of such an anticholinergic psychosis is increased if other drugs with anticholinergic properties such as aith tricyclics. An anticholinergic psychosis can be treated with 1-2 mg of physostigmine given IM or slowly IV. IV physostigmine should be used with caution since it can produce grand mal seizures. Physostigmine has a duration of action of only about 30 minutes.

A number of investigators have studied the incidence of birth defects in the offspring of mothers who have taken tricyclic antidepressants. As reviewed by Goldberg and DiMascio (1978), there is no substantial evidence that tricyclics produce birth defects.

The tricyclics have a quinidine-like effect that can cause some widening of the QRS and P-R intervals and some flattening of the T waves in the electrocardiogram. This quinidine-like effect can also suppress premature atrial and ventricular contractions and produce nearly every type of cardiac arrhythmia (Fowler et al., 1976; Sacks et al., 1968).

A possible neurological side effect of tricyclics is the worsening of tardive dyskinesia since any drug with anticholinergic activity has such potential (Baldessarini and Tarsy, 1978).

Kramer et al. (1961) have described symptoms of nausea, vomiting, malaise, myalgias, dizziness, and coryza occurring in some patients after the abrupt discontinuation of imipramine. Other withdrawal symptoms noted after discontinuation of tricyclics include abdominal pain, anorexia, insomnia, drowsiness, behavioral activation, anxiety, irritability, agitation, apathy, withdrawal, headaches, and recurrence of depressed mood (Dilsaver et al., 1983). Dilsaver et al. (1983) suggest treatment of antidepressant withdrawal symptoms with anticholinergic agents such as atropine. They postulate that since tricyclics have anticholinergic properties, a state of cholinergic overdrive develops when tricyclics are abruptly discontinued. Thus, it is advisable to taper the tricyclics rather than abruptly discontinuing them.

Flemenbaum (1976) has reported that a single bedtime dosage schedule of a tricyclic may produce an increased frequency of night terrors, or pavor nocturnus. In patients bothered by this side effect, Flemenbaum recommends a multiple dosage schedule rather than a single bedtime dosage.

Elderly depressed patients are often difficult to treat with tricyclics because of their susceptibility to anticholinergic side effects. Katon and Raskind (1980) have proposed using methylphenidate (10 mg b.i.d.) in elderly patients who are unable to tolerate the anticholinergic side effects of the tricyclics.

Tricyclic overdoses can be fatal. Lethal overdoses are usually in the range of 2 g and over (Biggs et al., 1977), although smaller doses can be fatal in children. Hence, prescriptions for tricyclics should be for less than a total of 2 g if the patient has any suicidal risk. Tricyclic antidepressant overdoses cannot be treated with dialysis because of the drugs' extensive protein binding. Serious tricyclic overdoses are usually associated with a widened QRS interval on the electrocardiogram of greater than 0.10 msec (Spiker et al., 1975). Sinus tachycardia is the most frequent cardiac arrhythmia associated with tricyclic overdose. Gastric contents should be removed by using Epicac or an Ewald tube as soon as possible following an overdose. IV fluids should be administered to promote excretion, and cardiac monitoring is necessary to alert the treatment team to potentially fatal arrhythmias.

There has been considerable controversy concerning whether a schizophrenic patient who develops depressive symptoms should be treated with a tricyclic antidepressant. There has been some concern that tricyclics might worsen schizophrenic symptoms. Prusoff et al. (1979) have reported that when tricyclics are added to antipsychotics in the treatment of depressed schizophrenic patients they help reduce depressive symptoms but may worsen schizophrenic thought disorder.

Tricyclic antidepressants should generally be avoided in patients with a history of significant urinary retention, angle-closure glaucoma, or increased intraocular pressure. They probably should be given concomitantly with monoamine oxidase inhibitors only with great caution. Hyperpyretic crises, convulsions, and death have occurred, although rarely, in patients taking a combination of these agents. It is safer to allow a minimum of ten days to elapse before beginning a tricyclic if a patient was previously taking a monoamine oxidase inhibitor. Because of the potential to produce cardiac arrhythmias, tricyclic antidepressants are not recommended during the acute recovery stages following myocardial infarction. Tricyclics may also impair both the mental and physical abilities necessary for operating machinery or driving a motor vehicle.

Bridged Tricyclic and Tetracyclic Antidepressants

Bridged tricyclic and tetracyclic antidepressants generally have the same indications as the tricyclics, i.e., depressive illness in patients with dysthymic disorder; major depression; and bipolar disorder, depressed phase. Maprotiline may also be effective for the relief of anxiety associated with depression. Due to the relatively lower atropinic effects of maprotiline, this agent may be more useful in geriatric depression and in patients with cardiovascular disease (Selvini et al., 1976).

Side effects that have been reported for the bridged tricyclics and tetracyclics include dry mouth, constipation, blurred vision, and rarely urinary retention. Cardiovascular complications include hypotension, hypertension, tachycardia, and arrhythmias; syncope may occur although the incidence is low. Drowsiness, dizziness, nausea, weakness, fatigue, and headache are other side effects. Limitations are generally the same as those for the tricyclics.

Monoamine Oxidase Inhibitors

The monoamine oxidase (MAO) inhibitors are not widely prescribed because of their potential to produce a hypertensive crisis. They are prescribed mostly for patients who are unresponsive to the tricyclics, who develop intolerable side effects with the tricyclics, or who give a history of previous response to an MAO inhibitor.

MAO inhibitors may also be the drugs of choice for a syndrome called "atypical depression." This syndrome is not related to the *DSM-III* classification "Atypical Depression," but is "atypical" because of the presence of symptoms such as increased rather than decreased sleep, increased rather than decreased appetite, somatic complaints, phobias, anxiety, and hysterical personality features.

Robinson et al. (1973) have reported favorable results with phenelzine in "atypical" depression. Quitkin et al. (1979) have reviewed eight studies, seven of which showed that phenelzine was statistically superior to placebo in "atypical" depression.

The MAO inhibitors have no significant anticholinergic activity (Snyder and Yamamura, 1977) and, hence, in contrast to the tricyclics, usually do not have troublesome anticholinergic side effects. However, dry mouth and urinary retention have been noted with phenelzine sulfate. MAO inhibitors may also cause hypotension.

As previously noted, combined tricyclic and monoamine oxidase inhibitor therapy may produce a central adrenergic syndrome characterized by hyperpyrexia and grand mal seizures. Ananth and Luchins (1977) contend, however, that it is less dangerous to start the two drugs concomitantly or to start the tricyclic first than to add a tricyclic once a monoamine oxidase inhibitor has been started.

A hypertensive crisis can be precipitated if a patient being treated with a monoamine oxidase inhibitor eats food rich in tyramine or other sympathomimetic amines. Monoamine oxidase inhibitors block the metabolism of tyramine by monoamine oxidase in gut, liver, and other tissues. The accumulated tyramine then enters the circulation and causes hypertension by releasing norepinephrine at the neuroeffector junctions. Some examples of foods rich in tyramine which need to be avoided during treatment with monoamine oxidase inhibitors include aged cheese, yogurt, chianti wine, foreign beer, liver, snails, pickled herring, cream, chocolate, broad beans, citrus fruits, raisins, soy sauce, yeast products, bananas, avocados, and canned figs, among others.

Since monoamine oxidase inhibitors interfere with the catabolism of sympathomimetic amines, patients being treated with MAO inhibitors should avoid medications containing sympathomimetic compounds such as diet pills and over-the-counter common cold preparations. Some medications that should not be used while patients are being treated with monoamine oxidase inhibitors include L-dopa, epinephrine, norepinephrine, methylphenidate, amphetamines, ephedrine, phenylephrine, antihistamines, non-MAOI antidepressants, and Demerol.

Since the monoamine oxidase inhibitors irreversibly destroy monoamine oxidase and the process of producing new monoamine oxidase takes about two weeks, patients should be instructed to wait two weeks before taking an incompatible drug or before eating tyramine-containing foods once they have discontinued a monoamine oxidase inhibitor.

If a hypertensive crisis does occur secondary to therapy with a monoamine oxidase inhibitor, it can be treated with an alpha-adrenergic blocking agent such as phentolamine or chlorpromazine (Byck, 1975). Of course, this complication is a medical emergency requiring intensive cardiovascular monitoring and support.

Generally, MAO inhibitors are to be avoided in patients with significant cerebrovascular or cardiovascular disease. They should not be used in the presence of pheochromocytoma since such tumors may secrete pressor substances. Combinations of MAO inhibitors should not be used.

Other Antidepressants

Trazodone, zimelidine, fluoxetine, fluvoxamine, nomifensine, alprazolam, and bupropion all have essentially the same indications as the tricyclics. Trazodone has low cardiovascular toxicity and no atropine-like effects. It does have hypnotic effects, however, and may be more effective in treating depressed patients with agitation, anxiety, and insomnia. Other side effects of trazodone include lethargy, headaches, confusion, nausea, and gastrointestinal discomfort. Trazodone may not exacerbate manic symptoms as described with the tricyclics (Larochelle et al., 1979; Friedman et al., 1977; Gershon et al., 1981). Zimelidine also has low cardiovascular toxicity but may cause nausea, diarrhea, headaches, tremulousness, hyperactivity, and restlessness. However, it is well tolerated by most patients. Fluoxetine and fluvoxamine may cause nausea, diarrhea, and restlessness as side effects. Since they lack anticholinergic and antihistamine effects, fluoxetine and fluvoxamine may be better tolerated by depressed geriatric patients, patients with significant cardiac conditions, and patients who do not tolerate atropine-like side effects. Side effects of nomifensine include dry mouth, tremulousness, restlessness, insomnia, and infrequently, fever (Poldinger and Gammel, 1978). Alprazolam has side effects of drowsiness and lethargy, while bupropion therapy may result in restlessness, insomnia, tremor, dizziness, dry mouth, diaphoresis, and nausea. Nomifensine, alprazolam, and bupropion all have low cardiotoxicity when compared with the tricyclics.

As previously noted, psychotropic uses of carbamazepine may include treatment of manic or depressive symptomatology, particularly in cases refractory to other standard agents. Side effects of carbamazepine include nausea, dizziness, and ataxia. Possible hematologic changes include leukopenia, reticulocytosis (Warren and Steinbook, 1983), and potentially irreversible aplastic anemia (Livingston et al., 1974). Thus, careful monitoring of blood counts is important. Carbamazepine should be stopped immediately if significant hematologic changes occur.

DEVELOPMENTAL AND AGE RELATED ISSUES

Children

The concept of childhood depression has been controversial for decades. Although discussed as a diagnostic entity in the psychiatric literature of the early 1950's, the existence of this diagnosis was doubted in the late 1950's and 1960's. However, work by Malmquist (1971), Carlson and Cantwell (1980), and Cytryn and colleagues (1980) helped bring the concept into acceptance.

While many children manifest classic *DSM-III* features of depression, there is a high frequency of so-called "masked depressions" in which symptoms are less apparent. In children, the typical features of depression are dysphoric mood and self-deprecatory ideation (Malmquist, 1971; Carlson and Cantwell, 1980; Cytryn et al., 1980; Petti, 1978; Weinberg et al., 1973; Poznanski et al., 1976). However, psychosomatic symptoms such as "bellyaches" and "headaches" frequently may be ascertained to be secondary to depression in children. So-called "aggressive children" have been studied and have a high frequency of overt depression on the basis of negative self-image, withdrawal, and crying (Poznanski et al., 1976). Also, many children described as "hyperactive," either with or without an attention deficit disorder, are subsequently observed to be depressed; and a significant number of these patients show dysphoria in response to stimulant medications. The frequent association between hyperactivity and depression in children has been shown by Brumback and Weinberg (1977).

Many laboratory markers of depression in adults are also noted in depressed children. Studies with plasma cortisol hypersecretion, urinary metabolites, and all-night sleep EEG analysis suggest a continuity of biologic changes similar to those seen in adults. (McKnew and Cytryn, 1979; Puig-Antich et al., 1979; Kupfer et al., 1979). Although an eclectic approach that includes an awareness of the family dynamics, environment, and stress factors in a child's life are essential to any psychotherapeutic process, many chronically depressed children also benefit from a psychopharmacologic approach.

Classic bipolar illness with distinctive manic and depressive episodes does not appear to occur in early childhood and is rare before middle adolescence (Gittelman-Klein, 1978). Some investigators, however, hypothesize (Annell, 1969; Schou, 1972) that bipolar illness may, in fact, exist in children but that it goes unrecognized because the symptoms and course differ from those found in adults. According to these authors, low doses of lithium (150-250 mg/day) have been effective treatment for children with mood swings accompanied by a variety of behaviors such as hyperactivity, temper outbursts, or poor school performance. Nevertheless, the discussion and methodologies relating to possible bipolar-like disorders in children leave much to be desired at this time, and the indications for lithium treatment in children remain questionable.

Many investigators, on the other hand, report beneficial effects of antidepressants, typically tricyclics, in treating unipolar depression in children. While the symptoms of the clinical populations studied show great variability (including somatic complaints, hyperactivity, enuresis, poor impulse control, headbanging, and psychosis), antidepressants seem helpful in 75 percent of the cases in which the child shows dysphoric mood (Gittelman-Klein, 1978). Puig-Antich (Gittelman-Klein, 1978), for example, identified 13 prepubertal children (eight boys, five girls) who met adult diagnostic criteria for depression upon admission as well as upon re-examination four weeks later. Eight of the children were treated with imipramine with a mean dose of 130 mg/day. Seven out of the eight children treated with imipramine showed improvement in mood within four weeks and sustained mood improvement during a three-month treatment period. Moreover, in a placebo-controlled crossover study of amitriptyline in 14 hospitalized depressed children, doses of 30-50 mg/day proved to be significantly superior to placebo (Lucas et al., 1965).

The Elderly

Affective disorders are common in geriatric populations. While the manic phase of bipolar disorder is similar to that observed in middle-aged populations, there are some manifestations of bipolar disorder, depressed phase, and of major depression more often noted in the elderly (Reynolds et al., 1983). Older patients frequently display prominent somatic concerns that are out of proportion to any demonstrable abnormality. They also frequently have memory or cognitive deficits that are out of proportion to any physical abnormalities present. Moreover, delusional thinking often accompanies the spectrum of depressive symptoms in the elderly. Lithium is most useful for treating manic-depressive illness in the elderly; however, caution in monitoring blood levels is warranted. Older patients generally have a decreased ability to clear and excrete lithium and, for this reason, are at a greater risk for side effects.

Antidepressants are lipid soluble and since the ratio of fat to other tissue increases with age, these agents accumulate more easily in elderly patients. In addition, the rate of metabolism of antidepressants decreases with advancing age. Some clinicians advocate the use of desipramine or nortriptyline for elderly patients since these agents should have fewer peripheral and central atropinergic side effects and because most of their metabolites are pharmacologically inactive (Reynolds et al., 1983). Therapy may be started at 25 mg of desipramine and gradually increased over one to two weeks to perhaps 50 to 100 mg daily. Nortriptyline has a higher per milligram potency and should, therefore, be started at a lower dosage and titrated accordingly. More serious side effects that should be monitored carefully include orthostatic hypotension, tachycardia, arrhythmias, confusion, urinary retention, and exacerbation of narrow-angle glaucoma.

As previously noted in this chapter, some of the newer antidepressants may have advantages for the elderly patient. Because of the reported low incidence of atropinergic side effects and cardiotoxicity, maprotiline and trazodone may be particularly useful.

Advanced age is still considered to be a relative limitation for using MAO inhibitors. However, in refractory depressions, moderate doses of MAO inhibitors can be used with good results.

PROFESSIONAL AND ETHICAL ISSUES

While a full review of all possible side effects of lithium and/or an antidepressant is not always practical in the clinical setting, ethically it is good medical practice to present the main side effects a patient might experience with a prescribed medication. In addition, if patients are prepared for the possibility of a side effect such as dry mouth, they may be less likely to discontinue their medication.

Tricyclic antidepressants have ironically been used successfully by many depressed patients to commit suicide, and the clinician, accordingly, should be extremely cautious in prescribing these medications to depressed outpatients. Patients with suicidal ideation are more safely treated as inpatients, of course, but when hospitalization is not possible, prescriptions should be given such that the maximum quantity that a patient could ingest (if he took all of the pills at once) equals less than 2 g.

FINANCIAL, LEGAL, AND SOCIAL/POLITICAL ISSUES

While cost is not a frequent limiting factor in the psychopharmacologic treatment of depression, the low-income patient all too frequently returns for follow-up reporting noncompliance with the prescribed medication regimen because of inability to pay for a given prescription or because of the desire to use the medication more sparingly than prescribed to make it last longer.

The encouraging results of pharmacotherapy in the treatment of affective illness have had significant social and political effects. The general public more readily accepts the idea of obtaining treatment for medical problems in which organic etiologies are understood (or at least strongly suspected) than functional emotional problems with no known cause. As chemical agents have proved effective in treating affective illnesses, governmental policies have shifted toward providing more funding for mental health centers on the assumption that more patients could be managed on an outpatient basis. The advent of antidepressants and lithium has also changed the psychiatrist's role. Economic pressures in many mental health centers have resulted in many psychiatrists' assuming more of a medical model role as manager of the pharmacotherapy of large numbers of patients. Although the past three decades have brought us far in the understanding and treatment of affective disorders, a frontier of research questions remains to be answered. New advances in the delivery of psychiatric care are likely to be affected more and more by socioeconomic and political issues.

REFERENCES

Alexander PE, Van Kammen DP, Bunney WE Jr: Antipsychotic effects of lithium in schizophrenia. Am J Psychiatry 136:283-287, 1979

Amsterdam JD, Winokur A, Caroff SN, et al: The dexamethasone suppression test in outpatients with primary affective disorder and healthy control subjects. Am J Psychiatry 139:287-291, 1982

Ananth J, Luchins D: A review of combined tricyclic and MAOI therapy. Compr Psychiatry 18:221-230, 1977

Annell A: Amitriptyline in childhood depressions. Acta Psychiatr Scand Suppl 207: 19-30, 1969

Asberg M, Bertilsson L, Tuck D, et al: Indoleamine metabolites in the cerebrospinal fluid of depressed patients before and during treatment with nortriptyline. Clin Pharmacol Ther 14:277-286, 1973

Asberg M: Relationship between plasma level and therapeutic effect of nortriptyline. Br Med J 3:331-334, 1971

Asnis GM, Asnis D, Dunnes DL, et al: Cogwheel rigidity during chronic lithium therapy. Am J Psychiatry 136:1225-1226, 1979

Baastrup PC, Hollnagel P, Sorensen R, et al: Adverse reactions in treatment with lithium carbonate and haloperidol. JAMA 236:2645-2646, 1976

Baastrup PC, Schou M: Lithium as a prophylactic agent: its effect against recurrent depression and manic depressive psychosis. Arch Gen Psychiatry 16:167-172, 1967

Bailey E, Bond PA, Brooks BA, et al: The medicinal chemistry of lithium. Prog Med Chem 11:193-272, 1975

Baldessarini RJ, Lipinski JF: Lithium salts: 1970-1975. Ann Intern Med 83:527-533, 1975

Baldessarini RJ, Tarsy D: Tardive dyskinesia, in Psychopharmacology: A Generation of Progress. Edited by Lipton MA, DiMascio A, Killam KF. New York, Raven Press, 1978

Beckman H, Goodwin FK: Antidepressant response to tricyclics and urinary MHPG in unipolar patients. Arch Gen Psychiatry 32:17-21, 1975

Biederman J, Lerner Y, Belmaker RH: Combination of lithium carbonate and haloperidol in schizoaffective disorder. Arch Gen Psychiatry 36:327-333, 1979

Bielski RJ, Friedel RO: Prediction of tricyclic antidepressant response. Arch Gen Psychiatry 33:1479-1489, 1976

Biggs JT, Spiker DC, Petit JM, et al: Tricyclic antidepressant overdose: incidence of symptoms. JAMA 238:135-138, 1977

Biggs JT, Ziegler VE, Clayton PJ, et al: Nortriptyline plasma levels and therapeutic response. Clin Pharmacol Ther 20:458-463, 1976.

Biggs JT, Ziegler VE: Protriptyline plasma levels and antidepressant response. Clin Pharmacol Ther 22:269-273, 1977

Braithwaite R, Goulding R, Theano G, et al: Amitriptyline plasma levels and therapeutic response. Clin Pharmacol Ther 19:795-801, 1976

Branchey M, Charles J, Simpson G: Extrapyramidal side effects with lithium therapy. Am J Psychiatry 133:444-445, 1976

Brogdon R, Heel RC, Speight TM, et al: Nomifensine: a review of its pharmacologic properties and therapeutic efficacy in depressive illness. Drugs 18:1-24, 1979

Brumback RA, Weinberg WA: Relationship of hyperactivity and depression in children. Percept Mot Skills 45:247-251, 1977

Brunswick DJ, Mendels J: Reduced levels of tricyclic antidepressants in plasma from Vacutainers. Commun Psychopharmacol 1:131-134, 1977

Bunney WE Jr, Mason JW, Roatch JF, et al: A psychoendocrine study of severe psychotic depressive crisis. Am J Psychiatry 122:72-80, 1965

Burrows CD, Davis B: Antidepressants and barbiturates. Br Med J 3:331-334, 1971

Burrows G, Scoggins BA, Turecek LR, et al: Plasma nortriptyline and clinical response. Clin Pharmacol Ther 16:639-644, 1974

Burrows G, Davies B, Scoggins BA: Plasma concentration of nortriptyline and clinical response in depressive illness. Lancet 2:619-623, 1972

Byck R: Drugs and the treatment of psychiatric disorders, in The Pharmacological Basis of Therapeutics. Edited by Goodman LS, Gilman A. New York, MacMillan, 1975

Cade JFL: Lithium salts in the treatment of psychotic excitement. Med J Aust 2:349-352, 1949

Carlson GA, Cantwell DP: Unmasking masked depression in children and adolescents. Am J Psychiatry 137:445-449, 1980

Carroll BJ, Feinberg M, Greden JF, et al: A specific laboratory test for the diagnosis of melancholia. Arch Gen Psychiatry 38:15-22, 1981

Cervi-Skinner SJ: Lithium-carbonate-induced hypercalcemia. West J Med 127:527-528, 1977

Cho JT, Bone S, Dunner DL, et al: The effect of lithium treatment on thyroid function in patients with primary affective disorder. Am J Psychiatry 136:115-116, 1979

Christensson TA: Lithium, hypercalcaemia, and hyperparathyroidism (ltr). Lancet 2:144, 1976

CIBA-Geigy Pharmaceutical Research Division: Summary for Investigation: Oxaprotiline. Summit, NJ, CIBA-Geigy, 1982

Cohen WJ, Cohen NH: Lithium carbonate, haloperidol, and irreversible brain damage. JAMA 230:1283-1287, 1974

Comfort A: Effects of psychotropic drugs on ejaculation. Am J Psychiatry 136:124-125, 1979

Coppen A, Noguera R, Bailey J: Prophylactic lithium in affective disorders. Lancet 2:275-279, 1971

Cytryn L, McKnew DH, Bunny WE Jr: Diagnosis of depression in children: a reassessment. Am J Psychiatry 135:22-25, 1980

Davis BM, Pfefferbaum A, Krutzik S, et al: Lithium's effect on parathyroid hormone. Am J Psychiatry 138:489-492, 1981

Davis JM: Overview: maintenance therapy in psychiatry, II: affective disorders. Am J Psychiatry 133:1-3, 1976

DePaulo JR Jr, Correa EI, Sapir DG: Renal glomerular function and long-term lithium therapy. Am J Psychiatry 138:324-327, 1981

Dewan MJ, Pandurangi AK, Boucher ML, et al: Abnormal dexamethasone suppression test results in chronic schizophrenic patients. Am J Psychiatry 139:1501-1503, 1982

Dilsaver SC, Feinber M, Greden JF: Antidepressant withdrawal symptoms treated with anticholinergic agents. Am J Psychiatry 140:249-251, 1983

Dinsmore PR, Ryback R: Lithium in schizoaffective disorders. Dis Nerv Sys 33:771-776, 1972

Ekbon K: Lithium in the treatment of chronic cluster headache. Headache 17:39-40, 1977

Evans DAP, Davison K, Pratt RTC: The influence of acetylator phenotype on the effects of treating depression with phenelzine. Clin Pharmacol Ther 6:430-435, 1965

Evans DAP, Manley KA, McKusick V: Genetic control of isoniazid metabolism in man. Br Med J 2:485-491, 1960

Evans DAP, White TA: Human acetylation polymorphism. J Lab Clin Med 63:391-403, 1964

Everett HC: The use of bethanechol chloride with tricyclic antidepressants. Am J Psychiatry 132:1202-1204, 1975

Fabre LF, McLendon DM: A double-blind study comparing the efficacy and safety of alprazolam with diazepam and placebo in anxious outpatients. Current Therapeutic Research 19:661-668, 1976

Fabre LF: Pilot open-label study with alprazolam (U-31, 889) in outpatients with neurotic depression. Current Therapeutic Research 19:661-668, 1976

Falk WE, Mahnke MW, Poskanzer DC: Lithium prophylaxis of corticotropin-induced psychosis. JAMA 241:1011-1012, 1979

Fawcett J, Maas JW: Depression and MHPG excretion: response to dextroamphetamine and tricyclic antidepressants. Arch Gen Psychiatry 26:246-251, 1972

Fawcett J, Simopoulos V: Dextroamphetamine response as a possible predictor of improvement with tricyclic therapy in depression. Arch Gen Psychiatry 25:247-255, 1971

Fieve RR, Platman SR, Plutchick RR: The use of lithium in affective disorders, I: acute endogenous depression. Am J Psychiatry 125:487-491, 1968

Flemenbaum A: Pavor nocturnus: a complication of single daily tricyclic or neuroleptic dosage. Am J Psychiatry 133:570-572, 1976

Folks DG, King LD, Dowdy SB, et al: Carbamazepine treatment of selected affectively disordered inpatients. Am J Psychiatry 139:115-117, 1982

Fowler NO, McCall D, Chou TC, et al: Electrocardiographic changes and cardiac arrhythmias in patients receiving psychotropic drugs. Am J Cardiol 37:223-230, 1976

Friedman E, Fang F, Gershon S: Antidepressant drugs and dopamine uptake in different brain regions. Eur J Pharmacol 42: 47-51, 1977

Frohman LA: Neurotransmitters as regulators of endocrine function. Hosp Pract 10:54-67, 1975.

Gerner RH, Post RM, Spiegel AM, et al: Effects of parathyroid hormone and lithium treatment on calcium and mood in depressed patients. Biol Psychiatry 12:145-151, 1977

Gerner RH, Psarras J, Kirschenbaum MA: Results of clinical renal function tests in lithium patients. Am J Psychiatry 137:834-837, 1980

Gershon S, Mann J, Newton R, et al: Evaluation of trazodone in the treatment of endogenous depression: results of a multi-center double-blind study. J Clin Psychopharmacol 1:395-445, 1981

Gershon S, Shopsin B: Lithium: Its Role in Psychiatric Research and Treatment. New York, Plenum, 1973

Gershon S, Yuwiler A: Lithium ion: a specific pharmacological approach to the treatment of mania. J Neuropsychiatry 1:229-241, 1960

Gershon S: Lithium prophylaxis in recurrent affective disorders. Compr Psychiatry 15:365-373, 1974

Gittelman-Klein: Psychopharmacological treatment of anxiety disorders, mood disorders, and Tourette's disorder in children, in Psychopharmacology: A Generation of Progress. Edited by Lipton MA, DiMascio A, Killam KF. New York, Raven Press, 1978

Glassman AH, Bigger JT Jr, Giardina EV, et al: Clinical characteristics of imipramine-induced orthostatic hypotension. Lancet 1:468-472, 1979

Glassman AH, Perel JM, Shostak M, et al: Clinical implications of imipramine plasma levels for depressive illness. Arch Gen Psychiatry 34:197-204, 1977

Glassman AH, Perel JM: The clinical pharmacology of imipramine. Arch Gen Psychiatry 28:649-653, 1973

Gleisinger B: Evaluation of lithium treatment in treatment of psychotic excitement. Med J Aust 41:277-283, 1954

Gold MS, Pottash ALC, Extein I, et al: The TRH test in the diagnosis of major and minor depression. Psychoneuroendocrinology 6:159-169, 1981a

Gold MS, Pottash ALC, Extein I, et al: Diagnosis of depression in the 1980s. JAMA 245:1562-1564, 1981b

Goldberg HL, DiMascio A: Psychotropic drugs in pregnancy, in Psychopharmacology: A Generation of Progress. Edited by Lipton MA, DiMascio A, Killam KF. New York, Raven Press, 1978

Goodwin FK, Cowdry RW, Webster MH: Predictors of drug response in the affective disorders: toward an integrated approach, in Psychopharmacology: A Generation of Progress. Edited by Lipton MA, DiMascio A, Killam KF. New York, Raven Press, 1978

Goodwin FK, Murphy DL, Bunney WE Jr: Lithium carbonate treatment in depression and mania: a longitudinal double-blind study. Arch Gen Psychiatry 21:486-496, 1969

Goodwin FK, Murphy DL, Dunner DL: Lithium response in unipolar vs bipolar depression. Am J Psychiatry 129:44-47, 1972

Goodwin FK, Prange AJ, Post RM, et al: Potentiation of antidepressant effects by L-triiodothyronine in tricyclic nonresponders. Am J Psychiatry 139:34-38, 1982

Grahame-Smith DG, Greene AR: The role of brain 5-hydroxytryptamine in the hyperactivity produced in rats by lithium and monamine oxidase inhibition. Br J Pharmacol 52:19-26, 1974

Hartigan GP: The use of lithium salts in affective disorders. Br J Psychiatry 109:810-814, 1963

Hekimian LJ, Gershon S, Hardesty AS, et al: Drug efficacy and diagnostic specificity in manic depressive illness and schizophrenia. Dis Nerv Syst 30:747-751, 1969

Hestbach J, Hansen HE, Amdisen A, et al: Chronic renal lesions following long-term treatment with lithium. Kidney Int 12:205-213, 1977

Himmelhoch JM, Forrest J, Neil JF, et al: Thiazide-lithium synergy in refractory mood swings. Am J Psychiatry 134:149-152, 1977.

Hirschowitz J, Casper R, Garver DL, et al: Lithium response in good prognosis schizophrenia. Am J Psychiatry 137:916-920, 1980

Hollister LE: Doxepin hydrochloride. Ann Intern Med 81:360-363, 1974

Hollister LE: Mental disorders - antipsychotic and antimanic drugs. N Engl J Med 286:984-987, 1972

Hullin RP, MacDonald R, Allsopp MNE: Prophylactic lithium in recurrent affective disorders. Lancet 1:1044-1046, 1972

Johnson F: Antidepressant effects of lithium. Compr Psychiatry 15:43-47, 1974

Johnson G: Differential response to lithium carbonate in manic depressive and schizoaffective disorders. Dis Nerv Syst 31:613-615, 1970

Johnstone EC, Marsh W: Acetylator status and response to phenelzine in depressed patients. Lancet 1:567-570, 1973

Johnstone EC: The relationship between acetylator status and inhibition of monoamine oxidase, excretion of free drug and antidepressant response in depressed patients on phenelzine. Psychopharmacology 46:289-294, 1976

Kane J, Rifkin A, Quitkin F, et al: Extrapyramidal side effects with lithium treatment. Am J Psychiatry 135:851-853, 1978

Katon W, Raskind M: Treatment of depression in the medically ill elderly with methylphenidate. Am J Psychiatry 137:963-965, 1980

Klein DF, Davis JM: Diagnosis and Treatment of Psychiatric Disorders. Baltimore, Williams & Wilkins Co, 1969

Klerman GL: Long-term treatment of affective disorders, in Psychopharmacology: A Generation of Progress. Edited by Lipton MA, DiMascio A, Killam KF. New York, Raven Press, 1978

Knapp S, Mandell AJ: Effects of lithium chloride on parameters biosynthetic capacity for 5-hydroxytryptamin in rat brain. J Pharmacol Exp Ther 193:812-823, 1975

Kragh-Sorenson P, Hansen CE, Asberg M: Plasma levels of nortriptyline in the treatment of endogenous depression. Acta Psychiatr Scand 49:444-456, 1973

Kragh-Sorenson P, Hansen CE, Baastrup PC, et al: Self-inhibiting action of nortriptyline's antidepressant effects at high plasma levels. Psychopharmacologia 45:305-312, 1976

Kramer JC, Klein DF, Fink M: Withdrawal symptoms following discontinuation of imipramine therapy. Am J Psychiatry 118:549-550, 1961

Kudrow L: Lithium prophylaxis for chronic cluster headache. Headache 17:15-18, 1977

Kupfer DJ, Coble P, Kane J, et al: Imipramine and EEG sleep in children with depressive symptoms. Psychopharmacology 60:117-123, 1979

Kupfer DJ, Spiker DG, Coble PA, et al: Sleep and treatment prediction in endogenous depression. Am J Psychiatry 138:429-434, 1981

Larochelle P, Hamet P, Enjalbert M: Responses to tyramine and norepinephrine after imipramine and trazodone. Clin Pharmacol Ther 26:24-30, 1979

Levy BF: Treatment of hypertension with pargyline hydrochloride. Current Therapeutic Research 8:343-346, 1966

Lipinski JF, Pope HG: Possible synergistic action between carbamazepine and lithium carbonate in the treatment of three acutely manic patients. Am J Psychiatry 139:948-949, 1982

Livingston S, Pauli L, Berman W: Carbamazepine (Tegretol) in epilepsy: nine-year followup study with special emphasis on untoward reactions. Dis Nerv Syst 35:103-107, 1974

Loosen PT, Prange AJ: Serum thyrotropin response to thyrotropin-releasing hormone in psychiatric patients: a review. Am J Psychiatry 139:405-416, 1982

Lucas AR, Lockett HJ, Grimm F: Amitriptyline in childhood depression. Dis Nerv Syst 26:105-110, 1965

Maas JW, Dekirmenjian H, Garver D, et al: Excretion of catecholamine metabolites following intraventricular injection of 6-hydroxydopamine in the macaca speciosa. Eur J Pharmacol 23:121-130, 1973

Maas JW, Landis DH: In vivo studies of metabolism of norepinephrine in the central nervous system. J Pharmacol Exper Ther 163:147-162, 1968

Maas JW: Clinical implications of pharmacological differences among antidepressants, in Psychopharmacology: A Generation of Progress. Edited by Lipton MA, DiMascio A, Killam KF. New York, Raven Press, 1978

Maggs R: Treatment of manic illness with lithium carbonate. Br J Psychiatry 109:56-65, 1963

Malmquist CP: Depression in childhood and adolescence. N Engl J Med 284:887-893, 955-961, 1971

Mandell AJ, Knapp S: A neurobiological model for the symmetrical prophylactic action of lithium in bipolar affective disorder. Pharmakopsychiatr Neuropsychopharmakol 9:116-126, 1976

Mannano E: The metabolism of C^{14}-noradrenaline by cat brain in vivo. J Neurochem 10:373-379, 1963.

Martin JB, Reichlin S, Brown GM: Clinical Neuroendocrinology. Philadelphia, Pa, Davis, 1977

McKnew DH Jr, Cytryn L: Urinary metabolites in chronically depressed children. J Am Acad Child Psychiatry 18:608-615, 1979

Mellerup ET, Lauritsen B, Dam H, et al: Lithium effects on diurnal rhythms of calcium, magnesium, and phosphate metabolism in manic-melancholic disorder. Acta Psychiatr Scand 53:360-370, 1976

Mendels J, Secunda SK, Dyson WL: A controlled study of the antidepressant effects of lithium. Arch Gen Psychiatry 26:154-157, 1972

Mendels J: Lithium in the treatment of depression. Am J Psychiatry 133:373-377, 1976

Merry J, Reynolds CM, Bailey J, et al: Prophylactic treatment of alcoholism by lithium carbonate: a controlled study. Lancet 2:486-488, 1976

Morris JB, Beck AT: The efficacy of antidepressant drugs. Arch Gen Psychiatry 30:667-671, 1974

Nies A, Robinson DS, Friedman MJ, et al: Relationship between age and tricyclic antidepressant plasma levels. Am J Psychiatry 134:790-793, 1977

Noyes R, Dempsey GM, Blum A: Lithium treatment of depression. Compr Psychiatry 15:187-190, 1974

Nurnberg HG, Coccaro EF: Response of panic disorder and resistance of depression to imipramine. Am J Psychiatry 139:1060-1062, 1982

Petti TA: Depression in hospitalized child psychiatry patients: approaches to measuring depression. J Am Acad Child Psychiatry 17:49-59, 1978

Poldinger W, Gammel G: Differences in effect between nomifensine and nortriptyline. Int Pharmacopsychiatry 13:58-62, 1978

Post RM, Gordon EK, Goodwin FK, et al: Central norepinephrine metabolism in affective illness: MHPG in the cerebrospinal fluid. Science 179:1002-1003, 1973

Poznanski EO, Krahenbuhl V, Zrull JP: Childhood depression: a longitudinal perspective. J Am Acad Psychiatry 15:491-501, 1976

Prange AJ, Wilson IC, Rabon AM, et al: Enhancement of imipramine antidepressant activity by thyroid hormone. Am J Psychiatry 126:457-469, 1969

Price LH, Yeates C, Nelson JC: Lithium augmentation of combined neuroleptic-tricyclic treatment in delusional depression. Am J Psychiatry 140:318-322, 1982

Prien RF, Klett CJ, Caffey EM: Lithium carbonate and imipramine in prevention of affective disorders. Arch Gen Psychiatry 29:420-425, 1973

Prusoff BA, Williams DH, Weissman MW, et al: Treatment of secondary depression in schizophrenia. Arch Gen Psychiatry 36:569-575, 1979

Puig-Antich J, Chambers W, Halpern F, et al: Cortisol hypersecretion in prepubertal depressive illness. Psychoneuroendocrinology 4:191-197, 1979

Quitkin F, Rifkin A, Klein DF: Monoamine oxidase inhibitors. Arch Gen Psychiatry 36:749-759, 1979

Quitkin F, Rifkin A, Klein DF: Prophylaxis of affective disorders: current status of knowledge. Arch Gen Psychiatry 33:337-341, 1976

Reichlin S: Neuroendocrinology, in Textbook of Endocrinology, 5th ed. Edited by Williams RH. Philadelphia, WB Saunders, 1974

Reynolds CF, Marin RS, Spiker D: Clinical considerations in prescribing antidepressants for geriatric patients. Ger Med Today 2:45-55, 1983

Richelson E: Are receptor studies useful for clinical practice? J Clin Psychiatry 9:4-9, 1983

Robinson DS, Nies A, Ravaris C, et al: The monoamine oxidase inhibitor, phenelzine, in the treatment of depressive-anxiety states. Arch Gen Psychiatry 29:407-413, 1973

Robinson DS, Nies A, Ravaris CL, et al: Clinical pharmacology of phenelzine. Arch Gen Psychiatry 35:629-635, 1978a

Robinson DS, Nies A, Ravaris CL, et al: Clinical pharmacology of phenelzine: MAO activity and clinical response, in Psychopharmacology: A Generation of Progress. Edited by Lipton MA, DiMascio A, Killam KF. New York, Raven Press, 1978b

Sachar EJ, Hellman L, Roffwarg HP, et al: Disrupted 24-hour patterns of cortisol secretion in psychotic depression. Arch Gen Psychiatry 28:19-24, 1973

Sacks MH, Bonforte RJ, Lasser RF, et al: Cardiovascular complications of imipramine intoxication. JAMA 205:116-118, 1968

Schanberg SM, Schildkraut JJ, Breese GR, et al: Metabolism of normetanephrine-H[3] in rat brain: identification of conjugated 3-methoxy-4-hydroxyphenylglycol as the major metabolite. Biochem Pharmacol 17:247-254, 1968

Schildkraut JJ: Norepinephrine metabolites as biochemical criteria for classifying depressive disorders and predicting responses to treatment: preliminary findings. Am J Psychiatry 130:695-699, 1973

Schou M, Juel-Nielsen N, Stromgen E, et al: The treatment of manic psychosis by the administration of lithium salts. J Neurol Neurosurg Psychiatry 17:250-260, 1954

Schou M: The range of clinical uses of lithium, in Lithium in Medical Practice. Edited by Johnson FN, Johnson S. Baltimore, University Park Press, 1978

Schou M: Depressive states, in Childhood and Adolescence. Edited by Annel AL. New York, John Wiley & Sons, 1972

Scully RF, Galdabini JJ, McNely BU: Case records of the Massachusetts General Hospital. N Engl J Med 304:1025-1032, 1981

Seager CP, Bird RL: Imipramine with electrical treatment in depression: a controlled trial. J Ment Sci 108:704-707, 1962.

Selvini A, Ross C, Belli C, et al: Antidepressant treatment with maprotiline in the management of emotional disturbances in patients with acute myocardial infarction: a controlled study. J Int Med Res 4:42-46, 1976

Settle EC, Ayd FJ: Trimipramine: twenty years' worldwide clinical experience. J Clin Psychiatry 41:266-274, 1980

Shopsin B, Johnson G, Gershon S: Cogwheel rigidity related to lithium maintenance. Am J Psychiatry 132:536-538, 1973

Shopsin B, Kim SS, Gershon S: A controlled study of lithium vs chlorpromazine in acute schizophrenics. Br J Psychiatry 119:435-440, 1971

Sletten IW, Gershon S: The premenstrual syndrome: a discussion of pathophysiology and treatment with lithium ion. Compr Psychiatry 7:197-206, 1966

Snyder SH, Yamamura HI: Antidepressants and the muscarinic acetylcholine receptor. Arch Gen Psychiatry 34:235-239, 1977

Sovner R, DiMascio A: Extrapyramidal syndromes and other neurological side effects of psychotropic drugs, in Psychopharmacology: A Generation of Progress. Edited by Lipton MA, DiMascio A, Killam KF. New York, Raven Press, 1978

Spiker DG, Weiss AN, Chang SS, et al: Tricyclic antidepressant overdose. Clin Pharmacol Ther 18:539-546, 1975

Spring G, Frankel M: New data on lithium and haloperidol incompatibility. Am J Psychiatry 138:818-821, 1981

Spring GK: EEG observations in confirming neurotoxicity (ltr to ed). Am J Psychiatry 136:1099-1100, 1979a

Spring GK: Neurotoxicity with combined use of lithium and thioridazine. J Clin Psychiatry 40:135-138, 1979b

Stallone F, Shelley E, Mendlewicz J, et al: The use of lithium in affective disorders, III: a double-blind study of prophylaxis in bipolar illness. Am J Psychiatry 130:1006-1010, 1973

Steiner M: Triiodothyronine, imipramine, and depression (ltr). Am J Psychiatry 137:383-384, 1980

Stokes PE, Kocsis JH, Arcuni OJ: Relationship of lithium chloride dose to treatment response in acute mania. Arch Gen Psychiatry 33:1080-1084, 1976

Stokes PE, Stoll PM, Shamoian CA, et al: Efficacy of lithium as acute treatment of manic-depression illness. Lancet 1:1319-1325, 1971

Strayhorn JM, Nash JL: Severe neurotoxicity despite "therapeutic" serum levels. Dis Nerv Syst 38:107-111, 1977

Sullivan JL, Maltbie A, Cavenar JO Jr, et al: Platelet monoamine oxidase activity predicts response to lithium in manic depressive illness. Lancet 2:1325-1327, 1977

Taska RJ, Sullivan JL, Cavenar JO Jr, et al: Recent advances in biological psychiatry. Current Concepts in Psychiatry 5:6-14, 1979

Taska RJ: Clinical laboratory aids in the treatment of depression: tricyclic antidepressant plasma levels and urinary MHPG. Current Concepts in Psychiatry 3:12-20, 1977

Taylor MA, Abrams R: The phenomenology of mania: a new look at some old patients. Arch Gen Psychiatry 29:550-552, 1973

Tupin JP, Schlagenhauf GK, Creson DL: Lithium effects on electrolyte excretion. Am J Psychiatry 125:536-542, 1968

Van Der Velde C: Toxicity of lithium carbonate in elderly patients. Am J Psychiatry 127:115-117, 1971

Van Kammen DP, Murphy DL: Prediction of imipramine antidepressant response by a one-day d-amphetamine trial. Am J Psychiatry 135:1179-1184, 1978

Van Scheyen JD, Van Kammen DP: Clomipramine-induced mania in unipolar depression. Arch Gen Psychiatry 36:560-565, 1979

Vendsborg PB, Bech P, RaFaelson OJ: Lithium treatment and weight gain. Acta Psychiatr Scand 53:139-147, 1976

Warren JA, Steinbook RM: A case report of carbamazepine-induced reticulocytosis. Am J Psychiatry 140: 247-249, 1983

Weinberg WA, Rutman J, Sullivan L, et al: Depression in children referred to an educational diagnostic center: diagnosis and treatment. J Pediatr 83: 1065-1072, 1973

Whyte SF, Macdonald AJ, Naylor GJ, et al: Plasma concentrations of protriptyline and clinical effects in depressed women. Br J Psychlomipramine-induced mania in unipolar depression. Arch Gen Psychiatry 36:560-565, 1979

Ziegler VE, Clayton PJ, Taylor JR, et al: Nortriptyline plasma levels and therapeutic response. Clin Pharmacol Ther 20:458-463, 1976a

Ziegler VE, Co BT, Taylor JR, et al: Amitriptyline plasma levels and therapeutic response. Clin Pharmacol Ther 19:795-801, 1976

Antipsychotic Agents

INTRODUCTION

Antipsychotic agents include a large and still growing number of compounds proven effective in the management of a broad range of psychotic symptoms. They are particularly useful in the treatment of schizophrenia and mania. Despite their chemical diversity, nearly all of the currently available agents produce similar neurological effects in animals and in human patients. The regular association between antipsychotic actions and extrapyramidal effects on posture and movement has suggested the term *neuroleptic* (producing signs of neurological disorder) for this class of drugs, a usage common in Europe. However, the recent discovery of several agents that have antipsychotic effects without neurological side effects supports the use of the more general term *antipsychotic* for this group of agents.

Although the usefulness of lithium salts for the management of excited or manic patients was described in 1949, the first antipsychotic drugs introduced into modern medicine were the phenothiazine chlorpromazine and the *Rauwolfia* alkaloid reserpine (1952-53). Reserpine is no longer used as an antipsychotic agent, but the phenothiazines and chemically related substances have been remarkably successful. It is often pointed out that the prevalence of hospitalization in U.S. public mental hospitals peaked at more than a half-million patients in the mid-1950's and then declined sharply to fewer than 200,000 patients in the late 1970's, despite the simultaneous rise in the population. The introduction of neuroleptic drugs in the mid-1950's represents an essential contribution to this dramatic change. Their use

119

permitted sociological and administrative changes that included a movement away from long-term institutional care of the severely mentally ill.

The references provided below include secondary reviews with bibliographies covering specific points made in this chapter. These include monographs or chapters by Appleton and Davis (1980), Baldessarini (1980, 1984a, 1984b), Barchas et al. (1977), Hollister (1978), Klein et al. (1980), Mason and Granacher (1980), Simpson (1984), and Van Praag (1978).

The tricyclic chemical nucleus of the phenothiazines was synthesized late in the nineteenth century with the development of aniline dyes. Such compounds were used clinically as antimicrobial agents. Their history is intimately related to the early development by Ehrlich and others of the theory of specific drug-tissue interactions. In the late 1930's, Charpentier, working at the Rhône-Poulenc Laboratories in France, noted that the phenothiazine derivative promethazine (Phenergan) had antihistaminic and sedative properties. Hoping to find molecules with similar properties, the company subsequently developed chlorpromazine. Antihistaminic sedative agents had been given to agitated psychotic patients in the 1940's with little benefit, so the eventual success of chlorpromazine was unexpected. Chlorpromazine was first tried clinically in 1950 as a preanesthetic sedative by the French surgeon Laborit, who described some of its peculiar effects on behavior as "artificial hibernation." In 1951-52 in Paris, several psychiatrists, prompted by Laborit, noted that the new agent increased the efficacy of barbiturate sedation in psychotic patients. In 1952-53, Delay and Deniker reported further promising experiences with low doses of the new agent used alone in psychiatric patients.

The drug was tried as an antiemetic, sedative, and hypothermic agent as early as 1954 in the United States, although its unique usefulness in psychosis was not appreciated initially. During the late 1950's, many reports of the antipsychotic efficacy of chlorpromazine appeared, including a steadily increasing number arising from rigorous, scientifically controlled therapeutic trials with adequate doses. Many pharmaceutical companies then rapidly developed chemically analogous compounds. By the 1960's, prototypes of most of the classes of antipsychotic agents currently in use were known.

PHARMACOLOGY

Types of Molecules with Antipsychotic Effects

The term *phenothiazine* is not a synonym for antipsychotic agent but refers only to those agents containing a tricyclic nucleus of two benzene rings (*pheno*) joined through a central ring containing a sulfur atom (*thio*) and a nitrogen atom (*azo*) to which is attached a carbon side chain terminating in a substituted tertiary amino nitrogen atom. Nearly 20 have reached the stage of clinical application since the introduction of chlorpromazine (Tables 1 and 2).

Several subtypes of phenothiazines exist which differ in the nature of the side chain (Figure 1). Thus, the terminal amine moiety may have methyl or other substituents with a straight chain of carbon atoms (*aliphatic* or *aminoalkyl* phenothiazines, such as chlorpromazine, and triflupromazine). The amino nitrogen atom may also be incorporated into a cyclic structure, as in the *piperidine* derivatives (such as thioridazine and mesoridazine) and the potent *piperazine* derivatives (such as trifluoperazine, perphenazine, and fluphenazine).

The tricyclic core of such molecules has also been altered without loss of antipsychotic effects. The nitrogen atom of the central ring of phenothiazines has been replaced with a carbon atom while leaving the sulfur atom. These sulfur-(*thio*)-containing structural analogs were designated *thioxanthenes* (Figure 1), the first non-phenothiazine antipsychotic agents. They include molecules with side chains of the aliphatic type (e.g., chlorprothixene) and piperazines (e.g., thiothixene). Further manipulation of the tricyclic structure produced the still experimental acridanes, with a nitrogen atom but no sulfur atom in the central ring (Figure 1).

The structure-activity relationships among these tricyclic antipsychotic agents include the requirement that a side chain of three carbon atoms (at position ten) separate the amino nitrogen from the central ring. The addition of an electronegative substituent in position two (such as Cl, CF_3, or SCH_3) usually markedly increases the efficacy of the molecule. Substitution of a piperazine group for an aliphatic or piperidine moiety on the side chain imparts markedly increased potency but *not* greater clinical efficacy. Higher potency is generally associated with less sedation and hypotension but an increased incidence of extrapyramidal reactions.

In 1959 Janssen in Belgium experimented with derivatives of meperidine (Demerol) and normeperidine, seeking a better analgesic. He developed the butyrophenones, neuroleptic compounds that can also be called phenylbutylpiperidines (Figure 2). The only butyrophenone routinely used in the United States as an antipsychotic agent is haloperidol (Haldol). Droperidol (Inapsine) is also a potent neuroleptic butyrophenone, even though it is approved in the United States only as a short-acting co-anesthetic agent. The butyrophenones share with the piperazine phenothiazines and thioxanthenes high potency and a strong tendency to affect the extrapyramidal motor system as well as a low tendency to produce sedation, hypotension, and anticholinergic effects at standard doses.

Several new compounds structurally related to the butyrophenones are currently undergoing clinical evaluation and include the *diphenylbutylpiperidines* such as pimozide, penfluridol, and fluspiriline (Figure 2). Pimozide is among the most potent neuroleptic agents known, and it is a relatively

Table 1. Approximately Equivalent Doses of Commonly Used Antipsychotic Agents by Chemical Type

Generic Name	Commercial Name[a]	Approximate Equivalent Dose (mg)[b]	Relative Potency
Phenothiazines			
Aliphatic			
Chlorpromazine	Thorazine, etc. (generic)	100	Low
Triflupromazine	Vesprin	30	Low
Piperidines			
Mesoridazine	Serentil	50	Low
Thioridazine	Mellaril	90-100	Low
Piperazines			
Acetophenazine	Tindal	15	Intermediate
Fluphenazine	Prolixin, Permitil	2[c]	High
Perphenazine	Trilafon	10	Intermediate
Trifluoperazine	Stelazine	5	High
Thioxanthenes			
Aliphatic			
Chlorprothixene	Taractan	75	Low
Piperazine			
Thiothixene	Navane	3-5	High
Dibenzazepines			
Loxapine	Loxitane, Daxolin	10-15	Intermediate
Clozapine	(Leponex, experimental)	60	Low
Butyrophenones			
Haloperidol (ester)	Haldol	2-3[c]	High
Droperidol	Inapsine (for injection)	1-2	High
Diphenylbutylpiperidines			
Pimozide	(Orap, experimental)	ca. 0.5-5.0	High
Penfluridol	(Semap, experimental)	2 (1 week dose)[c]	High
Indolones			
Molindone	Moban, Lidone	8-10	Intermediate
Rauwolfia			
Reserpine	Serpasil, etc. (generic)	3-5	High

[a] Trade names in parentheses are not yet licensed in the U.S. Many other agents used elsewhere are not available in the U.S. The commercial preparations are available as soluble salts (most are hydrochlorides; Loxitane or Daxolin is a succinate; Tindal is a maleate; Serentil is a benzylate: see Table 1). Other agents that are not commonly used now or are less effective in the treatment of psychoses are not included, e.g., butaperazine (Repoise), carphenazine (Proketazine), mepazine (Pacatal), promazine (Sparine), piperacetazine (Quide), and thiopropazate (Dartal). Droperidol (Inapsine) is an extremely potent, short-acting neuroleptic, now used mainly as a preanesthetic or coanesthetic agent i.m. or i.v., although it has powerful antipsychotic-sedative effects that might also be useful in psychiatric emergencies. In addition, prochlorperazine (Compazine) and thiethylperazine (Torecan), while having typical neuroleptic (and some antipsychotic) effects, are mainly used as antiemetic agents. Reserpine and other amine-depleting agents are inferior antipsychotic drugs but are sometimes used in the management of tardive dyskinesia. While the other tabulated drugs vary by over 100-fold in *potency*, they are very similar in their clinical *efficacy*.

selective antagonist of dopamine receptors in the brain. Penfluridol and fluspiriline act for a long time, about a week, even after oral administration. Other long-acting antipsychotic agents are long-chain aliphatic fatty-acid esters of fluphenazine: the enanthate (derived from a 7-carbon fatty acid) or the longer-acting decanoate (derived from a 12-carbon acid) (Figure 1). The fluphenazine esters are currently the only long-acting antipsychotic agents in general use in the United States. Such *prodrug* compounds, which are slowly converted to the active parent agent in the body, are useful in the management of chronically psychotic outpatients who are unreliable in taking oral medications, because the drug effects last from one to four weeks after a "depot" injection of an oily solution. Fatty acid esters of other phenothiazines as well as of thioxanthenes are available in Europe, and the decanoate of haloperidol may soon be available in the United States as a long-acting antipsychotic agent that can be injected once a month.

Another class of tricyclic antipsychotic compounds is the piperazine derivatives of *dibenzazepine* molecules (e.g., clozapine, a dibenzodiazepine, Figure 1) or their congeners. The latter include the dibenz*o*xazepine loxapine, which has an oxygen atom instead of a second nitrogen atom in the central ring (Figure 1), and the dibenz*othi*azepines metiapine and clothiapine with a sulfur atom replacing the same nitrogen atom. Clozapine has particular theoretical and practical importance as it is reported to lack the acute extrapyramidal side effects of other antipsychotic agents (including loxapine, metiapine, and clothiapine) in animals and human patients. Clozapine itself has been associated with bone marrow toxicity and remains experimental, its future uncertain. Similar analogues of clozapine, such as fluperlapine, are also being investigated.

Another group of experimental agents, the substituted *benzamides* (notably, sulpiride) is somewhat less likely to induce extrapyramidal side effects, at least at low doses, and may exert clinically useful antipsychotic actions at high doses (Figure 2). Some of these promising newer agents remain unavailable to American physicians at this time, but their discovery

---

b Data are summarized as averages from several sources, some of which vary greatly. These numbers are only an approximate guide, and dosage for each patient must be established by clinical response. In switching from high doses of one agent to a dissimilar one, it is well to proceed gradually over several days to decrease the risk of side effects from the newly introduced drug. It is also important to realize that these equivalent doses are *not therapeutic doses* (which are typically several times higher).

c Injectable fluphenazine esters are used in doses of 25-100 mg intramuscularly every one to four weeks. The enanthate (derived from a 7-carbon fatty acid) typically acts for two weeks, and the currently more popular larger decanoate (ester of a 12-carbon carboxylic acid) for about three weeks. An approximate equivalence is 25 mg (1 ml) of intramuscular fluphenazine decanoate every two to three weeks, which resembles in effectiveness about 10 mg of fluphenazine·HCl (orally) per day (or 500 mg of chlorpromazine). The decanoate ester of haloperidol is also under investigation and is given monthly in i.m. doses of 20 times the daily oral dose. Some long-lasting diphenylbutylpiperidines (experimental in the U.S.) can be used once weekly; penfluridol can be used as two percent of a *weekly* dose of chlorpromazine (i.e., 40 mg/week can replace 2,100 mg/week of chlorpromazine).

Figure 1. Tricyclic Antipsychotic Drugs

BUTYROPHENONES (PHENYLBUTYLPIPERIDINES)

Haloperidol (Haldol)

DIPHENYLBUTYLPIPERIDINES

Pimozide

Penfluridol

INDOLIC COMPOUNDS

Molindone (Moban)

BENZAMIDES

Sulpiride (Dogmatil)

AMINE-DEPLETING AGENTS

Rauwolfia Alkaloids

Reserpine (Serpasil)

Benzoquinolizines

Tetrabenazine (Nitoman)

Figure 2. Other Antipsychotic Drugs

supports the hope that other more selective drugs that retain desired antipsychotic effects but lack extrapyramidal effects can be developed.

Other types of molecules with demonstrated antipsychotic effects include indole derivatives (notably, molindone [Figure 2] and an experimental compound, oxypertine) known as *hydroindolones*. Their potency and pharmacologic activites are generally intermediate between the high and low potency agents of other chemical classes (Table 1). A large number of other agents have been partially evaluated and are not yet generally available.

Finally, several alkaloids prepared originally from the Indian snakeroot plant *Rauwolfia serpentina* and later synthesized, notably reserpine, rescinnamine, and deserpidine, have antipsychotic actions. Briefly in the early 1950's psychiatric interest in their clinical effects was considerable. Other entirely synthetic polycyclic compounds, such as tetrabenazine (Figure 2), benzquinamide, and oxypertine share with *Rauwolfia* alkaloids the ability to deplete amine stores from cells containing catecholamines and indoleamines, particularly in the brain. While most of these amine-depleting agents have some antipsychotic effects, they have not done well in controlled comparisons with the phenothiazines. Their limited efficacy; their side effects, especially sedation, hypotension, and diarrhea; and their association with clinical depression have led to their virtual abandonment for the treatment of psychosis. Reserpine had also been implicated as a contributor to risk of breast cancer, but recent controlled epidemiologic studies do not support this association. Despite its many limitations, it is worth bearing in mind that reserpine given in much higher doses (5-10 mg/day or more) than are used for the treatment of hypertension can be resorted to if side effects or allergic reactions preclude the use of standard antipsychotic drugs.

Most currently available antipsychotic agents induce many extrapyramidal neurological side effects, both acute and late. A few "atypical" antipsychotic drugs are much less likely to do so. The clearest example of an atypical antipsychotic drug is the investigational agent clozapine (Figure 1), which has little acute extrapyramidal activity. Thioridazine shares some of the pharmocologic properties of clozapine, resulting in a lower risk of acute extrapyramidal side effects. At low doses, the benzamides, such as sulpiride, have relatively little extrapyramidal action while their neuroendocrine actions are prominent; however, neurologic effects do appear at the high doses required for clinically useful antipsychotic activity. This pattern of activity probably reflects poor penetration of the blood-brain diffusion barrier rather than a high degree of pharmacologic selectivity as an antipsychotic agent.

The dosage forms of available antipsychotic agents are summarized in Table 2.

Table 2. Selected Antipsychotic Drugs: Chemical Structures, Doses, Side Effects, and Dosage Forms

Nonproprietary Name (Trade Name)		Dose			Side Effects			Dosage Forms	
		Antipsychotic Daily Dosage		Single IM Dose[a]	Sedative	Extra-pyramidal	Hypo-tensive	Oral	Injection
		Usual[b] (mg)	Extreme[b] (mg)	(mg)				T=tablet (mg) C=capsule (mg)	S=syrup E=elixer C=concentrate CS=Concentrated suspension / A=ampul V=vial S=syringe
Phenothiazines Main Structure (positions 1-9; S at 5, N at 10; R_1, R_2)	Side-Chain								
Chlorpromazine·HCl *Thorazine* $—(CH_2)_3—N(CH_3)_2$	$—Cl$	300-800	25-2000	25-50	+++	++	I.M.+++ Oral++	(T) 10,25,50, 100,200 (C) sustained release, 30,75, 150,200,300 (S) 10 mg/5ml (C) 30 mg/ml, 100 mg/ml[c]	(A) 25 mg/ml 50 mg/2ml (V) 25 mg/ml in 10 ml
Triflupromazine·HCl *Vesprin* $—(CH_2)_3—N(CH_3)_2$	$—CF_3$	100-150	25-300	20-50	++	+++	++	(T) 10,25,50 (CS) 50 mg/5ml[c]	(V) 10 mg/ml in 10 ml; 20 mg/ ml (S) 10 mg/ml
Mesoridazine Besylate *Serentil* $—(CH_2)_2—$ (piperidine, N—CH_3)	$—SCH_3$ ($\overset{O}{\|}$)	75-300	25-400	25	+++	+	++	(T) 10,25,50,100 (C) 25 mg/ml	(A) 25 mg/ml

Table 2. (contd.)

Nonproprietary Name (Trade Name) Phenothiazines (contd.)		Dose			Side Effects			Dosage Forms	
Main Structure	Side-Chain	Antipsychotic Daily Dosage Usual[b] (mg)	Extreme[b] (mg)	Single IM Dose[a] (mg)	Sedative	Extra-pyramidal	Hypo-tensive	Oral	Injection
Piperacetazine —(CH₂)₃—N◯—(CH₂)₂OH *Quide*	—COCH₃	20-160	5-200		++	++	+	(T) 10,25	
Thioridazine·HCl ◯ₙ—CH₃ —(CH₂)₂ *Mellaril*	—SCH₃	200-600	50-800		+++	+	++	(T) 10,15,25,50, 100,150,200 (C) 30 mg/ml 100 mg/ml (CS) 25 and 100 mg/5 ml[c]	
Acetophenazine maleate —(CH₂)₂—N◯N—(CH₂)₂—OH *Tindal*	—COCH₃	60-120	20-600		++	++	+	(T) 20	
Fluphenazine·HCl, enanthate, decanoate —(CH₂)₃—N◯N—(CH₂)₂—OH *Permitil, Prolixin*	—CF₃	2.5-20	1-30	1.25-2.5 (HCl) (25-50, deca-noate or enanthate q. 1-3 wks)	+	+++	+	(T) 0.25,1,2.5,5, 10 (T) sustained release, 1 (C) 5 mg/ml (E) 2.5 mg/5 ml	(V) 2.5 mg/ml in 10 ml (HCl) (S) 25 mg/ml (esters) (V) 25 mg/ml (esters) in 5 ml

Table 2. (contd.)

Nonproprietary Name (Trade Name) Phenothiazines (contd.)	Main Structure	Side-Chain	Dose			Side Effects			Dosage Forms	
			Antipsychotic Daily Dosage	Extreme[b] (mg)	Single IM Dose[a] (mg)	Sedative	Extra-pyramidal	Hypo-tensive	Oral	Injection
			Usual[b] (mg)							
Perphenazine —(CH₂)₃—N[ ]N—(CH₂)₂—OH *Trilafon*		—Cl	8-32	4-64	5-10	++	++	+	(T) 2,4,8,16 (T) sustained release, 8	(A) 5 mg/ml
Trifluoperazine·HCl —(CH₂)₃—N[ ]N—CH₃ *Stelazine*		—CF₃	6-20	2-60	1-2	+	+++	+	(T) 1,2,5,10 (C) 10 mg/ml	(V) 2 mg/ml in 10 ml
Thioxanthenes										
Chlorprothixene $\overset{\|}{C}$H—(CH₂)₂—N(CH₃)₂ *Taractan*		—Cl	50-400	30-600	25-50	+++	++	++	(T) 10,25,50,100 (C) 100 mg/5 ml	(A) 25 mg/2 ml
Thiothixene·HCl $\overset{\|}{C}$H(CH₂)₂—N[ ]N—CH₃ *Navane*		—SO₂N(CH₃)₂	6-30	6-60	2-6	+	+++	+	(C) 1,2,5,10,20[c] (C) 5 mg/ml	(A) 4 mg/2 ml

Table 2. (contd.)

Nonproprietary Name (Trade Name) Other Heterocyclic Compounds	Dose — Antipsychotic Daily Dosage Usual[b] (mg)	Extreme[b] (mg)	Single IM Dose[a] (mg)	Side Effects — Sedative	Extra-pyramidal	Hypo-tensive	Dosage Forms — Oral	Injection
Haloperidol *Haldol*	6-20	2-100	2.5-5	+	+++	+	(T) 0.5,1,2,5,10 (C) 2 mg/ml as the lactate	(A) 5 mg/ml, as the lactate (V) 5 mg/ml, as the lactate, in 10 ml
Loxapine succinate *Daxolin, Loxitane*	60-100	20-250	12.5-25	++	++	+	(C) 5,10,25,50 (C) 25 mg/ml, as the HCl	(A) 50 mg/ml as the HCl (V) 50 mg/ml in 10 ml as the HCl
Molindone·HCl *Lidone, Moban*	50-225	15-400		++	+	0	(T) 5,10,25 (C) 5,10,25 (C) 20 mg/ml	

[a] Except for the enanthate and decanoate forms of fluphenazine, dosage can be given intramuscularly up to every six hours for agitated patients; haloperidol has also been used cautiously intravenously.

[b] Extreme dosage ranges are occasionally exceeded cautiously and only when other appropriate measures have failed. Doses for elderly or infirm patients are typically ½ to ⅓ the usual daily adult oral dose.

[c] Chlorpromazine, U.S.P., is available as the free base in rectal suppositories in 25- and 100-mg sizes; the hydrochloride is also available in nonproprietary preparations. Thiothixene, U.S.P., is available as the free base in 1-, 2-, 5-, and 10-mg capsules. Triflupromazine is available as the free base in oral suspension, *equivalent to* 50 mg of the hydrochloride per 5 ml; thioridazine base is also available as an oral suspension (equivalent to 25 and 100 mg of the HCl per 5 ml).

Dose-Effect Relationships

Despite the clinical availability of antipsychotic drugs for more than three decades, quantitative pharmacological information from human studies is strikingly sparse. For example, a precise dose-response relationship has not been established for any antipsychotic drug in humans. Some useful information can be derived from a reanalysis of published "success rates" in studies comparing the antipsychotic effects of chlorpromazine with a placebo. These results suggested that the chance of success (particularly with patients called schizophrenic) was about 60 percent when less than 300 mg of chlorpromazine was given per day, 80 to 90 percent at doses of 300-500 mg, and virtually 100 percent at doses of 500 to 800 mg or more (Appleton and Davis, 1980). Doses as low as 100 mg/day may be effective in many acutely psychotic or elderly patients. The dose-response relationship of antipsychotic agents in humans is evidently broad. While minimum clinically effective doses can be estimated, maximally effective doses are not known. Standard recommended doses (Table 2) of potent antipsychotic agents, such as fluphenazine and haloperidol, are as effective as doses more than ten times higher, particularly when the comparison extends over two or three months (Klein et al., 1980).

In many early clinical studies of antipsychotic agents, serious problems obfuscated clinical dose-effect relationships. These included the application of broad diagnostic criteria as well as inadequate control of doses and short follow-up periods. In most studies patients were called "schizophrenic," but often mixed populations were evaluated. Recent controlled studies of fixed, moderate doses of neuroleptics suggest that doses effective in acute idiopathic psychoses may be as low as 100-200 mg of chlorpromazine per day or the equivalent. The dose-effect relationship in prolonged treatment aimed at reducing risk of exacerbations of chronic psychotic disorders is even less well studied. Evidence suggests that doses well below the equivalent of 200 mg/day of chlorpromazine may suffice for many chronically psychotic patients (Baldessarini and Davis, 1980). Currently recommended doses (Table 2) are set above estimated minimum effective doses. The maximum recommended doses are based on more limited research data and clinical experience.

An undetermined percentage of patients respond inadequately, even to doses equivalent to more than 1,000 mg of chlorpromazine a day. An occasional unresponsive patient may improve with a higher dose than usual, with injected medication, or after several months of continued treatment. Unique, but as yet ill-documented metabolic characteristics of unresponsive patients might account for their failure to respond to antipsychotic medications. Moreover, many clinicians believe that a major reason for poor response is failure to take medication as prescribed. Compliance can be increased by the use of injected medication or liquid oral preparations of antipsychotic drugs to avoid surreptitious disposal of pills.

Guidelines concerning approximate clinically equivalent doses of commonly prescribed neuroleptic agents are provided in Table 1. When these are used to guide changes between agents, the changes should be made gradually and cautiously. Thus, while 1,000 mg of chlorpromazine and 50 mg of trifluoperazine may be approximately equivalent in antipsychotic efficacy, suddenly switching from high doses of one to the other may result in severe reactions. These include dystonia in changing to a more potent agent or sedation and hypotension with a less potent drug.

Animal studies provide quantitative determinations of dose-response relationships, but these do not meaningfully predict clinical responses. Nevertheless, they do reflect what is also known clinically, namely that the *therapeutic index* (the ratio of a toxic or lethal dose to a dose that produces noticeable behavior effects) for most of the antipsychotic agents is extremely high. Lethal clinical doses cannot be ascertained. It is almost impossible to commit suicide with these agents unless medical assistance is unavailable, secondary complications of severe medical illness arise, other toxins have also been ingested, or there is pre-existing serious medical illness. More than 10 g of chlorpromazine has been ingested acutely by patients who survived.

The recommended agents and doses for use in children less than 16 years of age are more limited than for late adolescent or adult patients. A summary of current recommendations for children is discussed below (and in Table 5).

Absorption, Metabolism, and Excretion

The pharmacokinetics and metabolism of the antipsychotic drugs are being investigated actively. At present, however, few clinically relevant conclusions can be drawn. This situation is due in part to limitations of the laboratory techniques involved, the low plasma levels of most antipsychotic drugs (on the order of ng, or 10^{-6} mg per ml), the complex metabolism of some antipsychotic agents, and the many problems inherent in diagnosis and objective evaluation of clinical change in psychotic patients. Other problems have included the study of patients unlikely to respond clearly or rapidly to medication. Also, doses have often been inadequately controlled or so high as to minimize the range of clinical outcomes.

Nevertheless, a few generalizations can be made. Many antipsychotics have somewhat erratic and unpredictable patterns of absorption among individuals, particularly after oral administration; and blood concentrations of a drug vary widely among individual patients. Neuroleptics are highly lipophilic; highly membrane- or protein-bound; and accumulate in the brain, lung, and other tissues with a high blood supply. Accumulation may be particularly marked after repeated exposure to high doses of the less potent agents. The main routes of metabolism of the antipsychotic drugs are oxidative, mediated largely by hepatic microsomal drug-metabolizing enzymes. Conjugation with glucuronic acid is an important route of metabolism. Water-soluble, or hydrophilic, metabolites of neuroleptic agents are excreted in the urine and, to some extent, in the bile. Most oxidized metabolites of antipsychotic drugs are biologically inactive, but some are not (e.g., mesoridazine, 7-hydroxychlorpromazine, 7-hydroxynorloxapine) and may contribute to the biological activity of the parent substances. Active metabolites that form unpredictably in individual patients also complicate attempts to correlate chemical assays of drug molecules in blood with clinical effects.

In practice, attempts to correlate chemically measured plasma concentrations of neuroleptic agents or their metabolites with clinical response have not been especially successful. They indicate that plasma concentrations vary widely among individual patients. These variations may range from ten- to 100-fold and are not eliminated by controlling the dose, timing, and prior exposure to a drug, suggesting the involvement of genetic or other individual factors. Chemical assays of clinical plasma concentrations of chlorpromazine and of haloperidol, for example, have been reported typically to be on the order of tens of ng/ml, while levels of hundreds of ng/ml may be toxic. To complement chemical assays, a biological assay has been introduced. This method detects a drug and its pharmacologically active metabolites in blood. It depends on competition for binding of a radioactively labeled standard neuroleptic to "receptors" in animal brain tissue and so is known as a radioreceptor assay. Attempts to relate the levels of neuroleptic activity detected by such radioreceptor assays to clinical actions have met some success under controlled experimental conditions. These include fixed moderate doses of a neuroleptic given to acutely ill patients with a favorable short-term prognosis. Nevertheless, in general, assays of blood concentration of neuroleptics by any technique are not yet sufficiently well developed for routine use in guiding clinical practice, and plasma concentrations that best predict optimal clinical responses cannot yet be advised.

The less potent antipsychotic drugs may weakly induce their own hepatic metabolism or conjugation since concentrations of chlorpromazine and other phenothiazines in blood are often lower after several weeks of treatment with the same dosage. Alterations of gastrointestinal motility might be partly responsible for such changes.

Age is an important determinant of the rate of metabolism and excretion of antipsychotic drugs. The fetus, the infant, and the elderly have diminished capacity to metabolize and eliminate these agents and are more sensitive to them; while children eliminate them more rapidly than adults. Accordingly, relatively smaller doses are used for elderly patients.

Detailed comments on pharmacokinetics can be offered for only a few agents that have been well studied, such as chlorpromazine, thioridazine, and haloperidol. The low-potency phenothiazines are favored for such evaluations because they are used in large doses and relatively high concentrations of drug and metabolites are present for chemical assay. However, complex metabolism makes their evaluation more difficult.

The absorption of tablets of chlorpromazine is particularly erratic, and perhaps two thirds may be metabolized on the "first pass" through the gut and liver en route to the systemic circulation. The loss of haloperidol after oral administration is reportedly somewhat less marked and variable than that of chlorpromazine. The relatively strong anticholinergic effects of thioridazine can modify its intestinal absorption. Bioavailability of antipsychotic agents is increased somewhat by using liquid concentrates, but these preparations are relatively expensive and inconvenient to use. Peak concentrations of the phenothiazines and of haloperidol are attained in plasma about two to four hours after an oral dose. Intramuscular injection of neuroleptics avoids much of the first pass metabolism in the gut and liver which occurs after oral administration and provides measurable concentrations in plasma within 15 to 30 minutes. Bioavailability is increased up to ten-fold by injection, but a clinical guideline is to expect about a three- or four-fold increase in potency of injected over orally administered antipsychotic agents. The gastrointestinal absorption of chlorpromazine is modified unpredictably by food and is reported to be decreased by orally administered colloidal antacids. Early reports also suggested that anticholinergic drugs, such as antiparkinsonism agents, may decrease the gastrointestinal absorption of phenothiazines. This impression has not been supported by more recent, well-controlled studies.

Plasma concentrations of antipsychotic agents, as they are commonly assayed, are not equivalent to brain levels for all neuroleptics. Most neuroleptics are highly lipid soluble, pass the blood-brain diffusion barrier easily, and may be retained in brain tissue. Concentrations of some neuroleptics in brain are more than ten times those in blood. Total plasma levels of neuroleptic molecules by chemical assay or of neuroleptic activity by radioreceptor assay correlate closely with levels in brain tissue and with behavioral effects of the drugs in animals under laboratory conditions.

Neuroleptic drugs bind significantly and tightly in tissue membranes or to lipids and to plasma albumin; most are more than 90 percent bound in plasma. It follows that it is virtually impossible (and usually not necessary) to remove these agents by dialysis after an overdose. Technical difficulties have precluded meaningful attempts to evaluate the relationship between unbound or free levels of neuroleptics in plasma with corresponding brain levels in animals or with clinical effects in patients.

Thioridazine and its important active metabolite, mesoridazine, however, are exceptional agents. They are fairly polar or water-soluble molecules. They are much less extensively or firmly bound to plasma proteins than are other neuroleptics. Such properties of thioridazine as well as of the benzamides (e.g., sulpiride) contribute to their lesser ability to pass the blood-brain barrier than other neuroleptics. Evidently, in part for this reason, total plasma levels of thioridazine are typically ten to 100 times higher than those of many other antipsychotic agents.

A correlate of the ability of neuroleptic drugs to enter and accumulate in the CNS is their ability to enter the fetal circulation easily. It is not known whether those agents that enter the CNS with relative difficulty also have more limited access through the maternal blood-placental barrier.

The pharmacokinetics of all antipsychotic drugs follow a multiphasic pattern. The disappearance of neuroleptics from plasma includes a rapid distribution α phase (half-life, $t\frac{1}{2}$, about two hours) and a slower, true elimination β phase ($t\frac{1}{2}$, about 30 hours). Elimination from the plasma may be more rapid than from sites of high lipid content and binding, notably in the central nervous system (CNS). Markedly variable values of plasma half-life have been reported among agents and between individual patients. Since these rates are typically 20 to 40 hours, the biological effects of single doses of a neuroleptic persist for at least 24 hours. The large margin of safety of even relatively high peak tissue levels of neuroleptics, along with their slow elimination, supports the feasibility of taking the entire daily dose at one time. This practice is common once the patient has accommodated to the initial side effects of the drug.

The more prolonged, depot-like characteristics of fatty acid esters of neuroleptics are illustrated by the approximate half-lives of eliminations of preparations of fluphenazine. Whereas the orally administered hydrochloride is half-eliminated in ten to 20 hours, the enanthate requires three to four days and the decanoate, seven to ten days. On injection of the esters, however, sufficient free fluphenazine is commonly liberated to induce neurological side effects.

It is important to realize that the antiparkinsonism agents sometimes given with a neuroleptic are eliminated much more rapidly than the latter and have a low margin of safety. Accordingly, they are prescribed in divided daily doses and they are continued for several days after discontinuing a neuroleptic agent.

The half-life of elimination of neuroleptic molecules from the human brain is unknown. In animal studies, behavioral effects of neuroleptics persist after brain levels are no longer detectable by the most sensitive assays. Such effects suggest a slow dissociation of a small, critical pool of drug, possibly including specific receptor sites. Even slower phases of elimination probably occur, especially after repeated dosing; and neuroleptic molecules can accumulate in human lipoid and connective tissues, including the eye, skin, and probably the brain. Metabolites of some agents have been detected in human urine for as long as several months after the drug has been discontinued. Slow removal of drug may contribute to the typically slow exacerbation of psychosis after stopping drug treatment.

The most important site of metabolic alteration of antipsychotic agents is the liver, in which microsomal oxidation and conjugation mechanisms operate. The phenothiazines and thioxanthenes yield large numbers of metabolic products with various, largely unknown, pharmacologic activities. An example of a neuropharmacologically active metabolite is mesoridazine, which accounts for some of the neuroleptic activity of its precursor, thioridazine, and is itself marketed as the antipsychotic drug Serentil. Haloperidol and other butyrophenones are metabolically split into two inactive products but may also yield active hydroxy-derivatives. Many products of hepatic metabolism of neuroleptic agents are pharmacologically inactive. Most are also more water soluble and so are more easily excreted by the kidneys than are the "parent" substances.

In addition to the lack of lethality of the antipsychotic drugs, another special feature of their pharmacology is that they have a low potential for abuse and dependence. There is no craving for them, and they do not produce euphoria. Rebound excitation has been reported in animals after the abrupt discontinuation of high, prolonged doses of phenothiazines. A possibly analogous reaction can also occur in humans. Thus, abrupt discontinuation of ultra-high doses (hundreds of mg/day) of powerful neuroleptic agents, such as fluphenazine, can lead to severe, acute dyskinesias. Milder acute dyskinesias are sometimes also encountered after rapid discontinuation of more ordinary doses. Rapid discontinuation of moderate doses of neuroleptic agents following their prolonged use sometimes leads to symptoms of an apparent withdrawal syndrome, such as malaise and gastrointestinal dysfunction. Accordingly, withdrawal is ordinarily slowly graded by lowering the dose not more than ten percent a day, accompanied by even slower removal of more rapidly cleared antiparkinsonism agents.

Routine or early tolerance to the main effects of the antipsychotic drugs is not evident, whereas tolerance is found with many side effects of neuroleptics, including sedation, hypotension, anticholinergic effects, acute dystonic reactions, and possibly parkinsonism. Some tolerance to the antipsychotic effects appears to be possible, most likely after more than two years of continuous treatment. One recent study noted such adaptation in fewer than three percent of patients maintained on depot injections of an ester of fluphenazine.

Mechanisms of Action

The mechanisms of action of the antipsychotic drugs are only partially known. Moreover, the hope that such knowledge would provide important clues to the rational development of safer or more effective antipsychotic agents, let alone the pathophysiology of idiopathic psychotic illnesses, has not been realized. However, observations of the effects of most antipsychotic agents strongly suggest pathophysiologic mechanisms that underlie their neurological side effects.

While the antipsychotic drugs represent a wide variety of chemical structures, their pharmacology and clinical activities are remarkably similar. The antipsychotic agents in current use in this country all regularly produce a variety of disorders of the control of posture, muscle tone, and movement, presumably due to dysfunction of the extrapyramidal nervous system. A crucial question is whether the almost routinely encountered neurologic ("neuroleptic") effects of the antipsychotic drugs are essential to their actions. The fact that several apparently effective antipsychotic drugs only rarely induce acute neurologic reactions (dystonias, parkinsonism, and restlessness) challenges the inevitability of an association of neurologic and antipsychotic effects and encourages hope that more selective antipsychotic agents, with lesser neurologic side effects, can be developed.

As the pharmacologic basis of the selectivity of the so-called "atypical" antipsychotic agents remains obscure, the activity of an agent such as clozapine is not adequately predicted by current preclinical laboratory techniques. Some atypical antipsychotic agents, such as clozapine and thioridazine, are strongly anticholinergic, but molindone and sulpiride are not. Most of the atypical agents have weak activity in typical laboratory tests of antidopamine actions. They also fail to induce supersensitivity to dopamine agonists (such as apomorphine) in laboratory animals given clinically relevant doses—a putative predictive test of risk of tardive dyskinesia. Despite this partial understanding, there is no effective means of predicting the activity of atypical antipsychotic agents short of empirical clinical trials. The methods of screening new substances for potential antipsychotic activity which have led to most of the existing typical antipsychotic agents have essentially involved seeking neurologic reactions in laboratory animals because of the lack of satisfactory animal tests for psychosis. This impasse has contributed to repeated "rediscovery" over the past 30 years of agents with similar actions and limitations.

Various mechanisms have been proposed to explain the actions of the antipsychotic drugs. They differ from most other CNS depressants in several ways. Charpentier and Laborit first noted chlorpromazine's ability to reduce emotional reactivity without inducing somnolence or anesthesia as part of their description of the "neuroleptic syndrome" or "artificial hibernation." In general, neuroleptic agents have limited ability to induce sedative or hypnotic effects common to sedatives and other CNS depressants. Coma or respiratory depression is uncommon even after large overdoses. Dependence or addiction is unknown, and tolerance to their main (antipsychotic) clinical effects is not prominent. In further contrast to sedatives, neuroleptics are more capable of diminishing conditioned behavioral responses than of depressing unconditional responses. They selectively dampen neurophysiologic effects of peripheral stimuli in the forebrain while inhibiting to a much lesser extent the effects of direct stimulation of the brain stem. This difference may lie in actions of the antipsychotic agents at the level of the brain stem reticular activating system, which has a crucial regulatory action on forebrain activity and behavioral arousal. Also, antipsychotic drugs have striking inhibitory effects on autonomic and motoric expressions of arousal and strong affect in animals, presumably mediated by actions in the limbic forebrain and hypothalamus. The cellular and biochemical events underlying these behavioral and physiologic actions, however, have remained obscure until recently.

In the early 1960's European pharmacologists proposed that the neurologic, and possibly also the antipsychotic, effects of neuroleptic drugs may reflect their ability to interfere with synaptic transmission mediated by dopamine. This suggestion arose largely from the observation that among the biochemical properties of neuroleptic drugs, levels of the metabolites of dopamine consistently and selectively increased, drawing attention to the possibility of unique drug interactions with this monoamine neurotransmitter. Dopamine is prominent in the hypothalamus and in the nigroneostriatal tract, which links the midbrain and basal ganglia. In addition, there are dopamine-containing projections from midbrain nuclei to forebrain regions associated with the limbic system as well as temporal and medial prefrontal cerebral cortical areas closely interlinked with the limbic system. A somewhat simplistic, but attractive, concept has been that many extrapyramidal neurologic effects of the antipsychotic drugs may be mediated by antidopamine effects in the basal ganglia and that some of their antipsychotic effects may be mediated by the antagonism of dopaminergic neurotransmission in the limbic system, hypothalamus, and cortex.

In recent years, much information has accumulated to support the theory that the antagonism of dopamine-mediated synaptic neurotransmission is an important action of these drugs. Thus, antipsychotic agents, but not their nonantipsychotic congeners, increase the rate of production of dopamine metabolites in animal and human brain, as well as increasing both the rate of conversion of precursor amino acids to dopamine and its metabolites and the firing rate of dopamine-containing neurons in the CNS of animals. These effects have been interpreted as compensatory responses aimed at maintaining homeostasis in the face of an interruption of synaptic transmission at dopamine terminals in the forebrain.

Evidence that a crucial primary event may be the blockade of postsynaptic dopamine receptor sites includes the ability of small doses of antipsychotic agents to block behavioral or neuroendocrine effects of dopamine agonists. Examples are stereotyped behaviors in rodents induced by the dopamine agonist apomorphine, the locomotor excitement induced by the injection of dopamine into limbic sites, or the prolactin-decreasing response of dopamine agonists believed to be mediated by pituitary dopamine receptors. Such "tests" have been used as screening methods to detect even more agents of the kinds already available.

More direct evidence of a receptor blockade has been provided by the antagonism of dopamine-sensitive adenylate cyclase activity in forebrain tissue and the interference with electrophysiological responses to dopamine locally applied to receptive forebrain cells in animal brains. A more recent development is the application of experimental radioligand binding assays using homogenates of caudate nucleus or other forebrain tissues and low (nanomolar) concentrations of intensely radioactive, tritium-labeled butyrophenones or other neuroleptic drugs. Such binding is proposed to represent an interaction with dopamine "receptor" sites. Correlations between the clinical potency of most types of antipsychotic drugs and their ability to interfere with the binding of a butyrophenone are impressive. Clinically inactive analogs or isomers of the antipsychotic drugs compete only weakly for the binding sites. Neuroleptics generally interact with dopamine *agonist* receptor sites in poor correspondence with clinical potency, in contrast to binding sites defined by antagonists such as labeled butyrophenones.

These findings, taken together, strongly support the theory that antipsychotic agents interfere with the actions of dopamine as a synaptic neurotransmitter in the brain. Yet, they do not prove that antidopamine effects are either necessary or sufficient for antipsychotic efficacy. They strongly suggest that some of the extrapyramidal neurologic effects and neuroendocrine actions (prolactin elevation) of this class of agents may be produced by antagonism of dopamine receptors in the basal ganglia and pituitary, respectively. This theory, as it regards extrapyramidal effects, is based largely on analogy to Parkinson's disease with its demonstrated loss of dopamine in the caudate nucleus and putamen, and beneficial responses to L-dopa, the immediate precursor of dopamine. While it is plausible to assume that the antidopamine actions of neuroleptics play a role in mediating some of their neurological and neuroendocrine effects, there is no fully satisfactory way to account for the antipsychotic effects of these agents.

It is reasonable to suppose that limbic and cortical mechanisms are involved in the manifestations of psychosis and their suppression by neuroleptic drugs. Yet, progress beyond such a generalization has been difficult. Also, the selective effects of the atypical antipsychotic agents cannot be explained adequately by antidopamine actions. They are, generally, weak dopamine antagonists and do not exert impressive regionally selective actions, for example at limbic or cerebral cortical dopamine sites as opposed to the basal ganglia of the extrapyramidal system or the anterior pituitary. Thus, no coherent pharmacologic theory is available to guide future development of selective antipsychotic drugs free of neurologic or neuroendocrine side effects.

The dopamine receptor-antagonism theory may account for some neurological side effects of neuroleptic agents, such as signs of parkinsonism. It probably also contributes to their useful antidyskinetic actions, as in Huntington's disease and Gilles de la Tourette's syndrome. It almost certainly explains why most antipsychotic agents elevate levels of prolactin, whose release is tonically inhibited by actions of dopamine at receptors of the anterior pituitary. Antidopamine effects in the brain stem "chemoreactive trigger zone" or emesis center may also contribute to the antinausea and antiemetic actions of most typical neuroleptics. The dopamine theory does not, however, account for all effects of these drugs. Generally the less potent neuroleptics are less selective in blocking dopamine receptors and interact with many other systems as well. Some side effects, including sedation, hypotension, sexual dysfunction, and other autonomic effects which are commonly associated with the less potent compounds may reflect their ability to block adrenergic (especially α) and histamine receptors. Many apparent anti-parasympathetic actions of the antipsychotic drugs on cardiac, ophthalmic, gastrointestinal, bladder, and genital tissues have been ascribed to anticholinergic effects at muscarinic receptors. Antimuscarinic actions are more common with the less potent agents and are especially characteristic of clozapine and thioridazine. Finally, recent evidence suggests that some neuroleptic agents interact with sites thought to mediate actions of serotonin, particularly in forebrain regions other than the extrapyramidal motor system. Interaction with such so-called serotonin "type 2" receptors is characteristic of butyrophenones, but the physiological significance of this interaction is unknown.

In summary, effects of the antipsychotic drugs at the level of the limbic system, cerebral cortex, and reticular formation appear to correlate well with their observed behavioral and clinical effects, while other effects on the hypothalamus, pituitary, and basal ganglia seem to account for many of the autonomic, neuroendocrine, and neurologic side effects of these agents. Many of these local actions are probably mediated by the effects of these drugs at the surface of neuronal membranes—including sites of action of dopamine as a neurotransmitter in the CNS, but the precise local chemical changes and their neurophysiological consequences remain obscure. The basis of the apparently selective antipsychotic effects of the atypical agents such as clozapine is not known.

CLINICAL USE

Drug Selection

It can be difficult to choose among the large variety of antipsychotic compounds now available. The most important generalization that simplifies the problem is that most antipsychotic drugs are remarkably similar in their main actions and overall antipsychotic efficacy. A recent survey of thousands of patients in the Veterans Administration (VA) medical system indicates that the most commonly prescribed antipsychotics were chlorpromazine, thioridazine, haloperidol, fluphenazine, trifluoperazine, thiothixene, and perphenazine.

A practical consideration, especially regarding prolonged use of neuroleptic agents, is their cost. In a 1983 survey of costs of a typical month's supply of antipsychotic drugs (equivalent to 400 mg/day of chlorpromazine), prices ranged from about $10 to $30 a month. Since prices may vary in different regions, one should check with local suppliers for the best prices. It is worth noting that chlorpromazine and thioridazine have already outlived their patent protection and that chlorpromazine is available as a generic agent; other older drugs will soon follow, presumably with more competitive pricing. Finally, there are significant savings (by more than fivefold) by the use of unit doses of larger size (more mg per tablet).

Available data from controlled clinical trials of many drugs do not support rational selection of a class of agents, much less a particular drug, for a specific type of illness. Nonetheless, antipsychotic drugs may not all be equally effective for an individual patient. It is reasonable to try several dissimilar agents serially in adequate and increasing doses, even by injection, and to persist for several months, so that a patient who at first responds poorly may have the benefit of any doubt. Nevertheless, given adequate doses and duration of treatment, the chances of added success by a change in agent are probably small. The rate of "success" of treatment with an antipsychotic drug in terms of clinical improvement of psychosis or ability to leave a hospital has averaged 75 percent or more. For example, in a large National Institute of Mental Health-Veterans Administration (NIMH-VA) cooperative study, 75 percent of patients diagnosed as schizophrenic and given a phenothiazine improved within six weeks and only five percent became clinically worse; while of those given a placebo, only 25 percent improved and 50 percent were unchanged or worse.

The *potency* (effect per mg) of antipsychotic agents varies by more than 100-fold (Tables 1 and 2), but the overall clinical *efficacy* of most agents is remarkably similar, provided that adequate doses are used. This conclusion arises from controlled comparisons of agents given to many cases called "schizophrenia" prior to the early 1970's. Based on current diagnostic standards, many of these studies may have included several types of psychotic patients, although most patients were evidently severely and chronically ill. Studies done in the 1960's and early 1970's indicated that daily doses of an antipsychotic drug equivalent to 300 to 800 mg of chlorpromazine were needed for consistent benefit in such populations. Data based on large numbers of systematic comparisons of agents in groups of patients diagnosed by current methods are not available. Such comparisons are notably lacking among patients with acute or intermittent psychoses. A few recent studies suggest that some acutely psychotic or manic patients may do well with daily doses as low as the equivalent of 100 to 300 mg of chlorpromazine, and that many chronic schizophrenics can be maintained adequately on even lower doses, possibly as low as 50 to 100 mg a day.

There are a few exceptions to the rule that most neuroleptics are equally effective. For example, in about 60 percent of controlled studies, promazine (Sparine) and mepazine (Pacatal) were no better than a placebo, and reserpine failed to produce results better than placebo in about a third of its trials. Furthermore, prochlorperazine (Compazine) failed in about 22 percent of comparisons with a placebo and is associated with a high risk of acute dystonic reactions. It is not recommended for routine use as an antipsychotic agent and currently is more commonly used for nausea and vomiting. Loxapine, in a relatively small number of trials, has not been consistently as effective as other antipsychotic drugs. Yet, its chemical dissimilarity to the phenothiazines may provide a useful alternative, for example in cases of dangerous toxic reactions. The same advantage is offered by haloperidol, molindone, and possibly reserpine. To date, molindone has less often been associated with late dyskinesias than most other neuroleptics, although its efficacy is not as securely established as that of many older and more extensively evaluated agents. Nearly every other antipsychotic agent currently in common use produced better results than a placebo in at least 80 to 90 percent of comparisons (Appleton and Davis, 1980).

It may seem remarkable that chlorpromazine failed to be more effective than placebo in 17 percent of 66 controlled studies. These results cannot be taken as important evidence against the efficacy of chlorpromazine since they include very early studies of the 1950's using the drug in doses that were probably inadequate; moreover, in more than 100 studies that have made direct comparisons of antipsychotic agents in schizophrenia, no agent has been found to be more effective than chlorpromazine.

Sedatives such as phenobarbital, as well as normal or even high doses of diazepam (Valium), have nearly always failed to produce better results than an inactive placebo in the treatment of chronically psychotic patients. Nevertheless, sedative agents may have a specialized role in the management of acutely disturbed patients. For example, the early management of highly agitated, assaultive, or manic patients can be enhanced by administration of a benzodiazepine (e.g., diazepam in 5-10 mg doses or lorazepam in 1-2 mg doses) in frequently repeated (half-hourly to hourly) doses until sedation develops. Barbiturates and other sedatives are rarely used in this way now, in part due to their propensity to interact with the metabolism of other agents, including neuroleptics, and so complicate their use. Droperidol, a potent, short-acting, sedating butyrophenone neuroleptic, can also be used to sedate acutely agitated psychotic patients. A direct comparison of the short-term efficacy of rapidly repeated intravenous haloperidol or diazepam (2.5 to 10 mg every 30-60 minutes) showed similar benefits with both agents given to acutely psychotic patients after several hours or the next day. Selectivity of either type of agent in producing antipsychotic versus sedative effects in such short-term, high-dose treatment has not been shown. This apparent short-term similarity of sedative and antipsychotic agents does not, however, gainsay the conclusion that the former have not been proven effective in the treatment of chronic psychoses.

Sedative and antianxiety agents, particularly the benzodiazepines, are currently considered somewhat safer than neuroleptics in the management of psychotic and excited states associated with certain cerebral toxins, including phencyclidine (PCP), lysergic acid diethylamide (LSD), and strongly anticholinergic agents. Benzodiazepines are also agents of choice in the management of withdrawal from alcohol. Neuroleptic agents, particularly low potency phenothiazines, can increase the risk of grand mal seizures and may induce unpredictable changes in blood pressure and temperature in patients with delirium tremens. Neuroleptics may, however, have a place in the management of paranoid illnesses or hallucinosis occasionally encountered in alcoholics following detoxification.

It is also questionable practice to use antipsychotic agents for the routine treatment of anxiety. Neuroleptics are not particularly effective antianxiety agents, and their extrapyramidal side effects may even worsen anxiety as well as create neurological risks that can usually be avoided by alternative forms of treatment. The selectivity of action of the neuroleptic agents in psychosis refutes the idea that they are simply stronger ("major") "tranquilizers" than older sedatives. Neuroleptics are occasionally considered for anxious patients previously dependent on alcohol, sedatives, or anxiolytic agents.

Clinical folklore based on anecdotal experiences and perhaps on a misinterpretation of the significance of certain side effects has led to a widespread but probably erroneous impression that certain high-potency agents (particularly the piperazine phenothiazines and. the butyrophenones) are somehow more "incisive" in their ability to interrupt florid psychotic symptoms, or that the same agents are uniquely beneficial for more withdrawn and apathetic schizophrenics because of putative "activating" effects. Few firm data derived from controlled clinical trials support these concepts. Although there is no significant basis for these views, there is also no reason *not* to select the more potent antipsychotic agents either for floridly psychotic or withdrawn patients.

Attempts to "tailor" treatment to the individual patient's requirements are reasonable. One approach is to select a specific agent on the basis of side effects most likely to be encountered. For example, hypotensive or potential, mild cardiac depressant effects of some low-potency agents (such as the piperidine phenothiazines and aliphatic phenothiazines or thioxanthenes) might wisely be avoided in elderly, infirm, or cardiac patients. On the other hand, the early sedative effects of such low-potency agents may be desirable for a severely agitated, assaultive, manic, or sleepless patient. Such sedative effects would be undesirable in a school-aged child or an adult engaged in potentially hazardous work. High-potency agents may be especially poorly tolerated by young adult, male paranoid patients who may resent and misinterpret their neurological side effects. Such patients may also be disturbed by altered libido or orgasmic and ejaculatory function sometimes associated with low-potency agents. The risk of an acute dystonic reaction in an outpatient whose trust is still to be gained may also encourage caution in the use of a high-potency neuroleptic. In all cases early in treatment, the avoidance of long-acting depot preparations or of excessive doses of any neuroleptic, as well as the routine use of single daily doses, are sound practices. The usefulness of blood level assays to assure optimal doses of an antipsychotic agent or to monitor compliance with prolonged treatment has not been established.

In some instances, it may seem reasonable to consider combinations of agents during antipsychotic drug treatment, but there is rarely a rational basis for the use of more than one neuroleptic at a time. The short-term addition of a sedative agent to manage a dangerously acutely agitated patient has already been mentioned. On the other hand, the routine addition of a night-time sedative-hypnotic agent for sleep is almost always unnecessary. Sustained use of sedatives or hypnotics, especially of the barbiturate or other non-benzodiazepine classes, can complicate the determination of dosage requirements for an antipsychotic agent by inducing its increased hepatic metabolism and inactivation. The provision of an extra amount of a neuroleptic of any type at bedtime is often an adequate treatment of insomnia in psychosis. Sometimes it may seem desirable to counteract the sedative effects of a neuroleptic or to minimize the apathy of many schizophrenic patients by adding a stimulant or antidepressant. This tactic is rarely helpful, adds unnecessary complexity to treatment, and may increase psychotic agitation or the risk of cerebral intoxication.

Short-Term Use of Antipsychotic Agents

The antipsychotic drugs reduce and can even interrupt specific acute features of psychotic illnesses. These symptoms include delusions and hallucinations, often with a gradual disappearance of thought disorder. They are not specifically "anti-schizophrenic" agents, as the effects of antipsychotic drugs are not limited to schizophrenia and indeed have their least striking benefits in chronically psychotic patients. Rather, they exert beneficial actions in a number of severe psychiatric illnesses including schizophrenia, mania, agitated or psychotic reactions to stimulants, and even some aspects of organic dementia and acute brain syndromes. This class of agents is generally palliative rather than curative, and their antipsy-

Table 3. Indications for Short-Term Use of Neuroleptics

- Acute psychotic episodes
- Exacerbation of schizophrenia
- Acute reduction of manic excitement when the onset of lithium's action is slow
- Adjunctive therapy for depressions with prominent psychotic symptoms or when an antidepressant or ECT alone is not successful
- For agitation in delirium, dementia, or severe mental retardation while seeking to identify and treat the primary basis of the problem
- In certain chronic degenerative or idiopathic neuropsychiatric disorders with dyskinesias, such as Huntington's disease and Gilles de la Tourette's syndrome; or for ballism
- Childhood psychoses
- Miscellaneous medical indications, notably nausea and vomiting, or intractable hiccoughs

chotic effects are most readily observed in acute and florid psychotic excitement with considerable anxiety and agitation. Currently accepted short-term indications for antipsychotic agents are summarized in Table 3.

Target symptoms that consistently benefit from antipsychotic drugs include combativeness, hyperactivity, hostility, negativism, hallucinations, acute delusions, insomnia, poor self-care, anorexia, and sometimes seclusiveness. Improvement in insight, judgment, memory, and orientation are also likely in cases of acute psychosis or phases of acute exacerbation in recurrent psychoses, such as bipolar illness. In contrast, responses of the latter features of (chronic) schizophrenia and dementias are more variable and often unsatisfactory.

In addition to acuteness and excitation, many other factors also suggest that a patient will have a favorable response to antipsychotic drugs and a good prognosis. They include lack of insidious, prolonged onset or chronicity; history of a relatively healthy premorbid adjustment and of social, educational, and occupational accomplishment; current psychotic episode being the first; remissions between episodes; and previous favorable responses to similar medications or other medical treatments.

In an effort to maximize clinical benefit in the minimum time and to limit the total dose of antipsychotic agents, several uncontrolled trials and a few partially controlled trials of unusually high or rapidly increasing doses of antipsychotic agents have been made early in acute psychoses or acute exacerbations of schizophrenia. Due to the excessive sedation and hypotension associated with high parenteral doses of low-potency neuroleptics such as chlorpromazine, these trials have usually used a butyrophenone or the more potent piperazine phenothiazines or thioxanthenes. Such approaches can reduce some psychotic symptoms early, sometimes within a few hours.

However, the hope that aggressive early intervention might shorten or even prevent hospitalization has not been fulfilled, and outcome at one week or after several weeks did not differ when very intensive and more standard neuroleptic regimens were compared. A few studies failed to show consistent differences between high, rapid dosing versus more ordinary treatment, even within the first day. Whether the apparent benefits reported are due to the rapid induction of antipsychotic effects or sedation is not clear. At least one comparison of rapidly repeated intravenous injections of diazepam or haloperidol failed to find a significant difference in efficacy within the first day, suggesting that sedative or other nonspecific central depressant effects may have contributed to the outcome. Indeed, a clinical distinction between "sedation" and antipsychotic effect is often difficult in acutely disturbed and agitated patients, and the current impression that "real" antipsychotic effects (on disturbed, irrational thinking; delusions; hallucinations; and the like) may require several weeks to be manifest is based on experience with less acutely disturbed chronic schizophrenic patients for the most part. One final note concerning the use of "rapid neuroleptization" regimens is that they require close medical and nursing supervision as there are risks of inducing excessive sedation, occasionally with hypotension or compromised respiration. Rare fatalities have occurred.

There has also been a tendency to increase dosages of antipsychotic medications for more prolonged use in the hope that a greater percentage of favorable responses would be obtained. Controlled studies indicate that use of hundreds of milligrams of potent antipsychotic agents such as fluphenazine, trifluoperazine, or haloperidol probably does not increase the overall rate of favorable responses. Although a few cases may respond somewhat better, the overall effects of doses over ten times greater than those usually recommended are similar to ordinary doses at the end of several weeks, particularly with schizophrenic patients. The success of antipsychotic drug treatment may have raised expectations of rapid and dramatic responses in every case, even though this prospect is not realistic. Many psychotic patients, especially schizophrenics, respond gradually over many weeks. Early use of extraordinarily high doses is almost always unnecessary and increases the risk of toxicity as well as the expense of treatment.

Early uncontrolled studies also suggested that acute neurological side effects of high doses of antipsychotic drugs were no greater than were encountered with ordinary doses, and perhaps even less than usual (the "side effect breakthrough" hypothesis). However, the higher doses are not innocuous. There is an increased incidence of acute dystonic reactions with higher doses as well as other undesirable effects on the CNS. These include impressive akinetic and sedative effects that contribute to an apparent worsening of mental status in some cases. There may also be an increased risk of hepatic and autonomic toxicity. The consequences of *prolonged* exposure to high doses of these drugs are not known, but there is a suspicion that increases of the total dose and length of exposure may increase the risk of late neurological toxic effects. Thus, caution in the use of unusually high doses of antipsychotic agents is appropriate.

To summarize, unusually high doses of antipsychotic medication can be tried temporarily when responses to vigorous treatment with more ordinary daily doses, say up to 1,200 mg of chlorpromazine or 30 mg of fluphenazine or haloperidol or their equivalent, are unsatisfactory after several weeks. If higher doses do not bring about appreciable benefit within two or three months, they should be reduced or abandoned. Prolonged use of extreme doses is not established as safe and should be avoided unless a clearly demonstrable effect in an individual patient can be obtained in no other way. The unique value of very rapid increases to high doses within a matter of hours in the first few days of an acute psychotic illness has not been established.

In the early exposure of a psychotic patient to a neuroleptic agent, it is best to rely on *divided* doses for safety and to assure sustained availability of the drug throughout the day. Gradually, many patients can tolerate most or all of a day's medication in a single dose. The simplicity of this practice is especially attractive for treatment that extends for more than a few weeks. Typically, most of the day's dose is given at bedtime to minimize the risk of sedative and extrapyramidal side effects during the waking hours. Nevertheless, a reduction in the amount of drug required may be possible by dosing only in the morning or by relying on a two or three times per day schedule with doses that minimize side effects.

Sometimes, following initial improvement early in the use of an antipsychotic agent, the mental status of a patient may worsen. While the adequacy of dosage and of compliance should be reviewed, other explanations should also be considered. These may include worsening of the primary disorder under treatment or misinterpretation of worsening extrapyramidal or other CNS side effects. These may include akathisia, the neuroleptic "malignant syndrome," cerebral intoxication, or delirium. The latter neurotoxic reactions are especially likely if large doses of a neuroleptic or multiple centrally active medications are used.

In conclusion, evidence is abundant that currently available antipsychotic drugs are effective in treating relatively acute cases of psychosis, regardless of the cause or specific diagnostic type, at least in reducing symptom severity, facilitating clinical management, and supporting early rehabilitation (see Table 3). Controlled short-term studies using more than 300 mg per day of chlorpromazine or the equivalent of other drugs have consistently shown efficacy—for the most part in patients diagnosed as schizophrenic. Recent studies suggest that even lower doses may be adequate for many acutely psychotic patients. These results have led to the impression

Figure 3. Risk of Exacerbation in Schizophrenia vs. Treatment with Neuroleptic or Placebo

The 28 studies evaluated included controlled prospective assignment to a neuroleptic (usually a phenothiazine) (●) or a placebo (○) and clinical follow-up (typically for three to six months). Exacerbation included gross psychotic decompensation or rehospitalization. The mean differ-ence is highly significant. Based on data analyzed in Davis: Am. J. Psychiatry 132: 1237, 1975; and Baldessarini and Davis: Psychiatry Res. 3: 115, 1980.

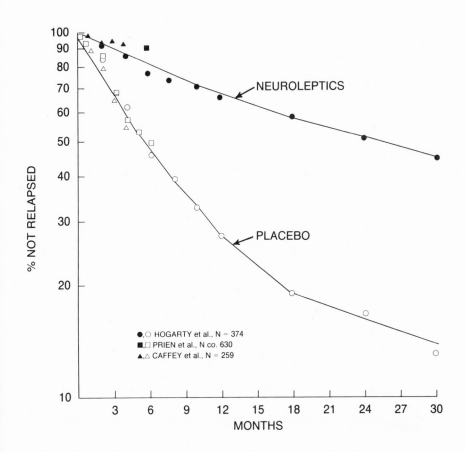

Figure 4. Clinical Maintenance of Schizophrenics Treated with a Neuroleptic or Placebo vs. Time

Data are from Caffey et al.: J. Chronic Dis. 17: 347, 1964; Prien et al.: Brit. J. Psychiatry 115: 679, 1969; and Hogarty et al.: Arch. Gen. Psychiatry 31: 604, 1974, and indicate rates of non-exacerbation ("survival") during follow-up after improvement of patients diagnosed schizophrenic and assigned to continued neuroleptic (phenothiazine) treatment or a placebo. The rate of "release" (worsening) is remarkably similar in all studies for the placebo groups over at least six months (about five to ten percent per month).

that it would be irresponsible not to treat acute psychosis or relatively acute exacerbations of schizophrenia with adequate doses of antipsychotic medication. The next question is how long to pursue the treatment.

Long-term Treatment

There is good evidence that sustained use of an antipsychotic agent prevents or delays exacerbations of psychotic illness in patients diagnosed as schizophrenic (Davis, 1975). (The term "exacerbation" is consistent with the current concept of schizophrenia as a chronic illness with sustained disability, with the possibility of acute worsening, but not a pattern of relapses and full remissions as may occur in manic-depressive, schizophreniform, or atypical psychotic conditions.) Most of this evidence has been obtained in controlled prospective studies in which patients who benefited from neuroleptic treatment in the short term were then treated with active medication or a placebo. Thus, patients who responded poorly to initial treatment would not even be candidates for such a study. The representation of such treatment-unresponsive patients among a general population of psychotic patients is not known, but an estimate would be perhaps 20 to 30 percent or more if only chronically psychotic schizophrenic or demented patients are considered. The available data indicate predictable risks of relapse or exacerbation following recovery from an acute psychotic illness or an acute phase of a chronic illness, especially after abrupt discontinuation of medication on discharge from the hospital. Neuroleptic agents can reduce this risk substantially, but many questions remain.

In nearly 30 studies, patients diagnosed as "schizophrenic" were followed for various periods, typically for three to six months, after initial improvement and aftercare with either active neuroleptic medication or an inactive placebo, presumably by random assignment. The overall results of an analysis of most of these studies (Figure 3) indicate a mean rate of clinical exacerbation (obvious worsening of psychosis or rehospitalization) of only 16.4 percent on active medication versus 58 percent on placebo. This difference, indicating a 42 percent sparing of exacerbation due to active medication, is highly significant statistically ($p < 10^{-100}$). Nevertheless, there has been striking variability in outcome across studies. Among cohorts of patients assigned to placebo (Figure 3), the rate of exacerbation ranged from 100 percent to less than 20 percent. Some of this variability among studies may reflect varying definitions of relapse as well as differences in the duration of follow-up or the average dose of medication. An additional important source of variance almost certainly has been the broad application of the term "schizophrenia" when most of these studies were carried out (mainly in the 1960's and early 1970's). It is probable that many cases would not meet current research criteria for schizophrenia or the standards of the American Psychiatric Association's *Diagnostic and Statistical Manual of Mental Disorders*, Third Edition *(DSM-III)*. Cases of acute psychosis, mania, psychotic depression, severe "neuroses," or character disorders as well as dementia, retardation, or pervasive developmental disorder might well have been included. Long-term outcome studies with different treatments among separate disorders formerly included among "schizophrenias" remain to be made. Such long-term trials based on currently accepted diagnoses might clarify the indications for prolonged, uninterrupted neuroleptic therapy. Also, long-term studies of agents other than phenothiazines (mainly chlorpromazine, thioridazine, or fluphenazine) are few.

At the present time, several conclusions are supported by adequate research or clinical experience. Risk of exacerbation is clearly high among schizophrenics who have recently improved in response to short-term treatment with a neuroleptic drug. Those maintained on a placebo, on the average, underwent exacerbation ("relapse") at the rate of about five percent to ten percent per month over the first six to 12 months of follow-up; about 50 percent relapsed within six months. This risk was reduced by a factor of two or three by continued medication (Figure 4). Little information is available about the risk of relapse after more than a year of follow-up in controlled studies. The available results are almost certainly contaminated by the statistical problem of bias in "drop-out" rates with increasing time as well as by inclusion of patients with differing degrees of illness.

Clinical experience indicates that the long-term benefits of indefinitely prolonged antipsychotic therapy become increasingly difficult to demonstrate in truly chronic "poor-prognosis" schizophrenia, especially as the duration of illness and of treatment increases. Long-term use of an antipsychotic agent thus requires repeated attention to an objective justification in each case. Such justification is required in view of the risks involved, particularly the potentially irreversible neurological sequelae, including tardive dyskinesia and subtle impairment of some higher cortical functions and psychomotor skills. These issues are matters of concern, not only among psychiatrists and other medical professionals, but also to the general public. Mutual agreements are required between clinician and patient or family based on judgments that weigh the possible benefits and risks of neuroleptic treatment continued longer than six months. There is wide agreement that patients with sustained psychotic symptoms and functional impairment are candidates for indefinitely prolonged treatment if re-evaluation indicates that the signs and symptoms are not only still present but also responsive to medication to a degree that justifies the risk of late toxic effects of the neuroleptics (APA, 1980).

At present, there is no scientific support for sustained use of neuroleptics in intermittent psychotic conditions such as bipolar (manic-depressive) illness; whereas, the long-term benefits of lithium salts in bipolar illness are indisputable, and the safety and efficacy of sustained antidepressant treatment for rapidly recurring, severe, unipolar major depressions are gaining

Table 4. Possible Indications for Continuous Long-Term Use of Neuroleptics
(for more than six months)

Primary indications
  Schizophrenia
  Paranoia[a,b]
  Childhood psychoses[a,b]
  Some degenerative or idiopathic neuropsychiatric disorders (notably, Hunting-
    ton's disease and Gilles de la Tourette's syndrome)[b]

Secondary indications
  Extremely unstable bipolar (manic-depressive) or other episodic psychoses (rare)[b]
  Otherwise unmanageable behavior symptoms in dementia, amentia, or other
    brain syndromes[a,b]

Questionable indications
  Chronic characterological disorders with neurotic or "borderline" characteris-
    tics[a,b]
  Recurrent major affective disorders[a,b]

[a] Efficacy has not been adequately demonstrated in controlled studies.
[b] Long-term neurological safety is not established.

It is important to clarify that there may be times when a neuroleptic drug is used in the short-
term management of exacerbations and crises of chronic or recurrent conditions such as those
outlined above. Moreover, there may be justification for even more prolonged uses based on
clinical judgment in individual cases and objective demonstration of important benefits. It is
also important to clarify that clinical research has not yet provided compelling support for long-
term uses in cases other than chronic schizophrenia, nor has it provided evidence that such
uses are contraindicated. Clinicians are left to rely on their evaluations of individual patients
and on their clinical experience as further research data are gathered and assessed. Thus, the
recommendations provided above can only be viewed as tentative and are based on an attempt
to balance the available research literature and clinical experience.

growing support. A summary of possible indications for prolonged (more
than six months) use of an antipsychotic medication is provided in Table 4.

Attempts to specify dosage requirements in prolonged maintenance
treatment of chronically psychotic patients are difficult, as most of the
available studies have been inadequate and poorly controlled. In a recent
analysis of nearly 30 studies that gave sufficient data to permit computations of mean daily antipsychotic drug doses in terms of the approximately
equivalent amount of chlorpromazine, doses ranged from 125 to 2,000 mg
daily (Baldessarini and Davis, 1980). The rate of presumed drug effect
(difference between the rate of exacerbation on placebo minus that of the
drug-treated cohort) ranged from about ten percent to 75 percent. The
correlation between these two measures was almost nil. One possible
explanation for this apparent lack of dose-effect relationship is that most of
the studies only partially controlled the dose of medication and allowed
some degree of dosage adjustment to meet clinical indications, thus obscur-
ing any relationship. Another interpretation is that even the lower range of

doses (daily equivalent of 100 to 300 mg of chlorpromazine) may exceed the requirements for many patients. A recent prospective study has been evaluating schizophrenics maintained on controlled doses of depot fluphenazine decanoate. Preliminary results suggest that doses below the daily equivalent of about 100 mg of chlorpromazine may be adequate for many patients. Further controlled prospective studies of other antipsychotic agents for more than a few months are required, with a particular emphasis on evaluating doses equivalent to the range of 25 to 250 mg/day of chlorpromazine.

In conclusion, guidelines for neuroleptic dosage for long-term use are hard to establish from research studies. Many patients are maintained with doses that are less than half of those used for management of acute psychosis. The selection of a low but effective dose for maintenance treatment is best worked out empirically and is a matter of clinical judgment. Good practice includes objective and repeated assessments of benefits and side effects and repeated attempts to reduce doses gradually or to try periods of time without medication. In this way, patients with acute psychoses who no longer require medication can be found, and those with relentless and unyielding chronic illnesses will also be better recognized. For both, risks of long-term side effects and toxicity would be minimized.

Influence of Age on the Use of Antipsychotic Agents

Use of antipsychotic agents in patients at the extremes of the age spectrum raises some special considerations. Many elderly patients have psychotic illnesses, including dementias, psychotic depression, paranoia (delusional disorder), or exacerbations of previously present schizophrenia or bipolar disorder. While the antipsychotic agents are useful in treating these conditions, it is common to prescribe doses about one-half or one-third those commonly used for younger adults. Nevertheless, a small number of controlled trials suggest that daily doses below 200 to 300 mg of chlorpromazine or the equivalent of another agent are not effectively antipsychotic for some patients. There is, however, a marked increase in the incidence of side effects and toxicity in the elderly which often limits the doses that can be tolerated. Thus, doses are initially small, divided, and increased slowly in small increments.

In the elderly, the low-potency antipsychotic agents tend to induce toxic CNS reactions, including confusion, disorientation, and lethargy, or restlessness and agitation. Thioridazine has been popular for older patients, partly because of its lower incidence of extrapyramidal reactions and its possible antidepressant effects. Nevertheless, owing to its strong anticholinergic and other actions on the autonomic systems, it is particularly likely to induce serious parasympatholytic side effects, toxic delirium, and possibly cardiac arrhythmia. Thioridazine and other low-potency agents are also associated with a high risk of postural hypotension. More *potent* agents in *moderate, divided* doses may be preferable for older patients with psychotic illnesses marked by agitation, delusions, hallucinations, and hostility. Alternatively, agents of moderate potency, such as perphenazine or acetophenazine, in moderate doses, may offer a compromise between the risk of anticholinergic autonomic and sedative effects of low-potency agents and the extrapyramidal effects of high-potency agents. More benign states of agitation which are not associated with psychoses or organic mental

Table 5. Antipsychotic Agents Recommended for Children

Agent (route)	Single Dose (mg/kg)	Typical Daily Dose (mg)	Daily Maximum (mg) <6 yrs	6-12 yrs
Chlorpromazine·HCl				
PO	0.5	10-50	—	—
IM	0.5	—	40	75
Rectal	1.0	—	—	—
Triflupromazine·HCl				
PO	0.5	10-50	—	—
IM	0.2-0.25	—	10 (>2½ yrs)	10
Thioridazine·HCl				
PO	0.25-0.50	5-50	—	—
Fluphenazine·HCl				
PO	0.05-0.1	0.75-5	0 (<5 yrs)	10 (≥5 yrs)
Perphenazine·HCl				
PO	0.05-0.1	1-5	4 (>1 yr)	6
Prochlorperazine·maleate				
PO	0.1	5-10	—	—
IM	0.05	1-2	—	—
Trifluoperazine·HCl				
PO	0.5	1-10	0	15
IM	0.05-0.10	1-2	0	2
Chlorprothixene				
PO	0.5-1.0	30-100	0	100

At the lower limit of age, there is little reported experience in infants. The preschool-age group is generally considered to be one or two to five or six years. For adolescent children aged 12 to 16 years, the lower range of adult doses can be used for most neuroleptic agents. For all children, *divided* daily doses are recommended (typically, TID). For late adolescents over 16, adult doses are used as required individually. Note that only eight agents are recommended for oral use, and only four for parenteral (i.m.) use; Thorazine can also be administered by rectal suppository; the liquid Compazine edisylate is not recommended for children. *Agents not included are not recommended for use in children.*

syndromes can often be managed by cautious use of short-acting benzodiazepines, but these have a high risk of inducing cerebral intoxication in the elderly. Other sedatives, especially barbiturates and long-acting benzodiazepines, are used cautiously, if at all, due to their tendency to induce ataxia and confusion and thus to worsen agitation. Paranoid delusional disorders in the elderly are particularly difficult to manage with any medication but, again, moderate doses of the more potent antipsychotic agents can be tried.

At the other end of the age range, the efficacy and safety of the antipsychotic agents have been shown consistently in the management of children with psychoses or with severe behavioral disturbances associated with brain damage. They are not used for neurotic or mild behavior disorders or for hyperactivity because of their potential to impair cognition and the risk of extrapyramidal reactions. They are used in the management of Gilles de la Tourette's syndrome and are sometimes included in the management of autistic children, with variable success. The greatest experience has been in the management of adolescent patients diagnosed as schizophrenic, in whom these drugs relieve psychotic thinking and disturbed (and disturbing) behavior, as they do in adults. Doses effective against psychosis in school-aged children are not much less than doses given to adults and so may be even higher than in adults on a mg/kg weight basis. The recent acceptance of relatively high doses of neuroleptic and other psychotropic agents for children reflects experimental evidence that rates of metabolism and clearance of these agents may perhaps be twice those in adults. Dosage in younger children is usually even lower and is determined partly by smaller body size but also reflects a greater awareness of side effects that may impair intellectual and other functions in school-aged patients. When antipsychotic agents are used for prolonged periods in young children, the patients are monitored closely for signs of impairment of their physical and scholastic development, in addition to the side effects typical of adult patients. Low potency agents are usually avoided, and the less sedating agents, such as trifluoperazine, fluphenazine, thiothixene, and haloperidol, have been preferred. Apart from the question of side effects, most antipsychotic agents in common use are probably as effective in childhood psychoses as they are in the adult illnesses. Nevertheless, current manufacturers' recommendations remain conservative regarding the agents, doses, and routes of administration recommended for children under age 12, as is summarized in Table 5.

TOXICOLOGY

The most important point to clarify about the toxicity and side effects of the antipsychotic agents is that they are among the safest drugs available in

Table 6. Neurological Side-Effects of Neuroleptic-Antipsychotic Drugs

Reaction	Features	Maximum Risk	Proposed Mechanism	Treatment
Acute dystonia	Spasm of muscles of tongue, face, neck, back; may mimic seizures; *not* hysteria	1-5 d	DA-excess?	Antiparkinsonism agents are di-agnostic and cura-tive (i.m. or i.v., then p.o.)
Parkinsonism	Bradykinesia, ri-gidity, variable tremor, mask fa-cies, shuffling gait	5-30 d (may persist)	DA-blockade	Antiparkinsonism agents help (p.o.)
Akathisia	Motor restless-ness; may experi-ence anxiety or agitation	5-60 d (commonly persists)	Unknown	Reduce dose or change drug; anti-parkinsonism agents or benzo-diazepines may help; low doses of propranolol
Tardive dyskinesia	Oral-facial dyski-nesia; choreo-athetosis, some-times irreversible, rarely progressive	mos.-yrs. (worse on withdrawal)	DA-excess?	Prevention best; treatment unsatis-factory
"Rabbit" syndrome	Perioral tremor (late Parkinson-ism variant?); usually reversible	mos.-yrs.	Unknown	Antiparkinsonism agents may help; reduce dose of neuroleptic
Malignant syndrome	Catatonia, stupor, fever; unstable BP, can be fatal	weeks	Unknown	Stop neuroleptic, antiparkinsonism agents usually fail, dantrolene or bromocriptine may help, general supportive care crucial

medicine. This safety, in no small measure, accounts for their widespread use. The overall incidence of important problems, other than extrapyramidal reactions, is a few percent; and some regularly occurring effects are more annoying than dangerous. The latter include feelings of heaviness, sluggishness, weakness, or faintness and a variety of mild effects presumed to be anticholinergic, including dry mouth and blurred vision. Postural hypotension can be a problem, especially early in treatment with low-potency agents and in elderly patients. Among the most common side effects characteristic of neuroleptic agents are those involving movements and posture. These are evidently mediated by effects on the extrapyramidal motor system.

Neurological Effects of Neuroleptic Drugs

The common and sometimes troublesome neurological side effects of most antipsychotic drugs represent a unique constellation of syndromes not associated with other psychotropic agents (APA, 1980). These reactions can be subdivided into five categories, as outlined in Table 6. Other classes of psychotropic drugs, including sedatives (e.g., barbiturates), tranquilizer-antianxiety agents (e.g., benzodiazepines), and even antidepressants and lithium salts, are more likely to induce toxic delirium and, eventually, coma and death. In contrast, CNS toxicity of the antipsychotic agents is expressed in several characteristic motor syndromes. Except for parkinsonism, the pathophysiology of these reactions is still poorly understood, although it is suspected that effects on dopamine mediated systems in the basal ganglia are involved. These syndromes are as follows:

   Acute dystonias typically occur within the first few hours or days of treatment and are most likely to be associated with the more potent neuroleptics. They involve sustained hyperkinesias of the muscles of the neck, jaw, and tongue, as well as the eyes and trunk. Signs may include trismus, opisthotonos, or tonic oculogyric movements or deviations of the eyes ("oculogyric crisis"). Facial grimacing, perioral spasms, protrusions or torsion of the tongue, and dysphagia are common. Laryngeal or pharyngeal spasm with dyspnea or life-threatening respiratory distress may develop, and a few fatalities have occurred. The reaction may be accompanied by sweating or pallor and fever. Severe anxiety is the rule. Such reactions seem to be especially common in young male patients. The pathophysiology of the condition remains obscure, in part due to the wide and inconsistent variety of agents reported to be of benefit. It has been reported that the period of maximum risk for neuroleptic-induced dystonias is during the phase of rapid decrease of blood levels of the drug. If dystonic reactions recur frequently, hypocalcemia may be present. Typically, tolerance to dystonias develops following days or weeks of treatment. Possible exceptions include the sudden change from a neuroleptic of low potency to relatively high doses of a potent agent, as well as the use of repeated injections of a fluphenazine ester, which may induce dystonic reactions repeatedly for many months.

The pattern of high risk when tissue levels are falling early during acute exposure to a neuroleptic, the greater risk of high-potency agents, and the tendency for tolerance to develop suggest that early responses of the nervous system to potent dopamine antagonism may be important in the pathophysiology of acute dystonias. Based on studies of laboratory animals, these responses include rapid, but possibly incomplete, blockade of dopamine receptors and a marked increase in the production and turnover or release of dopamine in the forebrain and in the synthesis and release of acetylcholine in the basal ganglia. If the availability of dopamine and of acetylcholine continues while the partial blockade of dopamine receptors is diminishing, it is possible that a temporary state of relative excess of both dopaminergic and cholinergic function may occur.

The main clinical problem with this syndrome is to recognize it and not to ascribe it to a seizure disorder, tetany or tetanus, or "hysteria." Patients in dystonic reactions are typically terrified and should be forewarned about them and treated immediately as a medical emergency. Treatment by injection of an antiparkinsonism agent is usually dramatically effective and virtually diagnostic. Diphenhydramine (Benadryl, 25 or 50 mg given intramuscularly or 25 mg intravenously) and benztropine mesylate (Cogentin, 2 mg intravenously) are currently popular choices. Some clinicians prefer to add an antiparkinsonism agent routinely when starting to treat a patient with a potent neuroleptic; and recent experience suggests that a protective effect against dystonia or other acute extrapyramidal reactions by such combined therapy may occur, especially when moderate or high doses of a potent neuroleptic are used. Thus, the probable benefits of routine use of moderate doses of an antiparkinsonism agent must be balanced against the possible added risk of peripheral autonomic or central neurotoxic complications of treatment. If an anticholinergic agent is given early to protect against dystonia, its need should be re-evaluated within two weeks.

Drug-induced parkinsonism is similar to other forms of the disease except that tremor is less prominent in the neuroleptic-induced form. The onset of the syndrome usually occurs within the first month of treatment. The risk increases with advancing age. There may be some "tolerance" to this effect, as the signs sometimes diminish over two or three months but with an unpredictable requirement for antiparkinsonism medication which varies among individual patients. In some cases, bradykinesia and inexpressive facies persist indefinitely and may be confused clinically with manifestation of the late "defect state" of schizophrenia or with depressed mood. Antipsychotic agents with higher milligram potency induce parkinsonism and dystonic reactions with greater frequency than less potent agents. Severe akinetic, catatonic reactions and mutism have also been associated

Table 7. Equivalent Doses of Antiparkinsonism Agents

Generic Name	Trade Name	Usual Dose Range (mg/day)
amantadine	Symmetrel	100-300
benztropine	Cogentin, Tremin, etc. (generic)	1-6
biperiden	Akineton	2-10
cycrimine	Pagitane	2.5-15
diphenhydramine	Benadryl	25-100
ethopropazine	Parisdol	6-10
orphenadrine	Disipal, Norlex	50-300
procyclidine	Kemadrin	5-30
trihexyphenidyl	Artane, Pipanol, etc. (generic)	5-15

These agents are commonly prescribed orally three times a day to provide the total daily adult doses stated above. Benztropine (2 mg) and diphenhydramine (25-50 mg) are commonly used intramuscularly or intravenously to reverse acute dystonic reactions to antipsychotic agents. Amantadine has been used to treat drug-induced parkinsonism and catatonia; it is relatively expensive and may lose effectiveness in a few weeks; overdoses may respond to physostigmine. Diphenhydramine and orphenadrine are antihistaminic and anticholinergic; ethopropazine is a strongly anticholinergic phenothiazine; the other agents are atropine-like. Most are available as soluble hydrochlorides, benztropine as the mesylate.

Note that because of the relatively short half-life and low margin of safety (therapeutic index) of these agents, they are not suitable for once-daily dosing. Also their short duration of action requires that they be continued for several days after discontinuation of a neuroleptic agent.

with relatively high doses of potent antipsychotics such as the piperazine phenothiazines and thioxanthenes, haloperidol, and loxapine. With such severe reactions, the temptation is to suspect worsening functional psychosis and give even higher doses of the offending agent, although improvement usually follows reduction in its dosage. The antiparkinsonism agents, including anticholinergics or amantadine (Symmetrel), may help. A similar but even more severe reaction ("neuroleptic malignant syndrome" or "hypothalamic crisis") is described separately below.

A variety of agents are now used for the treatment of idiopathic as well as drug-induced parkinsonism, and the differential effectiveness of various classes of agents provides strong support for the theory that dopamine deficiency (and perhaps a relative excess of cholinergic function) in the basal ganglia is an important aspect of the pathophysiology of both forms of the syndrome. In addition, there is excellent neuropathological and postmortem neurochemical evidence of dopamine deficiency in idiopathic parkinsonism. Antiparkinsonism drugs available for psychotic patients are listed in Table 7. L-dopa or dopamine agonists are considered too likely to produce agitation for routine use in such patients.

Most of the recommended antiparkinsonism drugs (except amantadine) are strongly antimuscarinic (atropine-like), so they can induce the syndrome of *anticholinergic poisoning*. This is characterized by restless agitation, confusion, disorientation, perhaps seizures, hyperthermia, dry and some-times flushed skin, tachycardia, sluggish and at least moderately dilated pupils, decreased bowel sounds, and often acute urinary retention. These effects are probably due to peripheral and central anticholinergic actions of these potent muscarinic blocking agents. The antiparkinsonism and cyclic (imipramine-like) antidepressant drugs are among the most potent centrally active anticholinergic agents used in medicine. Some antipsychotic drugs with relatively less tendency to induce acute extrapyramidal reactions (e.g., clozapine and thioridazine) are also strongly anticholinergic. The anticho-linergic intoxication syndrome is best managed by immediate removal of the offending agent. In addition, physostigmine (Eserine, Antilirium)—the only commonly available, centrally as well as peripherally active, reversible anticholinesterase agent—may be useful in moderate degrees of intoxica-tion. Its usefulness and safety in more serious and life-threatening intoxica-tions with coma and impaired vital functions (especially those associated with an acute overdose of an antiparkinsonism agent or an antidepressant) are less likely, and many emergency physicians avoid its use in comatose or otherwise dangerously intoxicated persons with unstable vital functions.

The potential to induce CNS toxicity is one of the problems associated with antiparkinsonism agents which indicates caution in their use, particu-larly in patients treated with neuroleptics of low potency or with cyclic antidepressants. Other problems include the added complexity and expense of routine "polypharmacy." Dependence may occur on these agents, which sometimes induce euphoria, an effect that may contribute to the common difficulty in discontinuing them. While the antiparkinsonism agents are sometimes given "prophylactically" to avoid acute extrapyramidal effects of antipsychotic agents, this practice is often unnecessary, especially given conservative dosing with the neuroleptics. It is a matter of clinical judgment to evaluate the urgency of indications and contraindications for their use. Furthermore, sound practice includes the attempt to withdraw these drugs gradually after several weeks, and certainly within four to 12 weeks after the onset of an acute extrapyramidal reaction. This practice is often possible due to the tolerance to early neurological effects of the antipsychotic drugs which evolves in many patients.

Akathisia (motor restlessness, fidgeting, pacing, "restless legs," and a drive to move about) is a common but often overlooked early motor symptom complex of obscure pathophysiologic basis. While the experience of anxiety is a part of the syndrome, it is often experienced as "alien" to the patient. It should not be mistaken for increasing primary psychotic anxiety or agitation or treated by increasing the dose of an antipsychotic drug. It can sometimes be managed by reducing the dose or changing to a different chemical class of antipsychotic agents. Antiparkinsonism drugs may have a beneficial effect, as may anxiolytic-sedative agents with putative muscle-relaxing properties, such as the benzodiazepines, or even moderate doses of propranolol. Unfortunately, some cases respond poorly to treatment, and the distress of the akathisia must be weighed against the need for antipsychotic medication. While the timing of this reaction is generally similar to that of parkinsonism, it may emerge as the symptoms of acute psychosis abate or may reoccur or persist indefinitely, because tolerance to akathisia is less likely than to dystonic reactions or parkinsonism.

Tardive dyskinesia (late and persistent dyskinesia) is a late-developing extrapyramidal syndrome that encourages reappraisal of the benefits and risks of uninterrupted and indefinitely prolonged neuroleptic drug therapy (APA, 1980). The syndrome consists of involuntary or semivoluntary movements of a choreiform (rapid, tic-like) nature, sometimes with an athetotic or dystonic component. These classically affect the tongue, facial, and neck muscles but often also affect the extremities and digits as well as the trunk and muscles that control breathing or swallowing. Early signs of tardive dyskinesia are unwanted movements of the tongue, face, or extremities. Oral-lingual-masticatory movements are well known, especially in older patients, but it is usual to find abnormalities of posture and choreoathetotic movements of the fingers as well, especially in younger patients. The movements of tardive dyskinesia are much less voluntary and purposeful and more classically choreoathetotic than the stereotyped mannerisms and posturing that may occur spontaneously in schizophrenia. The signs of tardive dyskinesia usually become worse if the antipsychotic agent is withdrawn and can be suppressed, at least temporarily, by increasing the dose, readministering a neuroleptic drug, or adding an amine-depleting agent such as reserpine.

Although tardive dyskinesias are painless, the syndrome can be embarrassing and distressing, especially in relatively well functioning outpatients. In some cases, the patient's skills in self-care, feeding, and swallowing, as well as vocationally important dexterity, can be impaired; and severe cases can be as disabling as Huntington's disease. A thorough neurological evaluation of cases of tardive dyskinesia should attempt to exclude other involuntary movement disorders such as Huntington's disease, rheumatic chorea, Wilson's disease, and other rare toxic or degenerative dyskinetic syndromes. The prevalence of the syndrome has varied in epidemiological studies from a few percent to as many as 40 to 50 percent of patients "maintained" on antipsychotic medications for many years. It is unusual to develop the syndrome in less than a few months. A recent study suggested an incidence of about five percent after a year of treatment with depot fluphenazine. Several surveys among the elderly indicate that spontaneous dyskinesias (especially oral-lingual movements) unrelated to neuroleptic treatment occur in perhaps five to ten percent of those evaluated. The prevalence of persistent dyskinesias, corrected for the occurrence of spontaneous dyskinesias, averages approximately 15 to 20 percent among those exposed to a neuroleptic agent for more than a year.

The risk of tardive dyskinesia and of spontaneous dyskinesias increases strikingly with age, especially after age 50, although children and adolescents sometimes develop severe and widespread dyskinesias. Generally, too, in elderly patients the severity increases, and chances for spontaneous remission diminish markedly. Women may be at a slightly higher risk than men, although younger men may be at somewhat higher risk of severe and generalized forms of the condition. Since most patients treated with neuroleptics do not develop late dyskinesias, it follows that unknown constitutional factors contributing to risk probably exist.

The cause of tardive dyskinesias remains mysterious. It is not even certain that it is reasonable to seek a unitary pathophysiology or etiology in view of the variable clinical manifestations and pharmacologic responses of conditions currently considered as tardive dyskinesia. Animal experimentation indicates that increasing sensitivity of dopamine receptors during prolonged neuroleptic treatment can lead eventually to a state of increased response to a dopamine agonist, even if the neuroleptic is not withdrawn. This observation has suggested a "dopamine supersensitivity" hypothesis for tardive dyskinesia, but this concept has not been proven to account for all features of the clinical phenomenon. Clinical support for this concept has, however, been provided by observations that tardive dyskinesia tends to be worsened by dopamine agonists and improved by antagonists. The observation that

Table 8. Suggested Guidelines for the Avoidance and Management of Tardive Dyskinesia

---

- Consider indications for prolonged neuroleptic therapy carefully; indications (chronic psychosis) should be compelling, with objective evidence of benefit

- Seek alternative therapies in neuroses and mood and character disorders

- Use lower doses in elderly patients and children, strive for minimum effective doses, avoid multiple drugs, and remove antiparkinsonism agents when possible

- Advise patients and families of risks and benefits; arrive at a mutual decision when use of neuroleptic exceeds one year. Note discussion and agreement in clinical record

- Examine patient regularly for early signs of choreoathetosis and oral-lingual dyskinesia. Consider alternative neurological diagnoses

- Reevaluate and document indications and response at least every three to six months and attempt to reduce dose

- At earliest sign of dyskinesia, lower the dose, change to a less potent agent, or ideally stop treatment and await remission as long as psychiatric status permits

- Treat dyskinesia with benign agents first (diazepam, deanol, or lecithin in high doses, possibly lithium or valproate); stay alert to new experimental therapies, if only to bide time and offer hope. Reinstitute reserpine or a neuroleptic only as an extreme measure for disabling dyskinesias, using lowest doses feasible

---

anticholinergic antiparkinsonism agents tend to worsen the movements is consistent with overactivity in the dopamine system as well.

No satisfactory treatment for tardive dyskinesia has been found. Many cases resolve slowly (months) after withdrawal of the neuroleptic treatment when the patient's psychiatric condition permits this course of management. Perhaps the best way to deal with the problem is through the thoughtful and conservative use of neuroleptic agents. Compelling indications (chronic psychosis that responds to the treatment) should be required to continue a neuroleptic for longer than six to 12 months. Other treatments are available for recurrent or chronic mood disorders, severe personality disorders, and conditions characterized by anxiety. Alternatives should be considered for conditions in which indications for a neuroleptic agent are not strong. The empirical search with each patient for the lowest effective dose of a neuroleptic for prolonged use in a "maintenance" program, as well as repeated attempts to remove the drug altogether, are sound practices. Additional suggestions for the management of tardive dyskinesia are provided in Table 8.

Sometimes transient tardive dyskinesia-like reactions occur for several days on the sudden discontinuation of a neuroleptic. These so-called "withdrawal-emergent" dyskinesias are especially common in young patients after discontinuation of relatively high doses of a potent neuroleptic. It is not known whether these temporary reactions are pathophysiologically identical to tardive dyskinesias or whether they represent early cases of the more prolonged variety.

"Rabbit" syndrome (perioral tremor) is another reaction associated with neuroleptic drugs which usually occurs late in therapy. This timing has led to its (probably erroneous) classification with the tardive dyskinesias. It may represent an atypical and localized variant of parkinsonism since the rate of the mouth movements (about five per second) is similar to more typical limb tremors of parkinsonism. Moreover, the reaction sometimes responds favorably to treatment with antiparkinsonism agents and is usually reversible after the neuroleptic treatment has been discontinued.

Other Neurological Effects of Antipsychotic Drugs

In addition to the common, neuroleptic-induced neurological syndromes already described, other effects of antipsychotic drugs on the central nervous system have also been described. They include the following:

Neuroleptic malignant syndrome or "hypothalamic crisis" is a group of reactions marked by *extreme* parkinsonism-like rigidity or catatonia and variable abnormalities of autonomic function, sometimes with striking hyperthermia. The reaction had been considered rare but is encountered increasingly commonly when large doses of the more potent neuroleptics are used. Additional risk factors may include youth or advanced age and elevated environmental temperature. It typically occurs early in treatment. The pathophysiology is not known, but it is reasonable to assume that effects that contribute to other acute extrapyramidal reactions as well as the poikilothermal or temperature-dysregulating actions of many neuroleptics are involved.

Features of this syndrome include persistent (sometimes high) fever, muscular rigidity, and catatonia (often with elevated plasma creatinine phosphokinase and myoglobin), coarse tremor, drooling, akinesia, stupor with fluctuating levels of consciousness, mutism or severe dysarthria, unstable blood pressure, and tachycardia. Dyspnea and seizures may also occur. There is a risk of myoglobinuria with renal impairment. This severe reaction has a significant mortality rate, possibly as high as 20 percent. Its treatment is unsatisfactory. Antiparkinsonism agents usually are not beneficial. There are a few case reports of beneficial effects with the muscle relaxant dantrolene sodium (Dantrium), typically in oral doses of 200 mg/day, by analogy to the use of intravenous dantrolene to interrupt the malignant hyperthermia rarely associated with general anesthesia and based on altered calcium transport in skeletal muscle that is not found in the neuroleptic syndrome. The dopamine agonist ergoline drug bromocriptine mesylate (Parlodel) in divided oral doses of 10-20 mg/day may also be helpful. Management of the malignant neuroleptic syndrome includes intravenous fluids, control of the fever, and other supportive measures. The reaction usually subsides gradually within a week or two. Especially prolonged and dangerous reactions have occurred following a depot injection of fluphenazine.

Seizures. Neuroleptic drugs, and perhaps especially low-potency phenothiazines and loxapine, may increase the incidence of seizures in epileptic patients. The piperazines and haloperidol possibly have less tendency to do this, and molindone may be especially unlikely to do so. (Antidepressants and lithium salts can also have this effect.) These impressions, however, are based on clinical anecdotes and indirect evidence from animal or other laboratory experiments rather than on controlled clinical studies. Usually, clinical judgment is required to balance the patient's need for antipsychotic medication with a need for an anticonvulsant. The dosage of the latter may need to be increased to counter the potentially increased risk of seizures. On the other hand, anticonvulsants often increase metabolic inactivation of neuroleptics and may diminish their effectiveness.

Acute Intoxication. In contrast to almost all other CNS depressants, the lethality of antipsychotic agents on acute overdose and their potential for inducing deep and prolonged coma and respiratory depression are limited. That is, they have a very high *therapeutic index* (ratio of toxic or lethal to therapeutic doses). The clinical half-maximally effective lethal doses (LD_{50}) for these agents are not known but can be ten to 100 times above behaviorally effective doses in laboratory animals. Patients have survived ingestions of many grams of chlorpromazine, and it is virtually impossible to commit suicide by taking an overdose of an antipsychotic agent alone. It is essential to consider the simultaneous presence of more lethal and treatable forms of acute intoxication since ingestions are often mixed. For example, comatose psychiatric patients may also have taken alcohol, a barbiturate, an agent with strong anticholinergic activity, or an antidepressant or lithium salt. Dialysis can be used to remove barbiturates, lithium, and some other central depressants; but it is not effective in removing antipsychotic or antidepressant agents because of their strong affinity for protein and lipids. The reversible anticholinesterase agent physostigmine (Eserine or Antilirium) penetrates the blood-brain diffusion barrier and can be administered cautiously for the central anticholinergic syndrome uncomplicated by coma or severe cardiovascular dysfunction. Attempts to induce vomiting after overdoses of antipsychotic agents may be unsuccessful, owing to the strong antiemetic effects of most of them (thioridazine and clozapine are exceptions). One implication of the limited acute toxicity, as well as the lack of addiction potential, of antipsychotic agents is that large quantities of these drugs can be prescribed with relative impunity, even for patients with impaired judgment or impaired impulse control.

General Toxicity of Antipsychotic Agents

Additive interactions may occur between neuroleptics and other agents acting on the central nervous system. Excessive sedation may thus occur upon mixing an antipsychotic agent with alcohol or a sedative or hypnotic agent. The risk of confusional states with an antidepressant or lithium salt is increased, particularly if an antiparkinsonism agent is also used.

Peripheral actions presumed to represent anticholinergic effects are modest with most antipsychotic agents and are usually limited to annoying symptoms, such as dry mouth and blurred vision, although ileus and urinary retention can occur, particularly in older patients. Precipitating an attack of acute glaucoma with any agent having anticholinergic activity is a possibility; but with antipsychotic agents and even with antidepressant drugs, this event is rare and is usually associated with "narrow angle" glaucoma, which itself is not common. Acute glaucoma is an emergency calling for immediate ophthalmologic treatment with a cholinergic or other miotic agent such as pilocarpine. Chronic glaucoma can almost always be managed with cholinomimetic eyedrops, even while anticholinergic psychotropic agents are used. Occasionally, cholinergic agents have also been given in eyedrops (such as pilocarpine nitrate, 1% ophthalmic solution) to overcome cycloplegia, in a mouthwash to increase salivation, or orally (in daily doses of 5 to 10 mg of pilocarpine, 5 to 15 mg of neostigmine, or about

75 mg a day of bethanechol [Urecholine]) to counter anticholinergic side effects of the antipsychotic or antidepressant agents. In general, however, this approach is not consistently effective and it is not usually used.

Other ophthalmologic problems can also occur with the antipsychotic agents. The most serious is a rare irreversible degenerative pigmentary retinopathy following large doses of thioridazine (above 900 mg/day) and possibly other low-potency neuroleptics. In addition, prolonged high doses of low-potency phenothiazines and thioxanthenes have been associated with deposits of drug substances and pigment in the cornea and lens as well as in the skin. The deposits in the eye can be visualized best with a slit lamp, rarely impair vision, and disappear over many months after withdrawal of the medication. Although penicillamine and other agents have been advocated to hasten the removal of phenothiazines from the eye or skin, there is little evidence that they help.

Skin reactions include photosensitivity early in treatment and later a blue-gray discoloration. The latter has most often been associated with prolonged high doses of chlorpromazine. Maculopapular rashes occur on occasion, and there is some risk of contact dermatitis among nurses handling solutions of antipsychotic agents.

The risk of severe cardiovascular toxicity due to antipsychotic agents is not high. Although sustained hypotension is not frequently encountered, orthostatic hypotension can be a problem, especially when the less potent phenothiazines are given to elderly patients. The hypotensive effects of these agents are rather idiosyncratic and inconsistently correlated with doses so that the formerly common ritual of giving small test doses of intramuscular medication is poorly founded. An important practical reason for avoiding large intramuscular doses, especially of the less potent agents, is that they are painful and may lead to elevated levels of transaminases or lactic dehydrogenase from local necrosis, *not* liver damage. If severe hypotension does develop, it can usually be managed by bed rest or elevation of the legs and use of elastic stockings. If a vasoactive agent is required, the rational choice is a purely α-adrenergic pressor amine such as metaraminol (Aramine) (rarely is the more potent agent *l*-norepinephrine, Levophed, required) to reverse the modest α-antagonistic effects of phenothiazines. The β-agonistic cardiac stimulants such as epinephrine or isoproterenol (Isuprel) would increase pooling of blood in the splanchnic and peripheral areas to worsen the hypotension and so are *contra*indicated. In addition to the unpredictable effects of antipsychotic agents on blood pressure, they may increase the risk of potentially lethal ventricular arrhythmias, partly because they prolong ventricular repolarization. These hazards may be greatest with thioridazine among the antipsychotic agents, but the risk with any antipsychotic agent appears to be small. Haloperidol, the potent piperazine phenothiazines, and molindone appear to be relatively safe for cardiac patients and unlikely to interact badly with digitalis and other cardiovascular and diuretic agents. Chlorpromazine may block uptake into sympathetic (noradrenergic) neurons and so reduce the antihypertensive efficacy of postganglionic blocking agents such as guanethidine (Ismelin). Because of their potential cardiovascular effects, as well as the possibility of undesirable drug interactions, it is considered good practice to reduce or omit the use of low-potency neuroleptics for a day or two prior to electroconvulsive treatment (ECT) with barbiturate anesthesia and prior to surgery. Alternatively, high-potency agents can be used when required in such circumstances.

Other annoying side effects of antipsychotic agents include presumably autonomic or hypothalamic effects such as changes in appetite, weight gain, fluid retention, breast enlargement and engorgement (in men as well as women), and even galactorrhea, decreased libido, and ejaculatory incompetence in men, and delayed ovulation and amenorrhea in women. These effects are most often associated with the less potent phenothiazines and particularly with thioridazine. Thioridazine has even been advocated as an adjunct in the treatment of premature ejaculation. Such sexual effects are sometimes overlooked by clinicians but can represent serious problems to patients.

A sustained prolactin-increasing action is characteristic of most antipsychotic agents (largely mediated by the antagonism of effects of hypothalamic dopamine on the anterior pituitary) and even small doses of reserpine as used to treat hypertension. This response represents a theoretical risk in patients with an occult or identified carcinoma of the breast. However, there is at present no compelling evidence that antipsychotic agents have a breast tumor-inducing effect or evidence that they increase the risk of any carcinoma. Nevertheless, regular breast examination should be a routine part of medical management of female patients treated with a prolactin-elevating agent for more than six months. Antipsychotic agents can mildly depress testosterone output, but this is of doubtful physiological or psycho-sexual significance. It has been reported that antipsychotic agents have inhibitory effects on the output of growth hormone, opposite to the releasing action of L-dopa. This effect is also of doubtful physiological importance, and antipsychotic drugs are not useful as a treatment of acromegaly. There is no evidence that antipsychotic agents retard to a clinically important extent the growth and development of psychotic children, although growth should be monitored closely in young patients exposed to any psychotropic agent for more than six months.

Although there has been a great deal of concern about jaundice and agranulocytosis due to antipsychotic agents, these problems are encountered infrequently. The jaundice is almost always of a cholestatic, presumably allergic, type and is usually transient. It was formerly more common, particularly in association with chlorpromazine, and it may have become less frequent (incidence not more than two percent) due to factors related to pharmaceutical formulation. It usually appears within the first month of treatment. Many CNS depressants can worsen hepatic encephalopathy, partly owing to their direct actions on the brain but also due to their tendency to diminish hepatic function by competition with hepatic microsomal oxidases. Subclinical biliary obstructive effects may be common, as a study of liver biopsies revealed an incidence of mild obstructive changes in as many as 25 percent of patients treated with an antipsychotic agent.

Agranulocytosis is rare (incidence less than 0.01 percent), has a peak incidence within the first two months of treatment, and has been encountered particularly in older women. This reaction has almost always been associated with low-potency phenothiazines and thioxanthenes and is virtually unknown with haloperidol, fluphenazine, or thiothixene. Agranulocytosis is a potentially catastrophic and often rapidly developing medical emergency with a high mortality rate. It can be predicted only in rare instances from occasional routine white blood cell counts and *must be suspected* and promptly evaluated in cases of malaise, fever, or sore throat that occur *early* in the course of antipsychotic chemotherapy. Leucocyte counts, repeated frequently in the first two months of treatment, may reveal a downward trend predicting agranulocytosis, although early, moderate, transient reductions in white cell levels are not unusual. Some hematologists advise weekly leucocyte counts for at least eight weeks after initiation of therapy, particularly with chlorpromazine, clozapine, or other low-potency agents.

Defensive rituals of little value have developed in the medical management of patients receiving antipsychotic agents for prolonged periods; these include occasional routine "liver function tests" and "blood counts," which contribute little other than a false sense of security and possibly some decreased risk of malpractice charges. Laboratory tests cannot substitute for an alert and well informed physician.

The safety of antipsychotic agents in pregnancy and lactation is not well established. These agents do pass the blood-placenta barrier as well as the blood-brain barrier, and they are secreted in human milk in very low levels. They can induce a mild degree of sedation followed by motor excitement in the newborn if the mother has recently been treated with a neuroleptic. Evidence of sustained neurotoxic actions in newborn laboratory animals born to mothers exposed to a neuroleptic is weak and inconsistent. There is no evidence that antipsychotic agents are responsible for an increased incidence of fetal malformations; and low, divided doses of the high-potency neuroleptics may be relatively safe during pregnancy. Nevertheless, the current consensus is that the use of antipsychotic agents should be avoided as far as possible in pregnancy and lactation, and especially in the first trimester of pregnancy. As a general principle, it is probably wise to avoid use of single high doses and of low-potency agents during pregnancy to minimize exposure to potentially toxic foreign molecules. Despite the need for a conservative approach to antipsychotic medication during pregnancy, clinical judgment must be exercised when the indications for medical treatment or psychiatric hospitalization during pregnancy are compelling.

Elderly patients treated with antipsychotic agents are particularly likely to be troubled by toxic effects of all types, and unwanted effects on the brain and behavior may be especially striking. Generally, except for the increased incidence and seriousness of effects in the elderly, the qualitative nature of the side effects of antipsychotic agents does not change with advancing age. Although there is a tendency to keep doses of antipsychotic agents low because of the intolerance of older patients to side effects, daily doses less than the equivalent of 200 or 300 mg of chlorpromazine are often ineffective in the control of psychotic thought, affect, and behavior. Thus, minimum effective doses of antipsychotic agents are probably not much less than those estimated for younger adults or adolescents, but the margin of safety is significantly reduced in the elderly. *Low*, *divided*, and *gradually* increased doses of the more *potent* agents are currently preferred over low-potency phenothiazines or thioxanthenes for elderly psychotic patients.

CONCLUSIONS AND SUMMARY

The availability of modern, effective, and safe antipsychotic drugs has contributed to an almost revolutionary change in the pattern of delivery of psychiatric care to the most severely disturbed patients. These agents have supported and reinforced the melioristic expectations of modern hospital and community psychiatry. Most psychotic patients can be managed in open psychiatric hospitals or in general hospitals, and the duration of hospitalization has been markedly reduced. Many psychotic patients can be maintained in day-care or foster-care programs or at home, and many incipient attacks of acute psychosis can be managed by psychiatrists or other physicians without the need for hospitalization.

Many antipsychotic drugs are now available to the physician; most are "neuroleptic" or more or less neurotoxic. Although there are several chemical types of antipsychotic drugs, they are pharmacologically similar, partly because the methods of predicting antipsychotic activity of new agents have usually depended on observing their neurological actions in animals or their interactions at dopamine receptors in laboratory tests. The main shortcoming of the available antipsychotic agents is their regular tendency to produce acute and sometimes long-lasting or even irreversible neurological disorders of the extrapyramidal motor system. A second shortcoming of antipsychotic drugs is that their efficacy is easiest to demonstrate in patients with the best prognosis; results are more disappointing as the chronicity of psychosis increases. There is reason to hope that better agents can be found to produce antipsychotic effects with minimal neurological toxicity. Despite the shortcomings of currently available antipsychotic agents, they are clearly effective in the treatment of a broad range of severe psychiatric and neuropsychiatric disorders.

REFERENCES

Appleton WS, Davis JM: Practical Clinical Psychopharmacology (second edition). Baltimore, Williams & Wilkins, 1980

Baldessarini RJ: Chemotherapy in Psychiatry. Cambridge, Mass, Harvard University Press, 1984 (in press)

Baldessarini RJ: Drugs and the treatment of psychiatric disorders, in The Pharmacological Basis of Therapeutics, seventh edition. Edited by Gilman AG, Goodman LS. New York, MacMillan, 1984 (in press)

Baldessarini RJ, Davis, JM: What is the best maintenance dose of neuroleptics in schizophrenia? Psychiatry Res 3:115-122, 1980

Barchas JD, Berger PA, Ciaranello RD, et al: Psychopharmacology From Theory to Practice. New York, Oxford University Press, 1977

Davis JM: Overview: maintenance therapy in psychiatry: I. schizophrenia. Am J Psychiatry 32:1237-1245, 1975

Hollister LE: Clinical Pharmacology of Psychotherapeutic Drugs. New York, Churchill Livingstone, 1978

Klein DF, Gittelman R, Quitkin F, et al: Diagnosis and Drug Treatment of Psychiatric Disorders: Adults and Children, second edition. Baltimore, Williams & Wilkins, 1980

Mason AS, Granacher RP: Clinical Handbook of Antipsychotic Drug Therapy. New York, Brunner/Mazel, 1980

Simpson GM (consultant): Antipsychotic drugs, in AMA Drug Evaluations. Chicago, American Medical Association, 1983

Task Force on Late Neurological Effects of Antipsychotic Drugs: Task Force Report 18: Tardive Dyskinesia. Washington, DC, American Psychiatric Association, 1980

Van Praag HM: Psychotropic Drugs: A Guide for the Practitioner, New York, Brunner/Mazel, 1978

3
Nutritional Therapies

3

Nutritional Therapies

INTRODUCTION

Nutrition is a branch of biology which studies organisms' requirements for foods, their composition, and the processes by which they are converted into energy and the tissue growth and repair required for health and life. Before 1750, nutrition was naturalistic and ethno-pharmacological. Plant and animal foods of unknown chemical composition were eaten in diets that varied greatly from culture to culture. Centuries of trial and error had demonstrated their value or danger. Certain foods were designated by Hippocrates to have special curative properties useful in the treatment of many human illnesses. Others were poisonous or taboo for unknown reasons. In the period from 1750 to 1900, as chemistry developed, foods were simply classified chemically as carbohydrates, proteins, fats, and the noncombustible ash. Attempts to raise animals on diets containing only these elements quickly showed the inadequacy of this simple classification.

The golden age of nutrition occurred between 1900 and 1950 when the discovery of the need for micronutrients launched a conceptual revolution based on the insight that many human illnesses resulted from the absence of significant dietary constituents. To the established infectious and toxic theories of illness were added the deficiency diseases. With the discovery of vitamins, essential amino acids, and trace elements, the nature of common diseases such as pellagra, beri beri, scurvy, nutritional anemia, and protein malnutrition was quickly understood. The development of quantitative standards for daily requirements of these nutrients for humans, animals, and plants stimulated revolutionary changes in food production and several major public health triumphs.

It is difficult to recognize that fewer than 50 years ago there were more than 200,000 cases of pellagra annually in this country. Mortality from this illness averaged 33 percent and about ten percent of the beds in state hospitals were occupied by demented patients with pellagra. In the South, where pellagra was endemic because of the staple diet of corn, fatback, and molasses, from one-third to one-half of the state mental hospital population had physical symptoms of pellagra and dementia (Roe, 1973). Pellagra was also common among sharecroppers and in prisons, orphanages, and other state institutions. The discovery in 1937 that vitamin B_3 (niacin) was the antipellagra vitamin and the subsequent fortification of most cereal products with this vitamin virtually eliminated pellagra in this country.

Clinical nutritional research was greatly accelerated during World War II because of the need to develop adequate military rations and led to the semi-quantitative determination of human needs for most nutrients. These efforts were so successful that World War II was the first war in which more combat troops died from war injuries than from malnutrition and infection (McNeill, 1982). The spin-offs to civilian nutrition were many. Today, nutritional science is sufficiently advanced that, in this country, malnutrition is uncommon and, when it does occur, is likely to be a function of poverty, alcoholism, or self-selected inadequate diets. This is not true in the Third World, however, where millions of children are stillborn, retarded, or die within the first few years of life because of the unavailability of adequate calories, protein, or micronutrients (Serban, 1975). In the world as a whole today, malnutrition remains as large a public health problem as infectious disease, with which it constantly interacts.

In the richer, industrialized world, research in nutrition has moved into more specialized areas. In medicine, there have been significant advances in the study of the nutritional needs of special populations such as pregnant women, premature infants, and the elderly. Vitamin requirements have been shown to increase when some drugs are administered for treatment of tumors, convulsions, or even for contraceptive purposes (Lipton and Kane, 1979). Great advances have been made in furnishing the nutritional requirements of post-surgical patients or those with severe burns by total parenteral feeding. Specialized nutritional needs have been found for some patients with ophthalmological or dermatological diseases. Genetic illnesses, such as phenylketonuria, have been found to be clinically responsive to minimizing the intake of the amino acid phenylalanine. And some rare genetic autosomal recessive illnesses characterized by mental retardation and multiple somatic defects can be prevented or cured by daily administration of large quantities of particular vitamins (Serban, 1975; Rosenberg, 1974; Scriver, 1973).

Nutritional theories of the etiology of common mental and behavioral disorders and treatments based on these theories are controversial. Nevertheless, new diagnostic methods have shown that several psychiatric illnesses may be complicated by nutritional deficiency and may respond to nutritional supplementation. These are all reviewed in the text *Nutritional Support of Medical Practice* (Schneider et al., 1983). A comprehensive review is offered in the six volumes entitled *Nutrition and the Brain* (Wurtman and Wurtman, 1983).

Many natural foods, especially those from plants, contain biologically active chemicals that may be either toxic or therapeutically useful. Many of these substances have been identified and isolated in pure form and now are useful products in our pharmacological armamentarium. In the industrialized world, food chemists supplement natural foods with nutrients and natural and synthetic additives to enhance the taste and appearance of foods and to diminish spoilage, thus facilitating their useful distribution. Residues from synthetic herbicides and insecticides used to increase crop production and steroids and antibiotics used to increase animal food production may appear in our food, however. Because of this occurrence, there has arisen a subspecialty of nutritional toxicology designed to protect the public from foods that might contain dangerous chemicals such as mercury in fish or selenium in wheat or foods to which chemicals are purposefully added during processing.

Interest in what might be called nutritional pharmacology has also increased. Selected, specific nutrients such as the amino acids tyrosine and tryptophan or the quaternery ammonium compound choline can be fed in doses far above their usual intake levels in order to elevate brain neurotransmitter levels. Such precursor therapy is actively under investigation, and its interest to psychiatry will be discussed below. Although the substances used are natural and even essential in our daily diet in small amounts, the quantities used in precursor therapy are so much greater than ordinarily required that we choose to call the use of the substances in these quantities "pharmacological." Moreover, their biological effects at high concentrations may be different from and unrelated to their primary action. For example, nicotinic acid and nicotinamide have nutritional value identical to that of vitamin B_3. In very high doses, nicotinic acid causes vasodilation and lowers blood cholesterol; nicotinamide does not. These actions of nicotinic acid at high doses are considered pharmacological (Lipton and Kane, 1983).

Also included under the rubric of nutrition is the study of food allergy and hypersensitivity either to specific foods or to commercial additives. Reactive hypoglycemia—generally attributed to high carbohydrate diets that result in the over-production of insulin which, in turn, leads to hypoglycemia—has also been studied in relation to clinical states as diverse as panic disorders, depression, and aggression leading to crime and delinquency (Gray and Gray, 1983; Gorman et al., 1983).

NUTRITIONAL PRINCIPLES

Humans, as evolutionary products of the animal kingdom, have nutritional needs similar to those of other mammals. The complex foods humans eat are digested to simpler molecules, which are then absorbed and resynthesized under genetic interactions to the multitude of compounds of which we are made. Maintenance of body temperature, movement, growth, repair, and reproduction require energy supplied mainly by the oxidation of carbohydrates and fat. Metabolic end products such as exhaled carbon dioxide or urinary nitrogen metabolites need constant replacement from dietary intake. Even the body minerals are constantly turning over metabolically and must be replaced by ingested food. For growth and development, a positive balance of calories and essential nutrients must be supplied. For adult maintenance the balance should be zero. Control of appetite and food intake involves a complex set of sensors and feedback systems in the brain and endocrine system which are beyond the scope of this chapter.

Despite the capacity of each species to synthesize the myriad of compounds unique to it, some needs must be supplied in the diet. These include water, the major anions and cations of the cellular fluids and skeleton; and trace elements such as copper, manganese, cobalt, fluorine, vanadium, selenium, and zinc. Ten amino acids, which cannot be synthesized and must be furnished, are needed for the synthesis of proteins and other nitrogenous compounds. Thirteen vitamins are required: Four of these are fat soluable; eight are members of the vitamin B complex; and the last is vitamin C, which is uniquely required by humans, primates, the guinea pig, an East Indian bat, and a bird. It is a remarkable testimony to the synthetic capacities of the body that the thousands of compounds of which we are made can all be synthesized from approximately two dozen organic compounds furnished in the diet.

Several features of human nutritional needs deserve comment. First, as mentioned previously, the human species is quite rare in requiring vitamin C. The evolutionary purpose of this need is not known. Second, the human is an omnivore who eats a greater variety of foods than any other known species except perhaps the rat. Undoubtedly, this characteristic offers a great evolutionary advantage since it permits humans to survive on the indigenous food of any region on earth. Third, the human being is apparently the only species whose choice of diet is determined by taste, smell, color, appearance, and even texture. The human is the only animal for whom eating is both a necessity and an aesthetic experience. In contrast to most animals who eat the same food every day of their lives, humans constantly seek variety. The aesthetic qualities of food have had interesting social consequences. For example, it may be argued that Columbus discovered America while looking for food additives, that is, the spices that help to preserve food and enhance its taste and color. In the industrialized United

States, food companies use food additives to compete vigorously in producing products that are more attractive than those of their competitors. Many food fads are based on presumed but unproven hazards created by commercial food processing. Humans still attribute to food magical properties that can hurt or help them.

Fourth, the precise nutritional requirements for humans are less well known than they are for the domesticated animals which supply their food. There are several reasons for this. Experiments can be done on food animals which cannot be done safely with human subjects. Animals are bred to be genetically homogeneous and efficient in their conversion of food to milk, eggs, or edible animal protein. Their daily activities and energy output are much more closely regulated than are those of humans. Finally, the economics of the food industry make it essential to know the minimum food requirements for maximum growth and marketability. Despite the difficulties in precisely determining the nutritional requirements of humans, reasonable estimates have been made since 1941 by the Food and Nutrition Board, National Research Council of the National Academy of Sciences. These are revised every five years; the ninth edition (NAS, 1980), offers recommended daily allowances (RDA) for calories, protein, minerals, and vitamins for men, women, and children. The RDA's are not minimal requirements. Recognizing substantial variance in human nutritional needs because of genetic heterogeneity and living habits, the RDA's are calculated by the board to exceed average nutritional needs by a "safe margin," allowing for individual differences in a basically healthy population. The magnitude of the safety factor is substantial. For example, the minimal requirement for folic acid is estimated to be about 50 micrograms per day; the RDA is 400 micrograms. The RDA's have been accepted by the American Medical Association (AMA, 1979) and are used by the Food and Drug Administration for food labeling. They are also the basis on which the Department of Agriculture and the United States Health Service established national food programs and nutritional educational programs. The RDA's can be found in most standard medicine, pharmacology, and biochemistry texts (Serban, 1975; Lipton and Kane, 1979; Schneider et al., 1983).

In an affluent society, man's omnivorous appetite and his wish for variety make it easy to obtain a nutritionally sound, balanced diet. RDA requirements are generally met by diets that offer a mixture of four food groups in adequate proportions: (a) fruits, vegetables, and fruit juices; (b) grains and grain products; (c) meats and meat products; and (d) milk and milk products. Such diets offer adequate nutrients as well as taste and variety. When they are consumed, vitamin or mineral supplementation is not required. Impoverished populations here or abroad who subsist largely on grain and who have no variety in their diets generally need supplementation with vitamins, minerals, and other proteins.

Under special conditions of illness, severe dieting, heavy alcohol consumption, stress, pregnancy, or lactation, supplementation with modest quantities of vitamins may be desirable. Massive supplementation with megadoses of vitamins is required only for three conditions: (a) in the genetic vitamin dependency or insufficiency illnesses; (b) when there are transport difficulties for nutrients in the gut or across other cell membranes; and (c) when antivitamin antimetabolites are used, as in the treatment of cancer.

Malnutrition generally produces mental changes along with somatic changes such as weight loss or anemia. In early or minimal nutritional deficiencies, mental changes may occasionally appear before readily observable physical changes ensue. But careful examination will reveal lowered blood or tissue levels of vitamins or minerals. Perusal of the literature shows that weakness, irritability, anxiety, anorexia, lassitude, depression, apathy, anergia, headache, dizziness, and inability to concentrate have been reported in subjects or patients with mild deficiency of any of the water soluble vitamins. When the deficiency is severe, memory loss, disorientation, delusions, hallucinations, and other signs of dementia may appear. Some orthomolecular psychiatrists believe that the brain may have nutritional requirements so much larger than those of the other body tissues that cerebral avitaminosis may exist and may account for much major mental illness.

Protein Calorie Malnutrition

Many studies conducted in impoverished societies have shown that severe, prolonged protein calorie malnutrition is especially devastating to infants and children and that the consequences are prolonged and likely irreversible. The results of such studies have been summarized in several monographs derived from international conferences on this subject (DeLicardi and Cravioto, 1973; Frankova, 1974). The reasons for this high vulnerability are the rapid growth of the human brain in infancy and the effects of malnutrition on that growth and development. Winnick (1964) has shown that, in humans, the number of brain cells increases linearly from gestation until birth and then more slowly until about ten months of age, at which time it virtually stops. Cell size, in contrast to cell number, continues to increase for several years. The weight of the brain increases rapidly from gestation through the first two years of life; its rate of growth diminishes thereafter, but adult weight is not reached until adolescence.

Studies of the brains of children who have died from marasmus in the first two years of life show 15 to 50 percent fewer brain cells than normal children of comparable age. Children with kwashiorkor who become malnourished after being taken off the breast in the second or third year of life have a normal number of brain cells but the size of the cells is diminished (Plum, 1974). Studies of the behavior of children who survive early malnutrition show that such children have profound disturbances in the acquisition of language, motor skills, interpersonal relationships, and adaptive and motivational behavior. Memory defects have also been found (DeLicardi and Cravioto, 1973; Winnick, 1964). Most of these studies have been limited to children studied only a few years after recovery from malnutrition. However, an ongoing longitudinal study by Cravioto and DeLicardi (Tizard, 1973) should ultimately answer the question of whether or not the damaging consequences of early malnutrition are truly irreversible. If they are, this fact would lead to a vicious cycle in which malnutrition during infancy results in a large pool of poorly functioning people, who, because of their poor level of functioning, rear their children under conditions destined to produce a new generation of malnourished people (Winnick, 1964; Tizard, 1973).

Children born into the poverty that leads to malnutrition also live in social and family environments that are themselves capable of retarding mental and behavioral development. Some ingenious experiments on rats, conducted by Frankova (1974), have shown that protein deficient rats raised with their mothers and litter mates show about a 20 percent decrement in exploratory activity. Rats that are on normal diets but have restricted optical and acoustical stimuli show about a 30 percent decrement in exploratory activity. Rats deprived of both protein and environmental stimuli show a 90 percent decrement. The effects of both types of deprivation simultaneously are thus more than additive; they are synergistic. The introduction of an "aunt," a nonpregnant virgin female, into the cages of protein deprived infant rats elevated their performance to that of normal rats, even though such a "mother's helper" did not lactate and was unable to offer food. She did, however, stimulate them by grooming and retrieving them.

DeLicardi and Cravioto have conducted experiments that led to similar conclusions in impoverished children from an agricultural community in Central America. In this population, 83 percent of the children showed no clinical signs of malnutrition, 11 percent showed mild and moderate malnutrition, and five percent showed severe malnutrition. Yet, the families of all the children had approximately equal incomes, land, and food. Therefore, no correlation could be established between the amount of food available to the families of these children and the level of malnutrition. However, a significant correlation was found by psychologists who studied this cohort of children while unaware of their nutritional antecedents. They found that the degree of psychological stimulation offered at age six months to those children who later developed severe malnutrition was significantly lower than that of controls from the same population matched by age and birth weight. Psychosocial deprivation in children whose diets are nutritionally marginal predisposes them to severe malnutrition, and malnutrition in turn to diminished activity, motivation, exploratory behavior, and those complex signals that ordinarily elicit a stimulating and gratifying response from parents. A vicious cycle is thus set up in which the effects of malnutrition synergize with those of environmental deprivation. The consequences may lead to irreversible emotional and mental disorders of development. The interaction between nutrition and psychosocial stimulation is not unique to rats or humans. All species that have been studied show the same interaction (Frankova, 1974).

VITAMIN DEFICIENCY STATES

Vitamin Requirements

Several methods have traditionally been used to determine the vitamin requirements of human subjects. One, commonly used with conscientious objectors during World War II, was the deliberate production of nutritional deficiency followed by the measurement of the quantity of nutrient required to eliminate the signs and symptoms of the deficiency and to maintain health. This quantity was then considered the recommended dietary allowance and was added to the K rations of U.S. troops. Variations on this strategy use populations in which nutritional deficiency is endemic. Another approach is to measure in the blood and urine abnormal metabolites of carbohydrate and protein known to exist in specific deficiencies. For example, elevated blood lactate and pyruvate occur in thiamine deficiency. The dose of a specific vitamin required to correct this biochemical abnormality is considered to be the daily requirement. The third approach is the direct measurement of the vitamin in the blood and urine by chemical or microbiologic means. "Normal" levels have been established. This strategy involves the use of large populations of healthy subjects of different ages, sexes, and races in order to obtain normative data. Recently a new approach to the measurement of vitamin requirements has been proposed, which is based on the assumption that the enzymes requiring cofactors should be fully saturated with cofactor at all times and that a vitamin deficiency exists if they are unsaturated. For example, serum or erythrocyte glutamic-oxalacetic transaminase activity is measured with and without added pyridoxal phosphate, the cofactor. If activity is greater with added cofactor, the enzyme is unsaturated and a deficiency is said to exist. This method is somewhat controversial, but it may be useful in detecting cases of vitamin deficiency and vitamin insufficiency illnesses (Kishi et al., 1975).

Using such methods, a number of vitamin deficiency states relevant to psychiatry have been found. Usually they are secondary to the use of pharmacological agents and most commonly follow the long-term use of antituberculosis drugs, anticonvulsants, oral contraceptives, and anti-tumor drugs (Lipton and Kane, 1983).

The functions of the water soluble vitamins in the nervous system, the manifestations of deficiency, and the vitamins' therapeutic utility have recently been reviewed in great detail (Wurtman and Wurtman, 1983; Lipton et al., 1979).

Vitamin B₆ (Pyridoxine)

Vitamin B_6 has many neurobiological functions. It is the precursor of a coenzyme required for more than 50 enzymes in the body. It is so widely distributed in our food supply that a deficiency in it has not been found to occur in populations throughout the world. Deficiency states have been produced experimentally, however. Mental symptoms associated with deficiency include lassitude, weakness, depression, anorexia, and confusion. Somatic symptoms include a microcytic anemia that fails to respond to iron but improves dramatically following treatment with small doses of the vitamin. Isoniazide and cycloserine form carboxyl addition compounds with pyridoxal or pyridoxal phosphate which make B_6 unable to function as a cofactor in the approximately 50 enzymes with which it is associated. The administration of vitamin B_6 supplement along with antituberculosis medication reveals that both neurologic and psychiatric symptoms disappear when supplementary vitamin is given in appropriate quantities (Cohen, 1969).

Estrogens have been shown to compete with pyridoxal phosphate for binding sites among its numerous apoenzymes. High estrogen levels, which occur during pregnancy or the use of oral contraceptives, seem to increase the requirements for vitamin B_6. In therapeutic trials on women who developed depression during pregnancy or while taking oral contraceptives, vitamin B_6 supplementation has been reported to improve mood and to correct the abnormal urinary excretion of tryptophan metabolites (Price et al., 1967; Price and Toseland, 1969; Winston, 1973). Based on such findings some investigators recommend the inclusion of supplemental B_6 in oral contraceptive preparations (Price and Toseland, 1969). In Spain, manufactured oral contraceptives contain 25 mg of pyridoxine, and the combination is reported to produce fewer side effects (Otte, 1969). The RDA for vitamin B_6 for adults is 2.0 mg/day. Doses ten times this are safe and can prevent deficiencies due to drugs administered for other purposes. Although vitamin B_6 is not very toxic, doses several hundred or thousand times the estimated daily requirement have been reported to cause convulsions and liver hypertrophy (Winter and Boyer, 1983). There is a recent report of severe sensory neuropathy from pyridoxine abuse at doses of 2-6 g for several months (Rudman and Williams, 1983; Schaumberg et al., 1983). These toxicities must be balanced against any presumed therapeutic utility from huge doses of vitamin B_6.

Vitamin B₃

Vitamin B$_3$ (niacin, niacinamide, nicotinic acid, nicotinamide) is combined with adenine, ribose, and phosphoric acid in the body cells to form nicotinamide adenine dinucleotide (NAD). NAD is a cofactor for many enzymes that catalyze oxidation-reduction reactions, which are involved in energy release from carbohydrates, the synthesis of fatty acids, steroid metabolism, etc. Niacin, in the judgment of some, is not truly a vitamin because limited quantities can be synthesized from the metabolism of the essential amino acid tryptophan (Smythies, personal communication). While this is correct, historical usage and the fact that niacin deficiency can be produced on diets ordinarily adequate in tryptophan seem to warrant its continued classification as a vitamin. Corn, which is deficient in both tryptophan and niacin, is the common food staple in countries where pellagra was common and where it continues to exist. Hartnup disease is an autosomal recessive disease characterized by diminished absorption of neutral amino acids, including tryptophan. Some of its symptoms resemble pellagra, and these respond to niacin (Dakshinamurti, 1977). The recommended daily allowance of niacin is 6.6 mg/1000 calories of food or about 10-20 mg/day. The requirement increases during pregnancy and lactation (Dakshinamurti, 1977).

Pellagra is characterized by a triad of symptoms—dermatitis, diarrhea, and dementia. In early deficiency, psychiatric symptoms are diffuse and include apathy, depression, anxiety, and memory deficits. In severe pellagra, mania, delirium, organic dementia, bulbar palsy, and visual field deficits may be present. The EEG has excessive theta and delta activity, which returns to normal after niacin treatment. Routine manufacture of wheat flour and all cereal products supplemented with niacin has caused pellagra virtually to disappear in the U.S. Niacin deficiency in the brain without deficiency in other tissues has been claimed by orthomolecular psychiatrists to account for schizophrenia and other mental disturbances. This theory will be discussed later.

In pharmacological doses of 10-30 g/day, nicotinic acid, but not nicotinamide, lowers blood cholesterol and causes transient cutaneous vasodilation manifested by a flush (Lipton et al., 1979). Nicotinamide, but not nicotinic acid, at doses of 250 mg/day, tranquilizes rodents and diminishes locomotor activity in gerbils (Beaton, 1976). At similar doses, it increases REM sleep and has been reported to be of benefit to some insomniacs (Beaton et al., 1974). Nicotinamide also binds weakly to the benzodiazepine receptor (Mohler et al., 1979). At ordinary dietary doses, the brain concentrations of nicotinamide are likely to be too low for biologically significant binding to this receptor; but at megadoses such binding might occur and niacinamide might have anxiolytic properties similar to those of the benzodiazepines. This theory has not been tested. Nicotinic acid and nicotinamide are identical as vitamins; the different properties of the two compounds occur only at pharmacological doses. Thus, there is no evidence to relate their pharmacological properties shown at high doses to their classical vitamin action as precursors of NAD. Niacin and niacinamide are not very toxic even in megadoses, but in view of their use in orthomolecular psychiatry at doses 100 to 500 times higher than the average nutritional requirement, it is worth noting that reported side effects include hepatoxicity (Winter and Boyer, 1973), hypotentsion, tachycardia, and hyperglycemia (Mosher, 1970).

Vitamin B_{12} (Cyanocobalamin)

Vitamin B_{12} (cyanocobalamin) is unique in three regards: It is the only vitamin containing a mineral (cobalt) as part of its chemical structure; it is not found in plants; and its absorption from the gut requires a highly specialized mechanism, the failure of which results in pernicious anemia. The RDA is about 0.3mg/day. One microgram daily causes remission of pernicious anemia. The vitamin is involved in transmethylation reactions and the synthesis of amino acids, purines, and pyrimidines. It is vital for blood formation and the maintenance of neuronal integrity.

A number of studies have shown that 25 to 30 percent of patients with untreated pernicious anemia have either major or minor psychiatric problems (Herman et al., 1937). These include depression and apathy, irritability, confusion, and paranoid states. Neurological symptoms result from demyelination of the dorsal columns of the pyramidal tracts, causing the syndrome known as combined system disease. As many as 60 percent of untreated pernicious anemia patients have been found to have an abnormal EEG (Herman et al., 1937; Cohen, 1975). Deficiencies of vitamin B_{12} may arise from strict vegetarian diets but more often follow failure to absorb the vitamin, as when there is lack of the gastric intrinsic factor or in ileitis and following bowel surgery. Pernicious anemia may also follow salicylic acid or colchicine. There is an increased requirement for vitamin B_{12} during pregnancy. Since folic acid is required for the absorption of B_{12}, folate deficiency may be accompanied by B_{12} deficiency (Ordonez, 1979; Carney and Sheffield, 1970).

Although a large percentage of patients with hematologic and neurologic findings of vitamin B_{12} deficiency also have psychiatric symptoms, in a significant number of patients the psychiatric manifestations may be the first symptoms and can antedate anemia or spinal cord disease. A recent report (Evans et al., 1983) presents two cases of organic psychosis without anemia or spinal cord symptoms which responded dramatically to the appropriate administration of intramuscular B_{12}. It is noteworthy that both patients had normal hematologic profiles. Diagnosis was made by finding low serum levels of B_{12}. With restoration of appropriate B_{12} levels, the presenting symptoms disappeared. Evans et al. (1983) recommend consideration of B_{12} deficiency and serum B_{12} determination in all patients with organic psychiatric symptoms whose cause is not clearly known. Even more recently, Van Tiggelen et al. (1983) have suggested that blood levels of B_{12} may not always correlate with cerebrospinal fluid levels and that the latter may be much lower.

Folic Acid

Folic acid (pteroylglutamic acid) is involved in hydroxylation reactions required for norepinephrine and serotonin synthesis; transmethylation reactions; and the synthesis of the purine bases, adenine and guanine, and the pyrimidine base thymine. Folic acid is, therefore, indispensible for the production of DNA and RNA. Transmethylation reactions are involved in myelin synthesis and in the inactivation of the neurotransmitters norepinephrine and serotonin. The RDA is less than 0.5 mg/day but doubles during pregnancy. Serum concentrations in humans range from 5 to 30 ng/ml. Folate deficiency has been produced in experimental animals, and diminished learning capacity and EEG changes have been reported in rat pups born of mothers with folate deficiency.

Folic acid, as the name implies, is present in leafy green vegetables and meats. In humans, folate deficiency occurs endemically in severely malnourished populations. It can be produced experimentally in volunteers on folate deficient diets and iatrogenically in marginally nourished people by the administration of anticonvulsants such as diphenylhydantoin, oral contraceptives, or the antifolates used in the treatment of malignancy. In experimental folate deficiency, forgetfulness and insomnia appear at the same time as megaloblastic anemia and can be quickly reversed by the vitamin. In less pure deficiency states, occurring among the aged or chronically institutionalized patients, the spectrum of mental disorders includes apathy, irritability, depression, psychosis, delirium, and dementia (Thornton and Thornton, 1978).

Folate deficiency can be readily determined by measurement of blood levels. When this is done, as many as 30 percent of psychiatric admissions have been reported to be deficient (Thornton and Thornton, 1978). Of a sample of admissions to a psychogeriatric ward, 67 percent have been reported to be folate deficient (Williams, 1971). Carney and Sheffield (1970) found that about 25 percent of 432 psychiatric admissions had low blood folate levels. Patients with organic psychoses, endogenous depression, and schizophrenia who were treated with folate had shorter hospital stays and left in better clinical condition than untreated patients.

An association between folate deficiency and gestational difficulties has been recognized for many years. Population surveys have shown that about 15 percent of women, especially among the poor, have marginal or deficient blood levels. Deficiency during pregnancy is associated with an increase in prematurity and teratogenicity.

In the last few years, evidence has accumulated which tends to relate folic acid deficiency during early gestation to neural tube defects and to the Fragile X syndrome of mental retardation. Both of these are polygenic illnesses in which the phenotypic expression of the genotypic defect is apparently determined by the nutritional state of the uterine environment. Smythells (1982) has found that when 493 women who had already given birth to a child with neural tube defect gave birth to a second child, 23 of these children also had such a defect. In 397 similar women who were given a vitamin supplement containing folic acid prior to conception and through the first missed menstrual period, only three had such recurrences. This strikingly significant difference cannot be readily explained except by a direct prophylactic effect of vitamin supplementation very early after conception.

The Fragile X chromosome is a relatively newly discovered cause of mental retardation. The fragility of the X chromosome can be rectified *in vitro* by folic acid (Southerland, 1979). Lejeune (1982) has reported that the administration of folic acid greatly reduced symptoms of autism and psychotic complications of mental retardation in seven out of eight patients.

Both of these interesting findings clearly require confirmation. If confirmed, they will represent a major advance in the understanding and treatment of two devastating illnesses of concern to neurologists, psychiatrists, and pediatricians through appropriate nutritional supplementation early in gestation. A series of studies has shown that folic acid can be added to staple foods, as nicotinic acid commonly is, and that such fortification is feasible, safe, and effective (Herbert, 1980). Until this is done, oral administration of folic acid tablets at a level of 0.5 mg/day to pregnant women, especially those living in poverty, appears to be prudent (Herbert, 1980).

A genetic vitamin dependency illness that requires about 20 mg of folic acid daily has also been reported. These rare cases presented with homocystinuria. One such patient showed mild retardation with symptoms of schizophrenia, which improved after folate administration and recurred six months after the supplementary vitamin was discontinued (Freeman et al., 1975).

PRECURSOR THERAPY

It is generally accepted that communication between neurons in the central nervous system is overwhelmingly chemical. Neurotransmitters synthesized in presynaptic neurons are extruded into the synaptic cleft when the neuron fires. They then engage specific receptors on post-synaptic neurons and initiate a series of metabolic steps which may excite, inhibit, or modulate their activity. More than 20 neurotransmitters are thought to exist;

they range in composition from simple amino acids to complex polypeptides. The classical neurotransmitters, dopamine, norepinephrine, serotonin, and acetylcholine, have been the most thoroughly studied. The paradigm for precursor therapy is the use of L-dopa in Parkinson's disease. The
enzyme for the conversion of tyrosine to L-dopa is lacking in the striatal
neurons of the brains of patients with this disease but the decarboxylation of
L-dopa to dopamine can still take place. Hence, L-dopa in pharmacological
doses permits the synthesis of sufficient dopamine to be therapeutically
effective for several years.

More than a decade ago, Wurtman and co-workers discovered that the
synthesis and release of several neurotransmitters in presynaptic neurons
can be influenced by the concentration of precursors offered to them. The
amino acids tryptophan and tyrosine are the precursors of serotonin and
norpinephrine, respectively. Choline is the precursor for the synthesis of
acetylcholine. The conversion of precursors to active neurotransmitters is
enzymatic. When saturating concentrations of the precursors are available,
the rate at which transmitters can be synthesized is limited by the enzymatic
capacity. But concentrations of the dietary precursors in the blood are not
constant and under some conditions the rate-limiting enzymes may not be
saturated but can become so if large doses of precursors are administered.
Precursor therapy is relatively safe because feedback inhibition and other
neuronal control mechanisms prevent the synthesis of more transmitter
than is needed by the neuron at any particular time. Consequently, few side
effects are noted when subjects are given pharmacological doses of tyrosine,
tryptophan (Wurtman, 1983), or choline (Cohen and Wurtman, 1975; Mohs
et al., 1979), that is, amounts much greater than the quantities usually
ingested in the diet. The finding that brain neurotransmitter levels can be
altered by experimentally manipulating the quantity of ingested precursor
has led to considerable basic research as well as clinical research on both
normal volunteers and patients in whom there is reason to believe that there
may be a neurotransmitter deficiency.

Dietary precursors must be absorbed from the gut, transported in the
blood, penetrate the blood-brain barrier, and finally enter into appropriate
neurons. These are complex processes that depend initially on the quantity
of the precursor in the diet, the effectiveness of the gut in absorbing them,
and the transport mechanisms within the blood. Circulating amino acids
then compete with each other for active transport through the blood-brain
barrier into the brain (Wurtman et al., 1980; Growden, 1979). The ratio of
plasma tryptophan, for example, to the sum of the concentration of other
neutral amino acids such as tyrosine, phenylalanine, leucine, isoleucine,
and valine determines the penetrability of tryptophan into the brain, hence,
the brain serotonin concentration. Thus, a high protein meal in which many
amino acids compete for transport into the brain depresses serotonin
synthesis in the rat brain (Wurtman et al., 1980; Fernstrom and Wurtman,

1972). A high carbohydrate, low protein meal raises brain serotonin because it elicits the secretion of insulin, which lowers the blood levels of other neutral amino acids without affecting tryptophan. Doses of tryptophan as large as 10-15 g would be more likely to diminish transport of other amino acids into the brain than doses of 1-3 g.

Tryptophan and Tyrosine

Tryptophan, administered at a dose of 50mg/kg to healthy young men in the morning, significantly increased self-reports of fatigue and inertia and reduced vigor and activity (Wurtman, 1983). It is interesting to note that in this same experiment, tyrosine at 100mg/kg had undetectable effects. It is also worth noting that tryptophan did not cause depression, anxiety, confusion, or anger in this experiment.

Tryptophan has also been used in treating insomnia with apparently favorable effects. Doses of 1-5 g before bedtime have been reported to reduce sleep latency without producing distortions of physiological sleep as measured by EEG recordings (Hartmann, 1977). Doses of 10-15 g cause EEG changes, but these are less pronounced than those resulting from the use of hypnotics. The mechanism for the effectiveness of tryptophan in insomnia is presumed to be due to its effects on serotonin levels in the brain stem (Hartmann, 1977). The use of L-tryptophan to treat insomnia is still experimental even though the amino acid is available for sale in health food stores. The current literature suggests that it would have substantial advantages over conventional hypnotics, but it appears not to be uniformly effective for insomniacs. Furthermore, the long-term effects of doses of 5-15 g per day require further investigation.

Serotonin deficits have been implicated in some depressions and mania, and clinical trials with tryptophan have yielded mixed results (Carroll, 1971; Prange et al., 1974). Since tryptophan is rapidly catabolized by liver pyrrolase, it was hypothesized that the concomitant administration of an inhibitor could more effectively raise brain serotonin. Nicotinic acid and nicotinamide are both pyrollase inhibitors; and in a preliminary report, encouraging results were obtained with the combination of tryptophan and nicotinamide in the treatment of depression (Chouinard et al., 1977). These results have not been confirmed. In very recent work, it has been reported that tryptophan diminishes sensitivity to mild pain and in people over 40 increases the likelihood of errors in performance tasks (Spring et al., in press).

The administration of tyrosine can, under certain circumstances, elevate levels of brain catecholamines (Wurtman et al., 1980; Growden et al., 1982). It has been reported to help some patients with depression (Gellinberg and Wurtman, 1980) and mild Parkinson's disease (Growden et al., 1982). Continued clinical research in which tyrosine or tryptophan is used with depressed patients might help to distinguish depressions in which norepinephrine is involved from those in which the defect may be in serotonin metabolism.

Choline and Lecithin

Several studies have shown that the administration of choline or lecithin, the precursors of acetylcholine, increased cholinergic function in the brain (Cohen and Wurtman, 1975). On the basis of this finding, clinical research has been conducted in conditions in which there is a possible disorder in acetylcholine metabolism. Tardive dyskinesia is one such disorder. Presumably the disorder arises because of prolonged administration of neuroleptics, which chronically block striatal dopamine receptors and cause these receptors to become supersensitive to dopamine (Gerlach et al., 1974). Some dopamine receptors are present on cholinergic neurons, and their supersensitivity probably causes a chronic decrease in the release of acetylcholine by decreasing the firing rates of the cholinergic neurons. Davis et al. (1975) reported marked clinical improvement after giving oral choline to a patient with tardive dyskinesia. Several additional studies have confirmed this finding (Growden et al., 1977; Tamninga et al., 1977). Unfortunately, large doses of choline have undesirable side effects, including a socially unacceptable odor which results from the degradation of ingested choline to trimethylamine by intestinal bacteria. Lecithin, a phosphatidylcholine, is the most common source of dietary choline. Lecithin is more effective than choline in raising plasma choline levels (Wurtman et al., 1977). Several reports suggest that it, too, is effective in diminishing symptoms of tardive dyskinesia (Jackson et al., 1979; Barbeau, 1978). A review of the literature suggests that there is modest improvement in the motor function of about one-half of the patients who receive lecithin. Interestingly, the antipsychotic action of neuroleptics has not been reported to be diminished by the administration of either choline or lecithin.

Choline has been administered to schizophrenic subjects and failed to modify their clinical symptoms (Davis et al., 1979). Lecithin has been administered to manic patients with encouraging results (Cohen et al., 1980). Disorders in acetylcholine function have been suggested in Huntington's disease, Friedreich's ataxia, and Gilles de la Tourette's syndrome. The results of therapeutic trials with choline or lecithin in those illnesses are equivocal. They have been reviewed by Growden et al. (1977).

Alzheimer's disease, the most common cause of dementia among the elderly, is characterized by impaired functioning of cholinergic neurons. On autopsy, the brains of such patients show a dramatic loss of brain choline acetyltransferase (Davies and Maloney, 1976; Davies, 1979; Wurtman et al., 1980). Memory deficits are characteristic of Alzheimer's disease, and many studies have been conducted to measure the effects of acetylcholine precursors in normal individuals and in patients with Alzheimer's disease (Mohs et al., 1979; Ferris et al., 1979). These studies have not convincingly shown any enhancement of memory after treatment with acetylcholine precursor. However, a preliminary report from an ongoing double-blind trial suggests that large doses of lecithin preparations containing high concentrations of phosphatidylcholine may have beneficial effects in some Alzheimer's disease patients (Levy et al., 1983).

Alternative methods for enhancing cholinergic activity include the use of cholinesterase inhibitors and cholinergic agonists. Physostigmine, a reversible short-acting cholinesterase inhibitor and arecoline, a short-acting cholinergic agonist, improve memory when given in low doses to healthy young adults (Davis et al., 1978; Sitaram et al., 1978). Physostigmine, in a double-blind experiment, enhanced the memory processes of patients with Alzheimer's disease for brief periods (Davis and Mohs, 1982).

It is curious that physostigmine, which enhances cholinergic function by inhibiting the enzyme that destroys acetylcholine, should be more effective than precursors that increase the concentration of this neurotransmitter. The reason is not known, but it immediately raises the question of whether a combination of a precursor and a choline agonist or cholinesterase inhibitor might be additive or synergistic. This idea has not yet been tested.

The precursor strategy with tryptophan, tyrosine, and choline has thus far yielded results that are of great research interest but have only preliminary and uncertain clinical utility. This type of research is young and vigorous. One might guess that greater clinical efforts from precursors may be achieved when they are combined with other types of psychotropic drugs. Tryptophan or tyrosine combined with tricyclics might accelerate the therapeutic process or decrease the required dose in depression. Stern and Mendels (1981) have reviewed the literature on the use of such combinations in the treatment of refractory depression. A recent report suggests that the combination of physostigmine and lecithin improves memory in Alzheimer's disease (Davis and Mohs, 1982).

Food Additives and Hyperkinesis

In 1975, the late Ben F. Feingold, M.D., a pediatrician and allergist, proposed that some children have a central nervous system variant that predisposes them to sensitivity to synthetic food additives, particularly to food colors and the antioxidants butylated hydroxyanisole (BHA) and butylated hydroxytoluene (BHT). He claimed that in such children hyperkinetic behavior results from the ingestion of these additives. Feingold based his findings on extensive clinical experience in open studies. He did not conduct controlled, double-blind trials to test his hypothesis. The Feingold dietary treatment gained considerable popularity among the lay public, and more than 20,000 families of hyperkinetic children were reported to adhere to the diet and to advocate its use (Morrison, 1978). Several uncontrolled clinical studies supported Feingold. Rigorous double-blind studies conducted in seven centers and involving about 200 children, however, have generally failed to replicate his findings (National Advisory Committee on Hyperkinesis and Food Additives, 1980; Consensus Development Conference Statement, 1982).

Food and Environmental Allergy and Hypersensitivity

The notion that hypersensitivity or allergy to foods or other environmental agents such as gasoline fumes, soaps, or hydrocarbons results in medical or psychiatric illness is subscribed to by what Brodsky (1983) calls a "medical subculture." It has been popularized extensively in books and in the media (Randolph and Moss, 1980; Bell, 1982; Randolph 1962; Gerhard, 1980). Symptoms that have been related to such sensitivity or allergy include lethargy, depression, palpitations, sleep disturbance, mood swings, poor concentration, anxiety attacks, aggressiveness, and delinquent behavior. The Feingold hypothesis (Feingold, 1975) that hyperactivity and learning disability in children are related to the ingestion of common synthetic food additives seems to be a specific variant of the food hypersensitivity thesis which focuses on synthetic food additives and natural salicylates. Hoffer (1979a) has claimed that many of his schizophrenic patients who failed to respond favorably to megavitamins do respond to five days of starvation followed by diets in which single items of food to which the patients are not sensitive are carefully introduced.

Pierson et al. (1983) recently sought objective evidence for the role of food hypersensitivity in 23 patients who attributed a wide variety of their physical and psychological symptoms to food allergies. These patients were seen independently for initial diagnosis by a psychiatrist who withheld his findings from the other investigating physicians. The allergists assessed the patients by medical and dietary history, a physical examination, and skin tests for common inhalant and food antigens. The patients were then put on exclusion diets consisting of uncommon foods to which they had no alleged hypersensitivity. All the patients improved. Single foods that the patients had themselves incriminated were then added openly. Many patients became ill with their initial complaints. Blind tests were then performed using the same foods, freeze dried, and in opague capsules. The investigators found that only four of the 23 patients had true food hypersensitivity. None of these four had significant psychiatric symptoms; and all of them had physical symptoms characteristic of atopy, i.e., allergic rhinitis, urticaria, asthma, or atopic eczema, which appeared even when the offending foods were given blindly. The 19 in whom food hypersensitivity could not be confirmed in the blind trials had physical and psychological symptoms not characteristic of the atopic syndrome. Eighteen of these 19 patients had been diagnosed by the intake psychiatrist as having significant psychiatric illness; ten were considered neurotically depressed, and the remainder had other neuroses and personality disorders although none were psychotic. The authors conclude that psychogenic reactions to food are common and that some form of double-blind testing is the only certain means by which the diagnosis of food hypersensitivity can be established. They note that "since the dangers of unwise dietary restriction are real, patients should not be encouraged to restrict their diet without specialist, dietetic advice and without objective confirmation of food hypersensitivity."

There have been claims that food allergies are responsible for delinquency and criminal behavior (Schauss 1980; Rimland, 1981; Hoffer, 1978), and statements have been made that food allergies are common in delinquents although prevalence rates are not given. The only reported double-blind studies of behavioral change in relation to food allergy have used sublingual testing, a method whose validity is considered doubtful (Grieco, 1982).

Clinical ecologists go further. Patients are initially tested for dietary sensitivity and are placed on elimination diets. If these are not helpful, they are placed in a "chemical free" environment in a hospital. If they improve in that environment, they are then treated by prescribed avoidance of environments that include such common substances as perfume, smoke, etc. to which they claim to be sensitive. Such avoidance inevitably leads to major changes in their lives, including a move to a "clean climate." Patients may also receive injections of the indicted substances in order to desensitize themselves. According to Brodsky (1983) they spend a great deal of their time on diets, conducting tests for sensitivity, and participating in a support group of similar patients. The views of clinical ecologists are not shared by most academic and practicing allergists and immunologists (Greico, 1982).

Schizophrenia and Gluten

In 1966, Dohan suggested that peptides derived from cereal grain glutens may play an important role in the pathogenesis of schizophrenia in genetically predisposed people. This proposal was based on the observations of considerably higher than chance occurrence of celiac disease in schizophrenics as well as schizophrenia among adults with celiac disease. In addition, both schizophrenia and celiac disease have been reported to be three times more prevalent in Ireland than in England and Wales. Dohan also found a strong correlation between a change in rates of admission of female patients with schizophrenia to psychiatric institutions and a change in wheat consumption during World War II among five countries (United States, Canada, Finland, Sweden, and Norway) variously affected by the war. Following these observations, he and his colleagues studied the effects of milk-free and cereal-free diet on schizophrenic patients. Forty-seven schizophrenic patients randomly assigned to a cereal-free diet showed a significant increase in rate of release from hospitals compared to 55 patients on a high cereal diet. No difference was found when wheat gluten was added to the cereal-free diet in a subsequent double-blind study (Dohan et al., 1969).

Singh and Kay (1976) found that schizophrenic patients who received neuroleptics and a cereal-free, milk-free diet showed a significant decline when challenged with wheat gluten in a double-blind manner. They suggested that clinical improvement on a gluten-free diet and subsequent deterioration on gluten challenge may be related to a gluten mediated decrease in neuroleptic absorption. In support of this theory, Fried et al. (1978) found that wheat gluten given to mice 20 minutes before a 1 mg/kg dose of haloperidol reduced the amount of neuroleptic absorbed into the blood stream. Recently, however, Osborn et al. (1982) found that five chronic schizophrenic patients did not improve on a gluten-free diet; furthermore, the gluten-free diet had no effect on blood levels of butaperazine, which had been administered in constant doses throughout the study. The study, however, selected patients who had failed to respond to traditional neuroleptic therapy and who thus might represent an atypical subpopulation. Also, as the authors note, their patients were on the special diet for only 36 weeks. Dohan and Grasberger (1973) stressed that chronic patients may require months or years of gluten-free diets before significant results are achieved.

Potkin et al. (1981) studied eight chronic schizophrenic patients who were maintained on a diet free of gluten, cereal grains, and milk and who were challenged in a double-blind manner with dietary wheat gluten and placebo. They found no deterioration in clinical status (as measured by the Brief Psychiatric Rating Scale) on gluten challenge; however, Singh and Kay (1983) have pointed out that with an N of eight, the authors' chances of detecting a true small or medium effect of gluten would be only seven percent and 15 percent, respectively.

Hallert (1982), who has studied many celiacs in Sweden, where the disease has a relatively high prevalence rate, found no schizophrenia in adult celiacs but did find significant depression. He suggests that celiac disease is not an appropriate model. Dohan (1983) recently reviewed the evidence supporting the model and suggests approaches for further study.

Recently, Zioudrou et al. (1979) reported that gluten peptides have naloxone-reversible endorphin activity at brain opiate receptor sites. This finding might explain a link between gluten-free diets and clinical response in a subpopulation of schizophrenics. However, such a relationship has yet to be demonstrated consistently, and the important observations of Dohan's group and of Singh and Kay merit exploration.

Reactive, Relative, or Postprandial Hypoglycemia

In animals and humans, food intake is intermittent and yet the blood sugar levels, except for transient rises after eating, remain relatively constant. Such homeostasis requires the synchronized participation of the liver, muscles, pancreas, other endocrine organs, and the central nervous system. Most body tissues can tolerate fluctuations in blood sugar; but the brain, which is unable to store glucose or glycogen in significant quantities and which uses glucose as its primary fuel, requires a constant supply. In the resting state, the brain accounts for 80 percent of the glucose consumed by the body.

Glucose homeostasis is remarkably effective. In a normal population, fasting levels of plasma glucose range from 50-115 mg/dc. Such levels occur five to six hours after feeding and do not change significantly overnight. In well nourished individuals, blood glucose levels change very little after several days of fasting. Many physical illnesses such as diabetes or islet cell tumors of the pancreas can either elevate or lower the fasting blood sugar (Williams, 1981; Davidson, 1982).

Reactive, relative, or postprandial hypoglycemia is an abnormal degree of depression of the extracellular glucose concentration reflected in the plasma, without a well defined cause. When plasma levels fall below 50 mg/dc or blood levels below 40 mg/dc, symptoms and signs of adrenergic hyperactivity, nervous system depression, or a combination of the two usually appear. Hypoglycemic activation of the adrenergic system causes tremulousness, anxiety, hunger, sweating, palpitations, and tachycardia. Central nervous system hypoglycemia causes perturbations of cortical and subcortical functions with symptoms of fatigue, headache, weakness, diplopia, confusion, amnesia, poor coordination, seizures, and coma. The cluster of symptoms of hypoglycemia varies substantially from patient to patient.

Several of the symptoms of hypoglycemia resemble those with which anxious, depressed, and hypochondriacal patients present. Consequently, some patients may diagnose themselves as having hypoglycemia. The tendency to do so is augmented by popular books in the lay press which have featured hypoglycemia as a global cause for a welter of illnesses and antisocial behaviors such as "nervous breakdown," alcoholism, juvenile delinquency, drug dependence, inadequate sexual performance, and overt aggression in prisoners (Schauss, 1980; Fredericks, 1969; Duffy, 1975). While most endocrinologists, psychiatrists, and criminologists have not accepted nutritional theories and dietary treatments of neurotic and antisocial behavior, these theories have, nonetheless, had an impact on prisons, probation departments, and school systems. The Los Angeles County Probation Department, for example, banned the consumption of chocolates, other sweets, and refined sugar products from juvenile facilities and is trying to reduce consumption of processed and additive-containing foods in prisons (Overend, 1973). There have also been malpractice suits in which patients have claimed that their physicians missed the diagnosis of reactive hypoglycemia and, therefore, treated them inappropriately.

The concept that postprandial or reactive hypoglycemia is common in the population has not been generally accepted by the medical profession. The American Diabetes Association (1973), in collaboration with other societies, has published statements to downplay the prominence of the misattribution of hypoglycemia as a cause of multiple illnesses. Yager and Young (1974) have referred to the epidemic proportions of the incorrect diagnosis of hypoglycemia as a cause for various other somatic and psychiatric complaints. Too often the diagnosis is made without a glucose tolerance curve at all. Diagnosis by questionnaires that attempt to relate symptoms to eating habits is inadequate. Many patients who have affective, somatization, or anxiety disorders report a relationship of symptoms to food intake which is not borne out in a glucose tolerance test (Williams, 1981; Leggett and Favazza, 1978; Lev-Rin and Anderson, 1981).

The reasons for the conflict between those who emphasize hypoglycemia as a major contributor to multiple psychiatric illnesses and those who discount it lie largely in the rigor with which a five-hour glucose tolerance test is conducted and in how it is interpreted. In this test, the patient should be prepared by eating a diet containing about 250 g of carbohydrate daily for three days. He then fasts overnight and is given 50-100 g of sugar orally in solution. Alterations in plasma or blood glucose are monitored at half-hour intervals for the ensuing five hours while subjective symptoms are recorded. The typical normal glucose tolerance curve shows a rise of 60-70 mg/dc in the first 30 to 60 minutes; this is the period when glucose enters the circulation from the gastrointestinal tract. In normal persons, increasing glucose concentration, abetted by cholinergic signals, stimulates insulin secretion. The increased circulating insulin, in conjunction with declining glucagon production, results in decreasing hepatic glucose output and a fall of blood glucose to levels approximating or slightly lower than the fasting state over the next four hours. By the fifth hour, there is usually recovery to base levels. At its peak, blood glucose levels in normal subjects seldom exceed 160 mg/dc. Higher levels suggest diabetes. At the nadir, glucose levels below 50 mg/dc should raise the suspicion of reactive hypoglycemia. For a definitive diagnosis to be made, the low blood sugar values should coincide in time with the symptoms of adrenergic activation and central nervous system hypoglycemia referred to above. The diagnosis should not be made on the basis of a low blood sugar without clinical symptoms or on symptoms alone without a low blood sugar. Many patients report symptoms and signs of anxiety with blood sugar levels above 70; others may have the blood sugar fall to levels of below 40 without manifest symptoms or signs of hypoglycemia (Leggett and Favazza, 1978). Since the glucose tolerance test may vary from day to day in any patient, borderline tests should be repeated.

The notion that hypoglycemia is related to panic attacks has recently been tested by Gorman et al. (1984). These investigators measured the blood sugar in ten patients who met *DSM-III* criteria for panic disorder or agoraphobia at the moment the patient experienced panic during an infusion of 0.5 molar sodium lactate under single-blind conditions. They found that, on the average, such patients had a fasting blood sugar of 98 mg/dc and at the moment of panic it was 94 mg/dc. None of these patients had serum glucose levels even close to hypoglycemic levels. These findings demonstrate that hypoglycemia is not a necessary condition for panic attacks but do not, of course, prove that hypoglycemia may not cause panic attacks. To determine the latter, it may be necessary to lower blood sugar experimentally in such patients by an insulin tolerance test and then determine whether it triggers panic and whether the blood sugar levels correlate well with the onset of panic. It is also now possible for patients who suspect that they have hypoglycemia related to panic, or to any other clinical symptoms, to screen themselves at home by collecting capillary blood on impregnated filter paper. They can measure the blood sugar levels themselves or send the tests to a laboratory for analysis (Marks, 1983). In either type of experiment, a close correlation between clinical symptoms and blood sugar values must be found in order to designate hypoglycemia as a proximate cause of the symptoms. It seems likely that such research will soon be conducted.

In summary, there is little evidence from carefully conducted research to support the concept that reactive hypoglycemia is a common condition and that it is causally related to psychiatric or behavioral disorders.

ORTHOMOLECULAR PSYCHIATRY

The theory, practice, and clinical value of megavitamin therapy and orthomolecular psychiatry have been the subject of debate for almost 20 years. An American Psychiatric Association Task Force (1973) reviewed the evidence thoroughly in 1973 and was very critical. Orthomolecular psychiatrists responded (Hoffer and Osmond, 1976), calling the task force report biased, unfair, and full of errors. Pauling (1974) was also critical; his criticisms were answered by Klein (1974) and Wyatt (1974). A book, *Orthomolecular Psychiatry: Treatment of Schizophrenia*, which details their theory and practice was published in 1973 (Hawkins and Pauling, 1973). A detailed update of the APA Task Force critique, which included a review of the role of the water soluble vitamins in the nervous system, was published in 1979 (Lipton et al., 1979). The present chapter summarizes some older reviews and adds material published since that time.

Orthomolecular Theory

The term "megavitamin therapy" was coined in the early 1950's to describe a treatment for acute schizophrenia that used vitamin B_3 (nicotinic acid or nicotinamide) in the dose range of 3-30 g daily. The theoretical basis for this treatment was initially pharmacological, not nutritional. The originators of megavitamin therapy attributed the pathogenesis of schizophrenia to the endogenous formation of adrenochrome and adrenolutein, which are hallucinogenic condensation products of oxidized adrenaline. Adrenaline is formed by methylation of noradrenaline and, in schizophrenia, the formation was thought to be excessive. The megavitamin therapists thought that these products caused perceptual distortions that were the primary causes of schizophrenia and that the perceptual defects could be detected and quantified by a psychological card sorting test called the Hoffer-Osmond Diagnostic Test (HOD).

The proponents of megavitamin therapy see schizophrenia as primarily a perceptual disorder. For example, Hawkins, co-editor of the book *Orthomolecular Psychiatry* (Hawkins and Pauling, 1973) says,

> Clinically, the illness begins as altered subjective experiences associated with changes in perception and these may or may not in time result in the observable changes upon which a diagnosis of schizophrenia has hitherto been based.... At this stage of the illness, the diagnosis may be made by interviewing techniques focused on detection of these subjective changes. The perceptual changes may also be detected by objective measures such as the HOD and EWI tests which parallel changes in the severity of the illness. The stage of the illness may be called metabolic disperception. It precedes the appearance of overt clinical schizophrenia—the signs and symptoms of schizophrenia are secondary to the perceptual disorders and these in turn precede the tertiary impairments in social functioning.

Hawkins then presents evidence to support the proposition that all of the manifestations of schizophrenia can be produced by perceptual changes alone. He describes the HOD score as being more accurate than the usual clinical criteria in evaluating the degree of the patient's illness and response to treatment. He says (Hawkins and Pauling, 1973),

> The majority of patients that we see with schizophrenia are not overtly psychotic. Although schizophrenia is technically classified as a psychosis, the development of irrationality indicates an advanced degree of the state of the illness. We, therefore, view schizophrenia as a disease process which is capable of producing psychosis.

He continues,

> The HOD test consists of 145 true-false questions, read and answered by the patient which are designed to measure visual, auditory, olfactory, touch, taste, and time perception as well as thought and mood disturbances. Underlying this work is the assumption now supported by substantial experimental evidence that there is a genetic predisposition in schizophrenics which under certain conditions leads to errors in metabolism resulting in the formation of chemicals that may interfere with

the function of the central nervous system which is responsible for maintaining perceptual abilities.

Kelm (Hawkins and Pauling, 1973) defines patients with metabolic disperception as "people who suffer from varying degrees of abnormal perception, with corresponding changes in thought, mood and behavior who respond favorably to megavitamin B_3 and allied therapy if treated before irreversible damage has developed." Subclinical pellagra is defined as:

> a deficiency syndrome characterized by the presence of perceptual changes affecting any or all of the five senses associated with neurasthenia. The HOD and related tests can measure the degree of perceptual abnormality and changes in thought and mood.

Hawkins (Hawkins and Pauling, 1973) continues,

> For routine use, the HOD test . . . is the most useful test, not only to confirm the diagnosis, but also to determine the degree of illness and to monitor the response to treatment. Beneficial measures are followed by a reduction of the HOD score and deleterious measures or an increase in the illness are followed by an increase. It can be administered and scored by anyone in the office. Shock treatment brings the most rapid reduction in the HOD score, the phenothiazines will also lower the score considerably, but usually not to within normal range. The patient can take the test retroactively; that is, he can answer the question according to how he felt when most ill or at any specified time in the past.

Hoffer remains committed to nicotinic acid deficiency as the primary cause of schizophrenia, which he sees as cerebral pellagra. He says (Hawkins and Pauling, 1973),

> If all the vitamin B_3 were removed from our food, everyone would become psychotic within one year. This pandemic psychosis would resemble pellagra and it would resemble schizophrenia. It could not be called pellagra, because none of the antecedents of that disease would exist.
>
> Schizophrenia and pellagra are not identical since they require different quantities of vitamin B_3. Most symptoms of pellagra are alleviated by doses of vitamin B_3 below 1 gram/day, but a small proportion may need many times as much. Most schizophrenia respond to 3 to 6 grams, but a small proportion may require more than 20 grams per day.

But Hoffer also believes in the use of ECT in the treatment of schizophrenics who do not respond to megavitamins. Commenting on the failure of others to confirm megavitamin therapy, he says (Hawkins and Pauling, 1973),

> Several experiments are underway, but they are testing only one part of the program. For example, they do not use ECT. It is, therefore, necessary to reiterate that the megavitamin program is not one which can be completed in a single month or six months or a year. Time alone is no criterion. One starts with the simplest therapy that is chemotherapy alone using megavitamin doses plus all the other

chemotherapies available to psychiatry as indicated in each case. The patients who recover are maintained on the program in order to keep them well. Patients who do not recover within three months are then given a series of ECT in addition to the chemotherapy. They may require a second or even a third series. With any acute series, using ECT if there is insufficient improvement within three months of beginning chemotherapy, one can expect a recovery rate of over 90 percent within one year and improvement in the other 10 percent.

He also says (Hawkins and Pauling, 1973),

All patients were treated with phenothiazines, megavitamins, accessory symptomatic medication, group therapy and all the other usual adjunctive measures. The exception was that 85 patients received ECT and 55 served as controls. When the results were tabulated and graphed, the very significant effect of ECT was observable. This was most marked in the younger age groups.

To prevent or treat schizophrenia, it was thought necessary to reduce adrenaline formation. Since adrenaline was formed by methylation of noradrenaline, a means to diminish methylation was sought. When nicotinic acid or nicotinamide is administered in large doses, n-methyl-nicotinamide is formed and is rapidly excreted; hence, both compounds are methyl acceptors. Since they are relatively nontoxic in large doses, they were chosen as competitive inhibitors of the methylation of noradrenaline. It is worth emphasizing that they were not chosen as nutrients; indeed, in a 1957 publication advocating the use of nicotinic acid in the treatment of schizophrenia, Hoffer et al. (1957) speculated about the mechanism of therapeutic action of nicotinic acid. They chose as the most likely mechanism the ability of nicotinic acid to be a methyl acceptor that would reduce the formation of the endogenous hallucinogen adrenochrome. They rejected its role as a vitamin, saying (Hoffer et al., 1957),

Psychosis [sic] association with pellagra does in many ways resemble the schizophrenia psychosis except that it contains qualities of toxic confusion. However, the incidence of avitaminosis among schizophrenic persons is no greater than among the general population. Doses adequate to treat any unknown deficiency are without affect on schizophrenia; it may, therefore, be concluded that this factor is unimportant.

In 1968, Pauling (1968) published a theoretical paper in which he suggested that some forms of mental illness might be due to deficiencies in essential nutrients occurring in susceptible individuals eating an ordinarily adequate diet. Man's genetic heterogeneity, he suggested, leads to biochemical individuality, with large variations in the need for essential nutrients, especially vitamins (Pauling, 1968). The brain might differ from other organs in its nutritional requirements so that localized cerebral deficiency could occur. Pauling named his concept "orthomolecular psychiatry," and he defined it as "the treatment of mental disease by the provision of the optimum molecular environment for the mind, especially the optimum concentration of substances normally present in the human body."

With the publication of this interesting theoretical paper, clinicians who had been practicing megavitamin therapy adopted Pauling's concept and claimed that what they had been practicing from 1952 to 1968 was, indeed, orthomolecular psychiatry. This conceptual shift from the transmethylation hypothesis in which nicotinic acid was a pharmacological methyl acceptor to a nutritional hypothesis in which schizophrenia was cerebral pellagra treatable by nicotinic acid functioning as a true vitamin was accompanied by the formation of the Academy of Orthomolecular Psychiatry and a name change of the group's *Journal of Schizophrenia* to *Journal of Orthomolecular Psychiatry*.

With this shift in theory, many other vitamins and hormones were added to the orthomolecular therapeutic armamentarium. The scope of the conditions that orthomolecular psychiatrists treat has also been expanded to include autism, hyperkinesis, depression, anxiety, alcoholism, drug addiction, and delinquency, among others. The current practice is perhaps best described by Hawkins et al. (1970):

> Clinicians practicing orthomolecular psychiatry are using a combination approach which varies from patient to patient depending upon the biochemical peculiarities of a given case and which often include high doses of niacin or niacinamide, ascorbic acid, pyridoxine, vitamin E, thyroid, vitamin B_{12}, hypoglycemic diets, cereal free diets, daily physical exercise, lithium, the phenothiazines, and also the commonly used tranquilizers and antidepressants.

Electroconvulsive therapy is still frequently used (Hoffer, 1978).

The change in the theory of schizophrenic pathogenesis from excessive transmethylation to nutritional deficiency broadened the therapeutic ingredients of orthomolecular practice greatly. With the first theory, there was a pharmacological need for nicotinic acid as a methyl acceptor and no special needs for other vitamins and nutrients. With the nutritional theory there is room for the addition of many other micronutrients to the therapeutic program. In current practice, many nutrients are added in megadoses simultaneously. Nonetheless, nicotinic acid always seems to be included in the therapeutic prescription for schizophrenia because that illness continues to be regarded as cerebral pellagra. Hoffer (1973) says, "It is clear that there are no clinical grounds for separating the two diseases. A distinction is artificial." He also says, "Schizophrenia is a vitamin B_3 dependent condition or an NAD deficiency disease" (Hoffer, 1973).Nonetheless, other water soluble vitamins and minerals are also used in megaquantities. The concept of reactive hypoglycemia and of food or environmental allergies as causative agents in many types of mental illness and behavioral disorders has also been adopted (Paterson, 1982).

The transmethylation hypothesis is testable and has been evaluated by many investigators over the past 20 years. No evidence of any excess transmethylation has been found. If anything, there may be diminished transmethylation (Smythies et al., 1979; Kelsoe et al., 1982). There is also neither clinical nor laboratory evidence for a metabolic defect similar to that found in pellagra in any of the schizophrenias. This subject was thoroughly reviewed a decade ago in the APA task force report (APA, 1973) and no evidence to the contrary has appeared since that time.

The Pauling statement that there is an optimal molecular environment for the neurons in the brain is probably true; but it is not testable, because optimal, especially for any single individual, cannot be defined or determined. Pauling noted that optimal intake of phenylalanine should be very low for the patient with phenylketonuria. But, in general, he tended to view optimum as very much larger than the RDA. He suggested that genetic variance in the transport of vitamins across the blood-brain barrier might, in selected individuals, result in a cerebral avitaminosis despite normal blood and other tissue levels of these nutrients. He also felt that the protein might be genetically defective so that much higher concentrations of apoenzymes for which vitamins or their derivatives function as coenzymes would be necessary in order for the enzymes to function. He stated that "the so-called gene for schizophrenia may itself be a gene that leads to a localized cerebral deficiency in one or more vital substances" (Pauling, 1974, 1968).

Roger Williams (1956), more than 30 years ago, presented evidence for a degree of variability within a species, which he called "biochemical individuality," which might account for differences in nutritional requirements. Pauling's hypothesis was an elaboration of Williams' thesis. And, while Williams' thesis is not arguable in principle, the quantitative aspects need empirical testing.

We all readily accept biochemical individuality for such areas as height, weight, hemoglobin, intelligence, caloric needs, metabolic rate, etc.; but, generally speaking, such variability is seldom more than 15 percent. Orthomolecular theory suggests that differences in vitamin requirements might be as great as several thousand percent. Some evidence has been found in rare genetic diseases to support this theory. There are about 25 known genetic "vitamin-responsive in-born errors of metabolism" (Rosenberg, 1974). These disorders are genetic autosomal recessives and are so rare that fewer than 1,000 cases have been described in the world literature. All of the water soluble B vitamins except niacin and riboflavin have been implicated. Vitamin dependency illnesses are characterized by an increase in the requirement for a specific vitamin that ranges from ten to several hundred times the RDA, due to mutant apoenzymes that require high concentrations of cofactor to function.

Vitamin dependency illnesses are manifest at birth or in early childhood, and they are generally associated with mental retardation as well as with multiple somatic disorders ranging from convulsions to severe anemias. Patients with these illnesses show demonstrable abnormalities in circulating amino acids or other metabolites. Unless they are treated with megadoses of the appropriate vitamin early in life, such patients show retardation in growth and development and usually die in childhood. Orthomolecular psychiatrists apparently believe that the large differences in nutritional needs that occur in the rare genetic vitamin dependency illnesses are common in psychiatric patients of all types. Hoffer (1973), for example, believes that schizophrenia is a vitamin B_3 dependent condition or an NAD deficiency disease. Since schizophrenia fails to meet the many other criteria established for the definition of autosomal recessive genetic diseases, it becomes necessary for him to postulate that the vitamin dependency characteristic is localized to the brain.

There is another genetic variant less severe than the vitamin dependency illnesses, which Blass and Gibson (1977) call "vitamin insufficiency illness" and which occurs in that small fraction of alcoholics who develop Wernicke-Korsakoff syndrome. Such patients are apparently able to grow normally to adulthood on ordinary daily requirements of thiamine and an average diet; but under the unusual circumstances of heavy alcohol consumption, when the vitamin intake diminishes and the vitamin requirement may increase, the syndrome develops. This condition can be detected by measuring a thiamine dependent protein apoenzyme called transketolase which in Wernicke patients requires a much higher concentration of thiamine pyrophosphate to function adequately. Folkers et al. (1978) have reported that patients with carpal tunnel syndrome may also have a vitamin insufficiency syndrome because their erythrocyte glutamate oxaloacetate transminase (EGOT) is unsaturated at normal dietary levels of pyridoxine. At megadoses the enzyme becomes saturated and new enzyme synthesis is induced. Of interest in this regard is a recent report by Harrison et al. (1983) of a patient who suddenly developed carpal tunnel syndrome, accompanied by low serum pyridoxine levels, while receiving the MAO inhibitor tranylcypromine. Presumably the amine group on the MAOI reacted with the aldehyde of pyridoxal phosphate, forming a physiologically inactive amine and a functional deficiency of pyridoxine. With the addition of pyridoxine (300 mg/day) to the treatment the symptoms subsided. Also of interest to psychiatry is the report of Rimland et al. (1978), who recently found that massive doses of pyridoxine could improve the symptoms of about 30 percent of autistic children and that in such children pyridoxine causes a drop in the urinary excretion of homovanillic acid, a major metabolite of dopamine. It is, therefore, possible that a subgroup of autistic children may have a vitamin B_6 insufficiency illness. Detection of this particular subgroup can thus far not be made clinically or biochemically. Moreover, even though some improvement occurs when these children are given pyridoxine, they are still far from being well.

The possibility that schizophrenia or even a significant subgroup of the schizophrenias is a vitamin dependency illness must be considered remote. Vitamin dependency illnesses have multiple somatic abnormalities which have not been found in schizophrenics. Patients with these illnesses are generally mentally retarded, and they have distinct biochemical abnormalities in the blood or urine which are detectable at birth or in early infancy. They respond quickly and dramatically to large doses of the single vitamin required to remedy their genetic metabolic abnormality. Schizophrenia fails to meet any of these criteria. Is schizophrenia a vitamin insufficiency illness which resembles the Wernicke-Korsakoff syndrome? Again, it is unlikely. A vitamin specific enzyme defect has not been found, nor is there any evidence of a metabolic abnormality.

RECENT STUDIES

Some literature has appeared in the last several years dealing with megavitamin therapy and orthomolecular principles in autism, learning disability, and mental retardation. Rimland et al. (1978), as already mentioned, conducted a double-blind crossover study of the effects of high doses of vitamin B_6 on autistic children. LeLord et al. (1982) have studied the effects of high doses of vitamin B_6 and magnesium on autistic children. Both groups have reported positive findings. The results suggest that in a heterogeneous illness such as autism there may be a subgroup of patients who respond to this treatment. The degree of response is modest but statistically significant.

Kershner and Hawke (1979) studied the efficacy of adding megavitamins to a low carbohydrate, high protein diet with 20 learning disabled children who carried diagnoses of hyperactivity, minimal brain dysfunctions, or both. After a double-blind six-month period of treatment, the addition of megavitamins failed to produce any significant improvement when compared to the diet alone on a variety of intellectual, school achievement, perceptual, and behavioral measures. The efficacy of the diet alone could not be assessed because no dietary control group was used. The parents of 18 of these children reported improvement in their children on this diet regardless of whether megavitamins or placebo was added. As the authors cautiously point out, this finding may reflect parent enthusiasm and/or the child's maturation rather than dietary effects.

In 1981, Harrell et al. (1981) reported the results of a study in which 16 children (age 5-15) with either Down's syndrome or unclassified mental retardation (IQ 17-70) received either placebo or a supplement containing 11 vitamins and eight minerals for a four-month period. All subjects were also placed on diets that restricted the intake of "sugary foods and soft drinks" and encouraged consumption of fruits and milk. All but one of the subjects were also given thyroid hormone because of low morning axial temperatures. At the end of four months, the children were evaluated by two of seven psychologists who did not all use the same IQ testing instruments. One of the psychologists, the principal investigator, was not blind to the conditions of the experiment. During the first four months of treatment, the five children who received supplemental vitamins increased their average IQ by 5-9.6 points and the 11 subjects on placebo showed negligible change. In a second phase of the experiment, all 16 subjects received vitamin supplements; the 11 subjects who had been on placebo in the first phase showed an average IQ increase of 10 points. The Harrell study has received considerable attention because of the implications of its conclusions. However, it has also received much criticism because of the weakness of its design and methodology.

Coburn et al. (in press) carried out a replication study using mentally retarded young adults. This experiment was conducted entirely on a double-blind basis with a uniform IQ testing procedure. None of the subjects, including those on the Harrell supplementation, showed any improvement in performance on the Stanford Binet test at ten to 20 weeks. Admittedly, the Coburn study examined mentally retarded patients who were older than those studied by Harrell et al. Possibly, improvement in IQ may be limited to very young subjects. However, given the methodological weaknesses in the Harrell study and the absence of confirmatory replication studies at this point, there is reason to be skeptical. Replication studies are required both for professional responsibility and in the public interest.

CONCLUSION

Nutritional research in relation to psychiatry continues at a steady, if not spectacular, pace. The pharmacological use of nutrients as in percursor therapy shows considerable promise. The special nutritional requirements of the early fetus and of geriatric patients are receiving constant attention, and it seems very likely that these will be better understood and treated. Unique nutritional requirements of most psychiatric patients have not been scientifically demonstrated. Nutritional treatments of the common major psychiatric illnesses and behavior disturbances remain questionable.

REFERENCES

American Diabetes Association: Diabetes statement on hypoglycemia. Diabetes 22: 137, 1973

AMA Concepts of nutrition and health: report of the Council of Scientific Affairs adopted by the House of Delegates. JAMA 242:2335, 1979

APA Task Force Report #7: Megavitamin and Orthomolecular Therapy in Psychiatry. Washington, DC, American Psychiatric Association, 1973

Beaton JM, Pegram GV, Smythies JR, et al: The effects of nicotinamide on mouse sleep. Experentia 30:926-927, 1974

Beaton JM: The sedative effects of nicotinamide on gerbil wheel-running activity. Experientia 32:1036-1037, 1976

Bell IR: Clinical Ecology: A New Medical Approach to Environmental Illnesses. Valenes, Calif, Common Knowledge Press, 1982

Blass JP, Gibson GE: Abnormality of a thiamine-requiring enzyme in patients with Wernicke-Korsakoff syndrome. N Engl J Med 297:1367-1370, 1977

Brodsky CM: Allergic to everything: a medical subculture. Psychosomatics 24:731-742, 1983

Carney MWP, Sheffield PF: Associations of subnormal serum folate and vitamin B_{12} values and effects of replacement therapy. J Nerv Ment Dis 154:404-412, 1970

Carroll BJ: Monamine precursors in the treatment of depression. Clin Pharmacol Ther 12:743-761, 1971

Chouinard G, Young SM, Hannibal LE, et al: Tryptophan nicotinamide combination with depression (ltr to ed). Lancet 1:249, 1977

Coburn SP, Schaltenbrand WE, Mahuren JD, et al: Effect of megavitamin treatment on mental performance and vitamin B_6 metabolism in mentally retarded adults. Am J Clin Nutr (in press)

Cohen AC: Pyridoxine in the prevention and treatment of convulsions and neurotoxicity due to cycloserine. Ann NY Acad Sci 166:346-349, 1969

Cohen BM, Miller AL, Lipinski JF: Lecithin in mania: a preliminary report. Am J Psychiatry 137: 242-243, 1980

Cohen EL, Wurtman RJ: Brain acetylcholine increase after systemic choline administration. Life Sci 16:1095-1102, 1975

Cohen MM: Nutritional disorders involving the nervous system, in Biochemistry of Neural Disease. Edited by Cohen MJ. Hagerstown, Md, Harper and Row, 1975

Consensus Development Conference Statement: Defined Diets and Childhood Hyperactivity. Bethesda, Md, National Institutes of Health, 1982

Dakshinamurti K: B vitamins and nervous system function, in Nutrition and the Brain, vol 1. Edited by Wurtman RJ, Wurtman JJ. New York, Raven Press, 1977

Davidson MB: Diabetes mellitus and hypoglycemia, in Endocrine Pathophysiology: A Patient Oriented Approach. Edited by Hershman JM. Philadelphia, Lea & Febiger, 1982

Davies P, Maloney AJ: Selective related enzymes in senile dementia of the Alzheimer's disease (ltr). Lancet 2:1403, 1976

Davies P: Neurotransmitter related enzymes in senile dementia of the Alzheimer type. Brain Res 171:319-327, 1979

Davis KL, Berger PA, Hollister LE: Choline for tardive dyskinesia. N Engl J Med 293:152, 1975

Davis KL, Hollister LE, Berger PA: Choline chloride in schizophrenia. Am J Psychiatry 136:1581-1584, 1979

Davis KL, Mohs RC, Tinklenberg JR, et al: Physostigmine: improvement of long term memory processes in normal humans. Science 201:272-274, 1978

Davis KL, Mohs RC: Enhancement of memory processes in Alzheimer's disease with multiple dose intravenous physostigmine. Am J Psychiatry 139:1421-1424, 1982

DeLicardi E, Cravioto J: Behavioral responsiveness of survivors of clinical severe malnutrition to cognitive demands, in Early Malnutrition and Mental Development, Swedish Nutrition Foundation XII. Edited by Cravioto J, Hambraeus L, Vahlquist B. Uppsala, Almquist and Wiksell, 1973

Dohan FC, Grasberger JC: Relapsed schizophrenics: earlier discharge from the hospital after cereal-free, milk-free diet. Am J Psychiatry 130:685-688, 1973

Dohan FC, Grasberger JC, Lowell FM, et al: Relapsed schizophrenics: more rapid improvement on a milk and cereal free diet. Br J Psychiatry 115:595-596, 1969

Dohan FC: More on celiac disease as a model for schizophrenia. Biol Psychiatry 18:561-564, 1983

Duffy W: Sugar Blues. New York, Warner Books, 1975

Evans DL, Edelson GA, Golden RN: Organic psychosis without anemia or spinal cord symptoms in patients with vitamin B_{12} deficiency. Am J Psychiatry 140:218-221, 1983

Feingold B: Why Your Child Is Hyperactive. New York, Random House, 1975

Fernstrom JD, Wurtman RJ: Brain serotonin content: physiological regulations by plasma neutral amino acids. Science 178:414-416, 1972

Ferris SH, Sathanathan G, Reisberg B, et al: Long term choline treatment of memory impaired elderly patients. Science 205:1039-1040, 1979

Folkers K, Ellis J, Watanabe T, et al: Biochemical evidence for a deficiency of vitamin B_6 in the carpal tunnel syndrome based on a crossover clinical study. Proc Natl Acad Sci USA 75:3410-3412, 1978

Frankova A: Interaction between early malnutrition and stimulation in animals, in Early Malnutrition and Mental Development, Swedish Nutrition Foundation XII. Edited by Cravioto J, Hambraeus L, Vahlquist B. Uppsala, Almquist and Wiksell. 1974

Fredericks C: Low Blood Sugar and You. New York, Constellation International, 1969

Freeman JM, Finkelstein JD, Mudd HS: Folate-responsive homocystinuria and schizophrenia. New Engl J Med 292:491-496, 1975

Fried WJ, Luchins DJ, Gillin JC, et al: Wheat gluten impedes absorption of haloperidol. Biol Psychiatry 13:769-772, 1978

Gellinberg AJ, Wurtman RJ: L-tyrosine in depression. Lancet 2:863-864, 1980

Gerhard JW: Food Allergy: New Perspectives. Springfield, Ill, Charles C Thomas, 1980

Gerlach J, Reisby N, Randrup A: Dopaminergic hypersensitivity and cholinergic hypofunction in the pathophysiology of tardive dyskinesia. Psychopharmacologia 34:21-35, 1974

Gorman JM, Martinez JM, Liebowitz MR et al: Hypoglycemia and panic attacks. Am J Psychiatry 141:101-102, 1984

Gray GE, Gray LK: Diet and juvenile delinquency. Nutrition Today, May 1983, pp 14-22

Grieco MH: Controversial practices in allergy. JAMA 247:3106-3111, 1982

Growden JH, Cohen EL, Wurtman RJ: Huntington's disease: clinical and chemical effects of choline administration. Ann Neurol 1:418-422, 1977

Growden JH, Hirsch MJ, Wurtman RJ, et al: Oral choline administration to patients with tardive dyskinesia. N Engl J Med 297:524-527, 1977

Growden JH, Melamed E, Logue M, et al: Effects of oral L-tyrosine administration on CSF tyrosine and homovanillic acid levels in patients with Parkinson's disease. Life Sci 30:827-832, 1982

Growden JH: Neurotransmitter precursors in diet: their use in the treatment of brain diseases, in Nutrition and the Brain, vol 3. Edited by Wurtman RJ, Wurtman JJ. New York, Raven Press, 1979

Hallert C: Psychiatric illness, gluten and celiac disease. Biol Psychiatry 17:959-961, 1982

Harrell RF, Capp RH, Davis DR, et al: Can nutritional supplements help mentally retarded children? An explanatory study. Proc Natl Acad Sci USA 78:574-578, 1981

Harrison W, Stewart S, Lovelace R, et al: Case report of carpal tunnel syndrome associated with tranylcypromine. Am J Psychiatry 140:1229-1230, 1983

Hartmann E: L-tryptophan as a hypnotic: a review. Waking Sleeping 1:155-161, 1977

Hawkins D, Pauling L: Orthomolecular Psychiatry: Treatment of Schizophrenia. San Francisco, WH Freeman, 1973

Hawkins DR, Bortin AW, Runyon RP: Orthomolecular psychiatry: niacin and megavitamin therapy. Psychosomatics 11:517-521, 1970

Herbert V: Nutrition, Cultism, Facts and Fiction. Philadelphia, George F Strickley, 1980

Herman M, Most H, Jolliffe N: Psychoses associated with permicious anemia. Arch Neurol Psychiatry 38:348-361, 1937

Hoffer A, Osmond H, Callbeck MJ, et al: Treatment of schizophrenia with nicotinic acid and nicotinamide. J Clin and Exper Psychopathology 18:131-158, 1957

Hoffer A, Osmond H: Megavitamin Therapy: In Reply to the American Psychiatric Association Task Force Report on Megavitamin and Orthomolecular Psychiatry. Regina, Saskatchewan, Canadian Schizophrenia Foundation, 1976

Hoffer A: Behavioral nutrition. Journal of Orthomolecular Psychiatry 8:169-175, 1979

Hoffer A: Some theoretical principles basic to orthomolecular psychiatric treatment, in Ecologic, Biochemical Approaches to Treatment of Delinquency and Criminals. Edited by Hippochen LJ. New York, Van Nostrand-Rheinhold, 1978

Hoffer A: Mechanism of action of nicotinic acid and nicotinamide in the treatment of schizophrenia, in Orthomolecular Psychiatry: Treatment of Schizophrenia. Edited by Hawkins D, Pauling L. San Francisco, W Freeman and Co, 1973

Kelsoe JR Jr, Tolbert LC, Davis DR, et al: Kinetic evidence for decreased methionine adenosyltransference activity in erythrocytes from schizophrenics. J Neurosci Res 8:99-103, 1982

Kershner J, Hawke W: Megavitamin and learning disorders: a controlled double blind experiment. J Nutr 109:819-826, 1979

Kishi H, Kishi T, Williams RH, et al: Human deficiencies of vitamin B$_6$, I: studies on parameters of the assay of glutamic oxaloacetic transaminase by the CAS principle. Res Commun Chem Pathol Pharmacol 12:557-569, 1975

Klein DF: Comment. Am J Psychiatry 131:1258, 1974

LeLord G, Callaway E, Muhs JP: Clinical and biological effects of high doses of vitamin B$_6$ and magnesium on autistic children. Acta Vitaminol Enzymol 404:27-42, 1982

Leggett J, Favazza AR: Hypoglycemia: an overview. J Clin Psychiatry 39:51-57, 1978

Lejeune J: Is the fragile X syndrome amenable to treatment? Lancet 1:273-274, 1982

Lev-Rin A, Anderson RW: The diagnosis of postprandial hypoglycemia. Diabetes 30:996-999, 1981

Levy R, Little A, Chuoqui P et al: Early results from a double blind, placebo controlled trial of high dose phosphatidylcholine in Alzheimer's disease. Lancet I:987-988, 1983

Lipton MA, Kane FJ: Psychiatry, in Nutritional Support of Medical Practice. Edited by Schneider HA, Anderson CE, Coursin DB. Philadelphia, Harper and Row, 1983

Lipton MA, Kane FJ Jr: The use of vitamins as therapeutic agents in psychiatry, in Psychiatric Complications of Medical Drugs. Edited by Shader RI. New York, Raven Press, 1979

Lipton MA, Mailman RB, Nemeroff CB: Vitamins, megavitamin therapy, and the nervous system, in Nutrition and the Brain. Edited by Wurtman RJ, Wurtman JJ. New York, Raven Press, 1979

Marks V: Hypoglycemic screening at home. Lancet 1:14445, 1983

McNeill WH: The Pursuit of Power. Chicago, University of Chicago Press, 1982

Mohler H, Pole P, Cumin R, et al: Nicotinamide is a brain constituent with benzodiazepine-like actions. Nature 278-563-565, 1979

Mohs RC, David KL, Tinklenberg JR, et al: Choline chloride in the treatment of memory deficits in the elderly. Am J Psychiatry 136:1275-1277, 1979

Mosher LR: Nicotinic acid: side effects and toxicity. a review. Am J Psychiatry 126:1290-1296, 1970

National Advisory Committee on Hyperkinesis and Food Additives. Final Report to the Nutrition Foundation. Oct 1980

Ordonez LA: Control of the availability of the brain of folic acid, vitamin B$_{12}$ and choline, in Nutrition and the Brain, vol 1. Edited by Wurtman RJ, Wurtman JJ. New York, Raven Press, 1979

Osborn M, Crayton JW, Javaid J, et al: Lack of effect of a gluten-free diet on neuroleptic blood levels in schizophrenic patients. Biol Psychiatry 17:627-629, 1982

Otte J: Oral contraceptives and depression. Lancet 2:498, 1969

Overend W: Health Foods vs Prison Fare in County Jails. Los Angeles Times, Oct 29, 1973

Paterson ET: Aspects of hypoglycemia. Journal of Orthomolecular Psychiatry 11:151-155, 1982

Pauling L: On the orthomolecular environment of the mind: orthomolecular theory. Am J Psychiatry 131:1251-1267, 1974

Pauling L: Orthomolecular psychiatry: varying the concentration of substances normally present in the human body may control mental diseases. Science 160:265-271, 1968

Pierson DJ, Rex KJB, Bentley SJ: Food allergy: how much is in the mind? A clinical and psychiatric study of suspected food hypersensitivity. Lancet 1:1259-1261, 1983

Plum F (ed): Brain Dysfunction in Metabolic Disorders. New York, Raven Press, 1974

Potkin SG, Weinberger D, Kleinman J, et al: Wheat gluten challenge in schizophrenic patients. Am J Psychiatry 138:1208-1211, 1981

Prange AJ, Wilson IC, Lynn CW, et al: L-tryptophan in mania. Arch Gen Psychiatry 30:56-62, 1974

Price JM, Thornton MJ, Mueller LM: Tryptophan metabolism in women using steroid hormones for ovulation control. Am J Clin Nutr 20:452-456, 1967

Price SA, Toseland PA: Oral contraceptives and depression. Lancet 2:158-159, 1969

Randolph TG, Moss RW: An Alternative Approach to Allergies: The New Field of Clinical Ecology Unravels the Environmental Causes of Mental and Physical Ills. New York, Lippincott & Crowell, 1980

Randolph TG: Human Ecology and Susceptability to the Chemical Environment. Springfield, Ill, Charles C Thomas, 1962

Recommended Dietary Allowance, 9th ed. Food and Nutrition Board, National Research Council of the National Academy of Sciences, Washington, DC, NAS, 1980

Rimland B, Callaway E, Dreyfus P: The effect of high doses of B_6 on autistic children: a double-blind crossover study. Am J Psychiatry 135:472-475, 1978

Rimland B: Innovative approaches to criminality, delinquency, and violence. Int J Biosoc Res 243-248, 1981

Roe D: A Plague of Corn: The Social History of Pellagra. New York, Cornell University Press, 1973

Rosenberg LE: Vitamin-responsive inherited diseases affecting the nervous systems, in Brain Dysfunction in Metabolic Disorders, vol 53. Edited by Plum F. New York, Raven Press, 1974

Rudman D, Williams PJ: Megadose vitamins: use and misuse. N Engl J Med 309:488, , 1983

Schaumberg H, Kaplan J, Weindelank A, et al: Sensory neuropathy from pyridoxine abuse: a new megavitamin syndrome. N Engl J Med 309:445-448, 1983

Schauss AG: Diet, Crime, and Delinquency. Edited by Ershman JR. Berkeley, Calif, Parker House, 1980

Schneider HA, Anderson CE, Coursin DB (eds): Nutritional Support of Medical Practice, 2nd ed. New York, Harper and Row, 1983

Scriver CR: Vitamin responsive inborn errors of metabolism. Metabolism 22:1319-1344, 1973

Serban G (ed): Nutrition and Mental Functions. New York, Plenum Press, 1975

Singh MM, Kay SR: The problem of type II error on the "gluten hypothesis." Am J Psychiatry 140:644-645, 1983

Singh MM, Kay SR: Wheat gluten as a pathogenic factor in schizophrenia. Science 191:401-402, 1976

Sitaram N, Weingartner H, Gillin JC: Human serial learning enhancement with arecoline and impairments with performance of placebo. Science 201:274-276, 1978

Smythells RW: Neural tube defects: prevention by vitamin supplements. Pediatrics 69:498-499, 1982

Smythies JR, Morin RD, Brown GB: Identification of dimethyl-tryptamine and O-methyl bufotenin in human cerebrospinal fluid by combined gas chromatography/mass spectrometry. Biol Psychiatry 14:549-556, 1979

Smythies JR: Personal communication, 1982

Southerland GR: Hereditable fragile sites on human chromosones, I: factors affecting expression in lymphocyte culture. Am J Hum Genet 31:125-135, 1979

Spring B, Maller O, Wurtman J, et al: Effects of protein and carbohydrate meals on mood and performance. J Psychiatry Res (in press)

Stern SI, Mendels J: Drug combinations in the treatment of refractory depression: a review. J Clin Psychiatry 42:368-373, 1981

Tamninga CA, Smith RC, Erisckson SE, et al: Cholinergic influences in tardive dyskinesia. Am J Psychiatry 134:769-774, 1977

Thornton WE, Thornton BT: Folic acid, mental function, and dietary habits. J Clin Psychiatry 39:315-320, 1978

Tizard H: Epidemiology of mental retardation: implications for research of malnutrition, in Early Malnutrition and Mental Development, Swedish Nutrition Foundation XII. Edited by Cravioto J, Hambraeus L, Vahlquist B. Uppsala, Almquist and Wiksell, 1973

Van Tiggelen CJM, Peperkamp JPC, Tertoolen HJF: Assessment of vitamin B_{12} status in CSF (ltr to ed). Am J Psychiatry 141:136-137, 1984

Williams R: Nutrition Against Disease. New York, Pittman, 1971

Williams RH: Disorders causing hypoglycemia, in Textbook of Endocrinology. Edited by Ensinck JW, Williams RH. Philadelphia, WB Saunders, 1981

Williams RJ: Biochemical Individuality: The Basis for the Genotypic Concept. New York, John Wiley & Sons, 1965

Winnick M: Malnutrition and the developing brain, in Brain Dysfunction in Metabolic Disorders. Edited by Plum F. New York, Raven Press, 1964

Winter SL, Boyer JL: Hepatic toxicity from large doses of B$_3$ (niacinamide). N Engl J Med 289:1180-1182, 1983

Winter SL, Boyer JL: Hepatic toxicity from large doses of vitamin B$_6$. Vitamin Horm 22:495-501, 1973

Wurtman RJ, Hefti F, Melamed E: Precursor control of neurotransmitter synthesis. Pharmacol Rev 32:315-335, 1980

Wurtman RJ, Wurtman JJ: Nutrition and the Brain, vols 1-6. New York, Raven Press, 1983

Wurtman RJ: Behavioral effects of nutrients. Lancet 1:1145-1147, 1983

Wyatt RJ: Comment. Am J Psychiatry 131:1262, 1974

Yager J, Young RT: Non-hypoglycemia is an epidemic condition. N Engl J Med 291:907-908, 1974

Zioudrou C, Streaty R, Klee WA: Opioid peptides derived from food proteins: the exorphins. J Biol Chem 254:2446-2449, 1979

4
Electroconvulsive Therapy

4

Electroconvulsive Therapy

INTRODUCTION

Since its introduction in 1938 by Cerletti and Bini (1938), electroconvulsive therapy or ECT (known also as electroshock therapy, electroplexy, or shock therapy, to mention but a few terms) has received a mixed reception. The attitudes toward it are deeply conflicted and reflect the struggle among the psychological, biological, and social philosophies that have rivaled one another in explaining and prescribing for the treatment of emotional and mental illness. Needless to say, rational discourse has not always prevailed either in practice or in the published literature (Frankel, 1975). Unlike insulin coma and leucotomy, treatment with ECT has survived and is, in fact, attracting renewed interest.

Clinicians who are closely associated with the dramatic improvements that attend the appropriate use of ECT have been perplexed by critics who have opposed the treatment on philosophical grounds. Others have been troubled by what they view as a preoccupation with its use in some centers. The reality is that ECT can be a safe and effective treatment—at times the most effective. Nonetheless, its benefits are clearly more apparent in some cases than in others. In light of these facts, a considerable effort is being directed toward learning how to predict who will and who will not benefit from its use, and studies are continuously underway to improve the technique of administration.

Any approach to an understanding of the contemporary use of ECT must recognize the refinements that have been wrought in the procedure. More than that, basic studies are underway which seek to understand its mode of action, and the body of clinical literature on ECT is growing. Where convincing data are not yet available, reliance must be placed on commonly accepted practices and the prevailing clinical wisdom.

HISTORICAL BACKGROUND

Clinical observation in the early 1900's favored the notion that epilepsy and schizophrenia were mutually exclusive. This led to the belief that seizures might have a therapeutic effect on schizophrenic behavior. Camphor was the first convulsant and was introduced by Meduna in Budapest in 1934, only to be rapidly replaced by the more dependable pentylenetetrazol (Meduna, 1937). Finally in 1938, electrical induction of the convulsive seizure was reported by Cerletti and Bini in Rome (Cerletti and Bini, 1938). This was the start of ECT. Cerletti understood well that it was the seizure, not the electrical current, that exerted the therapeutic effect.

The new method spread to other countries, including the United States, where its use was pioneered by Kalinowsky. His singular efforts contributed to its development in this country. Convulsant therapy was soon also applied to the treatment of depressive illness in addition to the general paresis and schizophrenia for which it was first tested.

At the outset, concerns about the danger of electrocution were surely understandable, given the crudity of the treatment in its original form. All in all, however, electrical induction seemed preferable to the use of pentylene-tetrazol, which was associated with a fearful sense of impending death just prior to the onset of the seizure. More than that, the violence of the seizure itself and its aftermath provoked considerable debate. Fractures, especially of the vertebrae, and dislocations were not uncommon. Memory loss and confusion following a course of treatment evoked concern, even though these appeared to improve after a few weeks. The notion of electricity being applied to the brain was accompanied by fear that sometimes amounted to panic. The public was disturbed, and many members of the psychiatric profession were thrust into taking sides for or against the use of the treatment. Allegations of inducing spontaneous seizures, cardiovascular complications, and damage to the brain were leveled at ECT, and papers were published representing both sides of the debate. The use of curare in the early 1940's (replaced later by other safer muscle relaxants such as gallamine triethiodide and then succinylcholine) did much to alleviate the stress on the musculoskeletal system; and with the introduction of barbiturate pre-medication and brief-acting anesthesia prior to the administration of succinylcholine and the electrical stimulus, considerable progress was achieved in lessening the physical risks associated with the treatment and in reducing the patient's anxiety.

Following World War II, large numbers of patients received ECT for the treatment of schizophrenia, depressive illness, and the neuroses, notably in treatment centers committed to the biological approach to psychiatry. However, objections were voiced alleging indiscriminate use of the treatment, and the strong reservations that were widely held were expressed in a report of the Group for the Advancement of Psychiatry, dated September 1947 (GAP, 1947). Here the membership acknowledged the probable value of ECT in the treatment of involutional melancholia, questioned its value in the treatment of schizophrenia, and considered it contraindicated in the neuroses other than for symptomatic relief in severe, resistant, neurotic depressions. The report emphasized the adjuvant nature of this form of intervention, recommended it only as part of a total psychiatric treatment program, and stressed the need for further studies.

The advent of the psychotropic drugs in the early 1950's, followed by the development of the antidepressants, had a major impact on the course of modern psychiatry. Among the changes was a shift away from the use of ECT, which survived but was practiced in only comparatively few centers. Whereas the use of insulin coma in the treatment of schizophrenia virtually ceased, some academic departments did undertake to examine the relative values of pharmacotherapy, ECT, and their combined use. Then, as the limitations and side effects of the drug therapies unfolded, interest in the value of ECT was renewed. The hope grew that improved techniques would provide a safer and more effective treatment that would also help reduce the duration and cost of hospitalization.

As was true during the earliest years of ECT, its recent history has continued to include innovative methods and studies. They have been prompted by the drive to understand the nature of the treatment and to achieve a more effective procedure with fewer side effects. In this regard the following contributions are noteworthy: Cronholm and Ottosson (1960) showed the importance of the cerebral seizure per se rather than the application of electrical energy in achieving clinical improvement. Although unilateral placement of electrodes was described in 1942 (Friedman, 1942), a more widespread and serious investigation of the possible benefits of placement over the nondominant hemisphere was publicized in the 1970's. D'Elia (1970, 1974), d'Elia and Raotma (1975), Sand-Stromgren (1973), and Squire (1977) reported favorably on the lessened average memory impairment following unilateral placement. Blachly and Gowing (1966) reported on their work with multiple monitored ECT. During one anesthesia session they administered multiple seizures. They also introduced the practice of monitoring the EKG and EEG throughout the procedure, thus restricting the risks. Murillo and Exner (1973), working with severely ill schizophrenic patients, refocused attention on the possible usefulness of multiple treatments per day. Finally, the significance of the seizure in convulsive therapy was conclusively shown by comparative studies of subconvulsive and convulsive therapies (Ulett et al., 1956; Fink et al., 1958). Subconvulsive treatments were found to be of limited therapeutic efficacy.

Perhaps related to the renewed clinical interest in ECT, but just as surely a consequence of the social and political climate of the late 1960's and 1970's, ECT has become the focus of considerable public attention in recent years. In the harsh denunciations of the involuntary incarceration and treatment of the mentally ill, the side effects of all forms of physical treatments were thrust into the forefront by groups organized to fight for civil liberties and consumer rights. Both the judiciary (*Wyatt* v. *Stickney*, 1973; *Wyatt* v. *Hardin*, 1975) and legislators (California Assembly, 1976) were persuaded to lay down requirements for the administration of ECT. The *Wyatt* v. *Stickney* decision was a consequence of the generally unacceptable standards of treatment and the inadequate medical care that prevailed at the time in state mental hospitals in Alabama. The act of the California legislature, on the other hand, attempted to regulate medical practice by statute. However, it contained inaccuracies and has created cumbersome, unrealistic, and unnecessarily restrictive requirements that must be met prior to the use of ECT in that state. Furthermore, during the time that this chapter has been in preparation, unsuccessful attempts have been made to ban the use of ECT in Berkeley County, California.

Within the climate of angry rhetoric, questioning, and doubt, local authorities began to establish committees (Frankel, 1973) to study and recommend standards for the administration of ECT. In 1974, the APA Council on Research and Development resolved to establish a task force on ECT, "with tenure of about two years, to have liaison with the Commission on Judicial Action and to include in its study consideration of legislative issues, consent, indications for its use and possible increasing use because of shortened length of stay in hospital." The report of that committee was published in 1978 (APA, 1978). Some of its contents will be summarized and presented in this chapter. In keeping with the results of other evaluations, its findings support the administration of ECT as valuable, effective, and safe in appropriate cases. In addition, the report of a conference on the psychobiology of ECT sponsored by the National Institute of Mental Health and New York Medical College, (Fink et al., 1974), the proceedings of a 1978 NIMH and Temple University-sponsored conference on the impact and efficacy of ECT (NIMH, 1978), and a detailed and scholarly volume on the subject by Fink (1979) provide additional supportive evidence. They attest to the earnest nature of the investigative studies in the field and to the clinical importance of the treatment.

THEORETICAL ISSUES

The APA task force report (APA, 1978) initiated a discussion of ECT theories as follows:

An explanation of any therapeutic process is limited by our knowledge of the etiology of the disorder which the treatment is found to resolve. In the four decades of its use, the convulsive therapy process has been explained according to the prevailing theories of the etiology of mental illness. The explanations in the 1930's reflected the strong emphasis on brain pathology, while in the 1940's the explanation focused on psychological and interpersonal mechanisms. Since the 1960's, explanations have been based on neurobehavioral, biochemical, and neuroendocrine factors. Considering the diversity of present theories of mental illness, we are not surprised that no single explanation exists for the efficacy of ECT in depressive, manic, and schizophrenic disorders; in endogenous and reactive subtypes; and among the elderly. If we seek to explain the process, we must develop different explanations for its effects in different populations.

Because of the clear success attending the use of ECT in depression, the data on that population are plentiful. In addressing the theoretical issues here, the APA task force report (APA, 1978) observes:

How ECT benefits depression is unclear, but many theories of the mode of action of ECT have been disproven because of evidence developed in the last 20 years. ECT does not produce this therapeutic benefit in depressed patients because of nonspecific stress or anticipatory fear, since sham ECT is ineffective. Also, unmodified ECT, which is much more stressful, is no more effective than modified ECT. In addition, ECT does not produce its effect through non-specific events such as anoxia, hypercapnia, etc., since well-oxygenated ECT is as effective as unmodified ECT. Furthermore, ECT does not produce its effects through memory disturbance since unilateral treatment with minimal memory changes is often as effective as bilateral treatment with a greater degree of memory change. The physical concomitants of the convulsion are not essential since modified treatment is as effective as unmodified treatment.

The convulsion, as a central electrical event, is critical to ECT's therapeutic action. Since ECT given with excess electrical current is not more effective than ECT given with minimal current to produce a convulsion, and since subconvulsive electrical current is not beneficial to depressed patients, the dose of electrical current is not essential to ECT's therapeutic effect.

The importance of the cerebral seizure was first shown by Cronholm and Ottosson (1960). They used lidocaine to reduce the duration and amount of EEG seizure activity and found that lidocaine-modified seizures were less effective than unmodified seizures in their antidepressant efficacy.

There is a growing literature dealing with the possibility that the cause of depression may lie in alterations of cerebral neurotransmitters. It is of interest that in humans ECT affects the metabolism of neurotransmitters, and its mode of action might parallel that of the antidepressant drugs. What remains conjectural, however, is how the electrical activity in the brain during and following the ECT relates to the changes in the central neurotransmitters.

Fink (1979) has suggested that ECT is a special intervention that increases the activity of central neurohumors and releases hypothalamic peptides. It is this action that leads to the relief of the primary depressive syndrome—a syndrome characterized by hypothalamic dysfunction.

Bidder (1982) points to the important and exciting findings on the subsensitivity of beta-adrenergic receptors and the effects on cyclic nucleotides, such as norepinephrine-stimulated adenylate cyclase; these appear to be characteristic of the *chronic* administration of clinically effective pharmacological antidepressants (Creese and Sibley, 1981; Crews et al., 1981; Sulser et al., 1979). Indeed, similar findings have been reported with electrically-induced convulsions in rats (Gillespie et al., 1979; Bergstrom et al., 1978). These receptor changes are particularly significant since their time-course parallels that of the clinically observable effects of antidepressant modalities.

THE PROCEDURE

Before consideration of the nature of the treatment, the procedure itself will be described. It must be emphasized that the outline suggested here is but one of several acceptable methods used by experienced psychiatrists to administer ECT and is included in the APA task force report (APA, 1979). Fink has described a similar technique (Fink, 1979). Procedures that differ in one or more details from that described here are frequently used and are equally acceptable.

Ideally, before a patient receives the treatment, the psychiatrist discusses it with him and reassures him that it will be given with care and concern for his welfare. He undergoes a careful assessment of his physical condition, especially his cardiovascular and pulmonary status.

1. Preparation of the patient

When ECT is to be administered in the early morning, nothing by mouth (including oral solid medications) is taken after midnight. If the treatment is administered in the afternoon, a non-solid breakfast is permitted. Careful supervision for the enforcement of these important restrictions is particularly necessary in the confused and unreliable patient—and doubly so if such a patient is being treated on an outpatient basis.

The bladder is emptied just prior to treatment.

2. Drugs and equipment

A. Drugs

It is recommended that the following drugs and solutions be available with dose instructions for immediate administration:

(1). Atropine sulfate - 0.4 mg/ml
(2). Calcium chloride - 10% solution - 10% ml
    vial (emergency syringe)
(3). Dexamethasone (Decadron) - 4 mg/ml and/or
    24 mg/ml
(4). Dextrose - 5% in water - 250 ml units

(5). Diazepam 5 mg/ml - 2 and 10 ml
(emergency syringe)

(6). Epinephrine - 1:10,000 solution - 10 ml vials

(7). Lidocaine (Xylocaine): special preparation
for use in cardiac dysrhythmias - 2%
solution = 5 ml = 100 mg in emergency
syringe

(8). Metaraminol (Aramine) - 1% solution -
10 ml vial

(9). Methylprednisolone (Solu-Medrol) - 125 and
1,000 mg/vial

(10). Sodium bicarbonate - 7.5% solution =
44.6 mEq. - 50 ml (emergency syringe)

(11). L-norepinephrine (Levophed) - 2 mg/ml-4ml ampuls.

B. Equipment to be available for immediate use:
(1). Suction—tested for proper function
(2). Needles
(3). Infusion sets
(4). Electrocardiograph
(5). Defibrillator. While rare cases of cardiac arrest occurring with ECT
can usually be managed by a blow to the precordium, the adjunctive use of a defibrillator may occasionally be necessary. This
apparatus should be reasonably accessible
for this contingency.

C. When ECT is administered in a hospital, the emergency (crash) cart
should be readily available. In other facilities, a comparably equipped
unit should be available.

3. The patient is placed on a cart or bed that is adequately insulated so that
the electrical current cannot be grounded through the patient.

4. Teeth are examined just before starting treatment to note dental appli-
ances (which should be removed if possible) as well as chipped and/or
loose teeth.

5. Syringes are loaded with anticholinergic agent (methscopolamine is
recommended), thiopental (Pentothal) or mexthohexital (Brevital), and
succinylcholine (Anectine, Sucostrin, Quelcin). Alternatively, some therapists treating several patients in succession use dilute solutions of anesthetic
and succinylcholine. These solutions are infused at rates sufficient to
produce the desired pharmacological effects.

6. If the patient presents special risks (e.g., heart disease, emphysema, bronchopulmonary disease, obesity, advanced age), the anesthetic mask is gently placed over the face and moderately deep breathing of 100% oxygen is encouraged for a two- to three-minute period prior to injecting the anesthetic agent.

7. Scalp-vein needle (21G butterfly infusion set) is inserted into an accessible vein. A vein on dorsum of hand (infiltration quickly detected) or a lateral vein in the antecubital fossa (artery lies medially) is suggested. The needle is threaded up the vein and secured to the skin with tape. This needle is left *in situ* until the treatment is completed and the patient is responding; it serves as an IV line for injecting medications used in the treatment and for drugs and solutions that may be required in the event of adverse responses.

8. After determining the pulse rate, increments of 0.25 mg methscopolamine or 0.5 mg of atropine are injected intravenously until a discernible increase in heart rate occurs (e.g., rate increases by 10 percent). The anticholinergic drug can be given subcutaneously 45 minutes prior to the treatment, but this procedure makes it difficult to titrate the dose so that adequate cardiac cholinergic block will be produced.

Some patients receiving ECT will be receiving agents (e.g., antipsychotic drugs, tricyclic antidepressants, antiparkinsonism compounds) which, singly or in combination, will have significant anticholinergic actions as manifested by tachycardia. It may be judged that additional anticholinergic medication is not required in these patients (Stoelting and Peterson, 1975).

A quaternary (charged) anticholinergic agent (e.g., scopolamine methylbromide methscopolamine, Pamine) is used. These drugs are effective peripheral anticholinergics.

9. The anesthetic agent is administered next through the IV line. A test minidose (e.g., 50 mg of thiopental) is injected. This dose should be sufficient to evoke anaphylaxis in hypersensitive individuals and produce pain in the event that intra-arterial injection has been made. In the absence of these responses administration of the anesthetic is resumed in 15-20 seconds.

The dose of anesthetic is individualized for each patient, and fixed doses are not relied upon to produce an adequate depth of anesthesia. The following signs are useful indicators of an adequate level of anesthesia:
   A. The patient does not respond to spoken commands (e.g., "Take a deep breath!");
   B. Yawning occurs;
   C. Airway obstruction occurs as manifested by noisy, snoring respiration;
   D. The eyelash (not eyelid) reflex disappears.

10. When the desired anesthetic end-point has been reached, the anesthetic mask is placed on the face and ventilation with 100% oxygen is started.

11. If the "tourniquet technique" is being used the blood pressure cuff is now inflated to 175-200 mm Hg. A tourniquet applied to one limb prevents access of the paralysant to that extremity.

12. The succinylcholine is now injected in doses of 0.5-1.5 mg/kg. In patients with "atypical" plasma pseudocholinesterase, marked prolongation of the duration of paralysis may occur, even with very small doses of succinylcholine. The possibility of atypical responses can be detected beforehand by a laboratory test available for patients whose personal or family histories suggest that they might be affected (Kalow and Lindsay, 1955).

13. Following the injection of the succinylcholine the syringe is left attached to the butterfly infusion set and taped to the arm.

14. The establishment of maximal muscle paralysis can be determined by the following methods:
   A. By cessation of muscle fasciculations in the lower extremity.
   B. When the "tourniquet technique" is used in the lower extremity, a method for establishing that maximal muscle paralysis has occurred becomes available. This method is particularly useful in cases where muscle fasciculations cannot be observed. The ventral surface of each foot is stroked in the manner used to elicit the Babinski sign. A withdrawal motion of the foot on the cuffed (i.e., unparalyzed) side should occur; whereas, no muscular response should take place on the uncuffed (paralyzed) side.
   C. By ascertaining that the lower jaw has become freely movable due to loss of muscle tone.

15. When it has been determined that maximal paralysis has occurred, preparations for administering the electrical current and for the seizure are undertaken in the following order:
   A. A mouth gag (made of gauze rolled into a 3/4" x 10" cylinder and wrapped with tape) is inserted between the teeth—and especially between the premolars and molars. Alternatively, a soft rubber bite-block can be inserted.
   After these devices are in place—and when care has been taken to ensure that the tongue and soft parts are not between the teeth—pressure is exerted at the tip of the mandible to approximate the teeth and to hold them in this position until the convulsion has ceased.

B. Electrodes with cotton pads moistened with a solution containing 25% sodium bicarbonate plus a few drops of dishwashing detergent in water are attached firmly in one of the following positions:
  (1). For bilateral or bitemporal ECT each electrode is placed 1 1/2" above the middle of a line extending from the external auditory meatus and lateral angle of the orbit (Figure 1).
  (2). For unilateral ECT, one or both electrodes are placed on the same side as the dominant hand. In the classical Lancaster electrode placement (Lancaster et al., 1958), the lower electrode is posi-

Figure 1. Bilateral or Bitemporal Electrode Placement

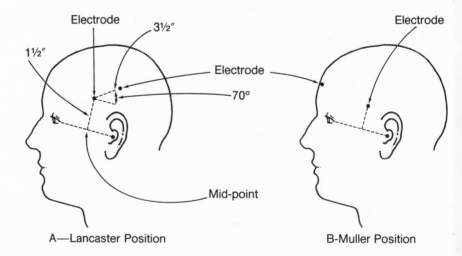

Figure 2. Unilateral Placements

tioned as described in (1) above (Figure 2A). The upper electrode is placed 3 1/2" higher than the lower one and at an angle of 70° to the line. In the Muller electrode placement, one electrode is placed as described in (1), above, while the other is positioned on the forehead anteriorly (Figure 2B). (There are other positions for electrode placement in unilateral ECT, but the above are commonly used.)

C. The individual holding the electrodes in place, if they are hand-held, is protected against electrical shock by suitable insulation and/or by wearing rubber or plastic gloves.

D. An attendant places one hand on each thigh near the knee. This support will prevent the patient from falling off the treatment cart in the event that a vigorous and essentially unmodified convulsion occurs unexpectedly.

16. The electrical stimulus is then administered in accordance with the directions for the machine being used.

17. The therapeutic adequacy of the seizure is determined by one or both of the following:

A. Occurrence of a characteristic major seizure pattern on the electrocorticograph tracing or oscilloscope image if this type of monitoring is being used;

B. Occurrence of a tonic muscular contraction in an extremity. This tonic contraction persists after the electrical stimulus has ceased and progresses into a clonic pattern.

Some psychiatrists favor the use of smaller doses of succinylcholine, sufficient only for a moderate reduction in seizure severity. They claim that with their method the occurrence of a generalized seizure is readily observable. Anesthesiologists generally tend to prefer the larger doses of succinylcholine to reduce not only the musculoskeletal effects but also the cardiovascular effects of the seizure.

18. In the event that a therapeutically adequate seizure has not been evoked, the electrical parameters are increased appropriately and the stimulus reapplied. Because of the refractoriness that follows the first stimulus, an interval of 60-90 seconds is allowed to elapse before the second is applied.

19. When a therapeutically adequate seizure has occurred, the following are carried out, sequentially:

A. The mouth gag or bite-block is removed;

B. The teeth are quickly checked and the hypopharynx is examined with the use of a curved-blade laryngoscope. Secretions should be removed at this time—while the patient is still paralyzed. When secretions are removed by necessity after the succinylcholine's action is terminated, vomiting and laryngospasm occasionally occur;

C. The anesthetic face mask is reapplied, and artificial and assisted ventilation are instituted and continued until spontaneous respiratory muscle movements are strong enough to maintain an adequate tidal volume;

D. If the "tourniquet technique" is used, the blood pressure cuff is deflated and removed, if this has not yet been done.

20. While awaiting the return of muscle activity, consciousness, and protective reflexes, the patient's abdomen is uncovered so that impending regurgitation can be detected promptly. Sufficient assistance is always close at hand in order quickly to turn the patient's body to one side to minimize the possibility of tracheal aspiration.

21. When spontaneous respiratory muscle activity commences, the anesthetic face mask is still held in place until there has been enough muscle recovery from the succinylcholine to permit the establishment of an adequate tidal volume. This serves two purposes: The movements of the anesthetic bag are a measure of the tidal volume, and inadequate ventilatory movements can be supplemented by squeezing the bag.

22. With the establishment of a normal tidal volume the anesthetic face mask is removed and the patient can be moved from the cart to a bed. The positioning of the patient depends on whether or not protective pharyngeal reflexes have returned as indicated by the presence of swallowing and the capacity to phonate. When reflexes are not vigorously present it is advisable to place the patient in the semi-prone position. In moving the unconscious or semi-conscious patient, care is taken not to twist the neck and to avoid hyperextending arms and damaging the brachial plexus. Consultation with an anesthesiologist is helpful in learning these standard positioning techniques.

23. Careful observation and monitoring of vital signs is essential during the immediate post-treatment period. Particular attention is paid to the adequacy of ventilation, the absence of cyanosis, and the pulse rate, volume, and rhythmicity. The awakening patient is systematically re-oriented and reassured—preferably by someone who is familiar.

24. Most individuals receiving ECT are confused and unsteady following treatment, especially during the first hour. Patients are carefully supervised, particularly during this interval, to prevent injury. Outpatients return home

in the company of a reliable individual and with clear admonitions against operating a motor vehicle or hazardous machinery.

25. Essential to safe and acceptable ECT are the following procedural details:
   A. The administration of an anesthetic agent,
   B. The administration of a muscle relaxant and,
   C. Oxygen supplementation.

PHYSIOLOGICAL CONSIDERATIONS

In attempting to understand the nature and effect of ECT in physiological terms, we are confronted by the need to separate specific therapeutic effects from the nonspecific changes that accompany any physiologic stress on the body. In this case, the stress can arise from the electrical current, the seizure, the convulsion, hypoxemia, hypercapnia, or the psychosomatic consequences of fear, panic, or anxiety. It has become clear that the nonspecific factors are not responsible for the therapeutic effect and that, in ways not fully understood, the generalized CNS seizure is crucial.

The physiological, neurophysiological, and neuropharmacological events that are known to occur when a therapeutic seizure is electrically induced can be described in two categories: central reactions and peripheral responses. The known peripheral consequences of an electrically-induced seizure can be eliminated without apparent detriment to the therapeutic response, and most of the acute adverse consequences result from peripheralization of the central seizure process.

Central Effects of an Electrically-Induced Seizure

Electroencephalographic Effects. Among the most striking manifestations of the typical induced seizure is the change in the electroencephalographic pattern from the desynchronized resting configuration characteristic of the level of anesthesia employed to a high-amplitude synchronized pattern (Holmberg, 1963). Depth recordings indicate that for bilateral ECT the seizure process is initiated in the central part of the brain and spreads centrifugally to the cortices (Bickford and Rome, 1949). Immediately after the electrical stimulus, the EEG is isoelectric for one to five seconds. Beginning in the frontal leads there is a rapid build-up of diffuse, bilateral, synchronous spike and multiple spike activity, which may last from ten to 25 seconds and which is associated with the typical tonic muscular contractions of the convulsion. Paroxysmal high voltage slow waves usually follow for ten to 20 seconds and are associated with the clonic motor movements.

The EEG seizure may terminate abruptly with the cessation of all muscular seizure activity, or there may be a gradual decrease in amplitude and an increase in frequency as slow waves are replaced (Small, 1974).

It is of interest that with each successive seizure, the duration of the slowing is longer, the mean frequency is lower, and mean amplitude greater. With greater numbers of seizures at shorter intervals, EEG slowing is greater and persists longer after the end of treatment. Following the last treatment, there is a progressive disappearance of slow wave activity. The mean frequency increases toward the normal alpha range within two to six weeks. In some patients, resolution may be slower, with abnormal frequencies persisting for months.

Effects on the Cerebral Circulation: Acute Responses. Studies in both animals and humans indicate a prompt increase in cerebral blood flow which reaches a maximum approximately three minutes after the seizure and progressively returns to normal during the ensuing 30 minutes (Plum et al., 1968; Lovett-Doust et al., 1974). The maximum increase in cerebral blood flow is 100 percent or more and is chiefly the result of the systemic hypertension that accompanies an electrically induced seizure. The increase in blood-brain barrier permeability during ECT has been attributed to the increase in cerebral blood flow (Bolwig et al., 1977a, 1977b).

Effects on the Cerebral Circulation: Sustained Responses. Lovett-Doust and Raschka (1975) have tried to find physiological and biochemical changes that have a time-course parallel to the therapeutic response. They have shown that the increased cerebral blood flow induced by each treatment persisted for at least one week, especially in patients with depressive disorders in whom a satisfactory response to ECT had been achieved.

Effects on Cerebral Metabolism: Acute Responses. Many early animal studies of the short-term changes in brain metabolism following electrically-induced seizures were complicated by the occurrence of varying degrees of hypoxia. Plum and his co-workers (Plum et al., 1968; Plum et al., 1974) adequately ventilated their experimental animals with oxygen-enriched mixtures that prevented hypoxemia and hypercarboxemia. This refinement in technique marked a significant advance in the study of the changes occurring with an electrically-induced seizure. Their findings indicate neither a significant brain hypoxia nor a shift to anaerobic metabolism in anesthetized and paralyzed animals adequately ventilated with oxygen-enriched mixtures.

Because substantial hypoxia is not a requirement for the therapeutic effect of ECT, there is no need to tolerate it. Furthermore, there are positive reasons for preventing it. These include the uncertain relationship of severe cerebral hypoxemia to the memory dysfunction and confusion that occur with ECT and the potent cardiac dysrhythmiagenic action of hypoxemia and hypercarboxemia.

Effects on Cerebral Metabolism: Sustained Responses. There is a growing literature exploring the possibility that the cause of depression may lie in alterations of central neurotransmitters; the response of this condition to antidepressant therapies has been widely studied. However, the few investigations aimed at directly assessing the role of biogenic amines in ECT fail to provide a clear picture. For example, some studies (Kety et al., 1967; Ladisich et al., 1969; Ebert et al., 1973) report an increased turnover of brain norepinephrine and increased tyrosine hydroxylase activity in norepinephrine-rich areas of the brains of experimental animals subjected to a series of electrically-induced convulsions. However, these changes are of comparatively short duration. Others (Pryor and Otis, 1970; Pryor et al., 1972) report more persistent changes. In a review of the basis for an amine hypothesis in affective disorder, Baldessarini (1975) concluded that the metabolic effects of ECT suggest that seizures can release catecholamines and serotonin acutely but that effects of repeated seizures are likely to be nonspecific in the case of serotonin and small and of short duration in the case of norepinephrine.

Depression is associated with a hypersecretion of cortisol. Because the administration of dexamethasone fails to suppress the hypersecretion, the dexamethasone suppression test (DST) has been used in confirming the diagnosis of depression (Stokes, 1972; Carroll et al., 1976). Levels of cortisol fall with treatment and recovery (Sachar et al., 1973).

Regarding acetylcholine, Fink (1979) concludes that with the technical difficulties attending the study of that substance, it is unclear what role, if any, it may play in the ECT process.

Peripheral Effects of an Electrically-Induced Seizure

Many of the effects occurring outside the central nervous system can be viewed as consequences of the peripheralization of the seizure process. Like the central effects, they consist of an intensification of normally occurring neuronal processes and the resulting end-organ responses.

Musculo-Skeletal Effects. The muscle movements that signify the occurrence of a grand-mal convulsion result from the involvement of the motor cortices in the seizure process. They can be obliterated by the use of muscle paralysants such as succinylcholine with no discernible effect on the therapeutic action of ECT.

The movements consist of a tonic contraction during the time that the electrical current is flowing, a tonic contraction continuing after the electrical stimulus has ceased, and then clonic contractions. The muscular movements provide useful information that the seizure process has been sufficiently generalized to lead to a therapeutic response. However, they are also responsible for the musculo-skeletal injuries that accompanied the treatment procedure before the introduction of muscle paralysants. As stated earlier, the use of a tourniquet on one limb to prevent access of the paralysant confines the informative movements to one extremity while the rest of the body remains immobilized (Bidder, 1962).

Parasympathetic Effects. The most visible evidence of the involvement of cardiac parasympathetic nerve circuits is the bradycardia that appears with the onset of the convulsion in unmedicated animals and humans (Lewis et al., 1955; Perrin, 1961; Anton et al., 1977). It can be severe enough to produce asystole of several seconds' duration; on the other hand, it can be completely eliminated by adequate cholinergic blocking with atropine or scopolamine.

Sympathetic and Adrenal Medullary Effects. Release of norepinephrine in the heart results from peripheralization of the seizure process over sympathetic nerves. The combined adrenergic effects of this norepinephrine and the catecholamines released by the adrenal medulla include hypertension (average increases of 50-100 mg Hg) and tachycardia (average increases of 20-50 beats per minute) (Anton et al., 1977). Within one minute after initiation of the seizure, plasma norepinephrine and epinephrine concentrations are markedly elevated (ten- to 50-fold). They then decline rapidly in the second minute with a more gradual return to pre-seizure levels over the next five minutes.

Adrenal Cortical Effects. During the two- to four-hour period following an electrically-induced seizure, blood cortical steroid levels are elevated. The clinical consequences are apparently not significant.

Pituitary and Hypothalamic Effects. Following convulsive treatments, adrenocorticotrophic hormone (ACTH) in the plasma has been found to increase eight-fold with or without the use of muscle relaxants. The concentration was shown to peak 2.5 minutes after the electrical stimulus was applied and returned to normal during the next 45 minutes (Allen et al., 1974; Ylikorkala et al., 1976).

Studies of human growth hormone disclosed no significant changes, nor were there any alterations in the plasma concentrations of thyrotropin stimulating hormone, (TSH) follicle-stimulating hormone (FSH), or luteinizing hormone (LH) (Allen et al., 1974; Ylikorkala et al., 1976; Ryan et al., 1970).

Fifteen minutes after an electrically-induced convulsion, a ten- to 50-fold increase in serum prolactin concentration was found to occur in eight of nine female patients (Öhman et al., 1976).

ADVERSE RESPONSES ASSOCIATED WITH ECT

No discussion of the nature of ECT is complete without reference to its adverse effects. While minimized in some quarters, these have been extravagantly described and exaggerated in others (Friedberg, 1976). Furthermore, while the refinements introduced into the technique have been aimed

at reducing the complications of the treatment, the modifications themselves demand that the psychiatrist learn more about the nature of the
anesthetic and relaxant drugs now used.

Acute Adverse Responses to the Electrically-Induced Seizure

There is substantial evidence that circulatory disturbances are the important
and dangerous complications of ECT (MacKay, 1953; Alexander, 1953) and
that their incidence and seriousness is disproportionately increased in older
individuals and in persons with cardiovascular disease. Dysrhythmias have
been reported in several studies; indeed, in a series of guarded-risk patients
given treatments with electrocardiographic monitoring and expert anesthetic management, 50 dysrhythmias were encountered in 75 percent of the
patients. Fifteen percent were mild, 50 percent were of moderate severity,
27 percent were severe, and eight percent were very severe. It is important
to note, however, that these dysrhythmias are almost always transient and
that patients with severe cardiac disease tolerate ECT considerably better
than they do high doses of tricyclic antidepressant medication. Understanding the mechanism whereby this complication of ECT is generated provides
the opportunity for prophylactic strategy, anticipation and early recognition, and effective therapy. The major mechanisms involved, singly or in
combination, are:

Those Involving Inhibition of S-A Nodal Activity. Cardiac contractions are initiated by the normal pacemaker, the S-A node. Inhibition of
nodal activity can result in take-over of pacemaker activity by the A-V node
or by irritable etopic pacemakers. S-A nodal activity can be inhibited by the
intense outflow over the cardiac parasympathetic nerves which accompanies the electrically-induced convulsion and by the cholinergic agonist
activity that precedes the cholinergic blocking action of certain drugs such
as atropine in smaller doses and succinylcholine. Atropine in adequate
doses effectively reduces or prevents the bradycardia characteristically
produced by the succinylcholine prior to its paralytic action.

**Those Producing Localized or Generalized Ventricular Myocardial
Irritability.** Here we have factors such as coronary artery disease or
insufficiency, increased cardiac sympathetic or adrenergic activity generated
by peripheralization of seizure activity, the hyperkalemic response with
succinylcholine occurring under certain circumstances, and, importantly,
hypoxemia and/or hypercarboxemia.

Acute Adverse Reactions Associated With Drugs Used in ECT

Excessive atropine dosage can combine with the adrenergic cardiac effects,
causing tachycardia, which increases the need for blood supply beyond the
capacity of the coronary vessels to deliver it.

Light levels of anesthesia produced with low doses of anesthetic agents are likely to be associated with laryngospasm.

Adverse reactions can occur with succinylcholine, such as increased duration of action, decreased duration of action, hyperkalemic response, and prolonged paralytic action when administered in the presence of lithium (APA, 1978).

LONG-TERM ADVERSE EFFECTS OF ECT

1. Despite persuasive comments that ECT leads to permanent and disabling memory impairment, few careful studies have been reported until fairly recently. These have been well reviewed and summarized in the APA task force report (APA, 1978) as follows:

a. bilateral ECT is associated with greater anterograde amnesia than right unilateral ECT, even when memory is assessed with tests known to be particularly sensitive to dysfunction of the right cerebral hemisphere;

b. bilateral ECT also produces more extensive retrograde amnesia for remote events than right unilateral ECT;

c. extensive ECT (e.g., more than 50 treatments) may lead to long-lasting or permanent impairment in memory capacity or cognitive function, but a definitive conclusion is not yet possible;

d. the activation of the memory for previously learned material just prior to ECT does not cause amnesia for that material;

e. new learning capacity substantially recovers by six to nine months after the completion of bilateral or right-unilateral ECT, but persisting memory complaints are common in individuals who receive bilateral treatment;

f. memory for events that occurred long prior to ECT substantially recovers by six to nine months after ECT. Memory for events that occurred days prior to ECT may be permanently lost.

Despite the persistent complaints about memory by some individuals, evidence of memory impairment six to nine months after the last treatment has not been demonstrated on formal testing. While this finding could result from the use of tests that are not sufficiently sensitive, it should be remembered that many professional and academic persons and business executives who had ECT complain minimally or not at all of a lasting memory disability. Further studies of the nature of the complaints and the life situations of the complainants might add to our knowledge of the problem.

2. Reports of other central nervous system sequelae in the early literature on ECT describe brain damage, spontaneous seizures, and organic psychosis. These reports of brain damage are based on autopsy findings and animal experiments, neither of which can be viewed as reliable. The association of cardiovascular disease, neurological disease that might well have preceded the ECT, and hypoxia obscure the etiology of the necrosis, neurophagia,

and gliosis reported in the brains that were studied.

The relevance of the early animal experiments is similarly difficult to determine since many of the parameters of the treatment (seizure rate and number, strength of the current, physiologic state, age, and anesthesia) are not comparable to ECT in humans. Furthermore, none of the studies involved the use of hyperoxygenation in conjunction with the procedure.

"Kindling," or the precipitation of spontaneous seizures following the use of ECT in patients who had reported no such seizures prior to the treatment, has been described but rarely. The evidence that kindling does indeed occur is not persuasive (APA, 1978).

An organic brain syndrome including disorientation, impairment of memory and intellectual functions, confusion, perceptual defects, and defective judgment has also been attributed to ECT. As noted in the section on memory impairment, at six to nine months following the moderate use of ECT, there is no objective evidence of cognitive impairment. Although in a technical sense all induced seizures are associated with some type of organic impairment, the severe organic psychosis described here has been reported in some subjects (Kalinowsky, 1945). Its appearance was not interpreted as an adverse sign, and it disappeared within a few days. Treatment was not discontinued.

In a process termed "regressive ECT" (Glueck et al., 1957; Murillo and Exner, 1973), schizophrenic patients were treated three times daily to induce an organic psychosis. In such instances recovery took longer, the mental functions and behavior requiring more than a year to improve (Regenstein et al., 1975).

In summary it can be said that the repeated induction of seizures elicits a specific though apparently reversible neurological syndrome. Evidence for persistent brain damage is limited, and death from cerebral causes is rarely reported. The severity of the neurological effects is related to the number, frequency, and mode of induction of seizures; the clinical diagnosis; and the patient's age. The frequency and the number of seizures are the most critical factors.

In assessing the relevance of the earlier reports of adverse effects, it should be remembered that when the techniques of ECT were being developed, cyanosis was considered to aid therapeutic efficacy. The current use of an anticholinergic agent, a short-acting anesthetic agent, adequate oxygenation, and a muscle paralysant has modified the treatment considerably. The psychological stress, the panic associated with a missed seizure, fractures, and cardiac complications have been brought under control.

The most provocative and ubiquitous adverse effect of the treatment is the memory disability. It should be noted that adequate oxygenation and unilateral electrode placement have reduced the extent of that disability. The memory loss that follows low energy wave forms (e.g., bidirectional brief pulses) is no less than that following conventional sine-wave stimulation, provided the two wave forms are equated for their seizure producing efficacy (Spanis and Squire, 1981).

CLINICAL ISSUES

When first introduced in the 1930's, ECT was viewed as a treatment for severe psychiatric illness, notably schizophrenia. Despite the complications and adverse effects of the unmodified treatment, it offered a clear advantage over sedation, restraint, seclusion, and whatever other methods were in use to contain and alleviate psychotic behavior. An understanding of the early clinical reports of ECT is hampered by the poorly defined diagnostic criteria in use at the time, the lack of a standardized treatment pattern (treatments involved varying methods of induction, numbers, and frequency), and the absence of controlled comparison.

Probably largely as a result of clinical experience with it and subsequently because of the publication of studies with improved designs, ECT became recognized as a valuable method in the treatment of depressive illness. With the advent of the psychotropic drugs, particularly the antidepressants of the 1950's and 1960's, many predicted the total eclipse of ECT. However, because the side effects and complications of high dosage antidepressant medication continue to present problems and because some patients are unresponsive to medication, ECT not only survives but commands the increasing respect and recognition of the mental health profession as an important treatment procedure. With the constantly growing number of good clinical studies, a more uniform and rational perspective on the subject has begun to emerge to replace the former disagreements.

Affective Illness

In order to evaluate the efficacy of ECT in the treatment of the affective disorders, the following material will review some of the important findings in comparison and outcome studies and will discuss the prediction of response and the value of unilateral ECT. Regarding the number and frequency of treatments in affective disorders, the average in most good studies is between six and nine at intervals of 48 hours.

Comparative Studies. A number of studies in the 1960's demonstrated the efficacy of ECT (Kristiansen, 1961; Wittenborn et al., 1962; Hutchinson and Smedburg, 1963; Wilson et al., 1963; DeCarolis et al., 1964; Greenblatt et al., 1964; Bratfos and Haug, 1965; Hordern et al., 1965; Medical Research Council in England, 1965; Angst et al., 1966; McDonald et al., 1966) in the treatment of the more severe disorders included in the Endogenous and Psychotic Depressions of *DSM-II*. The work of Greenblatt et al. (1964) and Wilson et al. (1963), as well as a study by the Medical Research Council in

England (1965), exemplify the quality of the investigations and attest to the effectiveness of the treatment and its probable superiority to antidepressant medications. Greenblatt et al. (1964) found that 78 percent of a severely depressed sample responded to ECT, compared with 59 percent who responded to tricyclic drugs. Signs of vegetative dysfunction involving sleep, weight, and libido were especially responsive. The Medical Research Council study (1965) not only confirmed these findings but showed that 50 percent of patients who had failed to respond to antidepressants did respond to subsequent treatment with ECT. Those who had initially failed to respond to ECT did not improve with drug treatment. The findings suggest that a population of depressed patients exists which is clearly ECT-responsive and not drug-responsive.

Despite evidence that is strongly in favor of ECT, the value of antidepressant medication demands appropriate recognition. The prescription of drugs is less burdensome for both patients and physicians than is the use of ECT; to date there is no reported adverse effect on memory. Reviews of the literature (Morris and Beck, 1974) attest to the value of tricyclic antidepressants in 66 percent of depressions. With insufficient evidence to date to support the dependability of predictive criteria, the general circumstances of the patient and the individual clinical experience and judgment of the physician tend to influence the decision regarding the best initial treatment in a particular case. In delusionally depressed patients, however, there are data (Glassman et al., 1975; Hordern et al., 1965) to support an early choice of ECT.

Outcome. Studying the course of patients after treatment with ECT provides valuable information. In the late 1940's and 1950's, before the introduction of modern psychopharmacology, the outcome of treatment with ECT was compared with treatments that were at best palliative. Investigators then, such as Huston and Locher (1948), concluded that ECT shortened the length of hospital stay and led to a fuller recovery. More than that, in the treated population death from suicide was considerably lower. More recent work by Avery and Winokur (1976) reaffirms the value of combined ECT and adequate antidepressant medication in reducing mortality among depressed patients.

In 1959, Sainz (1959) reported the outcome of a study comparing ECT with "mock ECT." Patients receiving mock ECT were anesthetized but were given no subsequent electrical stimulus. Nine of the ten patients receiving ECT recovered, and one was improved; in contrast, none of the mock group showed improvement. However, when they in turn were given ECT, seven achieved full remission and two were substantially improved.

The use of sham or "mock ECT" was again tested in recent years by Freeman et al. (1978), Johnstone et al. (1980), Lambourn and Gill (1978), and West (1981). In the first study, the sham group was exposed to a course that commenced with two sham treatments, followed by real ECT. The outcome, compared with that for patients who had received only real ECT, revealed a larger total number of treatments in the sham group and a slower reduction in scores for depression. Although Lambourn and Gill failed to confirm the superiority of real ECT, the studies by Johnstone et al. and West clearly demonstrated the value of real ECT when compared with simulated treatment.

Several aspects of outcome associated with ECT remain dubious and await further investigation. In some instances we appear to be closer to a definitive answer than in others. For example, a 1976 study in the treatment of mania by McCabe (1976) demonstrated the value of ECT when compared with no treatment. However, a controlled study comparing the value of ECT, lithium, and neuroleptic drugs remains to be done.

A not inconsiderable number of clinicians favor the use of "maintenance ECT" for patients who, despite the administration of antidepressant medication, rapidly relapse after a course of ECT treatments. This approach entails administering additional single ECT treatments on a regular but infrequent basis (at approximately four- to six-week intervals) once the full course has been given. Memory appears to be unaffected by this method, and the patients continue to lead full lives. There is as yet, however, little consensus on the acceptability of this method and no adequate literature to confirm or question its value. The subject requires study.

The effect of ECT on the natural history of depression is not yet completely understood. It is evident that symptoms are reduced more rapidly with ECT; however, its impact on the rate of relapse is not yet known. Furthermore, although there is no evidence to support the simultaneous use of antidepressant medication with the ECT, some clinicians claim that the adjunctive use of these drugs prevents relapse before the ECT effect has been established.

Predictors. Once the diagnosis of affective disorder is made, one of the most challenging clinical issues that must be grappled with concerns the choice of the initial treatment. Apart from the suggestion above that an early choice of ECT in delusionally depressed patients is supported by the available data, studies to date have not been able to differentiate criteria that predict a good response to ECT from those that predict a favorable outcome with antidepressant drugs (Bielski and Friedel, 1976; Mandel et al., 1977). While clinicians still must depend on their best clinical wisdom when they confront such decisions, the course followed by many when they encounter a seriously depressed patient entails an initial trial of medication in adequate doses. If the patient's response is poor, ECT is then recommended. Because the effects of most antidepressant medication become manifest only after two or three weeks, the presence of a serious preoccupation with suicide or debilitation signals the need for early recourse to ECT. The general circumstances of the patient might also influence the consideration of ECT early in treatment.

Work progresses at both the clinical and biochemical levels toward a greater understanding of the biological parameters of depression and how these relate to the choice of antidepressant medication; this work might pave the way to a similar approach to decisions regarding the choice of ECT.

Unilateral ECT. As indicated above, unilateral placement of electrodes was first introduced in the 1940's (Friedman, 1942) and reported from a contemporary perspective by Lancaster et al. in 1958 (Lancaster et al., 1958). Subsequent studies (Halliday et al., 1968; Sutherland et al., 1969; d'Elia, 1970; Cohen et al., 1974) have confirmed that there was less memory disability with unilateral treatments. A consensus, however, has not yet been reached regarding the comparative efficacy of bilateral and unilateral treatments. Whereas d'Elia (1970, 1974), d'Elia and Raotma (1975), Sand-Strömgren (1973), and others (Friedman, 1942; Sutherland et al., 1969; Bidder et al., 1970; Fleminger et al., 1970) have found both forms of treatment effective, other workers, including Halliday et al. (1968), Canicott (1962), Strain et al. (1968), Abrams and Taylor (1976), and Kalinowsky (1984), have suggested that bilateral ECT produces a more rapid improvement with fewer treatments, achieving a more marked change in the depression score. Fewer treatments mean less exposure to anesthesia.

Proponents of unilateral ECT contend that the alleged superiority of bilateral treatment in some studies could be attributable to the ease with which submaximal or inadequate seizures in unilateral treatments can pass for full seizures. In the presence of muscle paralysis, the diagnosis of a cerebral seizure without EEG monitoring is not always reliable. Although the seizure activity might fail to spread across the centrencephalic region in unilateral treatment, such failure might escape the observer, who then records the event as a treatment, adding to the total number of unilateral ECT's considered necessary for that particular patient.

In unilateral ECT, neither therapeutic benefit nor memory loss appears to be influenced by the position of the electrodes on the head, provided that they are placed far enough apart to ensure the induction of a seizure.

The APA task force report focused considerable attention on this issue (APA, 1978) and came out in favor of unilateral ECT, particularly since the memory disability following that method is considerably less than that following bilateral treatment. The task force recognized, however, that for any individual patient, his or her psychiatrist is in the most advantageous position to decide on the best mode of administration. It is of interest that while 71 percent of all psychiatric hospitals in Sweden which administer ECT use unilateral placement, 75 percent of the APA questionnaire respondents who use ECT prefer the use of bilateral treatment (APA, 1978). Bidder (1979) has reminded us that "the conclusions that unilateral ECT is equitherapeutic with bilateral ECT and produces less memory dysfunction are based on average responses obtained from groups of patients. Individual responses (which are what the psychiatrist really needs to be concerned with when dealing with any particular patient) may be significantly different from these average expectations."

Schizophrenia

When ECT was introduced in 1938, it was administered to a catatonic schizophrenic patient. Since that time results in the treatment of schizophrenia have been regarded at best as ambiguous. Its efficacy has been more noticeable in the affective disorders. Nonetheless, it has continued to enjoy enthusiastic support in some centers, and a few standard textbooks (Kalinowsky, 1980; Sargant and Slater, 1963) still endorse its use for schizophrenia.

The available literature on the subject is, with few exceptions, not helpful. The earlier publications relating to the era before the advent of the neuroleptic drugs contain variable diagnostic criteria, methods of treatment that were not standardized, poor controls if any, and inadequate follow-up. Outcome in chronic illness sometimes defies interpretation even under the best of circumstances; for, in addition to evaluating relapse rates, work record, and socialization, one is attempting to measure the quality of life. Several of the observations and impressions in those early clinical reports are still relevant. It was recognized that ECT was useful in the early stages of the illness, particularly in gaining relief from symptoms; that the relapse rate for all patients was high; and that symptoms of affective disturbance responded best. Two later publications in the early 1970's (Wells, 1973; Folstein et al., 1973) also attest to the clear-cut efficacy of ECT in the treatment of schizophrenia when affective symptoms are prominent.

Neuroleptic drugs, since their introduction, have been compared with ECT and have also been administered in combination with ECT. The studies that are probably regarded as among the best and that are widely quoted are those of May and his co-workers (May and Tuma, 1965; May, 1968; May et al., 1976). They compared ECT, milieu therapy, psychotherapy, psychotropic drugs, and psychotherapy in combination with psychotropic drugs in the treatment of middle prognosis schizophrenic patients. After a three-year and then a five-year follow-up, the overall conclusion was that ECT cannot be considered desirable as an alternative to drugs alone or drugs in combination with psychotherapy. Reports of the combined use of ECT and neuroleptic drugs (Witten, 1962; Smith et al., 1967; Weinstein and Fischer, 1971; Wessels, 1971) have generally been favorable and at times enthusiastic. The combination is reported to be most suitable in acutely ill patients. Despite the risk of hypotensive crisis as a result of the hypotensive properties of some of the drugs accentuating the drop of blood pressure induced by ECT, only a few authors have paid attention to it (Weiss, 1955; Foster and Gayle, 1955; Grinspoon and Greenblatt, 1963). Others (Turek, 1973; Abrams, 1975) have been critical of most of the studies and have emphasized the need for further investigation.

Treatment Numbers. The number of ECT sessions is generally considerably higher for schizophrenic patients than for those with depression. Apart from the smaller number sometimes used to intervene in catatonic behavior, few cases respond to fewer than 18 treatments, and not infrequently the number reaches 25 or 30. The long-term effect on memory of large numbers of treatments is as yet unknown, but the distinct impression prevails that 50 treatments or more are not without risk (APA, 1978). The role of unilateral ECT in schizophrenia has not been studied. In the selection of a treatment method for a young schizophrenic patient, the disadvantages of a cumulative memory disability following ECT must be weighed against the risk of tardive dyskinesia following the long-term administration of drugs.

"Regressive ECT" first reported in 1957 (Glueck et al., 1957) referred to the advantages of two to four ECT treatments per day in chronic schizophrenic patients. Treatment continued until marked memory loss, confusion, slurred speech, and even incontinence were reached, at which time neurological examination usually revealed pathological reflexes. The patient was then nursed and fed back to recovery over a period of a few weeks, when some improvement in the symptoms was reported. The drastic nature of the treatment was highly criticized by most observers, but it was revisited in 1973 by Murillo and Exner (1973), who reported significant improvement among chronic patients so treated. The accuracy of the diagnoses in their study has come under fire.

Multiple monitored ECT (Blachly and Gowing, 1966) is a technique also using several treatments in one day, administered during one treatment session during which the EKG and EEG are continuously monitored. The total number of treatments is similar to conventional ECT, but the duration of the course of treatment is shortened.

A recent study by Taylor and Fleminger (1980) of 20 less seriously ill schizophrenic patients revealed little difference after four months between those who had been given ECT and those who had received only anesthesia, although initially the ECT group showed a greater improvement. What is abundantly clear from that study (Taylor and Fleminger, 1980), from the reviews in the APA task force report (APA, 1978), and from Salzman's extensive review (1980) is the need for further investigation of the role of ECT in the treatment of schizophrenia.

Illness Other Than Affective Disorder and Schizophrenia

From surveys (APA, 1978; Small and Small, 1981) and occasional clinical reports, it is clear that ECT has been used in conditions other than the affective disorders and schizophrenia. Neurotic depressions, obsessive compulsive disorders, anxiety states, and a wide range of conditions including hypochondriasis and unexplained and intractable pain have been treated with ECT. Some authors have considered ECT of value in the treatment of physical illnesses when these have been associated with psychiatric disorders. Pressed to find a means for improving obstinate psychiatric and physical illness, physicians have turned toward ECT through the years in the belief that it might help. The reports, for the most part, lack any dependable methodology. While one cannot ignore the claims made, they provide insufficient grounds for recommending the use of ECT in most of the conditions described. In the wake of the attention focused on ECT over the past decade it is more than likely that in recent years few psychiatrists have resorted to these unproven uses. The frequency of such use was probably never high, and other than the rough estimates that were made in the APA task force report (APA, 1978) figures are not available.

Considering the information in print and their collective experience, the members of the APA task force recognized that a difference of opinion exists regarding the use of ECT in conditions other than schizophrenia and the affective disorders. Such a difference of opinion is not unknown in medical practice. The committee suggested that care be taken to consult with colleagues prospectively whenever possible when the use of ECT is considered for these unproven situations. They also suggested that the effectiveness of the treatment be carefully studied.

Situations Requiring Special Care

Although there has been outspoken criticism of the use of ECT in children, on rare and exceptional occasions its use in adolescents and even younger children has been acceptable to a small group of psychiatrists. Here again, the APA task force suggested consultation with colleagues ahead of time, particularly with colleagues who, though understanding the use of ECT, generally depend on a different type of treatment method. ECT in children should, in general, be considered an experimental procedure, not an established clinical one.

In the presence of serious physical conditions such as space-occupying intracranial lesions and recent myocardial infarction, as well as in advanced pregnancy, the APA report (1978) recommended that "the administration of ECT should be in the hands of a team of physicians who, collectively, have had considerable experience both with the use of ECT and with these conditions."

Recent studies have reported the successful use of ECT even in the presence of an implanted pacemaker (Abiuso et al., 1978) and have described the effective treatment with propranolol of ventricular arrhythmias following ECT (Weiner et al., 1979). In a thoughtful review of very recent developments, Small and Small (1981) point out that in the last five years there has been a discernible shift in medical and psychiatric attitudes toward ECT. Instead of regarding it as dangerous and potentially harmful, the profession has moved to viewing it as the safest treatment approach to take under many circumstances. This is particularly true in the presence of medical illness or other situations where there is reason for urgency and where drug treatment is hazardous or otherwise of restricted use. With the use of ECT the risks are limited to the period during which the treatment is administered and can be appropriately monitored. Those authors point to the need for investigative research into the influence of ECT on various conditions, including parkinsonism. A clinical report by Lebensohn and Jenkins (1975) discussed the improvement following the use of ECT in two patients suffering with severe Parkinson's disease and depression. The depressive symptoms cleared up, and the parkinsonian signs showed striking and sustained improvement. Small and Small (1981) also confirm that there is really no absolute contraindication to ECT. It can be used in the presence of serious medical disorders provided the treatment is given in facilities equipped to provide the necessary care.

PROFESSIONAL AND ETHICAL ISSUES

Over the past decade the professional and ethical issues relating to ECT have become interwoven with social and political factors. As reported above, much of the critical questioning leveled at the treatment of mental illness during this time has focused on ECT. The concepts and principles enmeshed in the arguments about civil commitment, mind-altering techniques, behavior modifying treatments, and informed consent have in several instances been highlighted by reports of cases involving ECT.

Bearing in mind the importance of the doctrines involved, namely, the right to treatment, the right to informed consent, and the right to refuse treatment, plus the fact that psychiatric illness can and does at times modify a patient's capacity to give informed consent, the APA task force report (APA, 1978) attempted in its recommendations to balance the individual's clinical needs with his or her civil rights. It paid particular attention to the equilibrium because it believed that a rigid emphasis on either legal rights or clinical demands leads to poor clinical management. The committee also recognized that its recommendations regarding consent procedures must ultimately mesh with or be influenced by local and state regulations and rulings.

Although from the theoretical standpoint there is a clear difference in the concern felt for patients who are competent to make decisions about treatment and those who are not, in practice competence is at times an elusive concept. Roth and his colleagues (Appelbaum and Roth, 1981) have conscientiously and carefully shown this. In addition, they have pointed out that informed consent is more often than not a developing process that has to be nurtured in supportive clinical interviews and encounters rather than a single event (Munetz et al., 1982).

In all cases, meticulous records should be kept by the psychiatrists and the facilities involved in the use of ECT—including patients who are adjudged competent to consent to ECT or to refuse it and cases in which patients are incompetent and either acquiesce to the treatment or protest its use. The task force recommended that records should include (APA, 1978):

a. the nature and history of the clinical condition leading to the consideration of ECT;

b. the details of previous treatments including therapeutic response and adverse reactions;

c. the reasons for selecting ECT;

d. the details of all discussions relevant to consent to treatment;

e. the signed consent form, with the signature of the patient and/or the relatives or guardian when appropriate;

f. the signed concurring and contradictory professional opinions where they exist; and

g. specifics of the treatment, e.g., unilateral or bilateral electrode placement, dates of treatment, characteristics of the current, drugs administered, etc.

The wisdom of such reporting is self evident. It not only reflects good medical care, but constitutes the best means of countering unwarranted criticism. In a sense it ensures that "justice is not only done, but can also be seen to be done."

Regarding informed consent, the task force report (APA, 1978) recommended that

the patient and/or his/her close relative or guardian should be competent to understand the following in simple language and, in agreeing, should sign a consent form indicating consent to the procedure:

a. the nature and seriousness of the disorder;

b. the probable course that is likely with or without ECT (without providing guarantees);

c. a description of the procedure;

d. the nature, degree, duration, and probability of significant risks and/or side effects and/or adverse effects. Special attention should be paid to post-treatment confusion and memory dysfunction;

e. a description of reasonable treatment alternatives and why ECT is being recommended;

f. the right of the patient to accept or refuse ECT, the right to revoke his/her consent at any time, and acknowledgment that the consent is for a specified maximum period of time. Additional treatments shall require a renewed written informed consent; and

g. the costs of the proposed treatment.

Furthermore, the following information should be entered in the patient's record in a standard form: that the information outlined above has been presented to the patient, and/or his/her relative or guardian; that the patient, relative or guardian is competent to understand and intelligently act upon this information; and that the consent for a course of treatment is being provided voluntarily, without coercion. The statement should appear before the signature of the attending physician.

CONCLUSION

Considerably greater sums of money will have to be spent in the future than in the past if we are to resolve the challenging questions associated with ECT. The Research Task Force of the National Institute of Mental Health reported (NIMH, 1975) that less than one percent of its total somatic therapy research grants from 1968 to 1973 were devoted to convulsive therapy.

Blind clinical studies of ECT are difficult to achieve because of the nature of the treatment. However, attentionostic groups, prospective studies with appropriate controls, and blind outside raters. Samples should be random and their numbers significant. Care should be taken in the design to acknowledge the importance of the number and frequency of the treatments, electrode placement, type of equipment used, evidence of a cerebral seizure, and adequacy of drug levels. Behavioral assessment should be detailed.

Some of the major needs in the field will be met by increasing our understanding in several areas. With regard to depressed patients there is a lack of knowledge about a possible pure ECT-responsive, non-drug-responsive group of patients and their characteristics; when ECT should be considered the preferred treatment; the value of simultaneous use of drugs and ECT; the long-term effect of ECT on the natural history of the illness; the comparative results of maintenance ECT and drug maintenance; and the comparative efficacy of unilateral and bilateral electrode placement in severe illness.

With regard to schizophrenic patients, we need to know more about the efficacy of ECT, the specific diagnostic categories that are most responsive, the value of unilateral electrode placement, the effectiveness of multiple treatments, whether the simultaneous use of drugs and ECT enhances outcome, and what the risks of the combined treatment are.

In the area of adverse effects we especially need to know more about the duration of memory loss for events occurring during the period of one month to three years prior to ECT, the importance to the patient of the memory loss, other possible factors related to persistent memory loss, and the comparative effects on memory loss of different kinds of electric current parameters.

Among the theoretical questions to be answered, we lack information regarding the role of acetylcholine in the ECT process, the effects of ECT on receptor function, the possible effects of direct stimulation of the brain stem in depressed patients, the relevance of personality variables to the outcome of ECT, and the differences in response between schizophrenic and depressed patients which may be related to CSF chemistry or cerebral electrophysiology. We require data that could lead to the formulation of an integrated biochemical and electrophysiologic hypothesis for the action of ECT in schizophrenia.

In appropriately selected cases, the beneficial and important effect of ECT on the hapless clinical course of a severely depressed patient can be dramatic and even exciting. It is this excitement that has prompted and encouraged the continued and intelligent use and investigation of ECT over the years; indeed many of those who have worked in the field have shown considerable courage in the face of professional disinterest, occasional disdain, and political opposition. Their efforts have led to an accumulating body of knowledge about the treatment procedure and its effects. We must now hope that future investigations and clinical studies with ECT will not only continue to cast light on how to achieve its beneficial effects with a minimum of risk and discomfort to the patient, but will also widen our understanding of psychiatric disorders.

REFERENCES

Abiuso P, Dunkelman R, Proper M: Electroconvulsive therapy in patients with pacemakers. JAMA 240:2459-2460, 1978

Abrams R, Taylor MA: Diencephalic stimulation and the effects of ECT in endogenous depression. Br J Psychiatry 129:482-486, 1976

Abrams R: ECT and psychotropic drugs, in Rational Psychopharmacotherapy and the Right to Treatment. Edited by Ayd FH Jr. Baltimore, Ayd Medical Communications, 1975

Alexander L: Treatment of Mental Disorder. Philadelphia, WB Saunders Co, 1953

Allen JP, Denney D, Kendall JW, et al: Corticotropin release during ECT in man. Am J Psychiatry 131:1225-1228, 1974

Angst J, Varga E, Shepherd M: Preliminary Report of a Retrospective Study of the Treatments of Depression. Excerpta Medica International Congress Series no. 129. Proceedings of the 5th International Congress of the Collegium Internationale Neuropsychopharmacologium, Washington, DC, March 1966, pp 28-31

Anton AH, Uy DS, Redderson CL: Autonomic blockade and the cardiovascular and catecholamine response to electroshock. Anesth Analg 56:46-54, 1977

APA Task Force on Electroconvulsive Therapy: Task Force Report 14: Electroconvulsive Therapy. Washington, DC, American Psychiatric Association, 1978

Appelbaum PS, Roth LH: Clinical issues in the assessment of competency. Am J Psychiatry 138:1462-1467, 1981

Avery D, Winokur G: Mortality in depressed patients treated with electroconvulsive therapy and antidepressants. Arch Gen Psychiatry 33:1029-1037, 1976

Baldessarini RJ: The basis for amine hypothesis in affective disorders. Arch Gen Psychiatry 32:1087-1093, 1975

Bergstrom DA, Troester S, Kellar KJ: Electroconvulsive shock and reserpine: effects on monoaminergic binding in rat brain, in Catecholamines: Basic and Clinical Frontiers. Edited by Usdin E, Kopin I, Barchas J. New York, Pergamon Press, 1978

Bickford RG, Rome HP: The electroencephalogram recorded during seizures produced by electroshock. Electroencephalogr Clin Neurophysiol 1:369, 1949

Bidder TG, Strain JJ, Brunschwig L: Bilateral and unilateral ECT: follow-up study and critique. Am J Psychiatry 127:737-745, 1970

Bidder TG: Personal communication, 1982

Bidder TG: Electroconvulsive Therapy (ECT) Psychopharmacology Module VII. Sepulveda, Calif, Veterans Administration Medical Center, May 1979

Bidder TG: Localized-convulsive electroconvulsive treatment Anesthesiology 23:266-267, 1962

Bielski RJ, Friedel RO: Prediction of tricyclic antidepressant response. Arch Gen Psychiatry 33:1479-1489, 1976

Blachly P, Gowing D: Multiple monitored electroconvulsive treatment. Compr Psychiatry 7:100-109, 1966

Bolwig TG, Hertz MM, Holm-Jensen J: Blood-brain barrier permeability during electroshock seizures in the rat. Eur J Clin Invest 7:95-100, 1977a

Bolwig TG, Hertz MM, Paulson OB, et al: The permeability of the blood-brain barrier during electrically induced seizures in man. Eur J Clin Invest 7:87-93, 1977b

Bratfos O, Haug JO: Electroconvulsive therapy and antidepressant drugs in manic-depressive disease, treatment results at discharge and 3 months later. Acta Psyhchiatr Scand 41:588-596, 1965

California Assembly Bill 1032, September, 1976

Cannicott SM: Unilateral electroconvulsive therapy. Postgrad Med J 38:451-459, 1962

Carroll BJ, Curtis GC, Mendels J: Neuroendocrine regulation in depression, II: discrimination of depressed from nondepressed patients. Arch Gen Psychiatry 33:1051-1058, 1976

Cerletti U, Bini L: Un nuevo metodo di shockterapie "L'elettro-shock." Boll Acad Med Roma 64:136-138, 1938

Cohen BD, Penick SB, Tarter RE: Antidepressant effect of unilateral ECT. Arch Gen Psychiatry 31:673-677, 1974

Creese I, Sibley DR: Receptor adaptations to centrally acting drugs. Ann Rev Pharmacol Toxicol 21:357-391, 1981

Crews FT, Paul SM, Goodwin FK: Acceleration of betareceptor desensitization in combined administration of antidepressants and phenoxybenzamine. Nature 290:787-789, 1981

Cronholm B, Ottosson JO: Experimental studies of the therapeutic action of electro-convulsive therapy in endogenous depression. Acta Psychiatr Neurol Scand Suppl 35:69-102, 1960

d'Elia G, Raotma H: Is unilateral ECT less effective than bilateral ECT? Br J Psychiatry 126:83-89, 1975

d'Elia G: Unilateral electroconvulsive therapy, in Psychobiology of Convulsive Therapy. Edited by Fink M, Kety S, McGaugh J, et al. Washington, DC, VH Winston & Sons, 1974

d'Elia G: Unilateral electroconvulsive therapy. Acta Psychiatr Scand Suppl 215:1-98, 1970

DeCarolis V, Giberti F, Roccatagliati G, et al: Imipramine and electroshock in the treatment of depression: a clinical statistical analysis of 437 cases. Sist Nerv 16:29-42, 1964

Ebert MH, Baldessarini RJ, Lipinski J, et al: Effects of electroconvulsive seizure on amine metabolism in the rat brain. Arch Gen Psychiatry 29:397-401, 1973

Fink M, Kahn RL, Green M: Experimental studies of the electroshock process. Dis Nerv Syst 19:113-118, 1958

Fink M, Kety S, McGaugh J, et al: Psychobiology of Convulsive Therapy. Washington, DC, VH Winston & Sons, 1974

Fink M: Convulsive Therapy: Theory and Practice. New York, Raven Press, 1979

Fleminger JJ, Horne DeL, Nair NPV, et al: Differential effect of unilateral and bilateral ECT. Am J Psychiatry 127:430-436, 1970

Folstein M, Folstein S, McHugh PR: Clinical predictors of improvement after electroconvulsive therapy of patients with schizophrenia, neurotic reactions, and affective disorders. Biol Psychiatry 7:147-152, 1973

Frankel FH: Reasoned discourse or a holy war: postscript to a report on ECT. Am J Psychiatry 132:77-79, 1975

Frankel FH: ECT in Massachusetts: a task force report. Massachusetts Journal of Mental Health 3:3-29, 1973

Freeman CPL, Basson JV, Crighton A: A double-blind controlled trial of electroconvulsive therapy: ECT and simulated ECT in depressive illness. Lancet 1:738-740, 1978

Friedberg J: Shock Treatment Is Not Good for Your Brain. San Francisco, Glide Publications, 1976

Friedman E: Unidirectional electrostimulated convulsive therapy, I: the effect of wave-form and stimulus characteristics on the convulsive dose. Am J Psychiatry 99:218-223, 1942

Gillespie DD, Manier DH, Sulser F: Electroconvulsive treatment: rapid subsensitivity of the norepinephrine receptor coupled adenylate cyclase system in brain linked to down regulation of beta-adrenergic receptors. Commun Psychopharmacol 3:191-195, 1979

Glassman A, Kantor SJ, Shostak M: Depression, delusions, and drug response. Am J Psychiatry 132:716-719, 1975

Glueck BC, Reiss H, Bernard LE: Regressive electric shock therapy. Psychiatric Quarterly 31:117-135, 1957

Greenblatt M, Grosser GH, Wechsler H: Differential response of hospitalized depressed patients to somatic therapy. Am J Psychiatry 120:935-943, 1964

Grinspoon L, Greenblatt M: Pharmacotherapy combined with other treatment methods. Compr Psychiatry 4:256-262, 1963

Group for the Advancement of Psychiatry: Shock Therapy, Report 1. Washington, DC, American Psychiatric Association, 1947

Halliday AM, Davison K, Browne MW, et al: A comparison of the effects on depression and memory of bilateral ECT and unilateral ECT to the dominant and non-dominant hemispheres. Br J Psychiatry 114:997-1012, 1968

Holmberg G: Biological aspects of electroconvulsive therapy. Int Rev Neurobiol 5:389-412, 1963

Hordern A, Burt CG, Holt NF: Depressive States. Springfield, Ill, Charles C Thomas, 1965

Huston PE, Locher LM: Involutional psychosis: course when untreated and when treated with ECT. Arch Neurol Psychiatry 59:385-394, 1948

Hutchinson JT, Smedburg D: Treatment of depression: a comparative study of ECT and six drugs. Br J Psychiatry 109:536-538, 1963

Johnstone EC, Lawler P, Stevens M, et al: The Northwick Park electroconvulsive therapy trial. Lancet 2:1317-1320, 1980

Kalinowsky LB: Personal communication, 1984

Kalinowsky LB: Convulsive therapies in Comprehensive Textbook of Psychiatry, vol 3 3rd ed. Edited by Freedman AM, Kaplan HI, Sadock BJ. Baltimore, Williams & Wilkins Co, 1980

Kalinowsky LB: Organic psychotic syndromes occurring during electric convulsive therapy. Arch Neurol Psychiatry 53:269-273, 1945

Kalow W, Lindsay HA: A comparison of optical and manometric methods for assay of human serum cholinesterase. Can J Biochem 33:568-574, 1955

Kety SS, Javoy F, Thierry AM, et al: A sustained effect of electroconvulsive shock on the turnover of norepinephrine in the central nervous system of the rat. Proc Natl Acad Sci 58: 1249-1254, 1967

Kristiansen ES: A comparison of treatment of endogenous depression with electro-shock and with imipramine. Acta Psychiatr Scand 37(Suppl 162):179-188, 1961

Ladisich W, Steinhauff N, Matussek N: Chronic administration of electro-convulsive shock norepinephrine metabolism after intracisternal injection with and without the influence of drugs in different brain regions and by 7-H-NE uptake in vitro. Psychopharmacologia 15:296-304, 1969

Lambourn J, Gill D: A controlled comparison of simulated and real ECT. Br J Psychiatry 133:514-519, 1978

Lancaster NP, Steinert RR, Frost I: Unilateral electroconvulsive therapy. J Ment Sci 104:221-227, 1958

Lebensohn ZM, Jenkins RB: Improvement of Parkinsonism in depressed patients treated with ECT. Am J Psychiatry 132:283-285, 1975

Lewis WH Jr, Richardson DJ, Bahagan LH: Cardiovascular disturbances and their management in modified electrotherapy for psychiatric illness. N Engl J Med 252:1016-1020, 1955

Lovett-Doust JW, Barchha R, Lee RSY, et al: Acute effects of ECT on the cerebral circulation in man. Eur Neurol 12:47-62, 1974

Lovett-Doust JW, Raschka LB: Enduring effects of modified ECT on the cerebral circulation in man. Psychiatr Clin 8: 293-303, 1975

MacKay WS: Death in treatment. Proc R Soc Med 46:13-20, 1953

Mandel MR, Welch CA, Mieske M, et al: Prediction of response to ECT in tricyclic-intolerant or tricyclic-resistant depressed patients. McLean Hospital Journal 2:203-209, 1977

May PRA, Tuma AH, Yale C, et al: Schizophrenia: a follow-up study of results of treatment, II: hospital stay over two to five years. Arch Gen Psychiatry 33:481-486, 1976

May PRA, Tuma AH: Treatment of schizophrenia: an experimental study of five treatment methods. Br J Psychiatry 111:503-510, 1965

May PRA: Treatment of Schizophrenia. New York, Science House, 1968

McCabe MS: ECT in the treatment of mania: a controlled study. Am J Psychiatry 133:688-691, 1976

McDonald IM, Perkins M, Marjerrison G, et al: A controlled comparison of amitriptyline and electroconvulsive therapy in the treatment of depression. Am J Psychiatry 122:1426-1431, 1966

Medical Research Council: Clinical trial of the treatment of depressive illness. Br Med J 5439:881-886, 1965

Meduna LJ: Die Konvulsions Therapie der Schizophrenie. Halle, Carl Marhold, 1937

Morris JB, Beck AT: The efficacy of antidepressant drugs: a review of research 1958-1972. Arch Gen Psychiatry 30:667-674, 1974

Munetz MR, Roth LH, Cornes CL: Tardive dyskinesia and informed consent: myths and realities. Bull AAPL 10:77-88, 1982

Murillo LG, Exner JR Jr: The effects of regressive ECT with process schizophrenics. Am J Psychiatry 130:269-273, 1973

National Institute of Mental Health, Clinical Research Branch, and Temple University: Proceedings of Conference on ECT: Efficacy and Impact, New Orleans, February 1978

Öhman R, Baldin J, Walinder J, et al: Prolactin response to electroconvulsive therapy. Lancet 2:936-937, 1976

Perrin GM: Cardiovascular aspects of electric shock therapy. Acta Psychiatr Neurol Scand 6(Suppl 152):1-45, 1961

Plum F, Howse DC, Duffy TE: Metabolic effects of seizures. Association for Research in Nervous and Mental Disease 53:141-157, 1974

Plum F, Posner JB, Troy B: Cerebral metabolic and circulatory responses to induced convulsions in animals. Arch Neurol 18:1-13, 1968

Pryor GT, Otis LS: Persisting effects of chronic electroshock seizures on brain and behavior in two strains of rats. Physiol Behav 5:1053-1055, 1970

Pryor GT, Peache S, Scott MK: The effect of repeated electroconvulsive shock on avoidance conditioning and brain monoamine oxidase activity. Physiol Behav 9:623-628, 1972

Regenstein QR, Murawski BJ, Engle RP: A case of prolonged, reversible dementia associated with abuse of convulsive therapy. J Nerv Ment Dis 161:200-203, 1975

Research in the Service of Mental Health: Report of Research Task Force of National Institute of Mental Health. DHEW publication (ADM) 75-236. Rockville, Md, NIMH, 1975

Ryan RJ, Sanson DW, Faiman CH, et al: Effects of convulsive electroshock on serum concentrations of follicle-stimulating hormone, luteinizing hormone, thyroid stimulating hormone and growth hormone in man. J Clin Endocrinol Metab 30:51-58, 1970

Sachar EJ, Hellmexcretion in psychotic depression. Arch Gen Psychiatry 28:19-24, 1973

Sainz A: Clarification of the action of successful treatments in the depressions. Dis Nerv Syst 20:53-57, 1959

Salzman C: The use of ECT in the treatment of schizophrenia. Am J Psychiatry 137:1032-1041, 1980

Sand-Strömgren LS: Unilateral vs bilateral electroconvulsive therapy. Acta Psychiatr Scand Suppl 240:1-65, 1973

Sargant W, Slater E: Physical Methods of Treatment in Psychiatry. Edinburgh, Livingstone, 1963

Small JG, Small IF: ECT update. Psychopharmacol Bull 17:29-42, 1981

Small JG: EEG neurophysiological studies of convulsive therapies, in Psychobiology of Convulsive Therapy. Edited by Fink M, Kety S, McGaugh J, et al. Washington DC, VH Winston & Sons, 1974

Smith K, Surphles WRP, Gynther G, et al: ECT-chlorpromazine and chlorpromazine compared in the treatment of schizophrenia. J Nerv Ment Dis 144:284-290, 1967

Spanis CW, Squire LR: Memory and convulsive stimulation: effects of stimulus wave-form. Am J Psychiatry 138:1177-1181, 1981

Squire LR: ECT and memory loss. Am J Psychiatry 134:997-1001, 1977

Stoelting RK, Peterson C: Heart rate slowing and junctional rhythm following intravenous succinylcholine with and without intramuscular atropine preanesthetic medication. Anesth Analg 54:705-709, 1975

Stokes, PE: Studies on the control of adrenocortical function in depression, in Recent Advances in the Psychobiology of the Depressive Ilnesses. Edited by Williams TA, Katz M, Shield JA. Washington, DC, US Government Printing Office, 1972

Strain JJ, Brunschwig L, Duffy JP, et al: Comparison of therapeutic effects and memory changes with bilateral and unilateral ECT. Am J Psychiatry 125:294-304, 1968

Sutherland EM, Oliver JE, Knight D: EEG, memory and confusion in dominant, non-dominant and bitemporal ECT. Br J Psychiatry 115:1059-1064, 1969

Taylor P, Fleminger JJ: ECT for schizophrenia. Lancet 1: 1380-1383, 1980

Turek IS: Combined use of ECT and psychotropic drugs: antidepressives and antipsychotics. Compr Psychiatry 14:485-502, 1973

Ulett GA, Smith K, Gleser GC: Evaluation of convulsive and subconvulsive shock therapies utilizing a control group. Am J Psychiatry 112:795-802, 1956

Weiner RD, Henschen GM, Dellasega M, et al: Propranolol treatment of an ECT-related ventricular arrhythmia. Am J Psychiatry 136:1594-1595, 1979

Weiss DM: Changes in blood pressure with electroshock therapy in a patient receiving chlorpromazine hydrochloride (Thorazine). Am J Psychiatry 111:617-619, 1955

Wells DA: Electroconvulsive treatment for schizophrenia: a ten year survey in a university hospital psychiatry department. Compr Psychiatry 14:291-298, 1973

Wessels WH: A comparative study of the efficacy of bilateral and unilateral electroconvulsive therapy with thioridazine in acute schizophrenia. S Afr Med J 46:890-892, 1971

West ED: Electric convulsive therapy in depression: a double-blind controlled trial. Br Med J 282:355-357, 1981

Wilson IC, Vernon JT, Guin T, et al: A controlled study of treatments of depression. J Neuropsychiat 4:331-337, 1963

Witten K: Efficacy of ECT following prolonged use of psychotropic drugs. Am J Psychiatry 119:79-80, 1962

Wittenborn J, Plante M, Burgess F, et al: A comparison of imipramine, electroconvulsive therapy and placebo in the treatment of depressions. J Nerv Ment Dis 135:131-137, 1962

Wyatt v Hardin, no 3195-N (MD Ala Feb 28, 1975, modified July 1, 1975)

Wyatt v Stickney, 325 F Supp 781 (MD Ala 1971); 334 F Supp 1341 (MD Ala 1971); enforced by 334 F Supp 373, 344 F Supp 387, appeal docketed sub nom Wyatt v Aderholt, no 72-2634, 5th Cir, filed Aug, 1973

Ylikorkala O, Kauppila A, Haapalahti J, et al: The effect of electric convulsion therapy on the circulating concentrations of pituitary hormones, cortisol, and cyclic adenosine monophosphate. Clin Endocrinol 5:571-574, 1976

5
Psychosurgery

5

Psychosurgery

INTRODUCTION

In the period of social unrest occurring between 1965 and 1975, the topic of psychosurgery assumed a position of national prominence, with the public and professional groups voicing their concerns about the possible abuse of the procedure, the ethics of its use, and the validity of its effects as a therapeutic measure. The Congress of the United States appointed the National Commission on the Protection of Human Subjects of Biomedical and Behavioral Research to investigate, study, and recommend policies governing the use of psychosurgery.

The American and Canadian Psychiatric Associations also appointed bodies with the same charge. Reports were submitted by the American Psychiatric Association Task Force in March 1976, the National Commission in mid-1976, and the Canadian Professional Standards and Practice Council in 1977. In content and recommendations, the three reports were similar, with one or two differences. Each body independently adopted a working definition that closely resembled that of the others in all important details, the definition of the APA Task Force being used here:

> Psychosurgery is surgical intervention to sever fibers connecting one part of the brain with another or to remove, destroy or stimulate brain tissue with the intent of modifying or altering disturbances of behavior, thought content or mood for which no organic pathological cause can be demonstrated by established tests and techniques. Such surgery may also be undertaken for the relief of intractable pain.

Psychosurgery falls into two categories, one therapeutic, the other experimental. Therapeutic psychosurgery includes neurosurgical intervention to treat psychopathological conditions, using techniques that have been shown to produce overall beneficial effects in psychoses, neuroses, behavioral, or mood disorders. The term "psychosurgery" does not include neurosurgical intervention to treat or correct a disease for which there is a demonstrable organic basis, for example, the removal of an epileptic focus. Experimental psychosurgery is neurosurgical intervention undertaken on the basis of tentative evidence that such intervention will result in overall beneficial effects to the individual suffering from psychosis, neurosis, behavioral, or mood disorder.

There are two sets of conditions in which the definition of psychosurgery as a therapeutic procedure presents questions. The first is in severe pain that is intractable to relief by medication or other intervention, and the second is in forms of epilepsy for which a pathological focus cannot be shown by physiological methods.

Severe intractable pain may be a concomitant of conditions in which an organic pathological cause may be shown but no other treatment is effective, for example, in inoperable cancer. Brain surgery in such patients may produce significant pain relief with or without significant changes in the personality of the patient. Intervention intended to modify the total organismic response to pain is considered to be psychosurgery. Surgical intervention intended to sever the pain pathways or to modify the transmission of impulses from the periphery which would lead to the experience of pain is considered to be neurosurgery rather than psychosurgery.

There occur, however, conditions of intractable pain in which no physical, pathological, or physiological cause can be shown. The experience of pain is variable from person to person, the degree being determined by subjective factors. In persons complaining of severe intractable pain for which a physiological or pathological cause cannot be shown, significant psychopathological conditions such as psychoses or conversion syndromes are often found to exist. In these patients, major relief from pain may be obtained by neurosurgical intervention, which thereby falls in the category of psychosurgery.

In attempting to define psychosurgery as different from neurosurgery, special problems arise with respect to epilepsy because of the relative lack of uniformity of classification of behavioral manifestations associated with the varieties of the condition. When objective evidence of epilepsy has been demonstrated, surgical intervention to remove the pathological focus or area is considered neurosurgery and not psychosurgery.

HISTORY

With the discovery in archaeological excavations of human skulls in which there were holes with rounded edges, indicating that the subjects survived many years after the holes were made, it was postulated that ancient peoples may well have performed psychosurgery. It is more probable, lacking evidence to the contrary, that these holes were the result of disease or injury, for example by clubbing, though they possibly were made intentionally for medical reasons. In the latter case, they may have been made to "let out" evil spirits rather than to gain access to the brain itself.

In more recent times, the first recorded neurosurgical interventions for therapeutic purposes in psychiatric patients were in 1890 when Burckhardt, a Swiss psychiatrist, reported a small series of neurosurgical procedures for assaultive patients. In 1935, Egas Moniz, a Portuguese psychiatrist, heard a presentation by F. Jacobsen, an associate of John F. Fulton, at the International Neurological Congress in London. The lecture described dramatic changes in the personality of monkeys effected by excision of the frontal cortex. With a surgeon, Almeida Lima, Moniz submitted a series of chronically disturbed patients to prefrontal lobotomy, at first by the injection of alcohol and later by cutting with a leucotome; he published his results in 1936 (Moniz, 1936). As an innovative therapy, the operation received world-wide attention, opened a new approach for treatment of hitherto untreatable patients, and culminated in the bestowal on Moniz of the Nobel Prize for Medicine in 1949.

The original alcohol injection procedure advocated by Moniz proved temporary in effect and was replaced by the use of a leucotome. This instrument, with an extrudible wire loop at the end, was introduced into the brain through burr holes in the skull. When in position, the wire loop was extruded and rotated to cut a core of white matter, producing bilateral isolation of the superior, middle, and inferior gyri of the pre-frontal lobes of the cerebrum from almost all their connections with the rest of the brain.

Introduced into the United States in 1937, Freeman and Watts (1937) modified this technique, replacing the leucotome with a scalpel, which was moved up and down in a coronal section just anterior to the horn of the lateral ventricle. The immediate effects of this approach were often to eliminate aggressive and assaultive behavior; and the operation was enthusiastically adopted, albeit prematurely, as an accepted procedure of inestimable benefit to thousands of chronically ill, disturbed patients hospitalized for long periods of time, for whom all other known therapies had been ineffective.

It is now universally recognized that the wave of enthusiasm for active intervention in the treatment of chronic psychoses which arose in the 1930's and 1940's was generated in part by the apparent success claimed for insulin coma and electroshock in schizophrenic and depressed patients. This enthusiasm was in part a reaction to the dreadful condition of hundreds of thousands of mentally ill patients for whom the then available alternative therapeutic modalities were recognized as almost totally ineffective. As with all innovative therapies, enthusiasm overrode the need for cautious scientific evaluation. One may well draw a parallel with the enthusiasm at that time for the use of prontosil, and later penicillin, in almost every kind of disorder known to man, or, still earlier in psychiatry, for the wholesale removal of "foci of infection" advocated by Cotton in the 1920's (Cotton, 1922).

In the late 1940's, when the benefits and unwanted sequelae of complete coronal section had been thoroughly evaluated, the limitations of this approach were widely recognized (Greenblatt, 1950). Many patients, depending on the extensiveness of the section, were transformed into individuals without initiative of any kind—not infrequently to a vegetative state requiring almost complete supervision. Since a large proportion were chronic schizophrenic patients, the deterioration in personality was severe. Diminution in intelligence and loss of previous skills were marked in some, and it was recognized that isolation of the superior and lateral frontal cortex gyri particularly contributed to this outcome.

Other complications included intracerebral hemorrhage, sometimes due to aberrant blood vessels, and the onset of post-operative epilepsy, usually controllable with anticonvulsants but sometimes not. Other physical sequelae included paralysis, incontinence, and excessive weight gain. In those early years, the mortality rate was as high as five percent.

On the basis of these clinical experiences, new, more limited procedures were introduced. Though still performed on the frontal lobes, these modified approaches produced smaller areas of destruction with fewer and less deleterious complications. Thus, Scoville (1948) introduced "cortical undercutting," sectioning the fibers connecting the orbital cortex to other parts of the brain. With this "open" approach, the surgeon was able to view the area of the brain undergoing surgery. In the same year, Penfield (1948) carried out gyrectomy—removal of portions of the frontal gyri, and Peyton (Peyton et al., 1948) performed bilateral frontal lobectomy. Topectomy—removal of specific areas of the frontal lobes—was carried out by Pool and Mettles (Columbia-Greystone Associates, 1949). Of these procedures, orbital undercutting survived and, with modifications, was adopted by neurosurgeons in a number of countries.

Special mention should be made of transorbital lobotomy, first reported by Fiamberti (1937) and later adopted in the United States by Freeman (1948). Using this technique, usually performed in the post-electroshock, unconscious anesthetic stage, the cranium and the cerebrum are penetrated via the orbital plate of the skull using an "icepick-like" instrument. Freeman claimed to have treated more than 3,500 patients in this way with very good outcomes. This procedure was sometimes performed as an office treatment.

ADVANCES IN TECHNOLOGY

In 1947, Spiegel (Spiegel et al., 1947) first described stereotactic instrumentation for localization within the brain, opening up the potential for placing small, discrete lesions in specific sites outside the frontal lobes.

With the head in a fixed plane and using three-dimensional maps of the cranium and brain together with additional aids such as x-rays, the lesion-producing devices can be placed, with some degree of accuracy, in a large portion of the brain through small trephine holes in the skull. To create small precise lesions, a variety of techniques were devised. These included electrocoagulation by Grantham (1951), freezing by LeBeau (1954), thermo-coagulation with heat by Herner (1961), ultrasonic irradiation by Lindstrom (1954), prognostic electrostimulation prior to electrocoagulation by Crow and colleagues (1963), and implantation of radioactive yttrium-19 seeds by Knight (1965). The ability to see the effects of stimulation of the area selected, including the autonomic concomitants of emotional arousal, prior to operation greatly increased the accuracy with which the lesions could be placed.

As a result of experience with results of surgery on different parts of the frontal lobes, the consensus developed that the best results with a minimum of adverse personality changes were obtained by section of fibers passing to and from the ventromedial and orbital portions of the cortex. As a result of animal experimentation, clinical experience, post-mortem examination, and increasing recognition of the connections of areas of the frontal cortex to parts of the limbic system, sites outside the frontal lobes were selected. Anterior cingulectomy was carried out in 1952 by Whitty and Cairns in England with favorable results (Whitty et al., 1952). There followed reports of the effects of operation on other parts of the cingulum, the amygdala, and parts of the thalamic and hypothalamic complexes.

A combination of factors led to a great reduction in the number of operations from the mid-1950's onward, with less and less attention to psychosurgery on the professional level. It was never a concern on the public level until the late 1960's and early 1970's. Then, during this time of general social unrest, charges by activists that psychosurgery was used as a political tool received high media visibility. As a consequence of the public controversy, the number of procedures in the United States dropped still further. In the past decade, new data about the effects of psychosurgery have largely been derived from its use abroad, particularly in England.

INCIDENCE OF PSYCHOSURGERY

In the early 1970's, charges were made that some 40,000 to 50,000 "lobotomies" had been performed in the United States. There is no way either to substantiate this figure or to make any reliable estimate. In 1951, Kramer reported this difficulty in a survey of psychosurgery (Kramer, 1954).

The most recent figures are those reported by Donnelly (1978), who, in 1974, surveyed the 1,901 active members of the American Association of Neurological Surgeons and the Congress of Neurological Surgeons. Out of

1,481 responses (78 percent), 110 U.S. and 19 Canadian neurosurgeons reported carrying out psychosurgery in 1971-1973.

A total of 972 procedures were reported in the U.S.—308 in 1971, 343 in 1972, and 321 in 1973. Based on statistical correction to include nonresponders, the number arrived at is 1,246 or an average of 415 each year. However, because of the variation in the numbers of procedures by each neurosurgeon, together with other methods of checking the nonresponders, these figures are, without doubt, in excess of the true numbers. A much more likely figure is 380 to 400 per year for each of the three years studied.

Several items were of note. A large percentage of the neurosurgeons responding performed one to five operations per year. When four neurosurgeons were eliminated, the number of procedures showed evidence of a decline from 1971 to 1973. It is believed that in the years since 1974 the number has declined rapidly, in part because of the adverse publicity, fear of legal suits, and possibly a decrease in the number of patients meeting the criteria for surgery.

Another item of note was the number of different lesion sites selected. Cingulotomies constituted the greatest percentage, with lesions in other areas of the limbic system making up most of the remainder. Similarly, a variety of techniques were used to produce the lesions. A similar distribution in lesion sites was reported by Gildenberg (1975) from a questionnaire aimed at ascertaining the extent of stereotactic psychosurgery in the United States and Canada.

In comparison with United States experience, it was reported by Tooth and Newton (1961) that 10,365 procedures were performed in England between 1944 and 1955, while 431 operations between 1974 and 1976 were reported by Barraclough and Mitchell-Heggs (1978). The latter stated that other estimates have placed the annual number in the 200 to 250 range.

It may be noted in passing that there was comparable distribution of the number of procedures per surgeon in the various centers in England. However, there are two major neurosurgical centers in London where collaborative pre- and post-operative assessment, including psychologic and physiologic studies, are carried out, with short- and long-term follow-up providing data superior to those otherwise available (Kelly et al., 1972; Mitchell-Heggs et al., 1976).

The number of psychosurgery procedures per year has dropped rapidly in recent years. In addition to recognition of the therapeutic limitations of neurosurgical intervention on the frontal lobes, there are two other significant reasons for the decline that started in the early 1950's. The first was the introduction of other, less drastic therapeutic modalities; and the second was advances in knowledge about brain anatomy and the organization of cerebral functions.

With respect to therapeutic alternatives, there were three developments.

The first was the increasing use of electroconvulsive therapy (ECT) under anesthesia following the administration of muscle relaxants. The second was the introduction in the 1950's of the phenothiazine drugs, which almost immediately provided new modalities for eliminating or reducing disturbed, aggressive, and assaultive behavior that hitherto had been untreatable except by neurosurgical measures. The third development was the introduction of antidepressants in the 1960's, further reducing the number of patients unresponsive to treatment.

With these psychotropic agents, the number of potential candidates for consideration for psychosurgery had precipitously declined by the 1960's. Following public controversy at the end of that decade, the number of operations fell further so that now only a very limited number of interventions are performed each year. There is, however, no information available as to current incidence.

BASIC SCIENCE ISSUES

The reasons advanced in support of psychosurgery are essentially of an empirical nature, based on outcome in patients undergoing such procedures. They have almost always been performed on patients whose conditions are of long duration; have not responded to other available treatments; and, from a prognostic viewpoint, are judged to be otherwise incurable.

From a scientific viewpoint, the physiological basis for psychosurgery is still largely conjectural. The reasons given rest on a number of arguments, in part derived from animal experimentation, in part from clinical effects and outcomes of particular procedures, and largely by extrapolations derived from data from both sources.

Moniz was influenced by the results of animal experimentation, reported by Jacobsen, of the calming effect of ablation of the frontal lobes of monkeys. In the early years of its use, lobotomy performed on assaultive patients eliminated the aggressiveness but at an unacceptable cost to the personality. Further experimentation on animals led to increased knowledge of the role of certain areas of the brain in stimulating and inhibiting emotional arousal and of concomitant autonomic changes.

Surgical intervention in selected areas of the brains of human patients followed. The effects of electric stimulation by implanted electrodes increased recognition of the involvement of specific cortical areas and their relationships to emotional arousal and inhibition. The orbital and ventromedial areas of the frontal lobes were recognized as having a role in the emotions of the individual. Tracing their connections led to appreciation of the involvement of the dorsomedial nucleus of the thalamus and of the hypothalamus. There followed recognition of the role of other parts of the limbic system, the cingulate gyrus, the hippocampus, the fornix, the thalamus, the amygdala, and their intricate interconnections.

A combination of animal experimentation, electric stimulation in human subjects by Heath (1971) and others (Valenstein, 1973), and imposed stress by psychologic and physiologic means resulted in hypotheses regarding the role of the hypothalamus in anxiety and of the amygdala in aggression. Apparent supporting evidence was derived from the effects of lesions placed in these sites. There evolved consensus that the limbic system plays a major part in the evocation of emotional phenomena and that the medial and orbital areas of the frontal lobes modulate these responses.

Psychosurgery was then directed to severing specific connections between different parts of the limbic system, the target areas including the anterior, middle, and posterior cingulum; the substantia innominata; the internal capsule; the amygdala; and portions of the thalamus and hypothalamus. In the absence of specific information to explain the effects of surgical intervention, most hypotheses center around the concept of fixed, stabilized, pathological circuits or reverberating circuits that sustain the emotional disorder. Expressed in a variety of ways, interruption of these circuits is postulated to destabilize them with resulting beneficial effects. Granting that the interconnections of the limbic system are complex, it is not clear why intervention in different sites results in similar benefits.

The physiological rationale for modern psychosurgery rests on the work of Papez (1937), who hypothesized that the rhinencephalic structures, namely the hypothalamus, the mammillary bodies, the anterior thalamic nuclei, the cingulate gyrus, and the hippocampus, together with their connections, constitute a harmonious mechanism that might participate in the functions of central emotion and in emotional expression. The cortical representation of the emotions included cortex of the cingulate and hippocampal gyri. In the Papez circuit, the cingulate bundle in the cingulate gyrus is a key element of the interconnections.

The Papez circuit has been modified over the years, mainly by the addition of connections with other cerebral structures, including the medial central portion of the frontal lobe. Kelly (Kelly, 1973; Kelly et al., 1973) termed a limbic circuit, described some ten years earlier by Hilton (Hilton and Zbrozyna, 1963), as the "defense reaction circuit." This circuit passed from the amygdala to the hypothalamus via the stria terminalis and back to the amygdala. With increasing intensity of electric stimulation of these structures and their connections in the cat, the animal manifests progressive stages of arousal from the resting state to that of attack in response to visual and auditory stimuli. Concomitantly, marked autonomic phenomena occur, including changes in respiration, heart rate, and muscle vasodilation.

Sites of Intervention

On the basis of these observations, lesions are made in the lower medial quadrant of the frontal lobes to interrupt some fronto-limbic connections and in the anterior portion of the cingulate bundle and, in some patients, in the rostral portion of the bundle.

Almost all current psychosurgical operations are directed stereotactically to place lesions in the limbic system. By far, the majority are cingulotomies to interrupt the cingulate bundle. Some are located in the anterior portion; fewer in the middle or rostral segment. Other sites are the subcaudate and ventromedial frontal areas. While single bilateral lesions in the cingulum have been the rule, there has been a trend toward locating bilaterally two or more targets within the limbic system. The improved benefits claimed for this approach may result from the interruption of more than one of the circuits within the limbic system.

Amygdalotomy, with the intent of modifying severe pathological and uncontrollable aggression associated with a psychiatric disorder, is sometimes carried out abroad but is no longer performed in the U.S. Hypothalamotomy and thalamotomy are rarely performed anywhere. Suborbital undercutting is occasionally undertaken but not by neurosurgeons who specialize in surgical treatment of psychiatric illness.

One of the difficulties in predicting outcome arises from the anatomical variation of the precise site of the intended ablation. Another arises from the smallness of the lesion—if sufficient interruption is not produced, the effect is then at least less than intended. This appears particularly true for single lesions in the cingulum and, for this reason, one or more subsequent operations have been undertaken in some patients.

CLINICAL ISSUES

Psychosurgery is primarily a method for relief of severe psychic distress. The clinical syndromes that have been responsive are severe depressive disorders, anxiety and phobic states, and obsessive-compulsive neuroses. The criteria for selection of all patients for psychosurgery include the severity of and the incapacity produced by the illness, the duration, and the intractability to adequate trials of all alternate forms of appropriate and available treatment.

Irrespective of the sites of the lesions within the limbic system, there is universal agreement that depressions are benefited most. Claims of success range from 56 percent to 80 percent recovered and improved in endogenous depressions (Mitchell-Heggs et al., 1976; Stromberg-Olsen and Carlisle, 1971; Goktepe et al., 1975; Knight, 1973). In bipolar depression, the results are far less clear. Few such patients have undergone psychosurgical procedures. At the same time, evaluation and comparison of effectiveness are difficult because different surgeons place lesions in different sites and differ in the number of lesions placed. The potentially different criteria with regard to severity of illness and the categories of benefit also make comparisons difficult.

Success rates reported in obsessive-compulsive conditions also vary, apparently for some of the same reasons. These range from 50 percent to 89 percent success (67 percent recovered or much improved) (Kelly et al., 1972; Mitchell-Heggs et al., 1976; Stromberg-Olsen and Carlisle, 1971; Goktepe et al., 1975; Knight, 1973; Tippin and Henn, 1982). It has been noted that, while depressive syndromes gain maximum improvement rapidly, obsessive-compulsive states continue to improve up to at least 16 months and longer after the surgery. Experience with chronic anxiety and phobic conditions indicates the degree of success as falling in the range of 40 percent to 50 percent, with some patients who do well at first but relapse later.

Perhaps the most specific statement of the indications for psychosurgery are those of a three-hospital group of neuropsychiatric centers in the United Kingdom. Working together, each team operates on a different site according to the clinical picture (Bartlett et al., 1981). The most favorable outcomes reported are in patients who have maintained an intact premorbid personality. This is perhaps a manifestation of the finding that the prognosis is best when the disturbance is mainly or totally a disorder of mood, though the requirement of a stable personality has been questioned (Bridges and Bartlett, 1977).

There is a consensus in the U.S. that psychosurgery is not effective in schizophrenia. Part of the basis of this opinion possibly arises from the results of prefrontal lobotomies performed on such patients and part on the selection of patients who have manifested "blunting" of affect. Claims of improvement in some schizophrenic patients following psychosurgery using modern approaches have been made abroad, particularly in the United Kingdom, where different diagnostic criteria are used. The benefit occurs in patients in whom depression is a significant feature and is attributable to modification of the affective component of the clinical picture. It is generally agreed that psychosurgery does not alter hallucinations, delusions, and other thought disorders. It may, however, be effective in reducing or even eliminating strong affective components associated with them, particularly those with paranoid ideation. Where these are of a distressing nature to the patient, diminution or elimination of the associated affect appears to modify the experience of the patient so that the paranoid phenomenon gradually assumes decreasing prominence. This effect is comparable with successful neurosurgery for the relief of severe intractable pain due to physical disease. Some such patients state that they still have the sensation of pain but are not distressed by it.

Psychosurgical intervention has been performed, mostly in other countries, in a number of other psychiatric diagnostic categories, including in psychopathic personalities and criminals and for alcoholism and other addictive disorders (Rieber and Sigusch, 1979). Claims of benefit are mixed, but the consensus is that the evidence is not supportive of its effectiveness in these conditions.

Prefrontal lobotomy was first undertaken to relieve and control assaultive and violent behavior, particularly in schizophrenic patients. With the abandonment of lobotomies and the introduction of antipsychotic medication, this indication disappeared. Controversy arose in the early 1970's over reported operations on mentally retarded minors. These were reported to be very disturbed, ineducable, assaultive individuals whose behavior was very dangerous to those responsible for their care and who were uncontrolled by psychotropic drugs. Though few in number, they presented a severe management problem. The alternate treatment was the administration of large doses of depot medication, producing states akin to those resulting from extensive prefrontal lobotomy. The risk of irreversible incapacitating abnormal motor movements from such drugs is substantial since long-term administration is necessary.

Animal experimentation using implanted electrodes, together with clinical investigations, has provided evidence that the amygdala is involved in aggressive emotions and behavior (Kiloh and Smith, 1978). Amygdalotomy (Kiloh et al., 1974) has been performed, particularly abroad, on some patients in attempts to relieve the assaultive condition. In the United States, the procedure is not used unless organic pathology in the amygdala has been shown, for example, physical trauma or an epileptic focus, in which case the operation falls outside the definition of psychosurgery.

A controversial issue concerns the age before which psychosurgery should not be undertaken. The consensus is that it should not be performed at least until the individual has completely passed beyond the maturational stages of development. For most patients, this is in the range of 25 to 30 years. Except for limitations based on physical impairment, there are no limitations with regard to age beyond 60 years.

Another issue arises with regard to the stage of the illness at which psychosurgery is indicated. Generally, an operative approach is not considered until adequate trials of every other available and indicated treatment have failed to be effective. These therapies include psychotropic medication, psychotherapy, behavior therapy, electroconvulsive therapy, etc. Such a pattern clearly consumes a long period of time. A few psychiatrists, on the other hand, base their opinion on the generally accepted belief that the longer a psychiatric illness persists, the more fixed and irreversible it becomes. They, therefore, recommend early surgery after about 12 months of treatment have proved unavailing.

Post-Operative Deficits

Prefrontal lobotomy was abandoned largely because of the adverse post-operative personality changes, particularly with section of the connections of the superior and lateral cortex. Decrease in tested intelligence, apathy, lability of affect with easily triggered irritability, lack of initiative, impaired concentration, and loss of previously manifested skills were prominent as well as obesity and decreased attention to personal hygiene. Of concern also were the cases of operative and post-operative deaths, intracerebral hemorrhage, and post-surgical epilepsy. With modern technology, the reported mortality rates are low (e.g., one in 800 cases) and in most series nonexistent. Similarly, the incidence of epilepsy is significantly lower—in one series of 100 cingulotomies, no cases occurred. Often the patient is placed on anticonvulsant medication for six months, after which it is discontinued. Should epileptic attacks occur, the medication is reinstituted. This, apparently, is seldom necessary.

With operations confined to segments of the limbic system, the absence of post-lobotomy deficits, such as blunting of affect, is repeatedly reported. In many patients, the intelligence quotient is increased (Mitchell-Heggs et al., 1976; Teuber et al., 1977), as is performance in the Hidden Figures Test (Corkin, 1979). While few or no overt permanent neurological or behavioral defects are evident, some deficits are present on testing. In some post-cingulotomy patients, for example, an apparently irreversible deficit in copying a drawing on the Rey-Taylor Complex Figure Test has been reported by Corkin (1980). These findings impinge on the issue of the therapeutic purpose of psychosurgery. Since all patients have long been suffering severe, incapacitating psychic distress and have been unresponsive to other therapies, the question has been posed: Is the purpose to restore the individual to a state judged to be "normal" and, if so, how is "normal" to be defined? Like the IQ, most variables tested in psychometrics are distributed over the bell curve, including such innate skills as musical, manual, and mathematical abilities. If, on the other hand, the objective is to relieve the distress and remove the incapacity, the question has been raised how such a result is to be weighed against one or more relatively minor functional changes, especially when both increases and decreases in different variables occur in the same patient.

A Treatment of Last Resort

When all the information regarding claims of effectiveness of psychosurgery, the conflicting opinions with respect to age and stage of maturational development, the indications and contraindications, and appropriate categories are considered, there emerges a conclusion that this approach is effective primarily in the treatment of affective conditions of a severe incapacitating nature which have failed to respond to all other alternative psychiatric therapies—in other words, as a treatment of last resort. In spite of the recent treatments, there are still a few patients who meet these criteria and for whom there is otherwise no hope for relief of their distress.

The term "treatment of last resort" has been raised as an issue by some critics of psychosurgery. The term implies that all known therapies have been tried. Availability is a function of the distribution of social resources. In the practice of medicine, and in psychiatry in particular, there is great variation with regard to the availability of specific treatments on geographic, economic, and professional grounds. Liver and kidney transplants, for example, are less available in many parts of the country compared to large metropolitan centers. Even within these cities, the levels of care available to patients with limited financial resources are substantially below those of others who are more financially endowed.

ETHICAL ISSUES

More than any other treatment in medicine, psychosurgery raises profound ethical concerns. The first is the scientific evidence justifying such a radical approach. Much of the opposition is emotional, originating in the adverse effects of extensive prefrontal lobotomy. There often appears to be a lack of awareness that lobotomy was discarded many years ago and that the outcomes of modern psychosurgery bear little resemblance to those of the former.

Scientific Validation

Over the past two decades, there have been far-reaching changes in medical research in general. Current scientific methodology is more rigorous than in the past. Valid evaluative instruments as judged by currently accepted standards were not then available. In psychiatry, adequate patient information regarding symptomatology and prognosis, both pre- and post-operatively, was not studied in the same way as today. Further, as evidenced by the recent development and broad use of *DSM-III*, uniformity of clinical diagnosis, the then-current knowledge about psychiatric illness, the specificity of clinical categories, and the life history of specific conditions was less detailed than today. The number of psychiatrists, each responsible for large numbers of institutionalized patients, was small. Importantly, psychotropic medications had not been discovered.

Even now, strict scientific evaluation faces almost insuperable difficulties. The variation within specific conditions in the same diagnostic categories is immense, a problem that becomes more complex as more and more detailed data are obtained. A further major difficulty arises from the relatively small number of patients on whom psychosurgery has been performed in the past decade and a half. The problems are still further complicated by the variety of sites of intervention and the range of extensiveness of the lesions at any one site. Thus, the number of patients in whom valid comparisons can be made is greatly reduced.

A criticism of the claims of success for psychosurgery is the absence of the kind of controlled studies that are now standard in evaluating therapeutic measures. The intrusive nature of the procedures and the criteria for selection of subjects have been advanced as ethical considerations to explain why controlled studies have not been undertaken.

In accepted medical treatment of severe illnesses in which the therapeutic benefits outweigh the risks, ethical problems seldom arise. When psychosurgery is contemplated, the ethical problems are not so clear-cut. The fundamental question is: Has it been shown that, all other treatments having failed, psychosurgery offers potential benefits to the individual greater than both the potential consequences of the operative risks associated with the procedure and the potential impairment of previously present psychological capacities? Earlier legitimate concerns resulting from lobotomy regarding overt impairment of social and occupational levels of performance or of creative potential do not appear to arise according to the reports of the outcome of limbic operations. It has also been pointed out that patients may already have been impaired by their disorders or by prior treatment. In cases of many brain tumors, for example, it would be difficult to find any rational objections. In psychosurgery, the risk/benefit ratio is more difficult to define. Even though, with current techniques, adverse effects rarely occur, some may and do. The question facing both physicians and patients becomes one of relativity—one patient may judge these to be of greater significance than the relief of intolerable distress, while another may hold the reverse.

Experimental Nature of Psychosurgery

Few therapies in the practice of medicine have been accepted solely on theoretical scientific grounds before empirical therapeutic trials. The vast majority have been accepted on experimental findings. In psychiatry, this is certainly true. The history of the efficacy of innovative therapeutic measures is replete with examples of high hopes and optimistic claims later modified by long-term experience. Such is the history of psychosurgery, the indications for which have been more specifically defined and restricted as the result of both practical experience and the introduction of alternative therapies.

Because of the variables mentioned earlier, consensus is still lacking in some areas. Nevertheless, for a small number of patients suffering from intractable affective disorders, this approach, at the present time, may offer the only hope for amelioration of psychic distress. For such patients, the approach, whatever the potential benefits, is still experimental.

The Brain as the Organ of the Mind

There is evidence that some of the opposition to psychosurgery is based on the belief that the essence of the human being, the distinguishing feature that separates humankind from other animals, is ensconced in the cerebral substrate. It is argued that surgical intervention that produces changes in the brain results in a different person and, thus, is unethical.

Opposition based on this belief appears not to consider whether the individual at risk himself wants to live in the same condition that psycho-surgery may alter in ways considered beneficial by and for him. Questions have been raised by some whether the brain alone is identical with the self. It has been pointed out that the endocrine systems perform a crucial role in the normal functioning of the personality, for example, the thyroid and the effects of cretinism.

It is generally agreed that the brain is the coordinating organ through which the personality develops, based on the outcome of the individual's interactions with the environment from birth onward. The self is highly dependent on the individual's interactions with others for all the pleasures, gratifications, and enjoyment of life. On this basis, the self is not a unitary entity but a vast array of activities for which the brain is the coordinating or-gan. Overt aberrant behavior or intense chronic emotional distress leads to the presumption that the brain is not functioning in a normal way.

Another criticism has been that psychosurgery is operating on healthy tissue. This view has been subjected to modification. Until recently, the position that physical pathology had not been demonstrated in so-called functional disorders could not be refuted. Modern biochemistry has re-placed anatomical pathology in the area of normal and abnormal function-ing with considerable evidence that biochemical "pathology" is present in some psychiatric illnesses.

It has been observed that total prohibition of psychosurgery, based on the inviolability of the self, would deny to others the right to choose to undergo this approach for themselves and is internally self-contradictory.

Irreversibility of Psychosurgery

The irreversibility of the profound personality changes produced by pre-frontal lobotomy was one source of opposition to psychosurgery. However, modern techniques, procedures, and outcomes are sufficiently different that comparison is questionable. Adverse effects are rare in the reports of limbic psychosurgery. There is evidence that aspects of the personality, e.g., intelligence, which suffered under prefrontal lobotomy, may actually, in some patients, improve, presumably by removal of the restraints of dis-turbed affect. When adverse personality changes can be demonstrated by psychometric methods, these are usually in areas of minor significance to the normal functioning of the individual. Given the absence of gross adverse personality changes, together with evidence that intellectual func-tioning may be improved, the issue of irreversibility becomes less powerful than in the past.

LEGAL ISSUES

Until a decade ago, under the doctrine enunciated by Judge Cardozo in 1914, doctors were obliged to inform patients of the risks involved in medical and surgical procedures, using as a standard the information given in similar cases by their peers in their community. Failure to do so gave rise to the risk of a charge of "assault."

In *Cobbs* v. *Grant* (California, 1972), the court ruled for the first time that lack of informed consent constituted not battery but negligence, thus bringing the issue into the area of professional malpractice. The physician became obliged to inform the patient of all the benefits and risks that a *reasonable man* would require to make a *rational decision* with regard to undertaking treatment. Despite the attempt by that court to spell out the guidelines for legally valid informed consent, considerable ambiguity remained about how much information was required. As the doctrine was adopted in other areas of jurisdiction, more attempts have been made to eliminate ambiguity; but these have failed to solve the problems particularly pertinent to the psychiatric patient. Some of these difficulties originate in the concept of a reasonable man. At the same time, it has been recognized that excessively detailed information may render an already anxious patient excludable under the concept of a reasonable man and lead him to a decision clearly not in his self-interest.

Since the psychiatric patients most likely to benefit from psychosurgery are those suffering from severe intractable emotional disorders, difficult decisions regarding adequate information to be given have to be faced. The prime issues are the impact of providing information about all the adverse effects, the competence of the patient to make a valid decision, and whether the patient may later claim that, because of his psychiatric condition, he was not competent to decide.

Of the few decided court cases involving psychosurgery, the court decided in favor of the defendant neurosurgeon. A 1973 Michigan County court case, *Kaimowitz* v. *Department of Mental Health* (1973), brought national prominence to the issues of social and public policy with regard to psychosurgery. The legal issue concerned the capacity of an institutionalized criminal sexual psychopath to give informed consent to undergo *experimental* psychosurgery as a condition of his release. He had been informed of all the potential benefits and risks and had been interviewed by members of a human rights review committee, which judged that his consent met the necessary standards. Prior to surgery, an attorney representing a Medical Committee for Human Rights intervened to prevent the proposed operation. Although the research project was abandoned, the court proceeded with the case and decided to prohibit the surgery on several grounds. The court concluded that an involuntarily confined individual cannot give legally valid informed consent to experimental psychosurgery. It held that "the three basic elements of informed consent, competency, knowledge and voluntariness, cannot be ascertained with a degree of reliability warranting resort to use such an invasive procedure." The court found that an institutionalized individual is exposed to influences increasing his dependency and diminishing his capacity to make decisions so important as agreeing to undergo experimental psychosurgery. Regarding knowledge, the high risks and the potentially low benefits were so uncertain as to make informed consent impossible. Regarding voluntariness, the prospect of release was so influential as to inhibit the individual from not agreeing to the operation.

This decision dealing only with experimental psychosurgery is not legally binding in other jurisdictions. It should be noted that this and other reasoning by the county court have been challenged by a number of legal authorities and rejected by the California Appellate Court as being in conflict with the rights of an individual under the U.S. Constitution (Slovenko, 1975; *Aden v. Younger*, 1976).

Application of these concepts to involuntarily hospitalized psychiatric patients has raised some questions, including the competence to agree to the other forms of therapy—or to refuse treatment. If the individual is incompetent to give a valid consent on these grounds, the question follows whether or not commitment automatically involves the incompetency of the patient regarding treatment decisions—a question decided in Utah by its recently enacted commitment law.

If the patient cannot give valid consent for psychosurgery as for other therapies, the question of proxy, that is, the person or body authorized to do so, arises. The answer to this has given rise to a number of proposals for different solutions, to each of which cogent objections have been raised. In some states, legislatures have already enacted statutes either prohibiting psychosurgery outright or creating procedures to be followed in order for legally valid informed consent to be obtained, usually removing control of clinical decisions from the hands of physicians.

In regard to informed consent with respect to psychosurgery, the physicians involved, both psychiatrists and neurosurgeons, are well advised to give the patient, the next of kin, and the legally authorized proxy, where one exists, the maximum amount of information about the potential risks and benefits, including the probable outcome of not undergoing the procedure—recognizing that doing so may well lead to refusal of consent. Needless to say, all alternative therapies should already have been tried and proved unavailing.

SOCIAL AND PUBLIC POLICY

In the past 20 years, there have been vast changes in the public and professional attitudes toward the practice of medicine. Before that time, the physician was regarded as an individual motivated to care for his patients in a selfless way, acting only in their interests. The doctor was held, by both the public and himself, to be a benevolent paternal figure with an armamentarium of therapeutic knowledge and skills. Although limited changes were occurring in some quarters following World War II, the paternalistic role of the physician was increasingly questioned in the 1960's. Whereas the civil rights of the individual had not previously been a concern of the public or of the medical profession, this issue became a general major question in the social unrest of the late 1960's and after. In the aroused social climate of the time, when violence was being used as an instrument of political action, psychosurgery became the focal point of many activists, who equated the then current techniques with those of prefrontal lobotomy and with the same adverse effects. Claims were publicized that this approach was being used as an agent of social control for racist and discriminatory purposes against minority groups, political activists, the poor, and women.

The National Commission on the Protection of Human Subjects of Biomedical and Behavioral Research (1977) studied this issue closely and did not receive evidence supporting such charges. It is true that more women than men have undergone psychosurgery, but this is probably because the number of women suffering from severe depressive conditions is greater than men. Moreover, the vast majority of these were white, middle-class women.

The charge that psychosurgery was used to control probably originated in observations of amotivational states produced by the extensive prefrontal lobotomy of the earliest psychosurgery and was "popularized" by opponents using the work of a prominent neurosurgeon. He and his co-authors, who had published reports on amygdalotomy in the treatment of violent patients with limbic lobe epilepsy, speculated in a letter to the *Journal of the American Medical Association* (*JAMA*) about the "subtle role in violent behavior of other possible factors, including brain dysfunction in the rioters who engaged in arson, sniping and physical assault" (Mark et al., 1967). About the same time, further publicity about two proposed research projects on violence, one in Michigan, the other in California, provided additional fuel for the opponents of psychosurgery. While benefits have been obtained by some patients in whom violence was associated with organic brain disease, there is no convincing data supporting the effectiveness of psychosurgery for modification of violent behavior in the absence of organic pathology.

The state has a compelling interest to ensure the health and welfare of its citizens and, equally, to assure that medical practitioners do not infringe upon the legal rights of their patients. Licensed physicians are, to some extent, agents of social and public policy insofar as health is concerned. The right to privacy and to private decision making of voluntary patients is also a social and public policy, although it may be in conflict with other principles of public policy. The doctor-patient relationship has been modified by judicial decisions and by legislation in specific circumstances, for example, the reporting of contagious diseases in the interests of the general welfare.

Psychosurgery involves matters of social and public policy in regard to voluntary as well as involuntary patients. Because of the invasive nature of this procedure, protection of the patient is a legitimate concern of the state. The particular process by which this protection is offered is for the legislature to decide. Oregon (1973) was the first state to enact comprehensive legislation for regulation of psychosurgery, establishing a Psychosurgical Review Board that must approve performance of the procedure in each case. The Review Board, appointed by the governor, is a multidisciplinary group, including medical, psychological, neuroscientific, and lay representatives. Its duties include deciding on the clinical merit, appropriateness, and need of the patient for the treatment; the validity of the informed consent and the legal appointment of a guardian in the case of incompetency of the patient; and the determination that all other therapies have been ineffective. Other states also have enacted protective legislation, establishing a variety of bodies to approve performance of psychosurgery. In some cases, the authority is placed in the hands of a court, in some in a committee composed of physicians, and in others of representatives of a number of disciplines.

EVALUATION AND RESEARCH

With the advances in scientific technology and increasing knowledge of brain anatomy and physiology, new techniques for surgical intervention produce results without the gross adverse psychological deficits that the general public usually associates with these procedures. However, in the medical literature covering psychosurgery, there is a dearth of articles of high scientific research merit (Valenstein, 1977). A number of valid reasons have been advanced to explain this lack. Only in recent years have there been changes in all areas of medical research, with emphasis on scientific evaluation of therapies using matched controls, standardized tests, independent objective evaluations, and post-treatment protocols, etc. In the mental health field, there have not yet been developed psychometric or other tests sufficiently sensitive to measure the subtle personality changes that may occur following psychosurgery, for example, in abstract thinking. While a number of measures have been developed, they do not cover most of the finer aspects of personality functioning.

With potential psychosurgical patients, as with other treatments, there arise ethical problems in the use of controls and withholding possible benefits from patients suffering from profound psychic distress. These problems are intensified because for these patients the procedure is an acknowledged treatment of last resort.

Following the widespread media publicity regarding charges by social activists of the abuse of psychosurgery, neurosurgeons have become aversive to carrying out the procedure for fear of malpractice suits. As a consequence, few operations are now performed each year in the U.S. Even when more procedures were carried out, the distribution of neurosurgeons was widespread, with most performing only a few operations a year so that adequate research protocols would not have been feasible for lack of resources. Further difficulties arise from the variety of techniques, sites of lesions, and clinical pictures involved so that the reliability, validity, and comparability of reports are defective.

For these and other reasons, the National Commission for the Protection of Human Subjects of Biomedical and Behavioral Research (1977), the APA Task Force on Psychosurgery, and the Canadian Psychiatric Association (Earp, 1979) each made detailed recommendations. Psychosurgery, as a treatment of last resort, should be performed only in a hospital or facility that includes a qualified team of psychiatrists, neurosurgeons, psychologists, skilled nurses, and behavioral scientists. There should be explicit protocols for careful assessment before and after the operation with complete short- and long-term follow-up studies.

Among the recommendations was the establishment of a National Registry for Psychosurgery, charged with the collection, correlation, and evaluation of the data. Because of physician concerns about the reporting of patient data to a governmental agency, the APA task force recommended that such a national registry be established under the auspices of one or more national medical organizations concerned with the problem. A hospital peer review committee and an informed consent committee, both with multidisciplinary membership, would be required. Involuntary psychiatric patients should be deemed capable of valid informed consent only after extraordinary safeguards involving assessment by an external review committee including lawyers, clergy, representatives of the community, and psychiatrists not professionally or otherwise related to the institution or the treatment team.

There were some differences. Whereas the APA task force recommended that psychosurgery not be performed on children, the commission concluded that the procedure should be available for them under all of the above safeguards plus court approval. With regard to confined criminals, both bodies concluded that psychosurgery should be available, subject to specified safeguards.

Future research, under the conditions outlined above, would be directed to the standardized collection of data, including pre- and post-operative assessment, the effects of specific lesions produced by specific techniques at specific sites in the brain, and short- and long-term follow-up studies. Only in this way will the many continuing questions be convincingly resolved.

REFERENCES

Aden v Younger, 57 California App 3d 662, 1976

Barraclough BM, Mitchell-Heggs NA: The use of neurosurgery for psychological disorder in the British Isles during 1974-76. Br Med J 11:1591-1593, 1978

Bartlett J, Bridges P, Kelly D: Contemporary indications for psychosurgery. Br J Psychiatry 138:507-511, 1981

Bridges PK, Bartlett JR: Psychosurgery: yesterday and today. Br J Psychiatry 131:249-260, 1977

Cobbs v Grant, 502 P2d 1 (Calif 1972)

Columbia-Greystone Associates: Selective Partial Ablation of the Frontal Cortex: A Correlative Study of its Effects on Human Psychotic Subjects. New York, Paul B Hoeber, 1949

Corkin S: A prospective study of cingulotomy, in The Psychosurgical Debate. Edited by Valenstein ES. San Franciso, WH Freeman and Co, 1980

Corkin S: Hidden figures-test performance: lasting effects of unilateral penetrating head injury and transient effects of bilateral cingulotomy. Neuropsychologia 17:565-605, 1979

Cotton HA: The etiology and treatment of the so-called functional psychoses. Am J Psychiatry 79:157-194, 1922

Crow HJ, Cooper R, Phillips DG: Progressive leucotomy, in Current Psychiatric Therapies, vol 3. Edited by Masserman JH. New York, Grune & Stratton, 1963

Donnelly J: The incidence of psychosurgery in the United States, 1971-1973. Am J Psychiatry 135:1475-1480, 1978

Earp JD: Psychosurgery: the position of the Canadian Psychiatric Association. Can J Psychiatry 24:353-365, 1979

Fiamberti AM: Proposta di una tecnica operatoria modificata e semplificata per gli interventialla Moniz sui lobi prefrontali in malati di mente. Rassegna di Studi Psichiat 26:797-805, 1937

Freeman W, Watts JW: Subcorticol prefrontal lobotomy in the treatment of certain psychoses. Medical Annals of the District of Columbia 6:267-271, 1937

Freeman W: Transorbital leucotomy. Lancet 2:371-373, 1948

Gildenberg PL: Survey of stereotactic and functional neurosurgery in the United States and Canada. Appl Neurophysiol 38:31-37, 1975

Goktepe FO, Young LB, Budges PK: A further review of the results of stereotactic subcaudate tractotomy. Br J Psychiatry 126:270-280, 1975

Grantham EG: Prefrontal lobotomy for relief of pain with a report of a new operative technique. J Neurosurg 8:405-410, 1951

Greenblatt M: Psychosurgery: a review of recent literature. In Studies in Lobotomy. Edited by Greenblatt M, Arnot R, Solomon HC. New York, Grune & Stratton, 1950

Heath RG: Depth recording and stimulation studies in patients, in The Surgical Control of Behavior. Edited by Winter A. Springfield, Ill, Charles C Thomas, 1971

Herner T: Treatment of mental disorders with frontal stereotaxic thermolesions: a follow-up of 116 cases. Acta Psychiatr Neurol Scand Suppl 158, 1961

Hilton SM, Zbrozyna AW: Amygdaloid region for defense reactions and its efficient pathway to the brain stem. J Physiol 165:160-173, 1963

Kaimowitz v Dept of Mental Health, civil no 73-19434-AW (Cir CT Wayne Co, Mich, July 10, 1973)

Kelly D, Richardson A, Mitchell-Heggs NA: Stereotactic limbic leucotomy: neurophysiological aspects and operative technique. Br J Psychiatry 123:133-140, 1973

Kelly D, Walter CJ, Mitchell-Heggs N, et al: Modified leucotomy assessed clinically, physiologically and psychologically at six weeks and eighteen months. Br J Psychiatry 120:19-29, 1972

Kelly D: Psychosurgery and the limbic system. Postgrad Med J 49:825-833, 1973

Kiloh LG, Gye RS, Rushworth RG, et al: Stereotactic amygdalotomy for aggressive behavior. J Neurol Neurosurg Psychiatry 37:437-444, 1974

Kiloh LG, Smith JS: The neural bases of aggression and its treatment by psychosurgery. Aust NZ J Psychiatry 12:21-28, 1978

Knight G: Further observations from an experience with 660 cases of stereotactic tractotomy. Postgrad Med J 49:845-854, 1973

Knight GC: Stereotactic tractotomy in the surgical treatment of mental illness. J Neurol Neurosurg Psychiatry 28:304-310, 1965

Kramer M: The 1951 survey of the use of psychosurgery, in Proceedings of the Third Research Conference on Psychosurgery. US Public Health Service publication no 221. Washington, DC, US Government Printing Office, 1954

LeBeau J: Psycho-Chirurgie et Fonctions Mentales. Paris, Masson et Cie, 1954

Lindstrom PA: Prefrontal ultrasonic irradiation—a substitute for lobotomy. Arch Neurol Psychiatry 72:399-425, 1954

Mark VH, Sweet WH, Erwin FR: Role of brain disease in riots and urban violence. Letter. JAMA 201:895, 1967

Mitchell-Heggs NA, Kelly D, Richardson A: Stereotactic limbic leucotomy: a follow-up at 16 months. Br J Psychiatry 128:226-240, 1976

Moniz E: Tentatives operatories dans le traitement de certaines psychoses. Paris, Masson et Cie, 1936

National Commission on the Protection of Human Subjects of Biomedical and Behavioral Research: Psychosurgery: Report and Recommendations. DHEW publication no (OS)77-0001. Washington, DC, US Government Printing Office

Oregon 35 Rev Stat § 426.700 (Repealed 1981 Chap 372, Section 2), 1977

Papez JW: A proposed mechanism of emotion. Arch Neurol Psychiatry 38:725-743, 1937

Penfield W: Symposium on gyrectomy, in The Frontal Lobes, vol 27. Edited by Fulton JF, Aring CD, Wortis SB. Baltimore, Williams & Wilkins Co, 1948

Peyton WT, Noran HH, Miller EW: Prefrontal lobectomy (excision of the anterior areas of the cerebrum): a new form of psychosurgery. Am J Psychiatry 104:513-523, 1948

Rieber I, Sigusch V: Psychosurgery on sex offenders and sexual "deviants" in West Germany. Arch Sex Behav 8:523-527, 1979

Scoville WB: Proposed methods of cortical undercutting of certain areas of the frontal lobes as a substitute for prefrontal lobotomy. Digest Neurol Psychiatry 16:534, 1948

Slovenko R: On psychosurgery. Hastings Center Report 5:19-22, 1975

Spiegel EA, Wycis HT, Marks M, et al: Stereotaxic apparatus for operations on the human brain. Science 106:349-350, 1947

Stromberg-Olsen R, Carlisle S: Bifrontal stereotactic tractotomy: a follow-up study. Br J Psychiatry 118:141-154, 1971

Teuber HL, Corkin S,Twitchell MD: A Study of Cingulotomy in Man in Psychosurgery: The Report of the National Commission for the Protection of Human Subjects of Biomedical and Behavioral Research—Appendix. DHEW publication no (OS)77-0002. Washington, DC, US Government Printing Office, 1977

Tippin J, Henn FA: Modified leucotomy in the treatment of intractable obsessional neurosis. Am J Psychiatry 139:1601-1603, 1982

Tooth GE, Newton RF: Leucotomy in England and Wales, 1942-1954. Reports on Public Health and Medical Subjects, no 104. London, Ministry of Health, Her Majesty's Stationery Office, 1961

Valenstein ES: The practice of psychosurgery: a survey of the literature (1971-1976), in Psychosurgery. Report of the National Commission on the Protection of Human Subjects of Biomedical and Behavioral Research. Appendix. DHEW publication no (OS)77-0002. Washington, DC, US Government Printing Office, 1977

Whitty CWM, Duffield JE, Tow PM, et al: Anterior cingulectomy in the treatment of mental disease. Lancet 1:475-481, 1952

6
Other Somatic Therapies

6

Other Somatic Therapies

DISULFIRAM (ANTABUSE) IN ALCOHOLISM

Tetraethylthiuram disulfide (TETD), more commonly known as disulfiram (Antabuse), was introduced as an effective agent in the treatment of alcoholism in Denmark in 1948. The history of its application in treating alcoholism is serendipitous. Disulfiram had long been used in the rubber industry as an antioxidant, and rubber workers knew that those exposed to the preparation for a long period of time developed hypersensitivity to alcohol. While investigating its potential use as an anthelmintic, it was ingested by two researchers who, in turn, became ill at a cocktail party. Their insight and studies led to its use as an adjunct in the treatment of chronic alcoholism (Hald and Jacobsen, 1948).

The drug was introduced into the therapeutic armamentarium for chronic alcoholism with great hopes. While the enthusiasm regarding its benefits has diminished, it is still a widely used drug in the treatment of alcoholics. However, disulfiram should be used only as an adjunct to a broad spectrum of therapies, both biologic and psychotherapeutic. The biologic treatment would include correction of nutritional deficiencies, and, when indicated, antidepressants. The psychotherapeutic techniques include active participation in Alcoholics Anonymous, individual therapy, family therapy, and group therapy.

To comprehend disulfiram's mechanism of action, one must understand the metabolism of alcohol in the body (Billet, 1968), which occurs primarily in the liver. Generally speaking, alcohol becomes acetic acid in the body in two stages (Bourne and Fox, 1973; Isreal and Mardones, 1971). Alcohol is oxidized to acetaldehyde by the enzyme alcohol dehydrogenase in the presence of nicotinamide adenine dinucleotide (NAD). This intermediate aldehyde is very toxic. The aldehyde is then oxidized to acetate in the presence of an NAD requiring aldehyde dehydrogenase. The acetate is eventually broken down into carbon dioxide and water.

This second enzyme, aldehyde dehydrogenase, is found not only in the liver but throughout the body, and is inhibited by disulfiram, resulting in an accumulation of acetaldehyde and a toxic reaction characterized by marked vasodilation and hypotension.

Because disulfiram is metabolized slowly (Billet, 1968), alcohol must be avoided totally if the patient is on the drug. The use of disulfiram requires a cooperative patient. In the early years after the introduction of disulfiram, it was thought advisable for the patient to have a demonstration of the reactions that would result from the combination of alcohol and disulfiram, but today this procedure is considered unnecessary.

Initially, a maximum of 500 mg daily is given in a single dose for one to two weeks. It is usually taken in the morning. However, some patients experience a sedative effect and prefer to take it at bedtime. After one or two weeks the average maintenance dose is 250 mg daily, with the amount ranging from 125 to 500 mg. The daily dose should not exceed 500 mg. Most patients do well with only 250 mg and experience fewer side effects with lower dosages. The drug should be continued until the patient has evidenced substantial long-term social and vocational improvement. Thereafter, maintenance therapy may be required for months or years.

The Disulfiram-Alcohol Reaction

Patients on disulfiram have an abnormal reaction to alcohol in five to ten minutes (Billet, 1968). Initially, the patients develop a sensation of heat over the face and a bright red flushing of the face, sclerae, upper limbs, and chest. They complain of a constriction of the neck, irritation of the throat, coughing, and labored breathing. If the patients have consumed a large amount of alcohol, they commonly become nauseated and markedly hypotensive. Profuse vomiting may occur; a painful feeling of apprehension is the most uncomfortable symptom.

In the presence of a disulfiram-alcohol reaction, the patient should be put in a shock position, and an intravenous infusion of dextrose and saline should be started. Oxygen and plasma may be indicated, and an antihistamine should be given either intramuscularly or intravenously.

The ingestion of disulfiram may itself produce some side effects. The minor ones include fatigue and decreased libido and potency. With larger doses an acute toxic psychosis may be produced. An exacerbation of psychotic symptoms in schizophrenic patients may occur. The chronic ingestion of excessive amounts of disulfiram may produce a syndrome characterized by an acute organic mental syndrome, depression, extrapyramidal deficits, and peripheral neuropathy.

The use of disulfiram should be avoided in a number of situations. These include coronary occlusion, acute psychoses, and hypersensitivity. The patient must assiduously avoid the use of alcohol, vinegar, cough mixtures, and in some instances, after-shave lotion. The drug should be given with caution in pregnant women and in individuals who have diabetes mellitus, hypothyroidism, epilepsy, nephritis, cirrhosis of the liver, or hepatic insufficiency.

The drug also decreases the rate at which other drugs are metabolized (Kissin, 1974). It should be used with caution in patients receiving diphenylhydantoin as an abnormal accumulation of this drug may occur in patients concomitantly receiving disulfiram. The patients in these instances must be followed closely, with frequent evaluations of diphenylhydantoin blood levels; and the physician must be prepared to shift to alternative anticonvulsants. Also, since disulfiram may prolong prothrombin time, it may cause problems when given to individuals taking oral anticoagulants (Kwentus and Major, 1979).

As noted above, the drug is only effective if the patient will take the prescribed dose consistently.

OPIOIDS

The opioid drugs have a mechanism of action that parallels that of morphine. Some are derived from the opium prepared from the pcppy, papaver somniferum; others are made synthetically. The drugs considered to be opiates include the purified alkaloids of opium such as morphine and codeine and the semisynthetic modifications of morphine such as hydromorphone (Dilaudid), nalbuphine (Neubain), oxymorphone (Numorphan), and oxycodone (found in Percodan). Included among the opioids are a number of purely synthetic compounds including:

A. Phenylpiperidine derivatives such as meperidine (Demerol), alphaprodine (Nisentil), and anileridine (Leritine);

B. Diphenylheptane derivatives: methadone (Dolophine) and propoxyphene (Darvon);

C. Phenanthrene derivatives: levorphanol (Levo-dromoran) and butorphanol (Stadol);

D. Benzomorphan derivatives in the form of pentazocine (Talwin); and

E. Propionamide derivatives in the form of propiran (Dirame).

A few other less frequently used preparations are also available (Winkler, 1977) and are primarily used as analgesics. The analgesia is considered to be part of a general protective action whereby not only pain but also dyspnea, bowel and bladder urgency, cough, and hunger pangs are reduced or eliminated (Schaumann, 1954).

Opioids, in nontolerant persons, may also produce distress in the form of pain, anxiety and anticipation of pain, dyspnea, etc. Most important, they produce a sense of euphoria or, in the language of the streets, "a high." The opioids are drugs of dependence. However, all persons receiving opioids do not become dependent. Few persons who receive opioids for the relief of pain, even if they are given repeated dosages in frequencies and amounts sufficient to produce dependency in a "street person," compulsively persist in seeking opioids after the pain has gone and an opioid abstinence syndrome has disappeared.

The profile of those who become addicts is as follows (Weppner and Agar, 1971): These individuals are usually teenagers and have peers who are opioid users. They are not in physical pain, and they administer the drug to themselves to satisfy curiosity. Most important for many, drug use is a means to become accepted in a swaggering peer group. Heroin is the opioid of the streets. With the guidance of their peers, these young people pass through the discomforts of the initial experiences with heroin and reach the promised land of the heroin "high."

This particular scenario is to be distinguished from other opioid dependencies such as:

A. Drug abuse—occasional use of nonmedically indicated chemical agents.

B. Single addictions—These are addictions caused by treatment for the relief of pain in patients with incurable illnesses or intractable pain.

C. Self-inflicted addictions by professionals and inadvertent iatrogenic dependencies.

D. Endemic addictions such as opium smoking in China in past generations.

Currently, heroin administered intravenously is the opioid most often associated with endemic addiction.

Highly stereospecific binding sites for labeled opiates and their antagonists were discovered only recently (Pert and Snyder, 1973; Terenius, 1973). At about the same time, it was found that focal electrical stimulation in the periaqueductal grey matter produced analgesia that could be blocked by the specific opiate inhibitor, naloxone (Mayer et al., 1971). These findings suggest that the pharmacological action of opiates probably stems from their mimicking of a central nervous system transmitter or modulator. This concept led to the isolation of two endogenous opiate-like pentapeptides (Hughes et al., 1975), which have been called leucine-enkephalin and methionine-enkephalin. Methionine-enkephalin proved to be sequence 61-65 of the pituitary hormone beta-lipotropin. The term *endorphins* (endogenous morphine-like factors) was coined for peptides with opioid activity. The larger endorphins are concentrated in the hypothalamic-pituitary region. Enkephalins and beta-endorphin have analgesic effects when injected into the appropriate brain areas (Kosterlitz, 1976). Most pharmacologic actions of endorphins studied to date can be counteracted by specific opiate antagonists such as naloxone.

The discovery of the enkephalins and endorphins ties in well with the concept of "reward transmitters." Rewards act in several ways to steer and eventually terminate the rewarded response. It has been proposed theoretically that the reinforcement of operant behavior is mediated by catecholamine systems in the brain. Rewards may be associated with increases and decreases in arousal levels. Agents that increase arousal include morphine and related opioid narcotics. Those substances that increase and decrease the level of arousal are both actively self-administered by animals and humans. This idea leads to the proposition that drive-inducing reward functions may be mediated by catecholamines, and that drive-reducing reward functions may be mediated by enkephalins or related opioid peptides.

In addition, endorphins were reported to reduce catatonic states associated with extreme generalized muscle rigidity, waxy flexibility, and absence of spontaneous movements when injected into the periaqueductal grey matter or into the cerebral spinal fluid of rats. This finding raised questions regarding possible roles of endorphins in patients with schizophrenia. While opiate antagonists, such as naloxone, have been administered to schizophrenic patients in a series of studies (Gunne et al., 1977; Volavka et al., 1977), the results have been inconsistent.

Detoxification

Between 1952 and 1955, more than 90 percent of opioid addicts who had been detoxified and institutionalized for various periods of time relapsed to heroin addiction within two years (Hunt and Odoroff, 1962). More than 90 percent became re-addicted within six months of discharge from the hospital. Provisions for aftercare following detoxification and release from an institution did not significantly alter the prognosis for relapse.

Use of Narcotic Antagonists to Prevent Relapse

The use of narcotic antagonists to prevent relapse is still an experimental field. The narcotic antagonists are synthetically derived from certain opioids (Kleber, 1973); they include naloxone (N-cyclopropylmethyl-noroxymorphone) and naltrexone (N-cyclopropyl-methylbenzomorphone), which exert almost no actions of their own other than competitively antagonizing the agonist effects of opioids. Nalorphine (N-allylnormorphine) and cyclazocine (N-cyclopropyl-methylbenzomorphan), in addition to competitively antagonizing opioid agonistic actions, may produce some physical dependence on their own. Ideally, a narcotic antagonist should be effective when administered by mouth, and a single dose should block opioid effects for at least 24 hours. Both naloxone and nalorphine are too short-acting to fulfill this purpose. Naltrexone is longer-acting. This treatment, theoretically, is optimal and works best when the detoxified opioid addicts challenge the opioid blockade (experimental extinction) by self-administration of heroin. As noted above, this program is still experimental.

Methadone

Methadone (Dolophine) is a diphenylheptane derivative that, contrary to morphine, is effective by mouth and has a long duration of effect.

The abstinence reaction associated with methadone is less intense than that caused by morphine; however, it may also produce muscular aches and insomnia. In general, it has been found that using a ratio of 1 mg of methadone for 3-4 mg of morphine or 1 mg of heroin or 0.5 mg of hydromorphone or 20 mg of meperidine will suppress the usual abstinence produced by these opioids.

The usual technique is to administer orally 10-29 mg of methadone two or three times a day (20-60 mg per day) (Dole and Nyswander, 1965, 1967). Commonly, after three to five days of maintenance on these dosages, the daily amount of methadone is gradually decreased over a period of seven to ten days until it is eliminated. Most commonly, this process is associated with only slight discomfort, which may persist for weeks in the form of anorexia, insomnia, aches and pains, feelings of weakness, and vague anxiety. In general, methadone substitution and withdrawal have proven to be a convenience, when compared to the rapid reduction techniques, for patients with a high degree of opioid dependence. These detoxification techniques are carried out in hospitals where there are adequate safeguards against the smuggling of opioids. Methadone substitution and withdrawal, according to federal regulations, must be completed within 21 days. Beyond that, it is considered to be "methadone maintenance," which is carried out on an outpatient basis in special facilities.

Methadone Maintenance

Methadone maintenance was introduced in 1965 (Dole and Nyswander, 1965, 1967). The procedure of methadone maintenance therapy is as follows: When administered in a special maintenance setting, the patient is placed on 10-20 mg per day of methadone, given orally, in divided doses. This amount is gradually increased as tolerance develops until a stabilization level is established. This dose may range from 40-160 mg. A daily oral dose of 50-80 mg is usually adequate, provided there is no evidence of an unusually low plasma level. With this technique the individual reports daily for his maintenance dose. Periodically, the urine is examined for the presence of heroin and other drugs. The methadone maintenance program is voluntary and is limited to addicts who are 16 years old or older. Methadone is dispensed orally in liquid form.

The rationale for methadone maintenance is that following detoxification, addicts experience "drug hunger," which is decreased by the taking of opioids and, therefore, leads to a relapse. Methadone reduces the "drug hunger" without producing significant euphoria. Allegedly, a cross-tolerance to heroin develops, and the addict maintaining a large daily dose of methadone will not experience heroin effects; heroin-seeking behavior decreases and is eliminated. It is claimed that in the absence of the heroin behavior, the addict is more likely to show a capacity for social rehabilitation.

There are a number of complaints with regard to the methadone maintenance program (Chambers and Brill, 1973; Martin et al., 1973). Methadone given intravenously produces severe physical dependence and euphoria; this fact has given rise to methadone addiction, with a large black market for methadone occurring in a number of cities. Even when given orally, methadone produces a physical dependence and may be associated with a prolonged abstinence syndrome. There is no clear-cut evidence to indicate that there will not be marked recidivism following methadone detoxification. Individuals in methadone maintenance programs show marked physiologic changes, including electroencephalographic changes, increased REM sleep patterns, autonomic changes, hyperhydrosis, aches and pain, and others.

In addition, a sizable percentage of children born to mothers on methadone maintenance therapy are premature and underweight. Approximately 80 percent of these infants will display methadone withdrawal symptoms.

The detoxification and maintenance treatment of a large number of drug dependent individuals is even more complicated than that described above since many patients have multiple drug addictions. Neither narcotic antagonists nor methadone is effective in the management of addictions to drugs other than opioids.

STIMULANTS

The stimulant drugs, particularly the amphetamines dextroamphetamine sulfate (Dexedrine), amphetamine sulphate (Benzadrine), methamphetamine hydrochloride (Desoxyn), methylphenidate chloride (Ritalin), pemoline (Cylert), denol (Deaner), and cocaine are effective in relieving fatigue, producing anorexia, elevating mood, and stimulating wakefulness. However, they have significant abuse potential, mainly related to their euphoric effects. The stimulants have wide appeal as illicit "street drugs," commonly referred to as "uppers." Their excessive use can produce significant physiologic problems. These drugs have a great potential to produce addiction and major psychotic disorganization.

Method of Action

The amphetamines potentiate adrenergic neurotransmission by release of norepinephrine and dopamine. They also block reuptake of amines and are weak inhibitors of monoamine oxidase (Baldessarini, 1972; Snyder, 1973). Release and reuptake blockade are closely related. While release seems to be more important, currently the extent to which each may account for the amphetamine effect is uncertain.

The neurotransmitters sustaining the amphetamine-induced behavioral response, especially in the acute stages of intoxication, are primarily dopamine and secondarily norepinephrine. Amphetamines and cocaine block reuptake but also release catecholamines from central dopamine and norepinephrine neurons. The action of amphetamines depends primarily on the release of newly synthesized catecholamines. Alpha-methylparatyrosine blocks amphetamine-induced behavior. The drug action is mediated by the newly synthesized catecholamines. In contrast, cocaine and methylphenidate are relatively uninfluenced by alpha-methylparatyrosine. It is believed that amphetamine-induced hypermotility in rats probably depends on norepinephrine, while dopamine plays a major role in the induction of stereotypy.

Single doses of amphetamine may selectively produce euphoria in patients who later display a favorable therapeutic response to tricyclic antidepressants. Patients who respond to amphetamine with euphoria and whose depressions are alleviated by imipramine have lower urinary MHPH levels before drug treatment than do patients who respond less well (Maas et al., 1973). Patients who have higher MHPH levels appear to respond better to amitriptyline (Beckman and Goodwin, 1975).

In humans, it has been found that patients with pre-existing psychotic symptoms usually react to acute injections of small doses of amphetamine or amphetamine-like psychostimulants with an intensification of psychotic symptoms associated with behavioral activation and a clear state of consciousness (Janowsky et al., 1973; Janowsky and Davis, 1976). In an opposite vein, some adult schizophrenics who had a childhood history of attention deficit disorders seemed to obtain symptomatic improvement with intravenous methylphenidate. High doses of virtually all amphetamine-like drugs, including methylphenidate, amphetamine derivatives, and cocaine, induce psychotic symptoms in presumably nonschizophrenic individuals.

"Speed freaks," the street name for amphetamine addicts, intravenously self-inject huge amounts of amphetamines. Organic brain syndromes, manic episodes, and catatonic phenomena frequently occur with high doses of psychostimulants (Angrist and Gershon, 1970). The most common psychotic reaction is a paranoid state closely resembling paranoid schizophrenia. These patients evidence persecutory and grandiose delusions; visual, auditory, olfactory, or tactile hallucinations; increased restlessness; agitation; panic; changes in affect; loss of insight; increased sexuality; and perseverative stereotyped behavior ("punding"). The schizophrenogenic patterns noted above, together with the appreciation that the psychostimulant drugs are potent dopamine agonists, reinforce the theory that the psychoses, such as schizophrenia, may be related to an overactivity of dopamine. Similarly, the fact that antipsychotic drugs are dopamine blockers and antagonize amphetamine and cocaine is considered by some to be consistent with the dopamine theory of schizophrenia.

Uses of Psychostimulants

Attention Deficit Disorder. *Attention deficit disorder* (ADD) is a more recent term than *hyperkinetic* syndrome and is associated with central nervous system dysfunction. An attentional deficit may be a frequent or even more commonly noted attribute of children with central nervous system dysfunction than is hyperactivity. Approximately one-third to three-quarters of the children in different studies have learning disabilities. In addition to attention deficits, other commonly found symptoms and signs are altered interpersonal relations, decreased separation anxiety, and refractoriness to reward and punishment. Deficits in impulse control with low frustration tolerance, social impulsivity, and social transgressions are common. Altered emotionality is also noted, with marked lability, over-excitement, low self-esteem, and decreased pain sensitivity. In addition, there may also be perceptual-cognitive abnormalities, but this finding is not as commonly noted as the other points listed above. Some observers have expressed the opinion that the hyperactive or hyperkinetic aspects of this syndrome have been exaggerated (Werry, 1976; Wender, 1978).

Central nervous system stimulants appear to be of benefit in hyperkinetic children with attention deficit disorders. Some observers believe the stimulants should be used as adjuncts to remedial education and behavior modification direction with the parents and teachers (Wobraich, 1977). Others have not found behavior modification to be effective. The major drugs currently used for ADD are dextroamphetamine, methylphenidate, and pemoline.

One can offer only rough guidelines as to how much of an individual stimulant should be given to children with attention deficit disorders: a high dose of 1.5 mg/kg per day of dextroamphetamine and a high dose of 4.6 mg/kg per day of methylphenidate (Wender, 1971). Others have found an improvement in behavior ratings (based on teacher ratings) with a high dose of 0.7 and 1.0 mg/kg per day of methylphenidate (Sprague and Sleator, 1973). It should be appreciated that a given child may require a larger dose of stimulant than would be expected on the basis of body weight. There are great individual differences in blood levels of stimulants for comparable doses of the same drug in children of the same body weight. A specific stimulant may have a therapeutic effect for a given child only at a particular blood level.

When they are effective, these drugs produce a calming effect on children. Long-term studies suggest that hyperactive children are prone to develop significant psychiatric and social problems in adolescence and later life. In adolescence, antisocial behavior, academic retardation, poor self-image, and depression are the most commonly seen clinical patterns. Sociopathy, acting out behavior, alcoholism, and even psychosis are the most frequently encountered disorders in adult life. The hyperactive child is best considered as a multi-handicapped child. Treatment must be individualized and based on a comprehensive assessment of the child and his or her family.

There does not seem to be a predilection for hyperactive children who have been treated with psychostimulants to become drug abusers. While it has been suggested that suppression of weight and height may occur with prolonged use of amphetamines and suppression of weight but not of height with methylphenidate, these findings require further investigation. However, weight gain and linear growth should be measured at intervals.

Some investigators have suggested that imipramine has been effective in hyperactive children, with benefits occurring at times within a 24-hour period (Rappolt et al., 1977). (It should be noted that imipramine may take as long as two to three weeks to work as an antidepressant drug.) However, imipramine does not appear to be as effective as the stimulants in the long-term treatment of children with attention deficit disorders. Over time, children appear to develop a tolerance to imipramine. Antipsychotic drugs have been used by other investigators. At the present time, however, the tricyclic and antipsychotic drugs should be used only in those patients who either have not responded or who cannot tolerate the psychostimulants. There have been reports of abnormal electrocardiograms in children treated with imipramine.

Lithium carbonate is not as effective as the stimulants in the treatment of these children. It may be of use in those rare instances in which mania is a part of a bipolar disorder occurring in children. Anticonvulsant drugs are also of use in the treatment of children with hyperactivity if they have concomitant seizure activity. In the absence of seizure activity, anticonvulsant medications do not appear to be of any significant benefit in hyperactive children who simply have abnormal electroencephalographic tracings. Diphenhydramine (Benadryl) has not been proven effective with hyperkinetic children.

Narcolepsy. Narcolepsy is a syndrome of unknown etiology with the following characteristics:

A. Recurrent attacks of an uncontrollable desire to sleep;

B. Sudden transient loss of tone in the muscles of the extremities or trunk (cataplexy) often precipitated by emotional stimulation;

C. Pathologic weakness of muscles during emotional reactions such as laughing (lachschlag) or crying;

D. Attacks of an inability to move developing in the transition period between sleep and arousal (sleep paralysis);

E. Hypnagogic hallucinations characterized by vivid visual, auditory, or even tactile sensations at the onset of sleep. At times, autonomic behavior reminiscent of epileptic absence attacks with retrograde amnesia may occur; these patients awaken frequently from nocturnal sleep. The electroencephalogram is frequently normal if taken when the patient is awake. The sleep episodes are characterized by the immediate onset of full-blown REM (rapid eye movement) sleep in a high percentage of patients in whom narcolepsy is associated with cataplexy.

The age of onset is usually between the second and fourth decades, but it has been noted in patients in the first or after the fifth decade. There is a strong propensity for familial occurrence, and it is postulated that narcolepsy may be transmitted by a single dominant gene with slight penetrance.

Narcolepsy is a chronic syndrome. It would appear that in most instances, the symptoms persist throughout the patient's life. The excessive daytime sleepiness and the precipitous episodes of falling asleep respond best to the amphetamines or methylphenidate. High doses of psychostimulant drugs may be necessary, with dosages of amphetamine ranging as high as 100 mg per day and methylphenidate in a range of 40-60 mg per day.

The cataplexy and attacks of generalized muscular weakness associated with laughing or crying usually do not respond actively to psychostimulant drugs. In these instances, imipramine should be added in small dosages and gradually built up to a range of 100-150 mg per day (Rechtschaffen and Dement, 1969). The antinarcoleptic action of imipramine is immediate, unlike its antidepressant action. Tolerance tends to develop for all of the drugs, and periodic "drug holidays" may be necessary.

A syndrome of hypersomnia and bulimia known as the Kleine-Levin syndrome may be related to narcolepsy (Levin, 1936; Gallinek, 1967). This syndrome is rare, occurs predominantly in young adolescent boys, and is characterized by periodic attacks of somnolence in which the patient may sleep for several days or weeks, awakening only for a short period during which time he eats ravenously and excessively. When awake, the patient's sensorium may be clouded; and there may be partial or total amnesia for aspects of the attack. The episodes may be followed by periods of depression; one report states that amphetamines may reduce the severity and frequency of the attacks.

Amphetamines may be helpful in some instances of patients with petit mal or absence epilepsy to counteract the somnolence that may be induced by anticonvulsant drugs (Critchley, 1962).

Patterns of Abuse. With oral administration, as tolerance develops, the individual gradually increases the dose of the psychostimulants over a period of months (Ellinwood and Cohen, 1970). Alcohol or sedatives are often used to enable the patient to sleep at night. The intravenous use of stimulant drugs is almost entirely relegated to the "street culture," whose members obtain the preparations illicitly. The intravenous use of amphetamines and cocaine produces a sudden ecstasy or "flash."

Nasal insufflation, or "sniffing" or "snorting," is the most widely practiced manner of cocaine use. Cocaine is not usually swallowed because it is rapidly destroyed in the stomach. The relatively short duration of cocaine action is also due to rapid liver metabolism.

Tolerance and Withdrawal Effects. Anorexia and hyperthermic responses are two effects of amphetamines to which chronic users develop marked tolerance. Most amphetamine overdose-related hyperthermic deaths are reported in nontolerant individuals (Ellinwood and Cohen, 1970; Ellinwood, 1972). There is marked tolerance to the lethal effects of high dose amphetamine and probably to high dose cocaine. Cocaine is both a local anesthetic and a stimulant; therefore, its lethality tolerance is complicated. Little or no tolerance develops with regard to the local anesthetic, seizure-inducing effect. Death due to overdose of local anesthetics, including cocaine, is usually an acute process following an injection or massive absorption from local application. It is usually associated with respiratory arrest and, on occasion, cardiac arrest. Cocaine-induced seizures can be effectively treated with intravenous diazepam or other parenteral anticonvulsants. After the seizures are under control, the toxic effects secondary to adrenergic mechanisms can be managed with propranolol (Rappolt et al., 1977).

It should be noted that cocaine psychosis, at the present time, is rare due to the massive cost of maintaining a habit strong enough to develop a psychosis.

HORMONE THERAPY

Neuroendocrinology, now a well established field of laboratory and clinical research, evolved in crescendo fashion during the 1960's and 1970's. Studies in this field have established that the central nervous system (CNS) is a major factor in endocrine regulation (Sacher, 1976). The development of neuroendocrinology has paralleled and in many instances has been interrelated with our understanding of the role of central nervous system neurotransmitters. Also, a large number of studies have been conducted which dealt with the effects of hormones on various types of behavior (Leshner, 1978).

Hormonal secretions, in general, are under the control of the pituitary gland, which is governed, in great measure, by central nervous system mechanisms mediated through the hypothalamus. Various factors such as psychologic stress, sleep versus waking, sleep-stage cycling within the sleep period, and changes in the central nervous system neurotransmitters through the use of psychotropic drugs all can influence pituitary hormone secretions (Selye, 1973; Rubin et al., 1974; DeWeid and de Jong, 1974).

There are three interrelated major hormonal systems: the hypothalamic-pituitary-adrenal axis (HPA), the hypothalamic-pituitary-gonadal axis (HPG), and the hypothalamic-pituitary-thyroid axis (HPT) (Selye, 1973). The secretion rates of the anterior pituitary hormones, largely depend on the balance between central nervous system activity driving the hypothalamus (open loop mechanisms) and the effects of the negative feedback on the pituitary and brain by the seven anterior pituitary hormones and their target organ hormones (closed loop mechanisms) (Galliger et al., 1973).

The hypothalamic-hypophysiotropic hormones have both releasing and inhibiting actions. Chemically speaking, they are small polypeptides that are secreted by cells in the hypothalamus into the portal vessels of the pituitary stalk. These in turn bathe cells of the anterior pituitary where they exert their tropic effects. Pituitary hormones that have negative feedback mechanisms exerted by target organ hormones (i.e., adrenocorticotrophic hormone, luteinizing hormone, follicle-stimulating hormone, thyrotropin-stimulating hormone) appear only to have a hypothalamic releasing factor (Schally et al., 1973). On the other hand, those pituitary hormones that do not have clearly defined negative feedback relationships with a target organ hormone (i.e., prolactin, MSH, growth hormone) seem to have both hypothalamic releasing and inhibiting factors.

A number of central nervous system neurotransmitters have been found to affect the secretion of the hypothalamic-hypophysiotropic hormones with both pituitary hormone releasing and pituitary hormone inhibiting factors (Rubin, 1975). It would appear that overall the secretion of the hypothalamic hormones is qualitatively and quantitatively directed by the changing balance among many competing neural processes mediated through a number of neurotransmitters (i.e., dopamine, norepinephrine, serotonin, acetylcholine, gamma amino butyric acid, and possibly others).

The influence of CNS activity on neuroendocrine secretion has had additional documentation from sleep research. Shifts in central nervous system activity during sleep are evidenced by changing patterns such as slow-wave stage III-IV "deep" sleep, REM sleep, etc. These changes are regular and are aspects of a basic rest-activity cycle present during the entire 24-hour period (Kleitman, 1969; Hartmann, 1973).

Different pituitary hormones appear to be related to different aspects of the circadian sleep-wake cycle and the ultradian rhythms. Prolactin is closely linked to the sleep-wake cycle. Increasing blood levels are recorded at the time of sleep onset. Peak levels are found approximately five hours into sleep. Sleep-wake reversal immediately shifts prolactin secretion (Sassin et al., 1973). Growth hormone seems to be closely related to slow-wave sleep, with the major secretion of this hormone occurring during the first entry into slow-wave (stage III-IV) sleep during the first one or two hours of sleep (Sassin et al., 1969). If slow-wave sleep is blocked, growth hormone secretion decreases.

Treatment with Hormones

It is of interest only from a historical basis to note that castration had been tried in the past in the treatment of patients with schizophrenia and various types of psychopathic behavior. In a similar view, thyroidectomies have been performed on schizophrenic patients and on individuals with manic-depressive disorders. In an opposite vein, various endocrine tissues have been implanted in patients with a variety of psychoses. Even pituitary irradiation has been tried in an attempt to influence psychotic behavior.

As far back as the late 1940's active hormone therapies of various types were attempted in the treatment of a wide spectrum of psychiatric illnesses. While there have been reports testifying to benefits secondary to hormones in individual patients, no significant series of controlled studies has shown consistent successes with any particular endocrine treatment. The exception to this general statement is that some patients with endocrinopathies in which severe hypofunctioning or hyperfunctioning has produced abnormal psychic behavior may respond to appropriate therapy. However, even if certain endocrinopathies are modified, the psychogenic abnormalities may still remain.

Endocrinologic treatment has had its widest application in the treatment of so-called "involutional" depressions. While individual patients have been reported to respond to estrogens or progesterone, in general, the results have been poor (Hawkinson, 1938; Klaiber et al., 1976).

The widespread use of synthetic progesteronal contraceptives has produced both depression and euphoria in patients with certain personality matrices (Weissman and Slaby, 1973). Some women, for example, have reported depression after using oral contraceptives that have high concentrations of estrogen (Winston, 1973); the administration of pyridoxine is said to alleviate the depression. Estrogens did not appear to augment the antidepressant effects of imipramine in unipolar depressed women, nor did testosterone improve the effects of imipramine in depressed men (Prange et al., 1976).

During the 1940's and 1950's attempts were made to combine estrogens and progesterone with various somatic therapies. These hormones were combined with electroconvulsive therapy in the treatment of severe delusional depressions and in patients with post-partum depressions. The addition of the hormones did not enhance the therapeutic results. Insulin coma therapy and progesterone were combined in uncontrolled studies in the treatment of female schizophrenic patients; the results varied widely. Large doses of androgens were given to depressed female patients, while large doses of estrogens were administered to depressed male patients (Bleuler, 1954). No consistent or significant benefits resulted. While some patients became euphoric, other patients became worse.

A number of hypotheses relating adrenocortical activities to schizophrenia have resulted in a variety of treatments. Bilateral adrenalectomies were performed on chronic schizophrenic patients but produced no beneficial results. There have been no systematic controlled studies of antidepressants in combination with adrenal cortical hormones. Although ACTH and corticoid preparations have been used in the treatment of schizophrenic patients, no significant benefits resulted.

In an opposite vein, a variety of psychogenic abnormalities may appear when corticoids are used in the treatment of somatic abnormalities. These include depression, acute organic mental reactions, and schizophreniform behavior. Usually these psychologic disturbances disappear when the corticoid treatment is stopped. In some instances psychotropic drug therapy and even electroconvulsive therapy may be necessary to ameliorate these corticoid precipitated psychoses.

Treatment with hormones had its widest application as replacement therapy in patients with involutional depressions before the advent of the antidepressant drugs. The results were poor. From a historic basis hormone therapy was also used widely in an attempt to control sexual dysfunctions such as frigidity (Andersen, 1958) and impotence (Seid, 1962; Margoles and Leslie, 1966; Borelli, 1967). These studies were not controlled, and the treatment was of little significant benefit. In a similar fashion, hormones were widely used in the treatment of premenstrual tension with inconsistent results in uncontrolled studies (Greene and Dalton, 1953; Rees, 1953).

Desiccated thyroid, thyroxine, and synthetic l-thyroxine (Synthroid) have been used alone and in combination with various antidepressant preparations, particularly in the management of depressed patients with decreased psychomotor activity. In depressed female patients 25 μg of triiodothyroxine (T_3) appeared to cause more rapid improvement when combined with imipramine (Prange et al., 1969). T_3 did not appear to enhance improvement in depressed male patients. Others have found that T_3 appears to potentiate the action of both imipramine and amitriptyline (Goodwin and Ebert, 1977; Wheatley, 1972).

Synthesized thyrotropin releasing hormone (TRH), a polypeptide found in the hypothalamus and other areas of the brain, has been reported to produce significant antidepressant effects in depressed patients (Kastin et al., 1972; Prange et al., 1972). However, these findings have not been confirmed by other studies (Coppen et al., 1974).

Hormones have also been used in the treatment of male sex offenders. Medroxyprogesterone acetate was first used successfully for this purpose in 1966 (Money, 1970). In males, medroxyprogesterone acetate, injected in its long-acting form (Depo-Provera, Upjohn) is an androgen-depleting antiandrogen (Money, 1980) and probably also serves as an erotic tranquilizer that has a direct effect on erotosexual pathways in the limbic system. The hyposexual effects are reversible when the hormone therapy is stopped, except that the paraphilic fantasy and the behavior it dictates no longer have the same tyrannical, addictive quality (Money and Bennett, 1981).

PSYCHEDELIC (HALLUCINOGENIC) DRUGS

Many different psychopharmacologic agents may produce hallucinogenic reactions, delusions, illusions, and mood and cognitive changes. These include bromides, antidepressants, opiate antagonists, stimulants, corticosteroids, anticholinergics, and antimalarial drugs. LSD (lysergic acid diethylamide) and the related hallucinogens differ from these drugs in that they produce profound changes in sensation and mood coexisting with a relatively clear, uncluttered sensorium and consciousness in doses that result in comparatively slight physiologic activity.

Types of Psychedelic Preparations

LSD and Related Hallucinogens. Lysergic acid diethylamide (LSD), psilocybin, psilocin, diethyltryptamine (DET), and dimethyltryptamine (DMT) are all indolalkylamines. Mescaline is a more simple phenelethylamine type. Several phenelethylamines appear to be a blend between amphetamine and mescaline. These include 2,5-dimethoxy-4-methamphetamine (DOM-STP), 2,5-dimethoxy-4-ethylamphetamine (DOE), and others. These drugs produce similar subjective effects in spite of differences in chemical structure.

The psychedelic drugs produce hallucinogenic effects in a clear sensorium and even in a state of hypervigilant consciousness. These effects are in marked contrast to those produced by anticholinergic hallucinogens and other deliriants. The clinical differences between the drugs usually are in terms of duration, psychologic effects, and the severity of somatic symptoms.

Psychologic Effects. Psychologic effects may develop after 20-30 μg of LSD. The effects of oral preparations begin in about one hour; peak in two to three hours; and return to normal, gradually, in six to ten hours. Some preparations such as DMT and psilocybin produce a briefer reaction. The effects appear to be dose related. All cause impairment of motivation, concentration, and attention. Cognitive testing may be impaired or unchanged, and perceptual motor functions may be impaired. Studies of enhancement of sensation and the effects of the hallucinogens on creativity are not clear-cut.

Severe psychologic effects may occur when these drugs are used (Freedman, 1968; Smart and Bateman, 1967; McGlothlin, 1967; McGlothlin and Arnold, 1971). The so-called "bad trip," consisting of panic and terror and resulting at times in impulsive acting out and even suicide, is legend. The adverse psychologic reactions may also include paranoid behavior, psychotic phenomena, and prolonged depressions. In many instances these reactions have been found to occur in patients who have these disorders in a subliminal form or who have a propensity for such syndromes. Many of these reactions may become chronic. Phenomena such as "flashbacks" may also occur (Shick and Smith, 1970).

LSD therapy was used in the 1950's and early 1960's and stimulated a large number of clinical reports. Two types of LSD therapy could be defined:

A. Psychedelic therapy involving the use of large doses (200 μg or more of LSD orally) in a single session. Its proposed purpose was to help alcoholics and criminals or to improve the lives of "normal" individuals.

B. Psycholytic therapy. In this technique, smaller doses, no larger than 150 μg of LSD, were given over many sessions; the purpose was to help neurotic individuals or persons with psychosomatic disorders. Psycholytic therapy was recommended by some to speed up psychoanalytic types of therapy.

The use of LSD in conjunction with various types of psychotherapy for a number of purposes has all but disappeared, primarily due to the lack of reports of any consistent beneficial results and partly because of the illegality of the drug in the U.S. after its brief period of widespread social use. For example, even though a number of reports suggested that LSD therapy was beneficial in the treatment of alcoholics, this promise was not borne out by careful clinical evaluation (Ludwig et al., 1970).

Aldous Huxley was a great enthusiast of the psychedelic drugs, which he took on a number of occasions. He was given LSD by his wife as he was dying, an event that stimulated the use of LSD as part of a psycho-thanatologic technique.

Recent surveys suggest that the therapeutic use of psychedelic drugs was not particularly dangerous.

Anticholinergic Hallucinogens. The anticholinergic hallucinogenic drugs are related to atropine and scopolamine (Ericksen, 1969; Davoisin and Katz, 1968). These drugs all produce a confusional picture characterized by apprehension, decreased alertness, and confusion. With larger doses, drowsiness, restlessness, motor incoordination advancing into deep confusion, and hallucinations occur. With even larger doses, the patient may have convulsions, hyperthermia, and may even lapse into coma. These patients do not respond well to phenothiazines, which also have anticholinergic effects.

Anesthetic Drugs. Phencyclidine was used for a while as a general anesthetic but was discontinued because of postanesthetic reactions characterized by hallucinations and agitation. This drug is now available on the "streets" illegally and is referred to by a number of names including "PCP," "angel dust," "rocket fuel," and so on (Showalter and Thornton, 1977). It may be sold in combination with LSD. Unfortunately, phencyclidine is a drug that can be readily synthesized. It may produce extremely violent hallucinogenic patterns as well as delusions and cataleptic reactions. At high doses, it produces severe autonomic side effects in addition to neurologic abnormalities such as ataxia, nystagmus, dystonia, and convulsions. Unlike most other hallucinogens, death from overdosages may occur, usually in association with recurrent convulsions.

Any anesthetic whose action is characterized by a prolonged Stage II can produce hallucinogenic effects with psychotomimetic features. These include nitrous oxide, ether, or even chloroform. While nitrous oxide inhalation has been used clinically in anxious and psychotic patients (Lehman and Bos, 1947), it has also become a popular deliriant. This usage may be considered as part of the recent phenomenon of abuse of psychoactive volitile substances (National Commission on Marijuana and Drug Abuse, 1973; Press and Dane, 1967a, 1967b). These drugs are used predominantly by adolescents and include such substances as varnish, gasoline, paint thinner, aerosol sprays, glue, amyl nitrate, toluene, nitrous oxide, and others. These substances are not all hallucinogens nor should all of them be considered psychedelic drugs. Nitrous oxide, however, can cause clinical phenomena such as those described for the other anesthetic hallucinogens. The main problem with these agents is overdosage, which results in respiratory and cardiovascular difficulties.

Cannabis. Cannabis can appear to be hallucinogenic or not, depending on drug concentration, the patient's personality, the setting, expectations, and other phenomena that would affect the response to any hallucinogen (Information Canada, 1972).

The source of cannabis is hemp. The term *marijuana* refers to the leaves and other parts of the hemp plant which are chopped up and usually smoked. The term hashish, which comes from the Arabic term meaning *assassin*, is the dried resinous exudate of the flowering tops of the plant and usually has the highest concentration of psychoactive chemicals. The major part of the plant's potency appears to be due to substances called cannabinoids, of which more than 20 have been isolated from various plant material. More than 100 noncannabinoid compounds have been identified from the plant.

There is general agreement that most of the psychoactive properties of cannabis are due to delta-9-tetrahydrocannabinol (THC) (Gaoni and Mechoulam, 1964; Mechoulam and Gaoni, 1965). Delta-9, delta-THC, and monodihydroxylate metabolites all have cannabis-like effects. There is some question as to the relative importance of the hydroxylate metabolites in the production of cannabis intoxication.

THC can be synthesized, but the process is expensive. On the illicit market, that which is claimed to be THC is usually phencyclidine or combinations of other drugs. Hashish oil containing high concentrations of THC is available. The cannabinoids are readily absorbed through the lung or gastrointestinal tract and have a long half-life of approximately 60 hours with material to be found in the feces and urine for more than eight days. The long half-life is due, in part, to the drug's recycling through the enterohepatic circulation and its remaining in body tissues. Absorption is rapid after smoking, with the effects appearing within a few minutes. THC is about three times more potent when smoked than when taken orally.

The dose is important in determining the psychologic effect of cannabis (Bloomquist, 1968). A mild and brief "high" follows a low-dose smoke. A prolonged hallucinogenic experience usually follows a large oral dose. An initial, relatively short period of stimulation, accompanied by euphoria or anxiety and exaggerated perceptions, is usually followed by a period of sedation characterized by a relaxed dream-like state. The reactions parallel those produced by other hallucinogens and may include paraesthesias; altered time sense; problems speaking, remembering, and concentrating; and visual illusions. Most cognitive functions can be altered by cannabis. Autonomic changes can appear with higher doses of THC. These include orthostatic hypotension, a slight decrease in intraocular pressure, and tachycardia. In addition, muscle weakness, nystagmus, tremor, problems with coordination, and even ataxia may occur; these effects are dose related.

Tolerance to marijuana develops in humans at certain dosage levels. There appears to be some cross-tolerance between alcohol and cannabis but not between THC and LSD. Adverse psychologic problems, including some of those associated with other hallucinogens, appear to occur with cannabis as well (Jones, 1973). "Flashbacks" such as those reported after LSD use have also been noted with cannabis (Information Canada, 1972). Acute episodes of panic, disorientation, depersonalization, and delusions may occur; these are often referred to as "freaking out" and seem to resemble the "bad trips" that may follow LSD. An "amotivation" syndrome has also been described; this is characterized by low self-esteem, introversion, apathy, and loss of interest. As in the case of the hallucinogens, it is difficult to differentiate on many occasions what is cause and what is effect.

Cannabis has been recommended for a number of therapeutic purposes. However, with the possible exception of its role in terminal cancer, there has been no consistent documentation as yet that it has a pertinent role in medicine.

HEMODIALYSIS

In 1977, Wagemaker and Cade reported their use of hemodialysis in four chronically ill, hospitalized schizophrenic patients (Wagemaker and Cade, 1977). This treatment program followed their observations of psychologic improvement in a schizophrenic woman who had received multiple hemodialyses for the management of a severe hypertensive state. Their patients were dialyzed on a weekly basis. The authors stated that after the patients reported a significant improvement in their clinical status, the dialyses were reduced in frequency to every two weeks and even less.

They indicated that four patients improved to the point that they could be discharged from the hospital free of the overt manifestations of schizophrenia. These patients did not receive psychotropic drugs during the course of hemodialysis. One patient, who failed to continue on the dialysis program, experienced an exacerbation of the illness.

Wagemaker and Cade's paper received a great deal of attention in neuropsychopharmacologic circles, especially since several other papers supporting a so-called "opioid concept" as a basic cause of schizophrenia appeared at about the same time (Termius et al., 1976; Kline et al., 1977). In keeping with this concept, Wagemaker and Cade and their associates wrote that they had discovered a new peptide, a leucine-5-β-END (Palmour et al., 1977). The authors claimed that the clinical benefits resulting from hemodialysis were due to the removal of this leucine-5-β-END from the plasma.

The theory behind these reports, the technique itself, and the results have been severely challenged (Stephen et al., 1979). There have been vigorous discussions with regard to the types of dialysis membranes used, the psychologic nature of the therapeutic environment, and the nature of the diagnosis of the patients treated. No definitive studies have duplicated the favorable results reported originally by Wagemaker and Cade or their associates, and no other laboratory has detected leucine-5-β-END in the hemofiltrate.

CONTINUOUS SLEEP THERAPY

The systematic use of continuous sleep therapy was introduced in 1922 by Klaesi (1922), although prolonged sleep for the treatment of emotional disorders had been used for a long time. Klaesi's technique was the first systematic procedure of organic treatment in the endogenous psychoses (Kalinowsky and Hippius, 1969). Various drugs have been used for this treatment, both individually and as mixtures. In some instances, the medication is applied rectally. In other instances, barbiturates have been administered intravenously.

The patient is kept in a state of narcosis for ten or more days. The sleep-like state is reduced temporarily at specific intervals during which time the patient is permitted to eat and to urinate or defecate. The medication is tapered off slowly at the end of narcosis to avoid convulsions. An abrupt acute organic mental syndrome can also occur following the sudden withdrawal of the narcosis producing drugs.

Continuous sleep therapy is an expensive procedure since it requires a well trained staff to be present on a 24-hour basis. Respiratory, cardiovascular, or renal complications may occur in the absence of close supervision.

Following the introduction of electroconvulsive treatment, continuous sleep therapy was used sparingly except in the Soviet Union. Russian physicians modified the deeper barbiturate narcosis by inducing sleep, partly with hypnotics, partly with conditioning. The Russian therapists reported that schizophrenics with florid symptomatology responded better to insulin, while those with bland symptomatology did well with continuous sleep therapy (Ivanov-Smolenskii, 1939). Benefits have been claimed for continuous sleep in the treatment of the manic phase of manic-depressive psychosis and in agitated unipolar depressions. Schizophrenic patients in a state of catatonic excitement have also been reported to respond well.

In some European countries, particularly in well staffed private hospitals, continuous sleep treatment is actively used as part of the psychiatric treatment armamentarium. This technique is rarely used in the United States. Overall, the neuroleptic drugs have replaced continuous sleep techniques.

Electric Sleep Therapy

Electric sleep therapy was introduced in the Soviet Union by Giljarowsky (1956). This technique is accomplished by placing an electrode over the occipital region of the head and over the base of the nose with extensions to both eyes. With the patient in a dark room, he or she is informed that sleep will occur in less than half an hour. The current is continuous for several hours, and the patient usually continues to sleep after the current has been removed. Several patients can be treated simultaneously with leads from a single machine.

The term "electric sleep" is considered to be a misnomer since sleep does not usually occur during the treatment session (Rosenthal, 1972). The treatment itself consists of a low milliamperage (0.4-2.0 mA) pulsed unidirectional current. A slight tingling sensation occurs but without sleep. The treatments are given for a total of five to ten sessions.

Double-blind continual comparison between this technique of "electric sleep" and placebo suggests that the active treatment is most effective in relieving anxiety, insomnia, and minor depression. It works adversely in psychotic depression (Rosenthal, 1972). In the Soviet Union "electric sleep" is also used in combination with insulin treatment during the precoma phase.

Polarization Therapy

Polarization therapy is similar to "electric sleep" (Lippold and Redfearn, 1964). In this technique, electrodes are applied over the orbits and one leg. Smaller currents (0.25-0.5 mA) are used. The patient experiences no sensations during the flow of current. The beneficial response is said to depend on the fact that the head is "electropositive" with respect to the leg. While polarization therapy has been found to be superior to a placebo in a controlled trial in depressed patients, a double-blind controlled study in normal subjects showed no difference between genuine and sham polarization (Lippold and Redfearn, 1964).

There is a question as to whether the electric currents used in polarization therapy and in "electric sleep" therapy are sufficient to produce a neurophysiologic effect. These techniques do not appear to have proven to be of significant value.

SLEEP DEPRIVATION THERAPY

Sleep deprivation therapy has been used in the treatment of depression. Initially, it was employed in response to isolated reports suggesting that sleepless nights exerted a beneficial influence on patients suffering from depression, particularly endogenous depression. Those proposing the use of this technique stated that the circadian periodicity of various body rhythms becomes desynchronized during states of depression. While the mechanism by which sleep deprivation therapy is supposed to occur is not clearly understood, a few general concepts have been proposed. One suggests that sleep deprivation serves as a synchronizer of desynchronized circadian rhythms (Pflug, 1975). Another is that it causes antidepressant effects by lowering arousal levels. (Kupfer et al., 1976).

In order to appreciate the theory of sleep deprivation therapy, it is necessary to understand the circadian rhythm phase-advance hypothesis of depression. The pattern of rapid eye movement (REM) sleep during a night's sleep is normally uneven, with more REM taking place toward the end of the night than at the beginning (Dement and Kleitman, 1957). This distribution of REM sleep is changed in depressed patients in that more REM sleep occurs in the first third of the night than in normals. Some investigators have suggested that these changes in the temporal distribution of depressives' REM sleep could result from a phase advance of the circadian rhythm in the propensity to have REM sleep. In depressives, its maximum frequency occurs closer to the onset of sleep, rather than near dawn (Gresham et al., 1965). At the present time there is considerable debate as to whether or not there is an advancement in the phase position of the circadian temperature rhythm associated with depressive episodes. While some observers have stated that such advancement occurs (Kripke, 1979), others question this viewpoint.

In addition, it has been suggested that there is a "phase advance of neurotransmitter metabolite circadian rhythms" (Riederer et al., 1974). These findings and others have suggested the concept of a "circadian rhythm phase advance" hypothesis of depression. The cause of the phase disturbance is unknown.

Different therapeutic sleep deprivation procedures have been employed: (a) sleep deprivation limited to one night (Paponsek et al., 1975), (b) weekly single night sleep deprivation (one to 14 weeks) (Bhanji and Roy, 1975), (c) multiple variously placed single nights of sleep deprivation (Pflug, 1976), (d) REM sleep deprivation over a period of four to six weeks (Vogel et al., 1973; Vogel et al., 1980), and (e) partial sleep deprivation whereby the patient is awakened during the second half of the night (Schilgin and Tölle, 1980).

In most instances, sleep deprivation therapy is combined with antidepressant drug therapy. It should be appreciated that REM sleep deprivation itself represents a selective sleep stage deprivation comparable to the procedure in which a therapist might decide to deprive a patient of slow wave sleep or deep sleep.

The treatment results secondary to sleep deprivation treatment vary widely. One observer reported that 40 to 60 percent of patients with endogenous depressions derived significant improvement secondary to this technique (King, 1980), others have reported that it had no beneficial effect in some patients (Pflug, 1976), and some observers have stated that sleep deprivation may worsen depression (Vogel et al., 1973).

The response to a single night's sleep deprivation may be immediate or gradual. Beneficial responses have been reported as being clearly evident as early as the morning following treatment. This improvement may last for days (Pflug, 1975). On the other hand, the benefits may disappear after the patient experiences one night of continuous sleep (Paponsek et al., 1975). Some patients show gradual improvement but relapse shortly after treatment is completed. Others are said to improve gradually and steadily (Bhanji and Roy, 1975). On occasion, patients who relapse after an immediate beneficial response may show longer periods of clinical remission after another series of sleep deprivation treatments (Pflug, 1975). One observer reported that seven of 15 patients with endogenous depressions maintained benefits for from three to six months (Bhanji and Roy, 1975).

Patients with endogenous depressions responded best with either single night procedures or REM sleep deprivation therapy. Depressed patients with histories indicating either insomnia, anorexia, or a marked increase or decrease in psychomotor activity were reported to be most likely to experience good results (Pflug, 1976). In one study there was a significant interaction between the response to sleep deprivation and MHPG levels in the cerebrospinal fluid; it was decreased in those who showed clinical improvement and increased in those who did not respond (Post et al., 1976).

A number of adverse responses to sleep deprivation have also been reported. These include (a) worsening of depression, particularly among patients with "neurotic" depressions (Pflug and Tölle, 1971); (b) transient somatic complaints, such as headache or gastrointestinal discomfort; (c) hypomanic or manic symptoms; and (d) exacerbation of psychotic manifestations (Pflug, 1975).

The original studies with sleep deprivation therapy were performed in a hospital setting. More recently, it has been used on an outpatient basis as well. It is recommended that the procedure be carried out in a hospital on at least one occasion. The patient's family may be called on to assist in the treatment when it is carried out in the home.

The overall value of the sleep deprivation technique still awaits careful, controlled study. It is difficult to provide double-blind conditions for sleep deprivation techniques if one uses an all night or partial sleep deprivation technique. The possible application in clinical trials of combined strategies appears warranted.

PHARMACOLOGIC CONVULSIVE THERAPIES

Metrazol and Other Parenterally Administered Drugs

The use of parenterally administered drugs to produce seizures is primarily of historic interest at the present time (Kalinowsky et al., 1982) since they have almost totally been replaced by electroconvulsive techniques. A number of preparations have been used to induce seizures, including pentamethylentetrazol (Metrazol), picrotoxin, coriamytrin, ammonium chloride, and cyclohexylethyltriazol (Triazol).

Metrazol was introduced by von Meduna and was used widely until the introduction of electroconvulsive treatment. It is injected rapidly intravenously, with the initial dose usually being 0.5 grams (5cc). If no seizure occurs within one to two minutes, repeat injections are given. The convulsion produced by Metrazol parallels that noted with Indoklon in that it produces some clonic movements prior to the appearance of the tonic seizure. This event was labeled the "first-clonic phase." After the first-clonic phase, the patient loses consciousness and has a tonic phase usually lasting about ten seconds and then goes into a clonic phase that may be 30 to 40 seconds in duration. Irregular clonic movements may occur after the convulsion has ended. These are thought to be due to direct cortical stimulation. On occasion, second convulsions may occur with Metrazol.

There is no indication that the clinical results produced by Metrazol are superior to those resulting from electroconvulsive treatment. It produces a post-ictal confusional state comparable to that secondary to ECT. The most unpleasant feature of Metrazol treatment is a precordial discomfort occurring before the patient loses consciousness. This sensation is terrifying and has been described by patients as a feeling of impending death. Failures to produce a convulsion, when they occur, are associated with feelings of apprehension that may last for hours. These disadvantages and the greater efficiency of ECT in producing seizures were the main reasons ECT replaced Metrazol.

Inhalation Convulsive Therapy

Hexafluorodiethyl ether (Indoklon) is one of the aliphatic fluorinated ethers which has some anesthetic properties but which also produces convulsions (Krantz et al., 1957).

This preparation is a colorless, nonflammable liquid which, when applied directly by means of a mask and vaporizer, produces a convulsion within 15 to 30 seconds. The general pattern is that the patient, after losing consciousness, is noted to have myoclonic movements paralleling those seen in Metrazol convulsions. The patient then slowly develops a tonic contraction followed by clonic convulsive movements.

One of the primary disadvantages of Indoklon treatment is the observation that it may be difficult to see whether the patient has had a true and complete convulsive reaction (Kalinowsky et al., 1982). In addition, if Indoklon is given in the absence of barbiturate anesthesia, the initial convulsion is often followed by one or more additional seizures after an interval of one or two minutes. Experience has shown that this repetition of seizures can usually be avoided by careful regulation of dosage and barbiturate anesthesia.

The technique of the Indoklon treatment requires careful cooperation between the psychiatrist and an anesthesiologist. The technique may be summarized as follows (Karliner and Padula, 1959): The patient is first anesthetized with an intravenous drip of a short-acting barbiturate. After the patient is appropriately anesthetized, succinylcholine (Anectine) is administered by intravenous drip until satsifactory muscle relaxation is obtained. This is usually evidenced by the appearance of fasciculations in the neck, upper limbs, and lower limbs. After the fasciculations have stopped, it can be assumed that the patient is adequately relaxed.

A mask is applied to the patient's face while the patient is receiving the intravenous anesthetic and the succinylcholine. After adequate muscle relaxation has been obtained, 0.25-0.5 cc of Indoklon is injected into the vaporizer through a rubber diaphragm. The oxygen is turned off and the bag repeatedly squeezed, forcing the Indoklon into the patient's lungs; the action is continued until a tonic phase of seizure is noted. After this has occurred, the mask is removed and all Indoklon is removed from the bag. Oxygenation is then resumed, and the patient is ventilated until he resumes spontaneous breathing.

As noted above, one of the problems with the use of Indoklon is the confusion of myoclonic movements with a true convulsion. A tonic phase of a seizure must be documented if the treatment is to be of any benefit. It would appear that convulsive treatment induced by Indoklon inhalation is as effective as electroconvulsive treatment. The early claims that it was superior in the management of schizophrenic patients in whom other therapies have failed has not been effectively documented.

Nausea frequently follows Indoklon administration, and it is almost routine to administer prochlorperazine (Compazine) intramuscularly or intravenously, the usual dose being 5 mg. Post-treatment confusion is approximately of the same intensity as that experienced following ECT.

While Indoklon inhalation convulsant treatment was effective in the treatment of severely depressed patients, the problems associated with its administration and its side effects severely restricted its use when compared with electroconvulsive therapy. It was recommended as an alternative technique for patients who required electrconvulsive therapy but who rejected ECT because of fear associated with the concept of "electroshock." Indoklon therapy is presently only of historic interest as Indoklon is no longer being produced.

INSULIN TREATMENT

Insulin coma therapy was the first active treatment program for the management of schizophrenia. Sakel (1938) reported on the benefits of this treatment in the 1930's. At the present time, the insulin coma technique is used in only a few psychiatric hospitals throughout the world. Insulin coma is an expensive procedure requiring a large staff of well qualified personnel. Its extensive use was first reduced to a limited degree by the introduction of electroconvulsive treatment. Its almost total disappearance occurred following the introduction of the neuroleptics in the 1950's. At the present time, if used at all, it is reserved for schizophrenic patients who do not respond to any other type of treatment.

Insulin coma is a hospital procedure. Its optimal application depends on a trained staff of physicians and nurses working in a well equipped, pleasant environment. In some institutions, patients receiving insulin coma remain on a special unit during their entire hospitalization. Ideally, the patients also concomitantly receive psychotherapy and occupational therapy. In some institutions these are further supplemented by conjoint family group therapy.

Patient Selection. As noted above, insulin coma therapy is now reserved for patients who have failed after being exposed to psychopharmacologic treatment, ECT, and various types of psychotherapy. Therefore, when it is used today, it is used in chronically ill patients with a poor prognosis. Paradoxically, the best results are obtained in patients who have been actively ill for less than six months (Sargent, 1972; Laqueur, 1969; Kalinowsky et al., 1982).

All patients considered for insulin coma should have a careful physical examination. Individuals with cardiovascular disease, significant kidney or liver disease, significant endocrinological ailments, active pulmonary disease, or a febrile illness of any kind should not be exposed to insulin shock therapy. Pregnant women also should not receive it. One must be particularly careful with individuals in their late 40's or older.

Technique. A number of technical variations are used by different psychiatrists (Laqueur and LaBurt, 1960). Due to the possibility of an allergic reaction or hypersensitivity to insulin, treatment is usually started with ten to 15 units of regular insulin. This amount is increased on a daily basis by five to ten units. One must appreciate that there is a marked fluctuation in sensitivity to insulin. Some patients reveal hypersensitivity to small doses, while some may not become hypoglycemic even after receiving excessive amounts of insulin. A coma is usually obtained with 100-200 units of regular insulin.

The injections are given deep intramuscularly with the sites of injection being changed on each occasion to avoid local tissue damage. The levels of hypoglycemia occurring as a result of insulin have been divided into five phases: The first, a pre-shock or pre-comatose phase, usually occurs about an hour after the injection or even sooner. During this phase it is often difficult to differentiate between hypoglycemic manifestations and the patient's psychotic symptoms and signs. The aim is to attain the second, or shock phase, at which time the patient loses consciousness. The desired depth of coma is arrived at when the patient ceases to show any response to painful stimuli. This level is usually attained at the beginning or during the early part of the third hour of hypoglycemia. The patient should be kept in coma for about 15 minutes on the first occasion. If no complications occur, the coma may be extended gradually up to one hour or longer. One must be cautious to avoid long periods of "deepened" coma in which spasms similar to those seen in decerebrate rigidity occur. Different diagnostic formulae have been developed to show the disintegration of brain functioning according to various levels of central nervous system activity descending from suppression of cortical activity, release of basal ganglia functioning, release of midbrain activity, and, finally, release of functions attributed to the medulla.

Termination of Hypoglycemia. Originally, the hypoglycemia was terminated by the administration of sugar in solution through a nasogastric tube. If this procedure was not fully successful after a 20-minute period, 33-50% glucose solution was given intravenously. These concentrated glucose solutions tended to cause local venous coagulation. More recently, the termination procedure has been simplified. The hormone glucagon is given in dosages of 0.33-1.0 mg either intravenously or intramuscularly (Laqueur, 1961). The patient usually awakens after ten to 20 minutes. If the individual does not react by that time, the dose is repeated.

Desired Number of Comas. Improvement, when it occurs with coma therapy, is gradual. It is advisable to continue treatment to what appears to be a maximum level of remission. Forty to 60 comas are considered a minimum. In some instances, individual psychiatrists have given patients 100 or more comas in a series over a period of four to five months.

Insulin coma can be an effective treatment if applied adequately in properly selected patients.

Complications. The most frequent and most severe complication of insulin coma is that of protracted coma in which the patient remains in coma after the hypoglycemia has been eliminated. In reality, this represents the development of an encephalopathy. The other serious complication is associated with acute cardiac insufficiency. (Before the introduction of glucagon, there was a mortality rate of approximately 0.25 percent due to protracted coma or cardiovascular complications. With the use of glucagon to control the hypoglycemia, fatalities became extremely rare.)

On occasion, an activation of the patient's psychosis may occur, but it is usually transient. Short-acting organic mental reactions may occur in protracted coma. Permanent brain damage is rare.

Subcoma (Ambulatory) Insulin Therapy

Subcoma insulin treatment was initially used in the 1920's before the introduction of insulin shock treatment (Klemperer, 1926). In this technique the patients receive small but slowly increased doses of regular insulin until they show signs of hypoglycemia without a loss of consciousness. Initially, this technique was used for sedating excited patients and in patients with delirium tremens, and it was extensively used during the withdrawal periods in morphine addicts.

In addition to its sedative effect, insulin aids in weight gain and, therefore, found extensive use in psychiatric patients who were malnourished. Later, during World War II, it was used in England in the treatment of combat neuroses. This technique was also used to treat schizophrenic patients. While positive benefits were described in a number of series, studies of controlled series are not available.

While subcoma insulin therapy may be combined with other somatic treatments, for example ECT (Sargent, 1972), there do not appear to be any significant benefits from this combined technique over those obtained with ECT alone. However, in France, subcoma insulin treatment was also combined with colloidal gold treatments and other colloidal solutions. These techniques are rarely used now.

In general, ambulatory insulin treatment is a safe procedure. However, complications may occur in patients who have insulin allergies or marked hypersensitivity reactions. The main danger is that the patient may go into a state of coma.

Subcoma, ambulatory insulin therapy is a very satisfactory means of attaining sedation. However, similar results may be obtained in most instances by using tranquilizers and sedatives.

INHALATION RESTITUTIVE THERAPIES

The inhalation techniques that will be described here are rarely used at the present time. They were all developed before the advent of the psychotropic drugs, and they do not appear to have a viable role in current psychiatric practice.

Restitutive therapies are those techniques that are used to produce an altered state of consciousness for therapeutic purposes. A wide range of pharmacologic agents can be used for these purposes, including alcohol, barbiturates, certain psychotropic drugs, and hallucinogens (these have been described in other chapters). The inhalation techniques that have been used include carbon dioxide, nitrogen, nitrous oxide, ether, and trichlorethylene. Broadly speaking, Indoklon, which is a hexafluorodiethyl ether, might fall into this categorization. However, it will be considered separately since it is a convulsant, in addition to having some anesthetic properties.

Carbon Dioxide

Carbon dioxide was initially used in the treatment of psychotic patients (Loevenhart et al., 1929). After some apparent success in the treatment of catatonic patients, further studies suggested that it was not beneficial; and it was given up for a period of time. Carbon dioxide inhalation had a rebirth in 1947, when it was applied to the treatment of psychoneurotic patients (Meduna, 1958). Statements appeared to the effect that the treatment was successful in patients with conversion symptoms, spastic colitis, alcoholism, stuttering, homosexuality, and personality disorders. It was claimed that carbon dioxide and oxygen inhalation were superior to psychotherapy in the treatment of phobias. The explanation given was that neuroses were caused by a low threshold to normal stimuli and that carbon dioxide normalized the threshold. It was found to work poorly in patients with obsessive-compulsive problems and hypochondriasis.

The technique consisted of inhalation of a mixture of 30 percent carbon dioxide and 70 percent oxygen. Initially, 20 to 25 respirations were given. After eight to 16 respirations the patient usually lost consciousness. At about that time, evidence of psychomotor excitement was often seen. Later carpal spasms similar to those seen in hyperventilation appeared. If the respirations were increased markedly, the pupils could become fixed and a decerebrate rigidity-like state could develop. The number of treatments necessary to achieve clinical results varied from 20 to 150. Some therapists used non-coma carbon dioxide, while others used coma doses.

Many conflicting reports appeared regarding the benefit of CO_2 therapy. Several studies concluded that it had no special effects in the treatment of psychoneuroses (Hargrove et al., 1954; Hawkings and Tibbets, 1956). Currently carbon dioxide treatment is rarely used.

Nitrogen and Nitrous Oxide

In a previous chapter, it was noted that nitrous oxide is one of the volatile psychoactive chemicals being used on the streets, particularly by adolescents. When used in this manner, the intoxication is short and characterized by an angry, drunken type of behavior.

Nitrogen inhalation was introduced in the late 1930's in the treatment of schizophrenia (Sillman and Terrence, 1943). It produced a brief anoxia that allegedly produced a depression of cerebral metabolism. It was reported that the patient went through the same changes as seen with the use of insulin, with the exception that the duration of the various stages of disintegration of cerebral functioning was limited to seconds rather than hours. The nitrogen was administered by an anesthetist at a rate of a six liters per minute for six minutes. The results of treatment with nitrogen inhalation were compared with those obtained with insulin and metrazol treatment. Nitrogen inhalation was found to be unsatisfactory. This treatment is not followed at the present time.

Nitrous oxide (N_2O) use was first reported in 1928, when it was suggested that it had some therapeutic value in the treatment of psychotic patients (Zador, 1928). In 1947, a report appeared suggesting differences between the effects of nitrous oxide and nitrogen inhalation (Lehmann and Bos, 1947). Nitrous oxide produced euphoria during the phase of induction; it did not produce the fear of loss of consciousness and shortness of breath noted with patients who inhaled carbon dioxide.

The drug is administered through an inhalator; the breathing bag is filled with nitrous oxide, until the patient's respirations become rapid, irregular, and autonomic. At this point, pure oxygen is administered, and after four to six respirations the mask is removed. Loss of consciousness occurs about one minute later, with the patient recovering in two to three minutes. A feeling of euphoria is experienced when the patient awakens. Nitrous oxide was reported to be of some benefit in manic excitements and was also used in narcoanalysis. It is rarely employed as a psychotherapeutic agent at the present time.

Ether and Trichlorethylene

Although ether was used as an "abreaction technique," in reality it served as an adjunct to psychotherapy. It was supposed to work by depressing the highest psychic centers, thus producing disinhibition and excitation to a greater extent than did sodium amytal (Shorvan and Sargant, 1947).

The technique was as follows: Ether was poured onto a mask which was held a distance away from the patient's face. Initially, the purpose was to cause a state of marked emotional excitement; thus, the patient was encouraged to talk about past experiences that would cause powerful feelings, particularly those of anger or terror. The mask was then brought over the patient's face. At the point at which the patient was slightly intoxicated, the therapist encouraged further emotional elaboration until the patient struggled and shouted. The patient had to be restrained, which added to the excitement. The procedure ended with the patient in a state of total exhaustion at which time he or she became limp and sometimes unresponsive. Ether was also used by a drip method in combination with glucose and saline over a period of two to three hours.

In 1950, a report appeared on the use of trichlorethylene as an aid to psychotherapy (Rees et al., 1950). This was said to be faster than other inhalation methods, and it produced no nausea. It was inhaled through a mask connected to a vaporizer, a technique that prodcued greater communication and at times marked emotional lability. Trichlorethylene was recommended for use in psychotherapy of various types, including narcoanalysis, narcosynthesis, abreaction, relaxation procedures, narcosuggestion, and reinforcement of reassurance.

In general, these techniques did not attain wide use and, as in the case of the other inhalants, are rarely used at the present time.

REFERENCES

DISULFIRAM (ANTABUSE) IN ALCOHOLISM

Billet SL: Antabuse therapy, in Alcoholism: The Total Treatment Approach. Edited by Catanzaro R. Springfield, Ill, Charles C Thomas, 1968

Bourne PG, Fox R: Alcoholism: Progress in Research and Treatment. New York, Academic Press, 1973

Hald J, Jacobsen E: A drug sensitizing the organism to alcohol. Lancet 2:1001-1004, 1948

Isreal Y, Mardones J: Biological Basis of Alcoholism. New York, John Wiley & Sons, 1971

Kissin B: Interactions of ethyl alcohol and other drugs, in Biology of Alcoholism, vol 3: Clinical Pathology. Edited by Kissin B, Begleiter H. New York, Plenum, 1974

Kwentus J, Major LF: Disulfiram in the treatment of alcoholism: a review. J Stud Alcohol 40:428-446, 1979

OPIOIDS

Chambers CB, Brill L: Methadone: Experience and Issues. New York, Behavioral Publications, 1973

Dole VP, Nyswander M: Heroin addiction: a metabolic disease. Arch Intern Med 120:19-24, 1967

Dole VP, Nyswander M: A medical treatment for diacetylmorphine addiction. JAMA 193:646-650, 1965

Gunne LM, Lindström L, Terenius L: Naloxone-induced reversal of schizophrenic hallucinations. J Neural Transm 40:13-19, 1977

Hughes J, Smith TW, Kosterlitz HW, et al: Identification of two related pentapeptides from the brain with potent opiate agonist activity. Nature 258:577-580, 1975

Hunt GH, Odoroff ME: Follow-up study of narcotic drug addicts after hospitalization. Public Health Rep 77:41-54, 1962

Kleber HD: Clinical experiences with narcotic antagonists, in Opiate Addiction: Origins and Treatment. Edited by Fisher S, Freedman AM. Washington, DC, Winston & Sons, 1973

Kosterlitz HW (ed): Opiates and Endogenous Opioid Peptides. Amsterdam, North-Holland, 1976

Martin WR, Jasinski DR, Haertzen CA, et al: Methadone: a reevaluation. Arch Gen Psychiatry 28:286-295, 1973

Pert CB, Snyder SH: Opiate receptor demonstration in nervous tissue. Science 179:1011-1014, 1973

Schaumann O: Analgetika and protekives system. Dtsch Med Wochenschr 79:1571-1573, 1954

Terenius L: Characteristics of the "receptor" for narcotic analgesics in synaptic plasma membrane fraction from the rat brain. Acta Pharmacol Toxicol 33:377-384, 1973

Volavka J, Mallya A, Baig S, et al: Naloxone in chronic schizophrenia. Science 196:1227-1228, 1977

Weppner RS, Agar MH: Immediate precursors of heroin addiction. J Health Soc Behav 12:10-18, 1971

Winkler A: Characteristics of opioid addiction, in Psychopharmacology in the Practice of Medicine. Edited by Jarvick ME. New York, Appleton-Century-Crofts, 1977

STIMULANTS

Angrist BJ, Gershon S: The phenomenology of experimentally induced amphetamine psychosis, Biol Psychiatry 2:95-107, 1970

Baldessarani RJ: Symposium: behavior modification by drugs, I: pharmacology of the amphetamines. Pediatrics 49:694-701, 1972

Beckman H, Goodwin FK: Antidepressant response to tricyclics and urinary MHPG in unipolar patients. Arch Gen Psychiatry 32:17-20, 1975

Critchley M: Periodic hypersomnia and megaphagia in adolescent males. Brain 85:627-656, 1962

Ellinwood EH, Cohen S (eds): Current Concepts of Amphetamine Abuse. Rockville, Md, National Institute of Mental Health, 1970

Ellinwood EH: Emergency treatment of acute reaction to CNS stimulants. J Psychedelic Drugs 5:147-152, 1972

Gallinek A: The Kleine-Levin syndrome. Dis Nerv Syst 28:1-8, 1967

Janowsky DLS, Davis JM: Methylphenidate, dextroamphetamine, levoamphetamine: effects on schizophrenic symptoms. Arch Gen Psychiatry 33:304-308, 1976

Janowsky DS, El-Yansef MK, Davis JM, et al: Provocation of schizophrenic symptoms by intravenous administration of methylphenidate. Arch Gen Psychiatry 28:185-191, 1973

Levin M: Periodic somnolence and morbid hunger: a new syndrome. Brain 59:494-515, 1936

Maas J, Dekirmenjian H, Jones SF: The identification of depressed patients who have a disorder of norepinephrine metabolism and/or disposition, in Frontiers in Catecholamine Research. Edited by Usdin E, Snyder SH. Elmsford, NY, Pergamon Press, 1973

Rappolt RT, Gay GR, Inaba DS, et al: Propranolol: a specific antagonist to cocaine. Clin Toxicol 10:265-271, 1977

Rechtschaffen A, Dement WC: Narcolepsy and hypersomnia, in Sleep: Physiology and Pathology. Edited by Kales A. Philadelphia, JB Lippincott, 1969

Snyder SH: How amphetamine acts in minimal brain dysfunction. Acad Sci 205:310, 1973

Sprague R, Sleator E: Effects of psychopharmacologic agents on learning disorders. Pediatr Clin North Am 20:719-735, 1973

Wender PH: Minimal Brain Dysfunction in Children. New York, Wiley Interscience, 1971

Wender PH: Minimal brain dysfunction: an overview, in Psychopharmacology: A Generation of Progress. Edited by Lipton MA, DiMascio A, Killam KF. New York, Raven Press, 1978

Werry JS: Medications for hyperkinetic children. Drugs 11:81-89, 1976

Wobraich ML: Stimulant drug therapy in hyperactive children: research and clinical implications. Pediatrics 60:512-518, 1977

HORMONE THERAPY

Andersen AP: Androgenic treatment of frigidity. Geburtshilfe Frauenheilkd 18:632-, 1958

Bleuler M: Endokninologische Psychiatric. Stuttgart, George Thieme, 1954

Borelli S: On the prescription of sex hormones in male sex disorder. Landarzr 43:476-477, 1967

Coppen A, Montgomery S, Peet M, et al: Thyrotropin-releasing hormone in the treatment of depression. Lancet 2:433-434, 1974

DeWeid D, de Jong W: Drug effects and hypothalamic-anterior pituitary function. Ann Rev Psychopharmacol Toxocol 14:389-412, 1974

Gallahger TF, Yoshida K, Roffwarg HD: ACTH and cortisol secretory patterns in man. J Clin Endocrinol Metab 36:1058-1068, 1973

Goodwin FK, Ebert MH: Recent advances involving treatment of affective disorders, in Psychopharmacology in the Practice of Medicine. Edited by Jerrick ME. New York, Appleton-Century-Crofts, 1977

Greene R, Dalton K: The premenstrual syndrome. Br Med J 1:1007-1014, 1953

Hartmann E: The Functions of Sleep. New Haven, Yale University Press, 1973

Hawkinson L: The menopausal syndrome: one thousand consecutive patients treated with estrogen. JAMA 111:390-393, 1938

Kastin AJ, Ehrensing RH, Schalch DS, et al: Improvement in mental depression with decreased thyrotropin response after administration of thyrotropin-releasing hormone. Lancet 2:740-742, 1972

Klaiber E, Broverman DM, Vugeli W, et al: The use of steroid hormones in depression, in Psychotropic Action of Hormones. Edited by Itil T, Laudahn G, Hermann WM. New York, Spectrum, 1976

Kleitman N: Basic rest-activity cycle in relation to sleep and wakefulness, in Sleep: Physiology and Pathology. Edited by Kales A. Philadelphia, JB Lippincott, 1969

Leshner AI: An Introduction to Behavioral Endocrinology. New York, Oxford University Press, 1978

Margoles R, Leslie GH: Review of studies on a mixture of Nux Vomica, Yohimbine and methyl testosterone in the treatment of impotence. Curr Ther Res 8:280-284, 1966

Money J, Bennett RG: Postadolescent paraphilic sex offenders: antiandrogenic and counseling therapy follow-up. Int J Ment Health 6:122-133, 1981

Money J: Love Sickness: The Science of Sex, Gender Differences, and Pair-Bonding. Baltimore, Johns Hopkins University Press, 1980

Money J: Use of an androgen-depleting hormone in the treatment of sex offenders. J Sex Res 6165-172, 1970

Prange A, Wilson IC, Rabon AM, et al: Enhancement of imipramine antidepressant activity by thyroid hormone. Am J Psychiatry 126:457-469, 1969

Prange A, Wilson I, Breese GR, et al: Hormonal alteration of imipramine response: a review, in Hormones, Behavior, and Psychopathology. Edited by Sacher E. New York, Raven Press, 1976

Prange AJ Jr, Lara PP, Wilson IC, et al: Effects of thyrotropin-releasing hormone in depression. Lancet 2:999-1002, 1972

Rees L: The premenstrual tension syndrome and its treatment. Br Med J 1:1014-1016, 1953

Rubin RT, Poland RE, Rubin LE, et al: The neuroendocrinology of human sleep. Life Sci 14:1041-1052, 1974

Rubin RT: Mind-brain-body interaction: elucidation of psychosomatic intervening variables, in Consultation-Liaison Psychiatry. Edited by Pasnau R. New York, Grune & Stratton, 1975

Sacher E (ed): Hormones, Behavior and Psychopathology. New York, Raven Press, 1976

Sassin JF, Frantz AG, Kapen S, et al: The nocturnal rise of human prolactin is dependent on sleep. J Clin Endocrinol Metab 37:436-440, 1973

Sassin JF, Parker DC, Mace JW, et al: Human growth hormone release: relation to slow-wave sleep and sleep-walking cycles. Science 165:513-515, 1969

Schally AV, Arimura A, Kastin AJ: Hypothalamic regulating hormones. Science 179:341-350, 1973

Seid B: Gonadotropic (HCG) treatment of impotence results in fifty-five cases. Va Med Mon 89:178-181, 1962

Selye H: The evolution of the stress concept. Am Sci 61:692-699, 1973

Weissman MM, Slaby AE: Oral contraceptives and psychiatric disturbances: evidence from research. Br J Psychiatry 123:513-518, 1973

Wheatley D: Potentiation of amitriptyline by thyroid hormone. Arch Gen Psychiatry 26:229-233, 1972

Winston F: Oral contraceptives, pyridoxine, and depression. Am J Psychiatry 130:1217-1221, 1973

PSYCHEDELIC (HALLUCINOGENIC) DRUGS

Bloomquist ER: Marijuana. Beverly Hills, Calif, Glencoe Press, 1968

Cannabis: A Report of the Commission of Inquiry Into the Non-Medical Use of Drugs. Ottawa, Information Canada, 1972

Davoisin R, Katz R: Reversal of anticholinergic syndrome in man by physostigmine. JAMA 206:1963-1965, 1968

Ericksen J: Atropine psychosis. Lancet 1:53-54, 1969

Freedman DX: On the use and abuse of LSD. Arch Gen Psychiatry 18:330-347, 1968

Gaoni Y, Mechoulam R: Isolation structure and partial synthesis of an active constituent of hashish. J Am Chemical Soc 86:1546-1648, 1964

Jones RT: Drug models of schizophrenia, in Psychopathology and Psychopharmacology. Edited by Cole JD, Freedman AM, Friedhoff A. Baltimore, Johns Hopkins Press, 1973

Lehman H, Bos C: The advantages of nitrous oxide inhalation in psychiatric treatment. Am J Psychiatry 104:164-170, 1947.

Ludwig AN, Levine J, Stark LH: LSD and Alcoholism: A Clinical Study of Treatment Efficacy. Springfield, Ill, Charles C Thomas, 1970

McGlothlin WH, Arnold DO: LSD revisited. Arch Gen Psychiatry 24:35-49, 1971

McGlothlin WH: Long lasting effects of LSD on normals. Arch Gen Psychiatry 17:521-532, 1967

Mechoulam R, Gaoni Y: A total synthesis of d1-delta-1-tetrahydrocannabinol: the active constituent of hashish. Journal of the American Chemical Society 87:3273-3275, 1965

National Commission on Marijuana and Drug Abuse: Inhalant, in Drug Use in America: Problems in Perspective. Washington, DC, US Government Printing Office, 1973

Press E, Dane AK: Solvent sniffing: physiologic effects and community control measures for intoxication from the intentional inhalation of organic solvents, I. Pediatrics 39:451-461, 1967a

Press E, Dane AK: Physiologic effects and community control measures for intoxication from the intentional inhalation of organic solvents, II. Pediatrics 39:611-622, 1967b

Shick JFE, Smith DE: An analysis of the LSD flashback. J Psychedelic Drugs 3:13-19, 1970

Showalter CV, Thornton WE: Clinical pharmacology of phencyclidine toxicity. Am J Psychiatry 134:1234-1238, 1977

Smart RG, Bateman K: Unfavorable reactions to LSD: a review and analysis of the available case reports. Can Med Assoc J 97:1214-1221, 1967

HEMODIALYSIS

Kline NS, Li CH, Lehmann HE, et al: β-endorphin-induced changes in schizophrenic and depressed patients. Arch Gen Psychiatry 34:111-113, 1977

Palmour RM, et al: Characterization of a peptide derived from the serum of psychiatric patients (abstract). Anaheim, Calif, Society of Neuroscience, November, 1977

Stephen RL, Velick SF, Kablitz C, et al: Dialysis/hemofiltration in schizophrenia:a journey by night and cloud. Artif Organs 3:31-37, 1979

Termius L, Wahlstrom A, Lindström L, et al: Increased CSF levels of endorphins in chronic psychosis. Neurosci Lett 3:157-162, 1976

Wagemaker H, Cade R: The use of hemodialysis in chronic schizophrenia. Am J Psychiatry 134:684-685, 1977

CONTINUOUS SLEEP

Giljarowsky WA, Liwenzew NM, Segal JJ, et al: Elecktroslaf. Berlin, VEB Verlag Volk u Gesundheit, 1956

Ivanov-Smolenskii A: Observations on insulin and prolonged narcoses therapy in schizophrenia. Sovet Psikhonverol 15:16, 1939

Kalinowsky LB, Hippius H: Pharmacological, Convulsive and Other Somatic Treatments in Psychiatry. New York, Grune & Stratton, 1969

Klaesi J: Uber die therapeutische anwendung der "dauernarkose" mittels somnifen bei schizophrenen. Ztschr fd ges Psychiat u Neurol 72:557, 1922

Lippold OCF, Redfearn JWT: Mental changes resulting from passage of small direct currents through the human brain. Br J Psychiatry 110:768-772, 1964

Rosenthal SH: Electrosleep: a double-blind clinical study. Biol Psychiatry 4:179-185, 1972

SLEEP DEPRIVATION THERAPY

Bhanji S, Roy GA: The treatment of psychotic depression by sleep deprivation: a replication study. Br J Psychiatry 127:222-226, 1975

Dement WC, Kleitman N: Cyclic variations in EEGs during sleep and their relation to eye movements. Electroencephalogr Clin Neurophysiol 9:673-690, 1957

Gresham SC, Agnew WF, Williams RL: The sleep in depressed patients. Arch Gen Psychiatry 13:503-507, 1965

King D: Sleep deprivation therapy in depressive syndromes. Psychosomatics 21:404-407, 1980

Kripke DF: Circadian rhythm phases in affective illness. Chronobiologia 6:365-375, 1979

Kupfer FG, Kupfer DJ, Coble P: Rapid eye movement sleep density. Am J Psychiatry 133:622-626, 1976

Paponsek M, Frank HP, Strohr H: Sleep deprivation therapy in endogenous depressions: effects on circadian rhythms, in Sleep 1974: Second European Congress on Sleep Research, Rome 1974. Edited by Levin P, Kroella WP. Basel, Karger, 1975

Pflug B, Tölle R: Disturbances of the 24-hour rhythm in endogenous depression and the treatment of endogenous depression by sleep deprivation. Int Pharmacopsychiatry 6:187-195, 1971

Pflug B: The effect of sleep deprivation on depressed patients. Acta Psychiatr Scand 53:148-158, 1976

Pflug B: Therapeutic aspects of sleep deprivation in Sleep 1974: Second European Congress on Sleep Research, Rome, 1974. Edited by Koella EP, Levin P. Basil, Karger, 1975

Post RM, Kotkin J, Goodwin FK: Effects of sleep deprivation on mood and central amine metabolism in depressed patients. Arch Gen Psychiatry 32:627-632, 1976

Riederer P, Birkmayer W, Neumayer E, et al: The daily rhythm of HVA, VMA, (VA) and 5-HIAA in depression-syndrome. J Neural Transm 35:23-45, 1974

Schilgen B, Tölle R: Partial sleep deprivation for depression. Arch Gen Psychiatry 37:267-271, 1980

Vogel GW, Thurmond A, Gibbons P, et al: The effect of REM deprivation on depression. Psychosomatics 14:104-107, 1973

Vogel GW, Vogel F, McAbee RS, et al: Improvement of depression by REM sleep deprivation: new findings and a theory. Arch Gen Psychiatry 37:247-253, 1980

PHARMACOLOGIC CONVULSIVE THERAPIES

Kalinowsky LB, Hippius H, Klein HE: Biological Treatments in Psychiatry. New York, Grune & Stratton, 1982

Karliner W, Padula LJ: Improved technique for Indoklon convulsive therapy. Am J Psychiatry 116:359-364, 1959

Krantz JC, Truitt EB Jr, Speers L, et al: New pharmacoconvulsive agent. Science 126:353-354, 1957

INSULIN TREATMENT

Kalinowsky LP, Hippius H, Klein EH: Biological Treatments in Psychiatry. New York, Grune & Stratton, 1982

Klemperer E: Versuch einer behandlung des delerium tremens mit insulin. Psychiatr Neurol Wehnschr 50:549-559, 1926

Laqueur HP, LaBurt HA: Coma therapy with multiple insulin doses. J Neuropsychiatry 1:135-138, 1960

Laqueur HP: Manfred Sakel, Karl Dussik, Max Rinkel and the development of Biological Psychiatry. In The Future of the Brain Sciences. Edited by Bogich S. New York, Plenum, 1969

Laqueur HP: Use of glucogen in insulin coma therapy. Dis Nerv Syst Monogr Suppl 22:1-3, 1961

Sakel M: The Pharmacological Shock Treatment of Schizophrenia. Neurosis and Mental Disease Mongraph Series, no 62. New York, Nervous and Mental Disease Publishing Co, 1938

Sargent W (ed): An Introduction to Physical Methods of Treatment in Psychiatry. 5th ed. New York, Science House, 1972

INHALATION RESTITUTIVE THERAPIES

Hargrove EA, Bennet AE, Steele M: An investigation of carbon dioxide as an adjunct to psychotherapy in some neuroses. Am J Psychiatry 110:844-847, 1954

Hawkings JR, Tibbets RW: CO_2 inhalation therapy in neuroses: controlled clinical trial. J Ment Sci 102:52-59, 1956

Lehmann HE, Bos C: The advantages of nitrous oxide inhalation in psychiatric treatment. Am J Psychiatry 104:164-170, 1947

Loevenhart AS, Lorenz WF, Waters RW: Cerebral stimulation. JAMA 92:880-883, 1929

Meduna LJ: Carbon Dioxide Therapy. Springfield, Ill, Charles C Thomas, 1958

Rees L, Annear MW, Crosse O: Trichlorethylene narcoses as a therapeutic aid in psychiatry. J Ment Sci 94:502-508, 1950

Shorvon HJ, Sargant W: Excitation reaction with special reference to its mechanism in the use of ether. J Ment Sci 93:709-732, 1947

Sillman LR, Terrence C: An analysis of shock therapy in schizophrenia on the basis of a nitrogen inhalation control series. Psychiatric Quarterly 17:241-245, 1943

Zador K: Der lachgas (NO_2) rausch in seiner bedeuting fur psychiatrie und neurologie. Arch v Psychiat 84:1-12, 1928

THE PSYCHOSOCIAL THERAPIES

**Part II of
The Psychiatric Therapies**

7

Psychoanalysis and Individual Psychotherapy

7

Psychoanalysis and Individual Psychotherapy

It is customary to divide psychotherapeutic procedures into two categories: the supportive and uncovering procedures. It must be borne in mind, however, that supportive measures knowingly or inadvertently are used in all forms of psychotherapy, and conversely some degree of insight is rarely absent from any sound psychotherapeutic approach.... In spite of this overlapping of uncovering and supportive effects in all forms of psychotherapy, one can differentiate between two main categories of treatment— between primarily supportive and primarily uncovering methods.

—Alexander and French (1946)

INTRODUCTION

When Alexander and French wrote these words, interest in psychological treatments was on the rise. Psychoanalysis was being applied, despite Anna Freud's (1954) caution, to an ever widening circle of psychiatric disorders, including schizophrenia and what even then were called "borderline conditions." In this unfamiliar territory psychoanalysts found that they had to modify standard analytic procedures (in Eissler's [1953] terms, to introduce "parameters"), a development that many conservative analysts viewed with concern. A battle ensued between those who made a sharp distinction between psychoanalysis and psychotherapy, viewing the latter as a baser metal that contaminated the purity of analysis itself, and those who saw analysis as only a special and limited case of the more general category of psychotherapy. The heat of the debate was not tempered by the fact that the Committee on Evaluation of Psychoanalytic Therapy of the American Psychoanalytic Association had been unable after three years of study to agree, in Rangell's (1954) words, on "exactly what constitutes psychoanalysis, psychoanalytic psychotherapy, and possible transitional forms."

If similar controversy has not entirely disappeared from the modern scene, clinical experience over the past three decades has greatly moderated its intensity. At least three factors are responsible for this change:

A. The diffusion of psychodynamic theory throughout the mental health field in America has produced thousands of psychotherapists who, while not trained to carry out psychoanalysis proper, have incorporated psychoanalytic principles into their practice. At the same time, trained psychoanalysts have devoted an increasing amount of their time to psychoanalytic psychotherapy rather than restricting their professional activities to formal psychoanalysis.

B. The rise of object-relations theory has broadened the view of psychotherapists through an expanded understanding of the ego and its functions, derived from the clinical observation of patients with character disorders and from the modern findings of developmental psychology.

C. Concern over the extended duration and expense of modern psychoanalysis has stimulated a number of clinicians to introduce briefer forms of dynamic therapy into the psychotherapeutic armamentarium. There is currently a widespread recognition that dynamic psychotherapy comprises a spectrum of techniques ranging from classical psychoanalysis to supportive measures. With the horizons thus widened, the psychotherapist of today is less rigidly restricted in his approach to treatment than his predecessors; he or she is better able to assess patients' psychological strengths and weaknesses and is more flexible in applying the specific therapeutic techniques that are indicated by the underlying psychopathology.

In what follows we shall examine four major focal points along the psychotherapeutic spectrum. We shall begin with an exposition of clinical psychoanalysis as the paradigm from which the modifications of psychotherapy take origin. We shall then examine psychoanalytic psychotherapy, with a special concern for the role that object-relations theory plays in determining its techniques. Next we shall review the nature of brief dynamic psychotherapy and shall conclude with a discussion of supportive therapy. It must, however, be clearly recognized that the seeming discreteness of these treatment categories (dictated by the formal requirements of didactic description) is not reflected in the realities of the consulting room. Especially in regard to uncovering and supportive techniques, as Alexander and French (1946) point out, there is a mixture of both in all psychotherapy; and the determination as to whether therapy will be labeled "supportive" or "uncovering" is based on the relative proportion of each modality to be found in any one specific course of treatment. A great deal of emotional support, for example, is provided by the relationship between doctor and patient in even the purest forms of classical psychoanalysis; and internal psychic change, the goal of uncovering psychotherapy, may occur in a patient undergoing supportive treatment as the result of identification with the therapist, even though the latter has not specifically attempted to effect such an alteration.

Psychoanalysis is the central and senior member of the family of uncovering therapies, variously called insight psychotherapies, dynamic psychotherapies, or analytically-oriented psychotherapies. Derived from the early psychoanalytic observations and theories advanced by Freud and his colleagues, uncovering therapies are based on the concepts of unconscious mental processes and psychological conflict, which determine the nature of the therapeutic techniques aimed at reducing conflict by altering psychic structure through the achievement of emotional insight, with the ultimate goal of enabling the patient to abandon infantile wishes and to develop new, more mature patterns of behavior and psychic integration. Psychoanalysis has had a major influence on the direction of psychotherapy in America. Its basic dynamic view of psychological functioning has been the central concept underlying not only the more classic Freudian approach to treatment but a wide variety of modern dynamic psychotherapies as well.

The prototypic embodiment of the psychodynamic theme is, of course, classical psychoanalysis. The variations on the dynamic theme reflect overt and covert modifications of theoretical conceptualizations as well as methodological and technical applications in practice. These include attempts to transcend, partially or completely, the biological focus of Freud with more interpersonal, social, ethical, and cultural considerations (e.g., Adler, Horney, Sullivan, Fromm, Fromm-Reichmann, Meyer, and Masserman); to extend or enhance the ego with earlier or more adaptive endowments (e.g., Federn and Klein); to enlarge man's temporality with a time focus on his primordial past (e.g., Jung), his present, and/or his future (e.g., Adler, Stekel, Rank, and Rado); to expand treatment procedures by altering the range and goals of treatment (e.g., Rank, Alexander, Deutsch, and Karpman); to revise the role of the therapist's personality and relationship to the patient by making the therapist a more direct, flexible, and active participant (e.g., Adler, Sullivan, Rank, Alexander, Stekel, Ferenczi, and Rosen); and to restore psychophysical balance by focusing equally on the physical half of the psychophysical split (e.g., Rado and Masserman) or by substituting an approach to therapeutic cure from the somatic side by trading the traditional mode of change through insight for the earlier catharsis by means of the bodily release of conflictual tensions (e.g., Reich) (Karasu, 1977).

Many other schools of individual psychotherapy have been developed which are based on theories of personality which do not deal with unconscious motivation. Some of these are briefly noted in the chapter entitled "Experiential Therapies." The most influential school of nonpsychoanalytic psychotherapy was developed by Carl Rogers. According to Rogers the only basic human drive is toward self-actualization. Emotional disorders develop when this drive is blunted as a result of negative experiences; Rogers' client-oriented approach works by creating a therapeutic climate in which the patient can fulfill his/her potentialities. This task requires that the therapists be psychologically mature people who show unconditional positive regard for their patients and can accurately empathize with the patient's feelings. The patient assumes considerable responsibility for treatment and receives a minimum of guidance from the therapist. Rogers' client-oriented therapy has had considerable influence in shaping educational, theological, and legal counseling. It has also supplemented the therapeutic rationale and techniques of many other psychotherapists.

CLASSICAL PSYCHOANALYSIS

Historical and Theoretical Considerations

When Freud gave up the use of hypnosis and turned to free association as the basic technique for eliciting psychological information from his patients, he effected a change in the nature of the therapeutic relationship which enabled him to observe the manifestations of resistance and the transference neurosis. The analysis of these phenomena rapidly became a central element in the psychoanalytic process and provided the basis for the later development of the analysis of the ego that characterizes modern analytic procedures (A. Freud, 1937; Hartmann, 1958). The latter are, of course, currently in the forefront of clinical and theoretical investigation (Kernberg, 1975; Kohut, 1971, 1977). Object-relations theory and the modifications in therapeutic approaches derived from it appear to be more applicable to the severe characterological problems of patients currently coming to the psychotherapist's office than are the more traditional psychoanalytic procedures, which have proved useful in treating neurotic symptoms and less severe personality disturbances. These recent developments in psychoanalytic techniques will be discussed below (see the section entitled "Psychoanalytic Psychotherapy"). In this section we shall describe the classical form of psychoanalysis (Glover, 1968; Greenson, 1967; Meissner, 1980; Nemiah, 1976; Stewart, 1980), fully aware that in actual practice it is often modified in a variety of ways depending on clinical exigencies.

The Nature of Psychoanalysis

The primary aim of psychoanalysis is to help the patient to achieve structural psychological changes through emotional insight into the unconscious dynamic and psychogenetic aspects of his mental life which are manifested in symptoms, characterological distortions, and disturbances in personal relationships. This change is achieved by techniques that promote a regressive transference in which id, ego, and superego forces dominate the doctor-patient relationship in the form of the transference neurosis, which recapitulates the infantile neurosis first appearing during the early years of the patient's psychological development. As the transference neurosis develops, the patient gradually becomes consciously aware of previously hidden primitive forms of psychic functioning, which become the central focus of analysis. The resolution of the transference neurosis is the primary task during the terminal phase of analysis, although it is generally not finally resolved until a significant time has elapsed after the last analytic session.

The development of the transference neurosis is enhanced by the following specific technical procedures:

A. The basic method of analysis is *free association*, i.e., the patient is asked to report, without editing or withholding, all that comes to mind, no matter how painful, frightening, distasteful, shameful, or humiliating. A special aspect of free association is the reporting of dreams and the associations stemming from the elements of the manifest content of the dream.

B. Free association is promoted through the use of the couch. The horizontal position of the patient, with the analyst out of sight behind him, exerts pressure on the patient's conscious and unconscious internal autistic processes to influence the flow and content of the associations.

C. This pressure is further augmented by the regularity and frequency of the analytic hours. In Freud's Vienna the usual practice was a daily hour six days a week. As Glover (1968) has commented, this routine did not survive the British weekend habit, and five hours a week became customary in both England and America. For a variety of reasons, economic and otherwise, the tendency in this country has been to drop the number of hours to four per week, and certainly any less than three would not entitle the procedure to be called analysis even if other technical procedures were maintained.

D. The analyst maintains a position of neutrality with respect to the patient's associations (without, however, losing his empathic concern) and often may remain silent for greater or lesser periods of time as he listens to the patient's productions. This technique encourages the flow and freedom of the patient's speech and avoids the possibility of contaminating his thoughts with those of the analyst.

In this kind of setting the patient is thrown very much upon himself, and the surfacing of irrational fantasies and feelings, derived ultimately from early life experiences and relationships, is encouraged. As these come into the open, they wind themselves around the patient's image of the analyst to form part of the developing transference neurosis. This is the patient's major contribution to the analytic process; it is met with and matched by specific activities on the part of the analyst:

A. The analyst must bring to the analytic situation (in addition to neutrality) a state of mind characterized by free-floating attention. Although seemingly a passive attitude, it is in reality a highly alert, active state of concentrated listening and immersing himself in the patient's associations without, however, a specific focus on or the singling out for attention of any one of the patient's associations over any other. In this way the analyst is able intuitively to perceive the forest of patterns of behavior and of personal relationships, and to detect significant connections between associations without becoming lost among the trees of the patient's individual thoughts. At the same time, the analyst subjects these empathically derived observations to disciplined, cognitive evaluation as a basis for assessing their significance and for making rational decisions about therapeutic maneuvers.

B. Although he is neutral and often apparently inactive, it is the analyst's task to become active in two ways: in making *clarifications* and in offering *interpretations*. Many of the patient's patterns of behavior and relationships are ego syntonic, and he does not initially see the pathological elements that may color them. The analyst, however, in the course of applying his free-floating attention, gradually becomes aware of the distortions in these complex patterns. As he does so, he proceeds to help the patient to gain distance from them and to perceive them more objectively. Initially *confronting* the patient with the nature of his behavior, he guides the patient, often by direct and focused questions, to an amplification and *clarification* of the details and circumstances of his behavior and relationships.

Gradually the patient begins to see himself in a new light as preconscious ego elements in his psychic structure become clearly illuminated in the spotlight of his observing ego. All of this is a pre-condition and prelude to a final understanding of the unconscious infantile roots of the attitudes and relationship patterns of which the patient has now become aware. As indicated earlier, these are prominently manifested in the transference neurosis. In the process of *clarification*, patient and analyst deal with conscious mental elements, whose preconscious connections become clear as they are explored. In *interpretation* the analyst introduces to the patient his, the analyst's, perceptions and understanding of the *unconscious* elements beneath the patient's surface behavior. If the proper groundwork has been laid through adequate clarification, the analyst's interpretation will strike a resonant note in his patient, who at that point becomes conscious of feelings, memories, attitudes, and fantasies previously hidden in the unconscious.

Two facts should be noted here. First, the development of the transference neurosis is usually gradual, slow, and often painful. The life-long defenses that, prior to the analysis, have contained the patient's impulses in the unconscious and have transformed them into derivative symptoms and behavior patterns operate strongly to impede the emergence of these same impulses in the transference relationship. This activity of the defenses within the analytic situation is manifested in the *resistance* of the patient to following the basic rule of free association and to conforming to the other requirements of the analysis. As a consequence, a significant portion of the analyst's activity is devoted to the analysis of the patient's defenses. Gradually, through clarification and interpretation, the defenses are modified to permit the emergence of the underlying impulses, which are now directed toward the analyst in the form of the transference neurosis. Interpretation bears a special relationship to the transference, for it serves as a tool with which the analyst can regulate his relationship with the patient and thereby control the transference neurosis.

Second, it should be emphasized that what we are describing here is a *process*. The ultimate changes brought about by psychoanalysis are not the product of a single, momentary flash of complete and curative insight. On the contrary, each pathological element must be dealt with by clarification and interpretation in a systematic and orderly sequence that uncovers one after the other of the unconscious psychic processes in the id, ego, and superego. Each unconscious defense, for example, must be brought into the open before the impulse behind it can be revealed and understood. Stubbornly persisting irrational patterns of behavior, as well as the defenses and impulses responsible for them, must be approached through *repeated* episodes of clarification and interpretation before permanent modification in the psychic structure takes place; this is the so-called process of *working through*. It is the necessity for working through that makes for the length of many analyses, which often go on for a number of years; at the same time it can lead ultimately to the successful resolution of the patient's transference neurosis and psychic conflicts, with resulting new, permanent, and healthier patterns of psychological functioning.

In reality, analytic treatment rarely conforms to the purity of the theoretically proper course of therapy described above. The analyst's complete neutrality is a goal that is approached more often than attained, and his everyday behavior in the treatment situation may include activities that are supportive rather than analytic in nature. Indeed, the relationship with the analyst in itself provides a basically and inescapably supportive environment for the patient. Furthermore, as we have noted earlier, the application of analysis to an ever wider number of psychiatric conditions, especially narcissistic and borderline character problems, requires more flexible *parameters* for those persons who cannot respond to more restricted analytic procedures. This broadened application has led to a greater understanding of ego functioning and its pathology and a better definition of supportive measures. Both of these topics will be dealt with below.

Indications and Limitations

In the early days of the analytic movement the indication for psychoanalysis was the presence of a psychoneurosis (hysteria, phobic neurosis, and obsessive-compulsive disorder) in which oedipal conflicts were regarded as central. Only patients with these disorders were viewed as being capable of developing the transference neurosis that was essential for successful analysis. The early recognition that both phobic and obsessional patients might require a modified treatment technique (Freud, 1955a, 1955b) and the increasing numbers of patients coming to analysis for characterological problems gradually led to the abandonment of choosing treatment on the basis of symptoms or a psychiatric diagnosis alone.

Instead, the emphasis shifted to criteria of analyzability based on personality characteristics and object relations. It is now generally agreed that those individuals who are suitable for analysis are well motivated for treatment, psychologically-minded, intelligent, give evidence of a capacity for good relationships, and manifest an availability of and ability to tolerate emotions without lapsing into disruptive regressive behavior.

In addition, it is felt that adults up to early middle age, whose personality features are less fixed by the aging process, have a greater capacity for internal change. These criteria are applicable whether or not the patients show symptoms or complaints of difficulties in interpersonal relationships resulting from characterological problems. In patients who fulfill the criteria for analyzability, this treatment is strongly indicated for those who do manifest such symptoms. Psychoanalysis has traditionally been advised against in patients with psychotic disorders because of the major deficits in their ego functioning and their inability to develop an analyzable transference neurosis. The use of psychoanalytic techniques in individuals with severe borderline character disorders is discussed in the next section.

PSYCHOANALYTIC PSYCHOTHERAPY

Historical and Theoretical Considerations

Two major factors underlie the modern practice of psychoanalytic psychotherapy: (a) the widespread dissemination of psychodynamic concepts and techniques and (b) the development of object-relations theory.

The rapid expansion of training in psychotherapy which followed World War II coincided with the rise of interest in psychoanalytic ideas, which, particularly in the United States, soon dominated psychotherapists' thinking and teaching. Influenced by the precepts of their supervisors, many of whom were formally trained in psychoanalysis, thousands of young psychotherapists were imbued with a psychodynamic approach to the diagnostic understanding and treatment of patients with emotional disorders. Though relatively few of this new generation of therapists underwent the rigorous psychoanalytic training that would allow them to practice psychoanalysis proper, the majority adapted psychoanalytic theories and techniques to their clinical activities and, in so doing, introduced numerous modifications that have transformed classical psychoanalysis into modern psychoanalytic psychotherapy.

Simultaneously with this huge increase in clinicians practicing psychodynamic psychiatry, the psychoanalytic approach was applied to a wider variety of clinical psychiatric conditions. Initially restricted to patients with psychoneuroses, the use of psychoanalytic techniques was gradually extended to patients with psychotic illness and complicated characterological disorders. The pioneering work of Harry Stack Sullivan (Mullahy, 1980) with schizophrenic patients focused attention on disturbances in early life experiences and the resulting distortions in adult interpersonal relationships. Similarly, clinical experience with patients with character problems arising from pre-oedipal conflicts led analysts such as Eissler (1953) to recognize the need to introduce parameters into psychoanalytic treatment in order to engage the patient in the therapeutic process. These clinical observations in adult patients have been matched by a growing body of related findings concerning developmental disturbances from the direct study of infants and their mothers (Greenspan and Lourie, 1981; Mahler and Furer, 1968).

Perhaps the most important influence on the course of modern psychotherapy is to be found in the current interest in narcissism—especially as it is related to borderline character disorders. Modern clinical investigation has delineated the borderline patient's disturbances in self-image and object-relations, his problems with aggression and dependence, his tendency to grandiosity and depression, and his use of primitive defense mechanisms such as splitting and projective identification, and has noted the turbulent transferences these disturbances induce in the therapeutic relationship (Gunderson and Singer, 1975; Kernberg, 1975, 1980a). Much of the concern of modern psychotherapy is centered on the techniques of managing the difficulties caused by these transference manifestations, and help in finding solutions has come from the area of object-relations theory. Originating in the creative early speculations of Melanie Klein (Kernberg 1980b), developed and expanded by the clinical and theoretical formulations of the British object-relations school (Bion, 1965, 1967, 1970; Winnicott, 1965), these concepts have had a profound effect on current American psychiatric thinking through the writings of Kernberg, Kohut, and their respective collaborators (Kernberg, 1975, 1976, 1980a; Kohut, 1971, 1977).

Despite the many questions and differences of opinion which remain unresolved, object-relations theory has already provided a useful conceptual basis for the treatment of borderline states; it has supplied psychotherapists with a rationale for selecting the appropriate specific techniques; and it has helped to clarify the nature of psychoanalytic psychotherapy and its relation to classical psychoanalysis.

The Nature of Psychoanalytic Psychotherapy

It is not possible to give hard and fast criteria that sharply distinguish classical psychoanalysis from psychoanalytic psychotherapy (Basch, 1980; Rangell, 1954; Wallerstein).* Like analysis, psychoanalytic therapy aims, when possible, to bring about structural psychological changes through insights arrived at by the use of free association, clarification, interpretation, and analysis of the transference. At the same time, psychoanalytic therapy allows the therapist to use a variety of supportive measures when these are required by the patient's clinical condition. Unlike analysis, psychoanalytic therapy is carried out with the patient sitting face-to-face with the therapist. The frequency of hours is usually once or twice a week, but (like analysis) therapy may continue for a number of years. The therapist is generally more active than the analyst in seeking information and focusing on specific areas of conflict.

In its uncovering mode, psychoanalytic psychotherapy is similar to classical psychoanalysis in its basic approach and therapeutic goals. The therapist aims to help his patient to resolve psychic conflict through an analysis of defenses and the underlying impulses. Such analysis, however, is more circumscribed than classical psychoanalysis. The therapist does not seek to resolve *all* areas of psychic conflict but limits his activities to effecting those changes in psychic structure which will be sufficient to enable the patient to overcome his major problems. Although the therapist may deal with transference issues, this area is balanced with equal attention to disturbances in current relationships and their genesis in early life experiences, without the emphasis that is central to classical psychoanalytic treatment on encouraging and analyzing a regressive transference.

As noted earlier, the flexibility of psychoanalytic psychotherapy permits the therapist to use a variety of supportive measures when indicated. Such measures are particularly useful and appropriate for patients with narcissistic and borderline character disorders—in strengthening unstable defenses and ego functions, in curtailing acting out, and in providing the "holding environment" (Winnicott, 1965) in which patients may safely express primitive affects and attitudes to an empathic and containing therapist.

Indications and Limitations

In the earlier periods of post-war psychiatry, psychoanalytic psychotherapy was used for a broad range of disorders of all degrees of severity. Particularly in those cases in which the patient was suffering from severe psychopathology, and when the therapy applied was too closely modeled on the

---

*Michels R: Conceptualizing the nature of the therapeutic action of psychoanalytic psychotherapy. Presented at the annual meeting of the American Psychoanalytic Association, Atlanta, May 7, 1978

pattern of silence and inactivity of classical psychoanalytic procedures, many patients suffered damaging regressions. Therapists are now generally more cautious, either reserving their treatment for emotionally healthier patients who fulfill the indications outlined earlier for psychoanalysis or, if they are dealing with narcissistic or borderline patients, modifying their techniques in accordance with the requirements imposed by the defects in their patients' ego structures.

Psychoanalytic psychotherapy in its uncovering mode is indicated for patients with a wide spectrum of symptomatic, characterological, and relationship difficulties who have a potential capacity for introspection and self-examination (psychological-mindedness) combined with an ability to tolerate the anxiety and depression that may accompany psychological exploration. Patients undergoing such psychoanalytic psychotherapy must, in addition, be able to deal with the possible problems posed by the longer time intervals between therapeutic hours—that is, they must be able to bear the therapeutic arousal of painful affects without the support of daily contact with the therapist and must be able to maintain therapeutic movement despite the extended period between therapeutic hours, which tends to foster a "sealing over" and regrouping of psychic defenses against the unconscious material mobilized by therapeutic probing. Although it often may not be possible within the limitations of psychoanalytic therapy to resolve the deepest and most primitive layers of the patient's conflicts, their derivative manifestations can generally be mobilized and modified by psychotherapeutic techniques.

As noted above, psychoanalytic therapy in its more supportive mode is usually indicated for patients with narcissistic and borderline character disorders—either in the early phases of treatment as a prelude to the use of uncovering techniques once the therapeutic relationship is firmly established or during periods of ego regression which occur in the course of more interpretive therapy. It should be pointed out, however, that there is no firm consensus among therapists as to the relative merits of uncovering and supportive techniques in patients with these characterological disorders. Analysts formerly leaned toward limiting their interventions to supportive maneuvers (Knight, 1954; Zetzel, 1971), but the trend in recent years has been more toward analytic, interpretive techniques (Kernberg, 1976, 1980). There are, however, differences of opinion even among modern clinical investigators who base their understanding of these disorders on object-relations theory. Kernberg (1976, 1980), for example, who views the character disturbances as pathological defenses, leans toward the use of an interpretive approach; Kohut (1971, 1977), on the other hand, sees behavior patterns as the reproduction of earlier phases of normally developing narcissism and avoids interpretations until the patient's ego has had the opportunity to grow to more mature levels within the "holding environment" provided by the therapist.

BRIEF PSYCHOTHERAPIES

Historical and Theoretical Considerations

Alexander's suggestion for shortening the analytic process (Alexander, 1954a, 1954b; Alexander and French, 1946) met with considerable resistance during the early post-war spread of analytic theory and practice. His ideas, however, subsequently came to flower in the work of a number of analytic clinical investigators, who during the past two decades have introduced a variety of forms of brief psychodynamic psychotherapy of demonstrated efficacy (Burke et al., 1979; Davanloo, 1978; Malan, 1976; Mann, 1973; Sifneos, 1975, 1979). Like classical psychoanalysis and psychoanalytic psychotherapy in its uncovering mode, the brief psychotherapies are aimed at bringing about internal psychological changes through engendering emotional insight into underlying psychodynamic conflicts. The techniques are applied to patients specifically selected for their capacity to respond positively in a relatively few treatment hours over a limited period of time.

The Nature of Brief Dynamic Psychotherapies

Although they share with other analytic psychotherapies the basic orientation of change through the development of emotional insight, brief dynamic psychotherapies have several characteristics that set them apart:

A. As the adjective "brief" implies, these therapies limit the number of hours devoted to the therapeutic work, a limitation that is made explicit to the patient before treatment begins.

B. Brief dynamic psychotherapies are focused on specific areas of conflict and do not attempt to bring about the more extensive psychological reconstructions aimed at by psychoanalysis and psychoanalytic psychotherapy.

C. Brief dynamic psychotherapies are confrontative—that is, the patient's attention is directed repeatedly to significant areas of psychic conflict, often with the arousal of painful anxiety and depression.

D. As is implied in the characteristics already listed, the therapist is far more active in carrying out brief dynamic therapy than when he is engaged in analysis or long-term psychoanalytic psychotherapy. As in other forms of insight-oriented therapy, he must, of course, listen to the patient's associations and reach an intuitive understanding of his conflicts. At the same time, he must actively direct the patient's attention to specific areas of conflict and solicit the related free associations.

E. Within the areas selected for observation and psychological analysis, emphasis is placed on systematically defining and examining the patient's conflicts in three areas: transference, current, and past relationships. In this regard, too, the therapist actively focuses the patient's attention on each of these areas and their interrelationships.

During the past decade a number of different forms of brief dynamic therapy have been described. We shall briefly review four of the better known modalities to illustrate the variety of different approaches that may be found in the general category defined by the criteria listed above.

Davanloo (1978) employs a highly confrontative form of psychotherapy in which the patient's defenses (especially obsessional isolation against aggression) are forcefully and directly challenged. Emphasis is placed on defining the patient's conflicts in terms of the triangle of related transference, current, and past relationships.

Malan (1976), a pioneer in the development of brief psychotherapy, adheres most closely to the analytic model by relying on extended guided free associations and on the analysis of the transference and its roots in the patient's relationship with his parents. Less focused than many of the other brief therapies, it is also longer, lasting as much as a year of weekly hours instead of the ten- to 30-session limit that characterizes the other modalities.

Time-limited therapy as proposed by Mann (1973) is restricted to exactly 12 hours of treatment extended over as long a period as needed. Because of the sharp limitation of time (of which the patient is apprised at the start) he begins treatment with an acute awareness of its termination and of the impending separation from the therapist. As a consequence, issues of dependence and loss are uppermost in the patient's mind and form the primary focus of the therapy.

Some 20 years ago, Sifneos (1975, 1979), another pioneer in the field, introduced short-term anxiety-provoking psychotherapy (STAPP). Aimed at patients selected because of circumscribed neurotic problems primarily oedipal in nature, STAPP actively forces the patient to examine and analyze his oedipal conflicts within the framework of the triangle of past, present, and transference relationships. The therapist focuses his and the patient's attention exclusively on oedipal material and consciously avoids dealing with regressive, pre-oedipal issues.

Indications and Limitations

As in the other forms of insight psychotherapy, patients must have the requisite psychological-mindedness, motivation for change, and capacity to bear emotional pain. However, when it comes to other criteria for the selection of patients, there is less consensus among the proponents of the various brief dynamic therapies. In the specific examples cited above, STAPP is the most restricted in its indications, being limited, as already noted, to patients with oedipal conflicts and a circumscribed clinical problem. For Malan, evidence of motivation for change is a central criterion for treatment and is, in addition, a key indicator of the potential for success.

Given adequate motivation, patients with a wide variety of symptomatic and characterological disorders are accepted for treatment; only a few clinical problems (e.g., addictions, alcoholism) are specifically excluded from the list of those considered treatable. Davanloo's method is similarly applicable to a wide range of disorders and appears to be particularly helpful in patients with highly structured and rigid obsessional defenses. Mann is less specific and selective in his criteria for treatment, limiting his indications to the presence of a clearly definable central problem.

SUPPORTIVE PSYCHOTHERAPY

Historical and Theoretical Considerations

In one sense, all psychotherapy is supportive, for no matter what specific therapeutic maneuvers the therapist uses, the relationship that develops between the patient and the therapist has a stabilizing effect on the patient's psychological functioning. Indeed, emotional support is a vital component in the relationships the patient develops with a wide range of care givers, physicians and otherwise. In supportive psychotherapy, such a relationship is the central element of the treatment. The modern era of supportive psychotherapy goes back to the period of "moral therapy" and the subsequent "nonrestraint" movement in the mid-nineteenth century treatment of psychotic patients, which was based on the use of human relationships rather than mechanical restraints to control psychotic symptoms and behavior. Since that time, the human milieu has been an important component of the management of patients with psychopathology resulting from serious disorders of ego functioning.

The Nature of Supportive Psychotherapy

The therapist-patient relationship is central to the process of supportive psychotherapy. The opportunity to be in the presence of and to reveal one's conflicts and suffering to a calm, attentive, concerned, and understanding therapist often has a beneficial effect on human anxiety, depression, and despair. This is particularly so in the face of acute emotional turmoil or crisis, but a longer-term relationship can be similarly supportive to individuals with chronic emotional problems. Such a stable, supportive relationship is central to the "holding environment" currently recommended for patients with severe narcissistic and borderline character disorders.

In addition to the central relationship itself, patients may be helped by several specific maneuvers (Bibring, 1954) that, in part at least, derive their effectiveness from the authoritarian role the supportive psychotherapist plays with the patient. *Abreaction* involves the discharge of and relief from painful emotions through their expression in the therapeutic session, such as the weeping that relieves delayed mourning or the sense of release from guilt which follows a confession to an accepting, nonjudgmental therapist. The therapist may use active *reassurance* by countering the patient's fear about a symptom with factual information or by helping him to see why he need not assume the guilt or responsibility for some putative wrongdoing. To strengthen the patient's *reality testing*, the therapist actively contravenes in the patient's fantasies or attitudes by presenting to him the facts of a situation or by voicing his, the therapist's, views and opinions concerning it. Through *clarification*, an extension and elaboration of reality testing, the therapist encourages the patient to look at all aspects of a conflict or problem as a means of getting him to arrive at his own solution. When using direct *suggestion* the therapist is more active and authoritative than when using the previously described elements of supportive therapy. Suggestion may be aimed directly at symptom suppression, or it may be used to encourage the patient to control troublesome behavior or to adopt new, constructive activities. *Advice* and directions for action are an extension of suggestion. Patients are given authoritative instructions that range from the use of medication, exercise, or relaxation techniques aimed at suppressing symptoms to complex directions concerning how to behave in every facet of their work, lives, and relationships.

One important aspect of this kind of therapeutic activity is limit-setting, aimed at preventing the patient from indulging in destructive behavior toward himself or others and at avoiding damaging regressive reactions. It should, furthermore, be noted that quite apart from what the therapist does, he lends himself as a model for identification, enabling the patient to acquire new and useful patterns of behavior based on his internalization of the therapist's image, attitudes, and strengths. And, finally, it should be emphasized that the therapist's dynamic understanding of the patient's conflicts, character structure, and needs forms an essential component of his ability to supply the appropriate supportive measures.

Supportive therapy must often be provided for long periods of time. Some patients, however, are able, through the process of identification, to deal with stressful situations without the explicit help and support of therapeutic sessions. In such cases, the number of psychotherapy hours may be reduced to a minimum, being reserved for an occasional follow-up visit. The frequency may, of course, be increased during periods when a flare-up of symptoms requires it.

Indications and Limitations

Supportive therapy is specifically indicated for and is most helpful in crisis situations in which painful external reality is too much to bear alone. Supportive therapy is most commonly used, however, in the treatment of emotional disorders in persons whose ego structure and conflicts contraindicate uncovering psychotherapy. As noted earlier, in some borderline patients supportive measures may be a prelude to the use of uncovering psychotherapeutic techniques after the supportive measures have sufficiently strengthened the individual's personality to allow him to deal with the anxiety and depression that accompany raising unconscious affects and fantasies. Supportive therapy, including help with developing social skills and advice about the practical details of daily living, is particularly valuable in conjunction with pharmacotherapy in the long-term management of patients with chronic psychotic disorders (Weissman et al., 1979), many of whom can live comfortably and safely in the community, provided they have adequate professional attention and guidance.

Since it forms a part of any psychotherapeutic process, one can hardly say that supportive psychotherapy is contraindicated. At the same time, it is clear that restricting oneself to the use of supportive techniques with a patient who could benefit from uncovering psychotherapy may not only deprive him of the opportunity for achieving significant psychological growth but may even lead him into regressive patterns of dependency.

AGE RELATED ISSUES

Children and Adolescents

Classical analysis has traditionally been viewed as a treatment for adults in the generative, active periods of their lives. Analytic principles, however, have been applied to the treatment of children with symptomatic and behavior problems. Because of the many special considerations of treating this particular subgroup of patients, however, the chapter of this volume entitled "Psychotherapy with Children and Adolescents" is devoted to the analytically-oriented treatment of children.

Unmodified classical analysis may be unsuitable for many adolescents because of their heightened struggle around autonomy and dependency issues and their lack of fully internalized and consolidated ego ideals (Ekstein, 1979; Scharfman, 1978). These features of adolescence do not rule out the suitability of the analytic process for adolescent patients, especially where there is evidence of a premature closure of personality development; but the analyst must be prepared to modify classical techniques as required by the patient's need for ego support. At the other end of the spectrum, the increasing psychological rigidity and inflexibility of persons of advanced age is felt to be a barrier to effecting favorable changes by analysis—a generalization that has not gone unchallenged by the favorable results brought about in selected older people by analysts interested in geriatric psychiatry (Kaufman, 1937; Segal, 1958).

Psychoanalytic psychotherapy, with its potentially greater focus on reality and its lesser degree of emotional intensity, may be specifically indicated for adolescent patients, especially those whose psychic structure is less mature, less stable, and less able to tolerate the buffeting of the more intensive classical psychoanalytic procedures.

The indications for the use of supportive techniques are more closely related to the ego structure of any given patient than to his or her age or developmental level. However, as has been pointed out in the discussion of uncovering psychotherapies, at certain life periods such as adolescence and advanced age, the age related instability of ego functions may require that the ego-supportive techniques be added to the more exploratory, analytic measures.

The Elderly

Twenty-five million Americans are now over age 65; and despite transitional crises and their experience of decremental depletion at a greater rate than at any other time in their lives, only four percent of them find themselves in psychiatric offices. As they cope with the decline and fall of their human empire, many of them undergo intense object hunger, at times associated with a recrudescence of various forms of sexuality called forth to compensate for loneliness and to restore self-esteem. Every day brings new biological, physical, and social threats to the cohesiveness and continuity of self. This is at the root of increasing numbers of accidents and high suicide rates, especially in men. In this phase of life, integrity of self is precariously balanced.

While many older people need a significant other with whom to share anxiety-provoking sensations from within or to reinterpret the body's responses or the feelings of worthlessness that retirement, emptying the nest, or just feeling less involved in life's mainstream create, the psychiatric profession has only begun to make available to this age group the benefits of dynamic psychoanalytic psychotherapy. While these years are not bereft of positive factors, psychoanalytic psychotherapy may help the elderly to cross the bridges to acceptance of an altered self-image and a changed relationship to others. A consistent error has been to attribute lack of vigor, hypochondriasis, and preoccupation with the past to immutable depletion and depression, implying the inability to work through problems in a dynamic setting. Frequently, the older person's potential for a revived sense of life, joy, and capacity for relating has been severely underestimated. Even benign memory loss has been confused with dementia in patients afflicted by the depletion-despair-depression syndrome.

The function of the psychoanalytic psychotherapist is to treat more than neurotic conflict. Interpretation is still the main mode of therapeutic intervention; but unification and empathic sharing are moving more to center stage. The threat of annihilation of self-hood, long before annihilation of physical self, may become quite real and is often verbalized. From mid-life on, the wish that one should not live long enough to outlive one's self-hood is frequently expressed. Psychoanalytic psychotherapy helps to prevent premature deflation of self-image; abandonment of relationships; and an empty, depleted old age. A person who feels extremely dependent may fear showing emotion to family and friends for fear of further abandonment by the few people left. At times this fear leads to flattening of affect and a seeming monotonous similarity in older people, even if they really are not. Difficulty in finding acceptable outlets for the accumulated bitterness, aggression, disappointment, and rage that burn within leads to a hunger for therapy which is little appreciated.

It is no longer tenable to assert that psychoanalysis with older people is not effective. A trial of analysis is frequently indicated, as long as the elderly patients satisfy the usual criteria of suitability (Cath, 1982; Muslin, 1983). The patient must have the capacity for prolonged introspection; the therapist must be able to immerse himself empathetically in the older person's self-object world. It would seem that the barrier to psychoanalysis with older people has been due to psychoanalysts' countertransference, which may include a bias based on their own fear of growing old. In cases that have been analyzed, the usual transferences emerge, although in men there is the likelihood of a reversed and enhanced negative oedipal configuration. Thus, the male analyst may find elderly male patients even more preoccupied with their intense need for an idealized male object on whom to lean (much like adolescent analyses) than are younger male patients. Part of the reason is that many older men find themselves "living in a woman's world," in which separation-individuation issues, usually characteristic of earlier phases of life, come to the fore.

In general, women survive seven years longer than their spouses and experience the depletion decline almost a decade later. Thus, more often than not, men find themselves dependent upon and dominated by a more intact and able spouse. This role reversal is correlated with physiological changes—"the androgenization of women" and "the estrogenization of men." The therapist must be able to withstand similar inevitable narcissistic injuries to his own aging body ego as he witnesses this decline. Many therapists have found themselves insufficiently insulated from these images to work comfortably with older persons, but with adequate support and supervision they can become effective therapists with this age group.

The goals of psychoanalysis remain essentially the same: to reduce neurotic conflict (although with increasing years, neuroses tend to fade into the background); and to facilitate more autonomous living, or if this is not reasonable, to accommodate a mutually interdependent existence. A consistent observation of analysts who have worked with older people is an appreciation of the late-life potential for resuming age-specific development, to move from self-preoccupation to greater object investment and to heal wounds that have habitually distorted close relationships. It is a serious error to think of all older people monolithically. Many are still engaged in struggles for power, success, and love. Some are able to achieve many of these goals. The self is held together by the cement of meaningful relationships, but these years are times of multiple object-loss. The psychoanalyst, then, is often working with a patient who is undergoing repeated bereavements and experiencing constant threats to self-cohesiveness and continuity. In these circumstances the analyst is not only a transference figure but the most significant primary object, providing understanding in the least critical of settings the patient has ever known. Accordingly, termination may not be as simple as in earlier years. The actual fullness of a patient's world, his self and mood regulation, as well as the analyst's sophistication and freedom from gerontophobia, will determine the appropriateness and degree of separation.

Lazarus and Gutmann, in a 1982 paper,* reported the process and outcome of brief psychotherapy with six elderly patients using a methodology based on the work of Malan and Horowitz with younger patients. Their most striking finding was that patients used the therapist to validate their normality and to restore their self-esteem. It was common for this group of patients to blame a place or person for current stress. They sought the therapist's permission to separate from or create distance between themselves and the source of their difficulties. A second major finding was that symptomatic improvement sometimes occurred with less improvement in major dynamic conflicts that the therapist originally thought were operative. Thus, some basics of brief psychodynamic psychotherapy for elderly patients may differ from concepts used to treat younger individuals. Since, for these elderly patients, the primitive defense mechanisms of externalization and projection served as way-stations with adaptive functions, these mechanisms should not be regarded as simply pathological in this patient group. Sustained improvement in symptoms seemed to be based on the use of the therapist to improve self-esteem and reaffirm the sense of continuity with a former positive self image. The patients were able to emerge feeling competent, psychologically more healthy, and able to master. These findings suggest a modification of the usual countertransference expectations for older patients.

Brief psychotherapy may also be especially appropriate when dealing with a particular kind of pseudoindependent elder who feels his integrity is assaulted by his need for help, from either children or a psychotherapist. These cases may do best with a predetermined number of "meetings," facilitating the psychotherapeutic contact. However, the possibility of a

*Lazarus LW, Gutmann D, et al: Process and outcome of brief psychotherapy with the elderly. Presented at the 35th annual meeting of the Gerontological Society, Boston, Nov 19-23, 1982

virtual crescendo of depleting disastrous events suggests that the therapist use an open door policy, for the patient's anchors may melt away faster than he can rebuild them. Still, his reluctance to reinvest emotionally in another important person only to suffer the loss of that person may take more energy than he feels he has in store. But should he change his mind, the therapist may still become the primary sustaining object who, even in brief therapy, should be available at all times. The length or the intensity of the session may be limited if the therapist senses that the patient can tolerate only so much. One should be not only less rigid in working with the elderly but also more willing to do home visits, hospital calls, or follow-through care should the patient need to go to a residential or nursing home.

A psychotherapist may, at times, be challenged by a patient's misleading concerns; that is, a patient may emphasize the psychological when he is really afraid he has an organic problem. The opposite may be equally true; he may hide behind physiological changes to conceal a depression. Such hypochondriacal preoccupation is distasteful to many physicians, who do not appreciate the body as a way-station, the care of which provides the patient with the needed nourishment—attention. Living long has its own deprivations, frustrations, and hardships. Thus, both patient and therapist share the awareness that over time development does not always progress to higher levels of integration. We have a built-in clock, "a mean time to failure," and are programmed to a destiny to which we all must yield.

In the especially creative, it is not just the passage of time or the incongruities between real achievements and the idealized self which create the "race against time" so characteristic of the middle and later decades of life. Those who have studied stress claim the loss of a spouse is most disruptive. Kohut's emphasis on the capacity of the self to remain cohesive and Cath's concept of the capacity for restitution in the face of loss of self-objects all along the life span seem appropriate. The notion of the existence of a sense of self-continuity formed in the early years which is ultimately shaken by the passage of time in a degree determined by a person's particular coefficient of tension related to self-annihilation has been an extremely important developmental construction. Finally, supportive therapies should be directed at the spouse of a patient who has developed an organic brain deterioration and is dying slowly before her eyes. The burden usually falls upon the wife because of her longer life span. This increasing population of women traditionally has been denied the benefit of psychotherapeutic understanding, and this area should be considered a valid one for psychotherapeutic work.

In some elders there is a tendency toward preoccupation with losses, depleting energies and skills, and dying which results in new forms of paranoia. The dynamics seem to be, "I really cannot be this incompetent person—someone must be interfering with my life, stealing my possessions, confusing my check book, or creating the chaos that exists around me." The age-specific supportive intervention needed is to share the intrapsychic world of such a patient and provide a protective other who relieves "depletion depression." The therapist does not take up paranoia directly but becomes available to talk about other issues that are really more significant, namely depletion depression, disease, despair, and death.

People over age 65 average four or five pathological organic diagnoses, usually accompanied by "benign memory loss" if not by more severe memory deficits. The elderly often tend toward repetitiveness and may experience a return of infantile-like phobias, such as fear of being alone or of being unable to handle unexpected situations by themselves. A person may have used the same defenses earlier; for example, a woman who felt abused, victimized, and tyrannized by her husband for 50 years or more may now accuse him of the same behavior. Only now her accusations are strengthened by deficits she feels but cannot tolerate as part of her self-image. The natural countertransference toward such defenses may prevent therapists from providing appropriate help. Sometimes without adequate understanding they negate a patient's reality in that they try to reason them out of their sense of loss and of something being taken. They fail to realize that the stolen object represents a part of the self symbolized in external space by possessions. Such countertransference confusion may make a therapist "give up," which he would not do with a younger person.

In order to do justice to their profession, clinicians must become involved with these patients, their families, and sometimes the staff of long-term care institutions. Should the therapist become the elixir of youth for an older person, he needs to permit the idealization to continue for some time, during which a transfusion of vital sense of worth from therapist to aged patient's self may alleviate much distress and paranoia.

FINANCIAL, PROFESSIONAL, AND ETHICAL ISSUES

In view of the time involved, psychoanalysis can be an expensive procedure for those for whom insurance benefits or low-fee analyses are not available. The variability in fees in different parts of the country and in the number of hours of analysis a week required of any given patient makes it difficult to give an absolute figure for the expense of psychoanalytic treatment.

Since psychoanalytic psychotherapy requires fewer hours a week than classical analysis, the fees for individual psychotherapeutic hours may in some cases be set higher than the customary hourly charge for the more intensive analytic procedure. However, given the fact that most health insurance plans cover at least some of the expense of psychotherapy and that the course of treatment usually is fairly well specified, the overall cost is a quarter to a third of that of psychoanalysis. Because of its limited duration, brief dynamic psychotherapy is less expensive than the longer forms of uncovering therapy. Its growing availability should make psychotherapy far more cost-effective for those whose problems can be dealt with by such measures and should make health insurance underwriters less dubious about including psychotherapeutic techniques among the benefits included in their plans.

Supportive therapy will, of course, vary in cost depending on the frequency with which therapeutic hours are scheduled. Many patients with chronic psychotic disorders can be treated successfully in therapeutic visits at a low annual cost, although there may be periods of crisis when more frequent contact with the therapist is required. Despite the expense involved in regularly scheduled hours for supportive therapy, a program of management carried out on an outpatient basis can be considerably less costly than the likely alternative of chronic hospitalization.

Analysis is an intensely personal and private procedure, and it is hard to monitor the quality of the clinician's daily practice. A considerable degree of clinical competence is assured in each analyst by virtue of the fact that his training is long (five to seven years of personal training analysis, seminars, and supervised performance of analysis) and is closely monitored by the faculty of the various analytic institutes, most of them located in large urban centers. Many candidates in training drop out before completing the prescribed course of work, either because they become aware that they have no vocation for an analytic career or because their teachers find them unsuitable for further training. As a result of such close and continued scrutiny, the graduates of analytic institutes have generally demonstrated competence, and the recent introduction of certification procedures by the American Psychoanalytic Association adds a further control over the quality of the work of those practicing psychoanalysts who have completed the training requirements of institutes approved by that association. Finally, continuing education through local institutes (including participation on a voluntary basis in clinical case study groups or paying for individual supervision) provides added assurances of clinical and intellectual competence in the field. Most of these institutes, however, are available only in large urban centers.

Two major potential ethical issues are related to analysis. Because of the requirements of free association, theoretically no information can be withheld from the analyst. Though this ideal situation is rarely, if ever, reached, it is still true that a wealth of highly personal facts and fantasies are revealed to the analyst. It is all the more urgently incumbent on the analyst, therefore, to keep the patient's trust inviolate.

Another set of potential problems has to do with the special relationship between doctor and patient. Because of the intensely personal and emotional nature of the interaction, the analyst is placed in a position of greater power to exploit his patients than are many physicians. At the same time, because of the unusual extent of his understanding of human behavior and psychology (including his own), the analyst is often able to recognize the nature of his own motivations and to eschew unethical behavior. When it does occur, such behavior is not only inherently more exploitative and reprehensible but potentially more damaging to the patient's mental health. Analysts, therefore, have a particular imperative to maintain a scrupulously ethical relationship with their patients.

Training in psychoanalytical psychotherapy follows the basic model of carrying out therapy under supervision. The trainees also receive seminars and courses in various aspects of psychotherapy and psychoanalytic theory. Experience indicates that many, if not most, individuals in training programs that teach dynamic psychotherapy develop a good degree of competence in the techniques by the time they have completed their formal training. Undergoing a personal analysis or analytic psychotherapy may help to develop the individual therapist's sensitivity, perceptiveness, and communication skills. Although highly desirable, personal analysis cannot be said to be a *sine qua non* for becoming a competent therapist.

Issues concerning quality control and ethical behavior are the same as those noted earlier in respect to classical psychoanalysis.

Training in the specific techniques of each of the brief therapies is a prerequisite to becoming skilled in their application. The attention paid to defining these techniques sharply has made them easier to teach and to learn, and the use of video tapes has similarly increased the efficacy of training. Special difficulties in learning may be encountered in therapists whose professional lives have been spent in doing psychoanalysis or long-term analytic psychotherapy. In particular, the active stance required of the therapist comes into conflict with the quiet and neutrality inherent in analytic techniques. As the teaching of brief dynamic therapy has become more widespread in training programs, the younger therapist, not yet set in a single mold, is able to integrate the various techniques into a more varied and flexible therapeutic armamentarium.

As the interest in short-term therapy has grown, it has come under considerable scrutiny. Both in teaching and in investigating its effectiveness, video tapes of individual sessions or an entire course of therapy have been used extensively. Brief dynamic therapy and those who do it are, therefore, highly visible in ways new to psychotherapy. This teaching technique ensures greater attention to the application of prescribed techniques and to the assessment of their therapeutic effectiveness—both central elements in providing quality control.

Like other forms of psychotherapy, supportive treatment must be learned through treating appropriately selected patients under supervision. Learning such therapy is an integral part of training. When a patient is accepted into treatment with supportive therapy, he should be given specific information about the extent of the support the therapist will provide, e.g., the frequency of sessions, the permissibility of extra sessions when the patient feels he needs them, and the availability of the therapist by phone. The limits set in this regard at the start of treatment are one important element in avoiding severe ego regressions. In supportive therapy the patient often becomes markedly dependent on the relationship for his mental well-being. The therapist, therefore, has a special responsibility to be consistent and reliable in his therapeutic role.

REFERENCES

Alexander F, French T: Psychoanalytic Therapy. New York, Ronald Press, 1946

Alexander F: Some quantitative aspects of psychoanalytic technique. J Am Psychoanal Assoc 2:685-701, 1954a

Alexander F: Psychoanalysis and psychotherapy. J Am Psychoanal Assoc 2:722-733, 1954b

Basch M: Doing Psychotherapy. New York, Basic Books, 1980

Bibring E: Psychoanalysis and dynamic psychotherapies. J Am Psychoanal Assoc 2:745-770, 1954

Bion W: Attention and Interpretation. London, Heinemann, 1970

Bion W: Second Thoughts: Selected Papers on Psychoanalysis. London, Heinemann, 1967

Bion W: Transformations. London, Heinemann, 1965

Burke JD, White HS, Havens LL: Which short-term therapy? Matching patient and method. Arch Gen Psychiatry 36:177-186, 1979

Cath SH: Psychoanalysis and psychoanalytic psychotherapy of the older patient. Journal of Geriatric Psychiatry 15:43-53, 1982

Davanloo H (ed): Basic Principles and Techniques in Short-Term Dynamic Psychotherapy. New York, Spectrum Publications, 1978

Eissler K: The effect of the structure of the ego on psychoanalytic technique. J Am Psychoanal Assoc 1:104, 1953

Ekstein R: Psychoanalysis, in Basic Handbook of Child Psychiatry, vol 3. Edited by Harrison S. New York, Basic Books, 1979

Freud A: The widening scope of indications for psychoanalysis, discussion. J Am Psychoanal Assoc 2:607, 1954

Freud A: The Ego and the Mechanisms of Defense. London, Hogarth Press, 1937

Freud S: From the history of an infantile neurosis, vol 17, in Complete Psychological Works of Sigmund Freud, standard ed. Edited by Strachey J. London, Hogarth Press, 1955a

Freud S: Line of advance in psycho-analytic therapy, in Complete Psychological Works of Sigmund Freud, standard ed, vol 17. Edited by Strachey J. London, Hogarth Press, 1955b

Glover E: The Technique of Psychoanalysis. New York, International Universities Press, 1968

Greenson R: The Technique and Practice of Psychoanalysis, vol 1. New York, International Universities Press, 1967

Greenspan S, Lourie R: Developmental structuralist approach to the classification of adaptive and pathologic personality organizations: infancy and early childhood. Am J Psychiatry 138:725,–735, 1981

Gunderson J, Singer M: Defining borderline patients: an overview. Am J Psychiatry 132:1,–10, 1975

Hartmann H: Ego Psychology and the Problem of Adaptation. Translated by Rapaport D. New York, International Universities Press, 1958

Karasu TB: Psychotherapies: an overview. Am J Psychiatry 134:851-863, 1977

Kaufman M: Psychoanalysis in late-life depressions. Psychoanal Q 6:308,–355, 1937

Kernberg O: Neurosis, psychosis and borderline states, in Comprehensive Textbook of Psychiatry, vol 1, 3rd ed. Edited by Kaplan H, Freedman A, Sadock B. Baltimore, Williams & Wilkins Co, 1980a

Kernberg O: Melanie Klein, in Comprehensive Textbook of Psychiatry, 3rd ed. Edited by Kaplan H, Freedman A, Sadock B. Baltimore, Williams & Wilkins Co, 1980b

Kernberg O: Technical considerations in the treatment of borderline personality organization. J Am Psychoanal Assoc 24:795,–829, 1976

Kernberg O: Borderline Conditions and Pathological Narcissism. New York, Jason Aronson, 1975

Knight R: Management and psychotherapy of the borderline schizophrenic patient, in Psychodynamic Psychiatry and Psychology. Edited by Knight R, Friedman R. New York, International Universities Press, 1954

Kohut H: The Analysis of the Self. New York, International Universities Press, 1971

Kohut H: The Restoration of the Self. New York, International Universities Press, 1977

Mahler M, Furer M: On Human Symbiosis and the Vicissitudes of Individuation. New York, International Universities Press, 1968

Malan D: The Frontiers of Brief Psychiatry. New York, Plenum Medical Book Co, 1976

Mann J: Time-Limited Psychotherapy. Cambridge, Harvard University Press, 1973

Meissner W: Theories of personality and psychopathology: classical psychoanalysis, in Comprehensive Textbook of Psychiatry, vol 1, 3rd ed. Edited by Kaplan H. Friedman A, Sadock B. Baltimore, Williams & Wilkins Co, 1980

Mullahy PF: Harry Stack Sullivan, in Comprehensive Textbook of Psychiatry, vol 1, 3rd ed. Baltimore, Williams & Wilkins Co, 1980

Muslin HL: Psychoanalysis in the elderly: self psychological approach. Presented at the annual meeting of American Psychiatric Association Meeting, New York, April 30–May 6, 1983

Nemiah J: Classical psychoanalysis, in American Handbook of Psychiatry. Edited by Arieti S. New York, Basic Books, 1976

Rangell L: Similarities and differences between psychoanalysis and dynamic psychotherapy. J Am Psychoanal Assoc 2:734, 1954

Scharfman M: Psychoanalytic treatment, in Treatment of Mental Disorder in Childhood and Adolescence. Edited by Wolman B. Englewood Cliffs, NJ, Prentice-Hall, 1978

Segal H: Fear of death: notes on the analysis of an old man. Int J Psychoanal 39:178-181, 1958

Sifneos P: Short-Term Dynamic Psychotherapy: Evaluation and Technique. New York, Plenum Medical Book Co, 1979

Sifneos P: Short-Term Psychotherapy and Emotional Crisis. Cambridge, Harvard University Press, 1975

Stewart R: Psychoanalysis and psychoanalytic psychotherapy, in Comprehensive Textbook of Psychiatry, vol 3, 3rd ed. Edited by Kaplan H, Freedman A, Sadock B. Baltimore, Williams & Wilkins Co, 1980

Wallerstein R: Introduction to panel on psychoanalysis and psychotherapy. Int J Psychoanal 50:117-126, 1969

Weissman M, Prusoff GA, DiMascio A, et al: The efficacy of drugs and psychotherapy in the treatment of acute depressive episodes. Am J Psychiatry 136:556-558, 1979

Winnicott D: The Maturational Process and the Facilitating Environment. New York, International Universities Press, 1965

Zetzel E: A developmental approach to the borderline patient. Am J Psychiatry 127:867,-871, 1971

Psychotherapy with Children and Adolescents

HISTORICAL BACKGROUND

Although isolated reports date to antiquity, early evidence of definable psychotherapeutic contact with children before the twentieth century is rare. Until this century, it appears that in those instances in which children's emotional and mental disturbances were recognized, they were handled primarily by advising parents of alternative means of dealing with their children or by other forms of environmental modification. The few experts rarely confronted the child directly in an effort to alter the clinical course. A noteworthy exception was the celebrated eighteenth century undertaking of the French otologist Jean-Marc Gaspard Itard (1962), who, with therapeutic intent, adopted Victor, a prepubertal boy who presumably had lived the bulk of his life as a savage with animals in the forest of Aveyron. Itard undertook to civilize and educate Victor in a manner that conceivably may be considered psychotherapy.

The modern era of child psychotherapy is generally thought to have begun with Sigmund Freud's (1955) case report in 1909 of "Little Hans," a five-year-old phobic child. Although the treatment of Hans should unquestionably be labeled psychotherapy, it was really filial therapy in that it was the boy's father, under Freud's direction, who was the psychotherapist. Indeed, Freud asserted that parental closeness was a prerequisite for the treatment.

It was more than a decade before psychoanalysts successfully undertook direct psychotherapy with children. The basis for this lag following Freud's supervision of Little Hans' treatment by his father is probably best illustrated by Sandor Ferenczi's (1950) report of the first attempt in 1913 of direct psychoanalytic treatment of a child without the use of a family intermediary. Ferenczi found that the psychoanalytic method, as then used with adults, was not feasible with his young patient, who readily became bored and wanted to return to his toys. It was only after analysts recognized that a child's play could be considered a valid means of communication that child psychoanalysis developed as a direct psychotherapeutic approach to the child.

Play was introduced to the treatment of emotionally disturbed children by women who had the benefit of experience with children as well as backgrounds in psychoanalysis. Hermine von Hug-Hellmuth (1921) published the first report following Ferenczi's abortive attempt. The major credit for the subsequent development of child psychoanalysis belongs, however, jointly to Anna Freud (1929, 1945) and Melanie Klein (1932). Melanie Klein's theoretical assumptions about the similarity of the child's and the adult's personality structure were reflected in the development of a therapeutic technique that considered the child's free play to be a substitute for the adult's free associations. Anna Freud assigned more credence to the child's inevitable dependence on parents and evolved a different technique that has exerted considerable influence on derivative psychotherapies.

Around the turn of the century, in addition to the significant focus on childhood in both Sigmund Freud's psychoanalysis and Adolf Meyer's psychobiology, other independent developments contributed to the subsequent flowering of psychotherapy with children. Among these were the development of psychometry by Binet and Simon in France and the concept underlying the creation of separate courts for juveniles in Australia, Colorado, and Illinois. The courts in Illinois are particularly noteworthy because Chicago was the site of William Healy's pioneering psychiatric work with youngsters who were brought to the attention of the juvenile court. This work foreshadowed the development of the child guidance clinic movement in the United States in the 1920's under the aegis of the Commonwealth Fund and Clifford Beer's National Committee for Mental Hygiene.

The first report of the psychoanalytic treatment of an adolescent was Freud's "Dora" case in 1905. Freud's difficulty with the transference and countertransference issues in that case proved to be characteristic of the experience of many who have followed him. His work was extended and applied in a more systematic fashion by Aichhorn (1948), who established a residential treatment program for "wayward youth" based on psychoanalytic principles. Aichhorn served as teacher and model for a generation of psychoanalytically trained educators such as Anna Freud, Erik Erikson, Peter Blos, Fritz Redl, Rudolph Ekstein, and others who brought with them the principles of analytically-oriented psychotherapy with adolescents when they left Vienna and have continued to contribute to its growth. More recently workers such as Masterson (1972), Bruch (1979), Laufer (1975), and others have expanded the range of adolescent psychotherapy to the borderline disorders, eating disorders, and "developmental breakdowns" that may characterize this phase. In addition, group (Berkovitz, 1972), family (Williams, 1973), and behavioral (Lehrer et al., 1971) methods have been developed for special application to adolescent patients.

THEORETICAL ISSUES AND PHILOSOPHY

Brody (1964) has characterized child psychotherapy as a "theoretical orphan"—that is, without its own readily identifiable body of theory. Historically, views of psychopathology and its treatment have shifted to either external (sociocultural, familial, and behavioral) or internal (biological and psychological) dynamic factors. For instance, Freud's original view, derived reconstructively from adults, emphasized external environmentally induced traumata in childhood, such as sexual seduction. Subsequent data compelled him to de-emphasize presumed experiences of seduction in childhood and to focus, instead, on fantasies of seduction, thereby shifting his view of causality from external to internal intrapsychic factors. More recently, increasing attention has been paid to both neurobiological vulnerability and family transactional influences, without necessarily diminishing the importance of other factors. At the current level of knowledge, attempts to assert that all psychopathology is either internally or externally determined are patently artificial.

The choice of intervention with an individual youngster should be based on the clinician's understanding of the child's problem, stemming from an individualized assessment of the child and his or her family. But, regardless of how individualized such an evaluation is, any rational assessment requires that the data from observation be organized within a coherent framework. Typically, such systematizing schemata are derived from the clinician's preferred theory of personality development and organization, rendering it vital that he or she be vigilant in assuring that these theories do not distort the clinical observations or inappropriately influence the therapeutic interventions. Currently, five major theoretical systems underlie the bulk of child psychotherapy: (a) psychoanalytic theories, (b) social-learning behavioral theories, (c) family systems-oriented transactional theories, (d) developmental theories, and (e) constitutional theories.

Psychoanalytic Theoretical Issues. According to psychoanalytic theory, exploratory and interpretive psychotherapy works with patients of all ages by retracing the evolution of psychopathological processes. A principal difference noted with advancing age is a sharpening distinction between psychogenetic and psychodynamic factors; the younger the child, the more the genetic and the dynamic forces are intertwined.

The development of pathological processes is generally thought to begin with experiences—the child's perception and interpretation of reality—which have proved to be particularly significant to the patient. The reason for this effect may reside in the nature of the experiences, their intensity, or both. Their influence may have been exaggerated because of their occurrence in the early, impressionable years of the patient's life or under special emotional or physical circumstances that rendered him vulnerable. Although in one sense the experiences were real, in another sense they may have been misinterpreted, imagined, or colored by fantasy. In any event, for the patient they were traumatic experiences that caused unconscious complexes to which the patient reacted in a manner that has been compared to the body's organic reaction to irritating foreign bodies. Being inaccessible to conscious awareness, these unconscious elements readily escape rational adaptive maneuvers and are subject to a pathological misuse of adaptive and defensive mechanisms. The result is the development of distressing symptoms, character attitudes, or patterns of behavior that constitute the emotional disturbance.

Increasingly, the psychoanalytic view of emotional disturbances in children has assumed a developmental orientation. Thus, the maladaptive defensive functioning is directed against conflicts between impulses that are characteristic of a specific developmental phase and environmental influences or of the child's internalized representations of the environment. In this framework the disorders are the result of environmental interferences with maturational time-tables or conflicts with the environment engendered by developmental progress. The result is difficulty in achieving or resolving developmental tasks and in acquiring the capacities typically correlated with ensuing phases of development. These phases can be codified in a number of ways, such as Anna Freud's (1965) lines of development and Erikson's (1950) concept of sequential psychosocial capacities. Each stage, however, is based on the integration of earlier stages, with their typical drive vicissitudes, stresses, nuclear conflicts, developmental tasks, social modes, growth potentials, and possible psychopathological resolutions.

Expressive and exploratory psychotherapy endeavors to retrace and correct this evolution of emotional disturbance through a re-enactment and desensitization of the traumatic events by free expression of thoughts and feelings in an interview-play situation. Ultimately, the therapist helps the patient understand and effect greater conscious control over the warded-off feelings, fears, and wishes that have beset him.

Although the patients may have varying degrees of desire to learn about themselves and, thus, to gain conscious control over maladaptive automatic processes, resistances are invariably manifested. These resistances are paradoxical tendencies that oppose therapeutic progress. For instance, patients experience an inertia grounded in the fact that the repressed material tends to perpetuate itself endlessly. Also, there may be advantages, real or imagined, in remaining emotionally disturbed. In addition, certain people, greatly burdened by conscience, develop a need to suffer which opposes psychic health.

At the center of these resistances to treatment are the psychic functions that facilitate forgetting and repetition, which lead the patient to re-experience certain feelings out of context without recalling their relevance. In the therapeutic setting the therapist becomes the object of these re-experienced thoughts, feelings, and reactions, a process that has been designated as transference. These feelings originated in a time that has passed and in relation to other people, notably parents. In such transferences, the therapist becomes the target of desires, loves, hates, or suspicions that make sense only when viewed in terms of relationships the patient experienced with other people. With the recognition that the patient misunderstands the present in terms of the past, the therapist attempts to use these transferred reactions to discover the genesis of the patient's problems and to formulate interpretations that will help the patient understand his enigmatic stance. The goal of these interpretations is to enable the patient to increase conscious control over heretofore automatic mental processes. The hoped-for result is a rearrangement of personality structure and an enhanced ability to realize his potential.

Whereas such an expressive-exploratory-interpretive approach seeks improvement by exposure and resolution of buried conflicts, suppressive-supportive-educative psychotherapy generally works in an opposite fashion: It aims to facilitate repression. The therapist, capitalizing on the patient's desire to please him, encourages the patient to substitute new adaptive and defensive mechanisms. In this type of treatment, the therapist uses interpretations minimally; instead, he emphasizes suggestion, persuasion, exhortation, operant or classical reinforcement, counseling, education, direction, advice, abreaction, environmental manipulation, intellectual review, gratification of the patient's current dependent needs, and similar techniques.

In recent years the contributions of psychoanalytic thinkers regarding narcissistic development and self psychology have been applied to therapeutic work with adolescents and children. This orientation suggests that in addition to the classically emphasized psychosexual and ego development, children also develop via critical "mirroring" relationships that help shape a sense of self. Distortions in this line of development may be seen in some severely disturbed young patients who often are difficult to treat in psychotherapy yet who may respond to an approach that is sensitive to the need for maintaining such a relationship. Marohn and co-workers' (1980) work with delinquent adolescents is an example of the application of this approach.

Learning-Behavioral Theoretical Issues. Although their roots are considerably older, today's behavioral approaches and their underlying learning theories stem directly from twentieth century developments (see Chapter 10 on "Behavior Therapy").

More than 60 years ago Watson and Raynot (1920) demonstrated the development of a phobia in 11-month-old Albert. After determining that Albert was not afraid of furry objects and that he had no previous experience with white rats, the researchers gave Albert a rat with which to play. Whenever Albert made an overture to the animal, the experimenters made a loud noise. After a short period of time, Albert appeared fearful whenever he saw the white rat. Fear was not the invariable response of all infants; some turned to scowl at the source of the noise while they continued to play with the animal. Albert's fear, however, proceeded to generalize to stimuli resembling the white rat, such as white rabbits, cotton, and other furry objects. This experimentally induced phobic reaction reportedly persisted for several months. Four years later, Mary Cover Jones (1924) demonstrated that another infant—who, like Albert, had been conditioned to fear furry objects—could be relieved of the fear by means of both social imitation and direct reconditioning. These landmark efforts have been supplemented by countless laboratory experiments that have contributed over the years to several learning theories that are relevant for all psychotherapeutic undertakings, not only those designated as "behavior therapy."

Originally derived primarily from laboratory experiments, the theoretical assumptions of behavioral therapy postulate that, inasmuch as disturbed behavior is acquired, its evolution and treatment can be understood within the framework of learning theories, in which value judgments regarding qualitative abnormality or deviance are de-emphasized. All behavior, regardless of whether it is adaptive or maladaptive, is a consequence of the same basic principles of behavior acquisition and maintenance. It is either learned or unlearned, and what renders behavior abnormal or disturbed is its social significance.

Although the theories and their derivative therapeutic intervention techniques have become increasingly complex over the years, it is still possible to subsume all learning within two global basic mechanisms. One is classical respondent conditioning akin to Pavlov's famous experiments; the other is operant instrumental learning, which has come to be connected with Skinner's name, even though it is basic both to Thorndike's law of effect regarding the influence of reinforcing consequences of behavior and to Freud's pleasure principle. Both of these basic mechanisms assign the highest priority to the immediate precipitants of behavior, de-emphasizing those remote underlying causal determinants that are assigned so much importance in the medical tradition. Some profess that this exclusive focus on classical and operant conditioning has obscured the amount of human learning that results from imitative modeling of behavior and the cognitive acquisition of attitudes, beliefs, values, and the like.

Regardless of the mechanisms of learning, however, the theory asserts quite simply that there are but two types of abnormal behavior: behavioral deficits that result from a failure to learn and deviant maladaptive behavior that is a consequence of learning inappropriate things.

Such concepts have always been an implicit part of the rationale underlying all child psychotherapy; however, the resurgence of interest outside of the laboratory in special systematized behavioral techniques developed to eliminate symptoms and to encourage positive behaviors in a wide range of childhood psychopathology has been relatively recent. Although these often ingenious multifaceted intervention strategies can be categorized under appropriately descriptive rubrics—such as systematic desensitization, operant conditioning (token economy, contingency management, and contracting), aversive control, emotive imagery, assertiveness training, covert reinforcement, modeling, feedback control, negative practices, implosion, flooding, and response prevention—much of their success, particularly with children, is derived simply from rewarding previously unnoticed good behavior and thereby highlighting it and making it more frequent.

Family Systems Theoretical Issues. Within the past few decades a major conceptual reorientation has been occurring in several sectors of the scientific community. Linear deterministic notions of causality have been enriched by a systems orientation that encompasses such concepts as circular reciprocal feedback mechanisms involving multiple factors and causing reverberating effects, so that the whole is different from the sum of its parts. Although families have long been an interest of children's psychotherapists, their understanding of transactional family processes has been greatly enhanced by conceptual contributions from cybernetics, systems theory, communications theory, object relations theory, social role theory, ethology, and ecology. A conglomerate of ideas has accumulated from multiple sources—observations of the effect of the parents' unconscious mental functioning on childhood psychopathology, the concept of a child's development reactivating parents' unresolved childhood conflicts, the delineation of scapegoating, the double-bind theory of schizophrenia (which has since been applied to other forms of psychopathology), the demonstration that the type and extent of the patient's psychopathology can be predicted from the parents' communication styles, and the frequently observed patterns of identification and projection between parents and children in which parental projection of self or part of the self to the child results in the parent's dealing with the child as though the child were a part of the parent.

The bedrock premise entails the family's functioning as a self–regulating open system that possesses its own unique history and structure. This structure is constantly evolving as a consequence of the dynamic interaction between the family's mutually interdependent subsystems and individuals who share complementary needs. From this conceptual foundation a wealth of ideas has emerged under rubrics such as the family's development, life cycle, homeostasis, functions, identity, values, goals, congruence, symmetry, myths, rules, structure, and so on. These concepts both stem from and contribute to the enhancement of the potential for understanding a wide range of therapeutic interventions. They constitute a vital underpinning of psychotherapy with children, whether that treatment is accomplished within the family system or with the child alone. In a provocatively challenging paper, Montalvo and Haley (1973) highlighted the extent to which individual child therapy inevitably represents a powerful intervention in the family system. Increasingly, it is being noted that appreciation of the family system sometimes explains why a minute therapeutic input at a critical juncture may result in far-reaching changes.

Developmental Theoretical Issues. Underlying child psychotherapy is the assumption that in the absence of unusual interferences, children mature and develop in basically orderly, predictable ways that are codifiable in a variety of interrelated bio-psycho-social sequential systematizations. The central role of a developmental frame of reference in child psychotherapy qualitatively distinguishes it from adult psychotherapy. Without necessarily possessing intimate knowledge of the intricate details, the therapist must be forever mindful of Werner's (1957) conception of organisms as naturally directed toward a series of transformations—whether in ontogenetic longitudinal development, in cultural organization, or in the contemporaneous development of a thought or perception—from a state of undifferentiated globality toward levels of increasing differentiation, followed by hierarchic integration of the interdependent parts. Thus, the therapist's orientation should entail something more than knowledge of age-appropriate behavior derived from such studies as Gesell's (1945) descriptions of the morphology of behavior. It should encompass more than psychosexual development with egopsychological and sociocultural amendments, exemplified by Erikson's (1950) epigenetic schema. It extends beyond familiarity with Piaget's (1972) sequence of intellectual evolution as a basis for acquaintance with the level of abstraction at which children of various ages may be expected to function or for assessing their capacity for a moral orientation, as has been delineated sequentially by Kohlberg (1963). It is more than recognizing that children of various ages react to hunger, frustration, injury, illness, separation, and death not in some uniform fashion resembling adult behavior but in ways representative of their stages of development.

Such normative data and an appreciation of the wide range of normal variation within interrelated developmental sequences are a vital foundation. Of central significance is the relevance of current states for later developmental phases and, conversely, the implications of future developmental tasks for current development. This information may be derived from a number of descriptions of child development; however, the information should be supplemented by personal knowledge and observation of children, with the resultant view of the child as a fluid, maturing, and developing organism who is not yet complete. The child's personality must be viewed in the perspective of the interrelationships of his or her past, present, and future; the focus must be on questions of regression-progression and transience-permanence rather than on static assessments, even if they are articulated in psychodynamic terms.

Special mention should be made of the developmental line, as Anna Freud (1965) conceptualizes it, from play to work. Children do not play solely for the recreational purposes that adults prefer to attribute to their own games and sporting activities. Play serves a number of important purposes for children such as facilitating the mastery of their inevitable developmental crises through playful transformation into activity of what was passively experienced. As a consequence, play has assumed a special position in child psychotherapy; it is simultaneously a medium of communication, a vehicle for expression, and a means of sublimation.

Constitutional Theoretical Issues. Thomas et al. (1968) point to the role of constitutional or other early developmental factors in contributing to temperament, early relationships, and the evolution of clinical problems. For instance, if they perceive maladaptive temperamental-environmental interaction as central in the development of a clinical disorder, they suggest focusing on parent guidance rather than parent treatment.

Over the past several years, child psychiatry has assigned credence to probable biological factors in many disturbances previously considered to be exclusively psychosocial in origin. Among these are autism, childhood schizophrenia, noctural enuresis, attention deficit disorder, major affective disorders, and some anxiety disorders. With this knowledge has come the recognition that some well intentioned psychotherapeutic interventions— e.g., focus on the "schizophrenogenic" mother—have generated iatrogenic difficulties. The role of psychotherapy is not being completely redefined, however. Psychodynamic, family, and behavioral factors typically are significantly involved in the form and extent of symptoms and in their responsiveness to biological interventions.

THERAPEUTIC AGENTS

Multiple classifications of child psychotherapy are possible, depending on various features of the process. A common framework for categorization is the global aim and mode of the treatment—that is, supportive-suppressive-directive or expressive-exploratory-ventilative. Psychotherapy can also be described in terms of its depth, duration, and intensity. Focusing on the therapist's approach, one can classify psychotherapy as being abreactive, interpretive, suggestive, persuasive, or educative. Eponyms such as Freudian, Kleinian, Rankian, and Rogerian refer to preferred theoretical concepts.

Identifying the element presumed to be helpful for the young patient is among the common bases for the classification of child therapy. The history of psychotherapy with people of all ages has been punctuated by emphasizing different factors or processes at one time or another as the ostensibly essential ingredient without which psychotherapy would not be effective. Before the ascendency of psychoanalysis, the most prominent ingredients were suggestion, persuasive exhortation, and reassurance. During the infancy of psychoanalysis, symptomatic relief tended to be attributed to the patient's rediscovery of a lost memory. Shortly thereafter, the abreactive release of dammed-up emotions was highlighted. With further development of psychoanalytic thinking, the emphasis shifted to modification of superego standards, identification with the therapist, resolution of the transference, development of increased emotional discipline in the working-through process, development of insight, analysis of defenses, and expansion of ego functioning.

Concurrent with this history, the prominence accorded learning-behavioral factors, such as motivating needs, stimulating cues, and the reinforcement of reward and punishment, has waxed and waned. Similarly, improvement has been perceived as developing from a deconditioning process that may involve systematic desensitization or a manipulation of the therapeutic relationship so as to provide a corrective emotional experience.

Although these elements are derived from different conceptual frameworks and expressed in markedly different languages, some of them overlap considerably. For example, subtle persuasion, operant conditioning, and the fostering of identification with the therapist often entail similar processes, although they are expressed in different frames of reference. Efforts to attribute therapeutic progress with all patients to a single factor have proved to be unconvincing, as all the therapeutic elements mentioned above are likely to assume varying degrees of significance under different circumstances. While none of these factors appears to be specific for any particular developmental stage, the therapeutic relationship itself and corrective emotional experiences generally exert a greater influence with children than with adults, whether they were specifically designed by the therapist or occur as the natural by-product of the therapist's empathic stance.

Isolating a single therapeutic element as a basis for classification tends to be an artificial exercise because most, if not all, of the factors are present in varying degrees in every child psychotherapeutic undertaking. For example, there is no psychotherapy in which the relationship between therapist and patient is not a vital factor; nevertheless, since John Levy's (1938) article, child psychotherapists commonly talk of *relationship therapy* to describe a form of treatment in which a positive, friendly, helpful relationship is viewed as the primary, if not the sole, therapeutic ingredient. Probably one of the best examples of pure relationship therapy is to be found outside of a clinical setting in the work of the Big Brother Organization.

Remedial, educational, and *patterning* psychotherapy endeavors to teach new attitudes and behavior patterns to children who persist in using immature and inefficient patterns, which are often presumed to be due to a maturational lag.

Supportive psychotherapy is particularly helpful in enabling a well adjusted youngster to cope with the emotional turmoil engendered by a crisis. It is also used with those quite disturbed youngsters whose less than adequate ego functioning may be seriously disrupted by an expressive-exploratory mode or by other forms of therapeutic intervention. At the beginning of most psychotherapy, regardless of the patient's age and the nature of the therapeutic interventions, the principal therapeutic elements the patient perceives tend to be the supportive ones, a consequence of therapists' universal efforts to be reliably and sensitively responsive. In fact, some therapies may never proceed beyond this supportive level, whereas others develop an expressive-exploratory or behavioral modification emphasis on top of the supportive foundation.

Release therapy, described initially by David Levy (1939), facilitates the abreaction of pent-up emotions. Although abreaction is an aspect of many therapeutic undertakings, in release therapy, the treatment situation is structured so as to encourage only this factor.

Pre-school-aged children are sometimes treated indirectly through the parent(s) (Furman, 1957). The therapist using this strategy should be alert to the possibility that apparently successful *filial treatment* can obscure a significant diagnosis (Harrison, 1971).

Psychoanalytically-oriented psychotherapy tries, through self-understanding, to enable the child to develop his potential. This task is accomplished by liberating for more constructive use the psychic energy that is presumed to be expended in defending against fantasized dangers. The child is generally unaware of these unreal dangers, his fear of them, and the psychological defenses he uses to avoid both the danger and the anxieties. With the awareness that is facilitated, the patient can evaluate the usefulness of his defensive maneuvers and relinquish the unnecessary ones that constitute the symptoms of his emotional disturbance.

This form of therapy is to be distinguished from *child psychoanalysis,* a more intensive and less common treatment, in which the unconscious elements are interpreted systematically from outside in, resulting in the orderly sequence of affect-defense-impulse. Under these circumstances the therapist anticipates unconscious resistances and allows transference manifestations to mature to a full transference neurosis through which neurotic conflicts are resolved.

Although interpretations of dynamically relevant conflicts are emphasized in psychoanalytic descriptions, this does not imply that elements

predominant in other types of therapies are absent. Indeed, in all psychotherapy the child should derive support from the consistently understanding and accepting relationship with the therapist, while varying degrees of
remedial educational guidance and emotional release are inevitably present.

The popular designation "play therapy" will not be accorded special
consideration here. Play is in fact often used as part of all the therapies
named above. Play creates a tolerable milieu for being with children and is
in itself a way of communication with them, in addition to and sometimes
instead of talking. It can help in establishing and maintaining a working
relationship with the therapist, often even an alliance. It can provide a field
for communicating sensitive issues and for experientially unfolding and
looking at a child's fantasies, wishes, thoughts, fears, and other feelings for
trying out possible mental scenarios. These often unfold largely in displacement, experientially, with the child assuming variable amounts of responsibility, and without his saying "I" or "my family" but rather something
such as "this dog hates his baby sister. . . . ," etc.

The therapeutic possibilities of play are many and flexible; to add a few to
those above, one could cite changing passive to active, taking a leave of
absence from the reality principle, identifying with the aggressor, exploring
the pleasure principle and its restraints and modulation, exploring aggression and/or abreaction, and exploring sublimation. Play in therapy can
also at times provide a retreat, a defense, or a cooling-down area.

Among the current tools of the trade are the following: clay, blocks, dolls,
puppets, doll houses (including toilet, stove, refigerator, sink, bed), paper
and pencil and crayons or paint, bits of costumes, trucks, cars, soldiers, toy
dishes, toy pistols, pipe cleaners, some games (e.g., checkers, table
pingpong, or basketball). Two currently widely used play techniques are
Winnicott's Squiggle game (Winnicott, 1977) and Gardner's (1971) mutual
story-telling technique. In general, however, play is such an integral aspect
of most psychotherapy with children that specifically designating "play
therapy" is almost as unspecific as referring to "verbal therapy" for adults.

An Integrative Approach

Witmer's (1946) *Psychiatric Interviews with Children* provides ten detailed
child guidance case reports by nine different therapists, many of whom
represent different schools of therapy. Witmer noted, however, that the
differences between the allegedly discrepant theoretical frames of reference
fade out when applied in actual practice. Observing that the several
therapists responded sensitively to what they perceived as the child's needs,
Witmer asserted that certain principles basic to all child psychotherapy
overshadow the influences of the therapist's theoretic inclination.

But the resurgence of interest and activity in behavioral techniques during
the 1960's was accompanied by an emphasis on the differences between

behavioral and psychodynamic approaches. Eysenck (1960) emphasized that treatment strategies that use behavior explicitly should be distinguished from psychotherapy that uses psychological methods. A comparable segregationist attitude was as evident on the psychodynamic side, where similar efforts to demarcate boundaries permeated the literature and educational programs. Treatments that focused on symptoms were actively criticized; it was assumed—inaccurately, as it happened—that such an emphasis could lead only to symptom substitution. Often enough, there was a valid basis for this segregation; nevertheless, too little attention was paid to the presence of psychological influences in even the most mechanistic behavioral techniques. And the inevitable presence of behavioral influences in the purest psychological therapies was similarly ignored.

The exaggerated emphasis on this segregation of theory led to a tendency to neglect noteworthy integrationist efforts. Mowrer (1950) and Dollard and Miller (1950) examined psychodynamic therapy from a learning-behavioral theory perspective and were able to document cross-fertilization. More recently have come discussions of behavioral therapy with children from a psychodynamic perspective in efforts to synthesize these apparently conflicting concepts without minimizing, demeaning, or sacrificing the essential richness of the contribution of each point of view (Kessler, 1966; Blom, 1972). Feather, cited by Aronson (1972), suggested that some of the effectiveness of systematic desensitization in behavior therapy may be a consequence of enhancing the patient's discrimination between fantasy and reality. On the other hand, the effectiveness of interpretation in psychoanalysis and related therapies may, in part, be derived from their desensitizing effects.

While the theoretical origins of behavioral treatment differ from those of psychodynamic psychotherapy and the approaches often appear quite different, if not antithetical, the theories and modalities can be integrated fruitfully. Symptoms from whatever source—psychodynamic, learned deviance, family dynamics, or biology—may seriously impair the development of supportive, empathetic relationships or crucial identification with parents and others. Further, symptoms can develop sufficient autonomy to persist even beyond the resolution of their etiological source (Rapaport, 1967). Thus, a behaviorally based amelioration of a symptom that has fueled tension, distance, and hostility in the parent-child relationship could lead to significant psychodynamic change (Blom, 1972).

Probably the most vivid examples of the integration of psychodynamic and behavioral approaches, even though they are not always explicitly conceptualized as such, are to be found in the milieu therapy of child psychiatric residential and day treatment facilities. Noshpitz (1971) noted what he referred to as a ping-pong effect in residential treatment. Behavioral change is initiated in the residential setting, and its repercussions are explored concurrently in individual psychotherapeutic sessions so that the action in one arena and the information stemming from it augment and illuminate what transpires in the other. Blom (1972) summarized this process succinctly by noting that change is "capable of being accomplished both from the inside out and the outside in."

Although some segregationists remain, integration of a family systems transactional model with the developmental and psychodynamic models (Kramer, 1968) is expanding on both the empirical and practical levels. McDermott and Char (1974) pointed out that, on the one hand, systems theory appropriately suggests that the sum of the parts does not explain the whole but that, on the other hand, the converse is also true—knowledge of the whole family system does not necessarily entail understanding of its parts, particularly those youthful parts that are developing most rapidly. They recalled that child psychiatrists struggled long and hard to establish the fact that treating children's difficulties often requires more than counseling and treating parents. Malone (1974) discussed the advantages of flexibly combining therapeutic work with individuals, family subsystems, and total families. He asserted that the "central concept involved is the inseparability of internal and external." This phrase strikes a chord remarkably reminiscent of Blom's (1972) observation about the interrelationship and interdependence of the behavioral and psychodynamic perspectives.

The issues of combining multiple treatments that affect different aspects of the same difficulty in the same person are illustrated most vividly by the relationships between the psychotherapies and the pharmacotherapies. Rationally, it is self-evident that prescribing medication should not preclude attention to intrapsychic and interpersonal factors, nor should the use of psychotherapy necessarily preclude using medication or environmental intervention.

HOW PSYCHOTHERAPY WITH CHILDREN AND ADOLESCENTS DIFFERS FROM THAT WITH ADULTS

Logic suggests that psychotherapy with children, who generally are more flexible than adults and have simpler defenses and other mental mechanisms, should consume less time than comparable treatment of adults. Experience does not usually confirm this expectation because of the relative absence in children of some elements that contribute to successful treatment.

A child or adolescent, for example, typically does not seek help. As a consequence, one of the first tasks for the therapist is to stimulate the child's motivation for treatment. Children commonly begin therapy involuntarily, often without the benefit of true parental support. Although the parents may want their child helped or changed, this desire is often generated by frustrated anger with the child. Typically, this anger is accompanied by relative insensitivity to what the therapist perceives as the child's need and the basis for a therapeutic alliance. Thus, whereas adult patients frequently perceive advantages in getting well, children may envision therapeutic change as nothing more than conforming to a disagreeable reality, which heightens the likelihood of perceiving the therapist as the parent's punitive agent. This is hardly the most fertile soil in which to nurture a therapeutic alliance.

Children and adolescents tend to externalize internal conflicts in search of alloplastic adaptations, finding it difficult to conceive of problem resolution except by altering an obstructing environment.

The tendency of children to re-enact their feelings in new situations facilitates the early appearance of spontaneous and global transference reactions that may be troublesome. Concurrently, the eagerness of children for new experiences, coupled with their natural developmental fluidity, tends to limit the intensity and therapeutic usefulness of subsequent transference developments. How the child's transference situation is recognized and handled by the therapist, in fact, determines its role and usefulness in the course of treatment.

Children have a limited capacity for self-observation, with the notable exception of some obsessive children who resemble adults in this ability. In the exploratory-interpretive psychotherapies, development of a capacity for healthy ego splitting—that is, simultaneous emotional involvement and self-observation—is most helpful. Only by means of identification with a trusted adult and in alliance with that adult are children able to approach such an ideal.

Although prior experience in treating adults is potentially both an advantage and an interference in initial psychotherapeutic efforts with children, the different qualities of strain on the therapist inherent in therapy with individuals at various developmental stages deserve attention. Regressive behavioral and communicative modes can be wearing on child therapists. Typically motor-minded, even when they do not require external controls, children may demand a degree of physical stamina that is not of consequence in therapy with adults. The age appropriateness of such primitive mechanisms as denial, projection, and isolation hinders the process of working through, which relies on a patient's synthesizing and integrative capacities, both of which are immature in children. Also, environmental pressures on the therapist are generally greater in psychotherapeutic work with children than with adults. Insofar as the therapist is able to recognize the many quantitative and qualitative differences between the child and the adult, his or her task becomes more manageable. The process of physical growth and the size differences among children and between child and therapist are important considerations. The developmental process itself, within which new functions are gradually emerging, must also be recognized. The cognitive-conceptual immaturity of the child, reflected in differing capacities to understand abstractions and language, must also shape one's therapeutic strategy. These factors, as well as a consideration of a child's natural dependence on real external parents, the child's more patent and intense regressive pull to more instinctual modes of experience and expression, and the child's natural tendency to externalize inner mental states by the use of play all constitute significant differences that, when recognized, aid in facilitating the therapeutic process.

Although children compare unfavorably with adults in many of the qualities that are generally considered desirable in therapy, children have the advantage of active maturational and developmental forces to propel them forward. The history of psychotherapy for children is punctuated by effrts to harness these assets and to overcome the liabilities. Recognition of the importance of play as valid communication constituted a major forward stride in these efforts.

Many of these characteristics of psychotherapy with children apply to adolescents as well, albeit inconsistently. Just as adolescents confront parents with a confusing patchwork of independence and dependence, progress and regression, psychotherapy with adolescents varies—between and within individuals—from something resembling play therapy to high levels of self-observation.

The question of who is seeking help is critical with adolescents. Perhaps even more than with children, parents' and schools' wishes to be helpful are frequently accompanied by anger and the wish to make the adolescent behave more compliantly. Thus, the therapist is readily perceived as an enemy rather than an ally in the developmental tasks of separation or sexual identity formation.

Adolescents frequently externalize conflicts, using the defenses of denial, projection, and distortion to a greater extent than adults. Frequently, conflicts are expressed through behavior to the extent that the therapist may feel compelled to intervene directly in the adolescent's life rather than remaining in the traditional psychotherapeutic position of working with the patient on his perceptions, thoughts, and feelings. This need may arise, for instance, with a dangerously delinquent patient or one with anorexia nervosa whose weight is becoming critical. While neutrality may be desirable for some aspects of psychotherapy, not acting in response to dangerous behavior or to a potential medical crisis may be experienced by the adolescent as neglect. Thus, the therapist must at times respond as a "real" object without abandoning the "therapeutic" perspective through which one helps the patient understand both his behavior and the response he has elicited from the therapist and others.

Communicating with Children and Adolescents in Psychotherapy. Some children participate in play activities immediately and verbalize spontaneously without assistance from the therapist, but others appear to require considerable help. Responsive to the child's apparent needs, the therapist either assumes a relatively passive, observing role or a more active, intervening one. Such activity may be of a superficial interpretive nature, focused on the child's reluctance; however, the therapist may find it necessary to assume a far more active stance, tantamount to a form of creative pump priming. For example, the therapist may speak with a puppet about why the very young child is afraid, thereby encouraging the child to communicate playfully though the puppet, or the therapist may pretend that he and the patient are on a television show, akin to Gardner's (1971) mutual storytelling technique.

Although there is general agreement that the ratio of play to verbalization in therapy shifts as children mature or even during the long-term therapy of the same youngster, there is no unanimity regarding the extent to which the therapist should participate actively in the child's play. Some advocate that the therapist invariably be an actively involved participant, appropriate to the child's developmental stage. Others advise therapists to sit consistently in one place and avoid all participation in the child's play, lest it contribute a parameter that later has to be analyzed. Therapists who advocate this position tend also to advise minimization—to the point of elimination, if possible—of contact with the parents. Neither extreme is appropriate for all children at all times. Although nonparticipating observation very likely enhances the therapist's capacity for free-floating attention while active participation risks interfering with such attention, it is inconceivable that therapists should rigidly adhere to one approach or the other unless they carefully select patients to conform with their preferred pattern. Different children under different circumstances with different therapists call for different approaches. Participation in play can be limited to playing roles assigned by the patient and in the manner directed by the patient; at the other extreme, particularly with young or regressed children, the therapist can see his or her involvement as a vehicle for therapeutic intervention.

Children generally are not as verbal as adults, so it is particularly vital that the child therapist appreciate the importance of nonverbal communication. The child's faces, gestures, posture, and mobility and the content, form, and configuration of his play and art may say more than his words. Indeed, therapists working with children must realize that verbalization is not essential for therapy. But, this is not to say that verbalization is insignificant. Many assert that one must have conscious recollections of one's own childhood in order to be able to talk comfortably with children. In addition, adults should consider the extent to which they view their own childhood and adulthood as interrelated aspects of a continuum and the extent to which they are considered to be separate, polarized, and discontinuous stages. In other words, each clinician must assess individually how, when, and why he or she views children as miniature adults and adults as larger children and the circumstances under which he or she thinks of children and adults as distinctly different.

Understanding the details of the varying connotations attached to the same words and phrases by people of different ages is a skill that can be re-learned and grows with practice. A striking example is the word "why," probably the most common word in psychotherapy with adults. Children, however, often seem to react to the question, "Why?" as if it were an accusation because children's previous experience with such inquiry has been limited to foci of disapproval. Thus, even if the child's capacity for abstract thinking is sufficiently mature to enable the child to appreciate that the therapist is interested in determining causal relationships, an evasive "because" may seem to the child to be a suitable and safe response.

Communicating with adolescents often requires particular sensitivity to the youngster's conflicts about dependency. An adolescent may assert his independence by demeaning his parents or teachers while appearing to have a trusting alliance with the therapist. As the therapeutic relationship develops, however, the adolescent may need to defend against his own wish to be dependent by repudiating the therapist. Thus, the child may re-enact a conflict with the therapist which is not only, or not necessarily, a specific transference but also an expression of a developmental phase-specific conflict.

Psychotherapeutic interventions with children encompass a range comparable to those used with adults. If the amount of therapist activity is used as the basis for a classificatory continuum, at the least active end are the therapist's questions requesting elaboration of the patient's statements or behavior. Closely aligned is the process of clarification of the patient's manifest productions by means of questions, recapitulation, and reorganization, which can arrange the child's productions in a logical, temporal sequence, so frequently neglected by children. Also, clarification can serve as a preliminary step toward the specific goal of the therapy by recapitulating the child's productions to highlight motivational possibilities, target behaviors, or whatever may be appropriate for the particular type of therapy. Next on the continuum of therapeutic activity are the exclamations and confrontations in which the therapist more pointedly directs attention to some data of which the patient is cognizant. Then there are interpretations designed to expand the patient's conscious awareness of himself by making explicit those elements that have previously been implicitly expressed in his thoughts, feelings, and behavior. Beyond interpretation, the therapist may educatively offer the patient information that is new because the patient has not been exposed to it previously. At the most active end of the continuum there is advising, counseling, and directing, designed to help the patient adopt a course of action or a conscious attitude.

There are vital differences in the way these interventions are used with children and with adults. The probable fate of broad, open-ended questions directed to children and adolescents can be illustrated vividly by citing the book title *Where Did You Go? Out. What Did You Do? Nothing.* To avoid such responses and to encourage verbal and nonverbal associations, the child therapist needs to be far more specific in focusing questions on what the child is just about ready to express. The best clues, of course, come from what the child has already communicated. In essence, the child is asked to elaborate on what he has already said or done. It is important to avoid sounding as though the adult is quizzing the child and invading his privacy. The more the therapist can imply curiosity, not unlike that of another interested youngster, the greater the likelihood of a fruitful response. This apparent naiveté should be tempered with awareness of the risk of asking questions that may seem devious to the child, such as those to which the therapist obviously knows the answer. For example, if the clinician, in the initial contact with the child, inquires as to the reasons for the consultation, the child, who assumes rightfully that his parents have already told the therapist, may perceive the therapist as dishonest. It can make a great deal of difference to the child if the therapist prefaces the question by indicating that he or she already knows the parents' ideas. Similarly, the therapist who inquires as to what dolls are doing in an effort to have the child elaborate on the fantasy underlying the observed doll play will very likely get a minimal response and may evoke suspicion because, from the child's point of view, what the dolls were doing should have been as obvious to the therapist as to the child. It is more productive for the therapist to express running commentary describing the dolls' activities, not unlike a television announcer at an athletic event. Under those circumstances the child often responds by elaborating on the therapist's description, thereby facilitating the approach to the underlying fantasy. Melanie Klein (1929), who initiated the interpretation of play in therapy, was the first formally to describe such an approach.

Certain interventions vital in therapy with children would be superfluous, if not insulting, to most adults. For example, to tell an angry adult that he is angry would be confrontation that could readily prove offensive. With an angry child, however, the identical intervention—that is, telling the child that he is angry—may be a necessary interpretation of affect, inasmuch as everyone may know about the child's anger except the child himself. Also, there are many more occasions with children than with adults in which clarification of misconceptions can be helpful.

It is generally advisable for therapeutic interventions to begin at the surface before proceeding deeper. Thus, attention is usually directed first to superficial behavior and affects, followed by defenses and other resistances, before dealing with conflict and impulses. Children, however, may present an important exception to this general guideline of attending to defenses and resistances before interpreting impulses. It may be unwise to undo the defensive projection into play that is characteristic of child therapy. Accordingly, when a child with adequate reality testing causes two dolls to fight, the therapist's running commentary might be limited to a description of the dolls' affect—namely, that the dolls are angry with one another. Although the displacement of the child's own feelings to one or both dolls may be obvious, it may be wisest to communicate about the anger within the context of the dolls' feelings and not attribute the anger to the child, thereby addressing the impulse without attending to the defensive projection into play. Under these circumstances, this playful displacement to the doll is viewed as an age-appropriate, adaptive mechanism rather than as a pathological, defensive maneuver. If the therapist had told the child that he had the dolls fight because of his own anger, the child's resistance and defensiveness might have increased to the point that he would stop the activity, thereby interrupting the communication. It is as if the therapist and the child with adequate ego strength had agreed to the significance of play without spelling it out specifically each time. Bornstein (1945) noted other disadvantages in interpreting play directly—for example, repeated interpretations of the symbolic meaning of play can impede the child's use of play in the service of the development of sublimations because such interpretations may facilitate libidinization of play.

Also from a psychoanalytic perspective, Fraiberg (1965) considered it "both a requirement and an impediment to treatment" that the therapist sometimes has to communicate with the child's imaginary characters and that therapeutic interventions may have to be intertwined in the child's dramatic play, in which the therapist may be playing roles. She asserted that it is vital that the fictional bad actor and his accusers eventually be acknowledged explicitly by the patient as stemming from his own impulses and conscience. Obviously, a prerequisite to this acknowledgment is the establishment of an initial understanding with the patient that his play and fantasies will be viewed by the therapist as communications about his problems. Without such a therapeutic contract, the patient may justifiably experience the therapist's intervention as an intrusive attack, although such an agreement does not guarantee that there will be no resistance.

Compelling clinical data are presented by those who have used both methods—sometimes not interfering with the displacement of psychic content into play; at other times assisting to undo that displacement by helping the child acknowledge explicitly the psychic content. Better results have been reported when the child's playful representations of his conflicts are eventually acknowledged directly by the patient. Nevertheless, questions should be raised about the outcome of those youngsters who appear to progress just as satisfactorily without ever verbalizing that acknowledgment and who do not return for further therapy because a second course of treatment is generally the source of the data cited to emphasize the advantage of verbal acknowledgment. But there is no direct evidence suggesting that those young children who never acknowledged responsibility for their play and have not returned for an additional course of psychotherapy have a less secure future. Is it conceivable that direct acknowledgment is indicated for some children and not for others? Clearly, additional knowledge is needed to resolve these questions and perhaps to delineate which approach is best suited for which patients.

With children whose ego functioning is so defective that they confuse play and reality, caution is called for in dealing with psychic content displaced in play. In such instances the therapist may have to devote some effort to educating the child about the distinction between play and reality before it is judicious to deal with the content of play. But this type of educational intervention is not supportive and, indeed, may be counterproductive for those children who do not have difficulty in distinguishing fantasy and reality.

In formulating and communicating therapeutic interventions, many therapists find the psychoanalytic structural system to be a helpful organizing framework. In that context the therapist's orientation is one of alliance with the patient's ego functioning, equidistant from superego and id unless there is a thoroughly reasoned justification for another stance. This advice should not stultify spontaneity, although therapists in training tend to find this inhibition difficult to avoid. With the accumulation of knowledge and experience, therapists establish an emotional set related to the goals of therapy following which their interventions are largely spontaneous within that set but subject to critical post hoc review.

Children typically evoke a protective, helpful, and educational, i.e., parental, attitude from most adults. Obviously, this attitude has considerable positive potential; however, in certain types of psychotherapy, it may encompass a potential liability about which therapists should be alert. A common example may be found in the special tone of voice that many adults assume in addressing children. If this special tone were used with another adult, it would likely be considered condescending or pedantic, a reaction that some children share, particularly as they become older. These typical adult attitudes toward children can combine with the therapist's emotional reaction to the child who rejects the clinician's valued therapeutic interventions to produce an excess of zealousness. If the patient does not accept the therapist's superficial interventions about manifest content, it is generally fruitless to proceed to latent content. Many therapists interested in the exploratory therapies tend to assign greater value to unconscious latent content than to conscious manifest psychic content. In consequence they may cite only that aspect of the ambivalent feelings of which the patient is unaware. For example, the youngster who verbally expresses love for his sibling but communicates nonverbally that he also feels significant unconscious hostility may be told by his therapist that he is *really* angry with his sibling, ignoring the patient's important conscious reality. Not only would it be far more palatable for the youngster but it would also be inestimably more accurate if he were told that, in addition to loving his sibling, he is also angry with him, which is not easy to recognize and accept.

Nurturing and maintaining a therapeutic alliance may require some education of the child regarding the process of therapy. Another educational intervention may entail assigning labels to affects that have not been part of the youngster's past experience. Rarely does therapy have to compensate for a real absence of education regarding acceptable decorum, playing games, and so on. Usually, children are in therapy not because of the absence of educational efforts but because repeated educational efforts have failed. Therefore, therapy generally does not need to include additional teaching efforts, despite the frequent temptation to offer them.

Adults' natural educational fervor with children is often accompanied by a paradoxical tendency to protect them from learning about some of life's realities. In the past, this tendency contributed to the stork's role in childbirth, the dead having taken a long trip, and similar fairy tale explanations for natural phenomena about which adults were uncomfortable in communicating with children. Although adults are more honest with children today, therapists can find themselves in situations in which their overwhelming urge to protect the hurt child may be as disadvantageous to the child as was the stork myth.

The temptation to offer oneself as a model for identification may stem also from helpful educational attitudes toward children. Although there are instances in which this may be an appropriate therapeutic strategy, therapists should not lose sight of the potential pitfalls of this apparently innocuous technique. Adolescents, with their transient identity confusions, may be particularly tempting in this regard. Many appear to need only a "big brother" or "big sister" with whom to identify. While this is certainly true at times, such an impression may conceal greater needs and conflicts.Often this becomes apparent as the therapist finds himself changing from feeling helpful and supportive to feeling angry or provoked.

Children can derive ego strength from any activity that provides gratification for achievement rather than for attention-seeking. The dependent child who, for instance, repeatedly indicates that he cannot perform a simple task, such as putting his shoes on, correctly needs to discover that there can be gratification in an accomplishment as well as in getting the assistance of an adult. Psychic growth is similarly promoted by the development of internal controls, rather than reliance on the adult's external controls, and by deriving gratification from work, as opposed to accomplishing the same tasks by cheating.

Issues Specific to Adolescence

Adolescence is, by definition, a transitional period. Its onset can, for most purposes, be arbitrarily defined as concurrent with puberty; but its end point is vague and indeterminate, shading off into whatever a particular culture defines as adulthood (Blos, 1976). Rapid and kaleidoscopic change in every sphere of life characterizes the period—physical, cognitive, affective, and social. Accordingly, techniques of psychotherapy must also vary as the adolescent progresses in the subphases of this protean and mercurial stage of growth. A developmental approach that correlates the therapeutic principles to the developmental needs and tasks of the growing person is, therefore, appropriate. The basic indications, principles, and objectives of the various therapeutic approaches—psychoanalysis, psychoanalytic psychotherapy, and supportive therapy—are the same as those outlined for adults but with significant technical nuances (see Esman, 1983).

Early Adolescence (12-14). The early adolescent is in the throes of puberty and its psychological repercussions. A major portion of the adolescent's attention, conscious or unconscious, is directed toward the bodily changes, with their exciting and frightening consequences and attendant changes in self-image and relations with parents and peers. Because of the intensity of these experiences the adolescent tends to maintain the integrity of the personality with relatively rigid defenses, relying heavily on externalization and rationalization. Profoundly self-involved, he or she tends to see adults in general, and parents in particular, as threats to the shaky sense of autonomy and as potentially seductive, since the earlier oedipal conflicts, incompletely resolved, are now reactiviated. The early adolescent tends to turn to peers, both defensively and adaptively, as sources of values and primary companionship. Cognitively, the early adolescent has not yet attained Piaget's stage of formal operational thought and thus tends to think concretely and to be present-oriented, relatively unconcerned for the future, and uninterested in the past.

For all these reasons, the early adolescent is typically difficult to engage in psychotherapy of any kind. The intense demands of psychoanalysis, even in a form more akin to child than adult approaches, will prove acceptable only to the more passive, immature patients; consequently, less intensive psychotherapies are more commonly employed. The therapist must be more active than with a typical adult patient; the young adolescent is intolerant of silences and requires a more conversational approach. Since he tends to be suspicious of adults, he is likely to engage in considerable testing, and the therapist must steer a careful line between ignoring or unconsciously sanctioning "acting out," defiant, or passive-aggressive behaviors and assuming an authoritarian role that will serve to confirm the patient's expectations. At times, where communication is difficult and resistance intense, the use of child therapy techniques, including game playing, may be necessary to maintain therapeutic contact.

The young adolescent is typically intensely involved with, curious about, and confused by his new sexual feelings, fantasies, and behaviors. He or she is rarely comfortable in talking about them with anyone. It is particularly difficult for him—and especially for her— to do so with an adult of opposite gender. Early adolescence is, therefore, one of the few situations in which there is a strong indication for taking the sex of the therapist into serious account.

Mid-Adolescence (15-17). In this period, roughly corresponding to the high school years, the rapid changes of the preceding stage have slowed and become better consolidated; the adolescent is more comfortable in his post-pubertal body. In addition, many adolescents, at least among the better educated, will have progressed cognitively into the stage of formal operational thought, which will promote their ability to think conceptually and to plan for the future. The propensity for action remains but is attenuated, and defenses are less rigid. Sexual interests are intense and experimentation is rampant, not only in behavior, but in thought, with a whole realm of values, ideals, and aims being opened up to exploration and testing. Adults are regarded with more tolerance and less suspicion, and relations with parents are generally less tumultuous in this subphase than in the earlier one (although mother-daughter relationships are still frequently stormy).

Many adolescents are more accessible to psychotherapeutic intervention at this time than formerly. They are better able to examine their behavior, to acknowledge subjective distress, and to tolerate the reduction of autonomy which is inherent in accepting the position of patient. Indeed, for the more reflective adolescents, psychoanalysis may be feasible, although for many, the enforced passivity of the supine position is still too great a threat and the analytic situation may require considerable modification from the standard adult technique.

For most, however, therapy will be experienced as a way of dealing with specific current "problems." Typically, when these acute symptoms or maladaptations have been remedied, adolescents' interest in therapy wanes and they tend to detach themselves from the therapist in favor of the various other pressing activities in their lives. Accordingly, adolescent therapy is often, perforce, a short-term situation. The therapist may be called on at times to express explicitly his views and beliefs on moral and ethical issues if the adolescent is foundering and needs support from a "neutral" figure. He must, however, avoid seeking to impose his views or adopting a judgmental stance. Adolescents have the capacity to arouse intense countertransference responses, especially where the therapist has not fully resolved his own adolescent conflicts.

Late Adolescence (18-21). By the end of high school the modal adolescent will have assumed adult roles in many aspects of his life; indeed, in most nonindustrial societies, he is expected to function fully as an adult. In our culture, with its demands for ever more advanced technical training, many remain in a phase-inappropriate dependent status and enter into what Erikson (1956) called a "psychosocial moratorium," delaying full assumption of adult status until extended educational programs are completed. Late adolescents' basic character organization (Blos, 1968) is fairly well established, however; and they are usually firmly committed to sex role identities.

Such late adolescents can, in most cases, be treated essentially as adults, with whatever modifications are required by the fact that they are rarely financially responsible for their treatment and by their geographic mobility incident on their attending colleges at some distance from their family home.

INDICATIONS AND LIMITATIONS

The present level of knowledge does not allow a simple list of indications for psychotherapy for children and adolescents. This limitation stems in part from the inadequacy of existing diagnostic classifications in both specificity and comprehensiveness. More basic, however, are the limitations to the notion that the diagnosis alone prescribes the treatment. Even the more specific and reliable diagnoses (e.g., Attention Deficit Disorder with Hyperactivity, Anorexia Nervosa) are still clusters of symptoms without linear relationships to etiology or treatment. While homogeneous in some respects, groups of children with the same diagnosis may be heterogeneous regarding the differential role of many contributing etiological factors such as neurophysiological factors, parental interaction, early psychosocial experience, cognitive capacities, family psychodynamics, psychosexual level, secondary reinforcers for maladaptive behavior, level of object relations, and capacity for a therapeutic alliance.

Even with increasing specificity, however, the prescription of psychiatric treatment, including psychotherapy, will require an assessment of factors that are independent of the diagnosis, though perhaps related. These include the global severity and temporal chronicity of symptoms, the extent to which symptoms are circumscribed or pervasive, the family's strengths and psychopathology, socioeconomic realities, the individual's psychosexual level, intrapsychic conflicts, cognitive capacity, level of object relations and capacity for a therapeutic alliance, and the contribution of neurophysiological factors. Wise clinicians currently consider these factors in assessment and treatment planning, yet their complexity makes it unlikely that there will ever be simple formulae for the prescription of treatment.

The optimal protocol for the prescription of psychotherapy may involve two levels. The first would be a consideration of the contributions of the diagnosis, using the most specific, valid diagnoses available. For instance, at our present level of knowledge, the diagnosis of Attention Deficit Disorder with Hyperactivity raises certain issues that must be addressed. There may be a neurophysiological dysfunction that may respond to medication; a structured, nonstimulating environment may enhance concentration; parents may need help with structuring and supporting the child; self concept and other internal factors should be addressed; and so on. The more specific the diagnosis, the clearer these common denominators of treatment tend to be.

The second level in the prescription of treatment would be a consideration of the cross-diagnostic factors described above—i.e., individual, family, socioeconomic, psychological, and physical factors about which a given diagnostic group may still be quite heterogeneous. For example, because the children might differ on these variables, one methylphenidate-responsive hyperkinetic child might be prescribed individual and/or family psychotherapy while another might not. In general, the factors that would suggest a trial of individual psychotherapy for a child or adolescent who has the potential for developing a therapeutic alliance are disorders of relatively long standing which are so pervasive that they impede maturational and developmental forces or induce pathogenic reactions in the environment.

Limitations for *individual* psychotherapy might include situations in which serious family pathology has designated one youngster as the "identified patient" and psychotherapeutic focus on that child would solidify the negative identity. Another might be a case in which reparative forces can be brought to bear with which psychotherapy would interfere. A difficult question is posed by situations in which the forces mobilized by individual psychotherapy might cause additional negative effects because of a precarious family equilibrium.

Certain elements in psychotherapy induce complications that militate against a particular variety of psychotherapy for a given child. For many neurotic children a form of exploratory-interpretive psychotherapy aimed at uncovering intrapsychic conflicts may be indicated. But if the youngster's ego functioning, particularly in the area of reality testing, is borderline, such an approach calls for considerable caution, lest it induce destructive ego regressions.

Psychoanalytically derived individual psychotherapy seems most applicable to youngsters who have internal, self-sustaining, neurotic conflicts that did not originate earlier than the phallic stage of development and that have resulted in circumscribed, ego alien symptoms. These clinical aggregations encompass more than symptomatic neuroses, which are relatively infrequent in childhood, as compared to the frequency with which neurotic conflicts underlie other childhood disturbances involving behavior and learning. Such expressive-exploratory-interpretive therapy is generally less helpful for those children whose disturbance has not caused them much immediate discomfort. Frequently, the syndromes are a consequence of conflict derived from prephallic phases in which the resulting disturbance tends to permeate the child's entire character structure. Psychoanalytically-oriented therapy is least applicable when the therapist cannot establish a therapeutic alliance with the child, as in those cases in which ego development has been arrested, resulting in diminished capacity for abstract thinking and object relationships.

The delineation of specific predictive diagnostic indicators to suggest when brief, focused, time-limited therapy is the treatment of choice has been handicapped by a long-standing tendency to conceive of short-term therapy as a less than desirable, unfinished fragment of what might be long-term treatment under better conditions. This bias has persisted despite well known, highly regarded reports demonstrating the value of brief therapy, some of them published 40 years ago. Among these are Allen's (1942) book and the many cases in Witmer's (1946) book reported by prominent child psychoanalysts with whom long-term intensive therapy is typically associated. Positive interest in short-term therapy, however, has been growing steadily, spurred by the theory that views crises as inevitable and as constructive opportunities rather than simply as traumatic events. This concept has been elaborated by Caplan (1964), Parad and Parad (1968), and Berlin (1970), among others.

Rosenthal and Levine (1970, 1971) and Proskauer (1969, 1971) wrote that brief therapy is of value in children with other than reactive disorders. They reported encouraging results for a wide range of difficulties in which the child possesses sufficient basic trust to develop a positive working relationship with the therapist and to perceive early termination, discussed at the beginning of therapy, as a positive growth experience rather than an abandonment. Indeed, most authors agree that time-limited, focused therapy is highly effective in helping children deal with situational crises, particularly those that entail separation or loss. This effectiveness is thought to be a consequence of the rich opportunity to rework the separation or loss in the termination phase of brief therapy, which may encompass a major portion, if not all, of time-limited therapy.

In undertaking brief therapy, the therapist is advised to formulate rapidly the child's difficulty, particularly in a family context; to define a specific dynamic focus for therapeutic intervention; and to establish specific realistic goals, such as the relief of immediate anxiety, the clarification of a conflict, the facilitation or encouragement of specific behaviors, or the maintenance of psychic balance. Obviously, the child's defenses regarding the focal issue should be sufficiently flexible so that such a focus has a constructive potential. Deeply entrenched rigid defensive operations can render brief therapy useless; and primitive brittle defenses, such as massive denial of parental divorce, may signal that brief, focused therapy will engender additional primitive defenses or leave the child vulnerable to major ego disruption. In other words, brief therapy requires active recognition of the child's and the family's strengths and weaknesses. There are distinct advantages in having the family participate by consciously endeavoring to change behavior and in having the family continue at home, with the therapist's guidance, discussions of certain issues raised in therapy. Increasingly, the family's participation in the therapeutic sessions has been used to advantage in short-term crisis intervention.

Therapeutic intervention requires a capacity for effective problem solving in complex situations. The problem is usually multidimensional, with mixed causes, and with the unique idiosyncratic features of the child or the family always present. As a bio-psycho-social synthesis, a child suffering from a disturbance in one aspect of his integrated human system often experiences it as being reflected in other parts of the system. Thus, the system manifesting the most disturbance is not necessarily the one in which the basic problem resides. Consequently, clinicians are inevitably faced with the interesting challenge of systemic interrelationships that demand multifaceted therapeutic modes.

PROFESSIONAL, ETHICAL, AND LEGAL ISSUES

Therapist's Use of Self. Sometimes the same clinician treats a child with individual exploratory psychotherapy, undertakes a combination of parent counseling and personal psychotherapy with the parents, and engages the entire family in focal family therapy. Such a regimen requires a degree of dexterity in the clinician's use of self which may not be within the capacity of all therapists. It is incumbent upon clinicians to be cognizant of their capabilities and limitations in this regard. Despite all the advances in psychopharmacology and in the therapeutic use of behavioral, social, milieu, and other external agents and instruments, the clinician's personality remains a potent and important psychodiagnostic and psychotherapeutic instrument. Consequently, this type of clinical work encompasses individualistic styles of practice requiring the clinician to achieve a considerable degree of self-understanding, self-realization, and self-actualization as a vehicle for sensitivity, empathy, and intuition. This use of self calls for a change in the detached approach model that characterizes most other types of medical practice. In addition, using different clinical approaches tends to require further differentiation in the therapeutic use of the self.

Many psychodynamically-oriented approaches postulate that the patient changes by cognitive-affective re-experiencing of the introjected past. This re-experiencing takes place in the course of a special kind of encounter with the therapist. To achieve it, the clinician is taught to keep personal reactions under control while observing his own internal process. The goal is to discriminate between objective professional reactions, reactions stemming from his own past, and reactions stimulated by the patient. Meanwhile, the patient is encouraged to look at himself, to explore the past, and to study its effect on the present. The result is a deep and powerful interaction that can approach aspects of the religious-magical contact between shaman and client (Frank, 1973). It places enormous demands on the therapist, who, in a sense, experiences the patient through himself as though the therapist were a part of the other's phenomenology.

A systems orientation and the related social intervention modes, such as family therapy, postulate that change stems from the therapist's affiliation with the family or other social system. He uses his relationship to alter individual roles in the dysfunctional transactional processes of the family and in its total structural organization. Therefore, the clinician is usually taught not to guard against spontaneous personal responses. It is assumed that those responses will be system syntonic; even if they are not, however, they can serve as valuable exploratory probes, contributing to the establishment of an affiliation with the family and experiencing its pressures.

Parents. Psychotherapy with children is characterized by the need for parental involvement. This involvement does not necessarily reflect parental culpability for the youngster's emotional difficulties but is a reality of the child's dependent state. This fact cannot be stressed too much because of what would be considered an occupational hazard shared by many who work with children. This hazard is the motivation to rescue children from the negative influence of their parents, sometimes related to an unconscious competitive desire to be a better parent than the child's or the clinician's own parents.

In practice, there are varying degrees of parental involvement in child psychotherapy. With preschool-aged children, the entire therapeutic effort may be directed toward the parents, without any direct treatment of the child (Furman, 1957). At the other extreme, children can be seen in psychotherapy without any parental involvement beyond the payment of fees and perhaps transporting the child to the therapeutic sessions. Most therapists agree that only relatively rare neurotic children who have reached the oedipal phase of development can sustain therapy by themselves. Even in such instances, however, most practitioners prefer to maintain an informative alliance with the parents for the minimal purpose of obtaining additional information about the child.

Probably the most frequent arrangements are those that were developed in child guidance clinics—that is, parent guidance focused on the child or on the parent-child interaction or therapy for the parents' own individual needs concurrent with the child's therapy. The parents may be seen by the child's therapist or by someone else. In recent years there have been increasing efforts to shift the focus from the child as the primary patient to the concept of the child as the family's emissary to the clinic. In such family therapy all or selected members of the family are treated simultaneously as a family group. Although the preferences of specific clinics or practitioners for either an individual or family therapeutic approach may be unavoidable, the final decision as to which therapeutic strategy or combination to use should be derived from the clinical assessment.

Sensitivity to the relationship of adolescents with their parents is critical. Adolescence poses certain developmental tasks for parents and families as well as for adolescents, and these can be critical pathogenic or healing forces. Adults, including therapists, tend to think stereotypically about adolescents as excessively aggressive, sexual, or in need of nurturance and may project their own concerns and conflicts onto the developing adolescent (Anthony, 1970). Adolescents, in turn, are willing recipients of such projections and stereotypes, often finding great power in their ability either to frustrate or to exceed adults' wildest expectations. These projections may be potent in the shaping of the adolescent's identity (Zinner and Shapiro, 1972).

It is rare that an adolescent referred for treatment fails to show some manifestations of his difficulties within the context of the family. Frequently, rebellious behavior conflict with parents or between parents is a major presenting issue. Parents are frequently frustrated and baffled about their child's behavior, and failures in communication are often blatant. It is important, indeed often essential, for the therapist to address these family issues; but discriminating judgment must be used in developing the appropriate mode for doing so. In cases where such conflict seems to be the dominant feature, formal family therapy may be indicated as the primary mode of treatment. In others, however, where internalized pathology is clear, occasional family sessions directed at specific conflicts can be usefully interspersed with individual sessions. In no case is it desirable for an adolescent's therapist to meet separately with parents without the patient's knowledge and assent; and the commitment to confidentiality is normally treated as a one-way rule; i.e., the therapist does not communicate the adolescent's revelations to the parents, but he is free to tell the patient what the parents discuss with him.

Confidentiality. Consideration of parental involvement likewise highlights the confidentiality question in psychotherapy with children. There are advantages to creating an atmosphere in which the child can feel that his words and actions will be viewed by the therapist as simultaneously serious and tentative. In other words, the child's communications do not bind him to a commitment; nevertheless, they are too important to be communicated to a third party without the patient's permission. Although such an attitude may be conveyed implicitly, there are occasions in which it is wise to discuss confidentiality explicitly with the child. It can be risky to promise a child that the therapist will not tell parents what transpires in therapeutic sessions. Although the therapist may have no intention of disclosing such data to the parents, the bulk of what children do and say in psychotherapy is common knowledge to the parents. Therefore, should the child be so motivated, it is easy for him to manipulate the situation to produce circumstantial evidence that the therapist has betrayed his confidence. Accordingly, if confidentiality requires specific discussion during treatment, the therapist may not want to go beyond indicating that he is not in the business of telling parents what goes on in therapy, as his role is to understand children and to help them.

It is also important to try to enlist the parents' cooperation in respecting the privacy of the child's therapeutic sessions. This respect is not always readily honored, as parents quite naturally are not only curious about what transpires but may also be threatened by the therapist's apparently privileged position (Burlingham, 1935).

Routinely reporting to children, especially older children and adolescents, the essence of all communications with third parties regarding the child underscores the therapist's reliability and respect for the child's autonomy. In certain types of treatment, this report may be combined with soliciting the child's guesses about those transactions. Also, it may be fruitful to invite children, particularly older children and adolescents, to participate in discussions about them with third parties.

FINANCIAL, LEGAL, AND SOCIO-POLITICAL ISSUES

The adolescent is rarely in a position to assume financial responsibility for his own treatment. As a result, he is dependent on parents and/or third-party payors; and the communication between the therapist and these authorities is often a matter of considerable delicacy and complexity. This may be particularly true where the patient and his family are concerned—often legitimately so—about the consequences of revealing to such institutions as schools, colleges, employers, and insurance companies the fact that the adolescent is receiving psychiatric treatment. The situation may be all the more sensitive when the adolescent is involved in delinquent or even criminal activities such as drug dealing. At times, such illicit behaviors may pose a threat to the treatment; the therapist may be confronted with difficult ethical choices and may at times be drawn into complex medical-legal situations. Consultation with colleagues is often in order in such circumstances.

Although the recent legal reassessment of the traditional parental right and responsibility to speak on behalf of their children's therapeutic needs has tended to focus on cross-sibling organ transplantations and hospitalization of the severely mentally ill or retarded, both the legal and the dynamic issues involved appear to be pertinent to psychotherapy. The pendulum is swinging from yesteryear's extreme of the courts' reliance on the psychotherapeutic professions to care for all troubled children to the apparently opposite position of legally protecting children from psychotherapeutic ministrations by questioning and overruling parental decisions. Recently some state legislatures have enacted statutes formalizing the traditional common law permitting emancipated minors living apart from parents and managing their own affairs to consent to medical care of all types.

Although legislatures and courts are not granting children younger than 12 years old the right to speak for themselves in therapeutic matters, their parents' rights to do so are increasingly being limited. This limitation has taken the form of the interposition of third parties empowered either to replace the parents as decision makers or to review parental decisions. The most evident effect has been on the parents' and guardians' traditional right to seek hospitalization for their disturbed children. Thus far, the major effect in outpatient psychotherapy has been on the nebulous issue of who is the rightful owner of the therapist's recorded notes and who should have access to them.

Whether that right of access pertains to the child patient, to his parents, or to both remains an uncertainty. That uncertainty is not confined to the legal issues; the developmental lines regarding the child's and the adolescent's expanding rights to privacy and to independent decision making have been insufficiently explored and explicated in all contexts (Guyer et al., 1982).

The right of adolescents to object to hospitalization has become a major part of the process of inpatient treatment. While this may in some cases frustrate parents' legitimate attempts to obtain treatment for their adolescent children, at times it can provide a forum for working through issues of dependency. Another legal area, beyond the scope of this report, is that of adolescent status offenders. While the involvement of the legal system may pose considerable problems, often it is critical in bringing to treatment an adolescent who has been dealing with conflicts in an externalized, alloplastic manner. While such therapy ostensibly may be involuntary, legal involvement (e.g., probation requiring psychotherapy) may provide an adolescent with a face-saving way to develop a therapeutic relationship.

REFERENCES

Aichhorn A: Wayward Youth. New York, Viking Press, 1948

Allen FH: Psychotherapy with Children. New York, WW Norton & Co, 1942

Anthony EJ: The reactions of parents to adolescents and to their behavior, in Parenthood. Edited by Anthony EJ, Benedek T. Boston, Little, Brown & Co, 1970

Aronson G: Panel report: learning theory and psychoanalytic theory. J Am Psychoanal Assoc 20:622-637, 1972

Berkovitz I: Adolescents Grow in Groups. New York, Brunner/Mazel, 1972

Berlin IN: Crisis intervention and short-term therapy. J Am Acad Child Psychiatry 9:595, 1970

Blom GE: A psychoanalytic viewpoint of behavior modification in clinical and educational settings. J Am Acad Child Psychiatry 11:675-693, 1972

Blos P: When and how does adolescence end? Adolesc Psychiatry 5:5-17, 1976

Blos P: Character formation in adolescence. Psychoanal Study Child 23:245-263, 1968

Bornstein B: Clinical notes on child analysis. Psychoanal Study Child 1:151-166, 1945

Brody S: Aims and methods in child psychotherapy. J Am Acad Child Psychiatry 3:385-412, 1964

Bruch H: Island in the river: the adolescent in treatment. Adolesc Psychiatry 7:26-40, 1979

Burlingham DT: Child analysis and the mother. Psychoanal Q 4:69–92, 1935

Caplan G: Principles of Preventive Psychiatry. New York, Basic Books, 1964

Dollard J, Miller N: Personality and Psychotherapy. New York, McGraw-Hill, 1950

Erikson E: The problem of ego identity. J Am Psychoanal. Assoc 4:56-121, 1956

Erikson EH: Childhood and Society. New York, WW Norton & Co, 1950

Esman A: The Psychiatric Treatment of Adolescents. New York, International Universities Press, 1983

Eysenck HJ: Behavior Therapy and the Neuroses: Readings in Modern Methods of Treatment Derived from Learning Theory. London, Pergamon Press, 1960

Ferenczi S: A little Chanticleer, in Contributions to Psychoanalysis, vol 1. New York, Robert Brunner, 1950

Fraiberg S: A comparison of the analytic method in two stages of child analysis. J Am Acad Child Psychiatry 4:387, 1965

Frank JD: Persuasion and Healing: A Comparative Study of Psychotherapy. Baltimore, Johns Hopkins University Press, 1973

Freud A: Normality and Pathology in Childhood. New York, International Universities Press, 1965

Freud A: Indication for child analysis. Psychoanal Study Child 1:127-149, 1945

Freud A: Introduction to the Technique of Child Analysis: Nervous and Mental Disease, Monograph 48. New York, Nervous and Mental Diseases Publishing Company, 1929

Freud S: Fragment of the analysis of a case of hysteria, in Complete Psychological Works of Sigmund Freud, vol 7, standard ed. Edited by Strachey J. London, Hogarth Press, 1955

Furman E: Treatment of under-fives by way of their parents. Psychoanal Study Child 12:250, 1957

Gardner RA: Therapeutic Communication with Children; the Mutual Storytelling Technique. New York, Science House, 1971

Gesell A: The Embryology of Behavior. New York, Harper & Row, 1945

Guyer MJ, Harrison SI, Rieveschl JL: Developmental rights to privacy and independent decision making. J Am Acad Child Psychiatry 21:298-302, 1982

Harrison SI: Symbiotic infantile psychosis: observation of an acute episode, in Separation-Individuation: Essays in Honor of Margaret S Mahler. Edited by McDevitt JB, Settlage CF. New York, International Universities Press, 1971

Itard J-MG: The Wild Boy of Aveyron. Edited by Humphrey G, Humphrey M. New York, Appleton-Century-Crofts, 1962

Jones MC: The elimination of children's fears. J Exp Psychol 7:302, 1924

Kessler JW: Psychopathology of Childhood. Englewood Cliffs, NJ, Prentice-Hall, 1966

Klein M: Personification in the play of children. Intl J Psychoanal 10, 1929

Klein M: The Psychoanalysis of Children. London, Hogarth Press, 1932

Kohlberg L: The development of children's orientation toward a moral order: sequence in the development of moral thought. Vita Humana 6:11-33,1963

Kramer CH: Psychoanalytically Oriented Family Therapy: Ten-Year Evolution in a Private Child Psychiatry Practice. Chicago, Family Institute of Chicago, 1968

Laufer M: Adolescent Disturbance and Breakdown. London, Penguin Books, 1975

Lehrer P, Schiff L, Kris A: Operant conditioning in a comprehensive treatment program for adolescents. Arch Gen Psychiatry 25:515-521, 1971

Levy D: Trends in therapy, III: release therapy. Am J Orthopsychiatry 9:713-736, 1939

Levy J: Relationship therapy. Am J Orthopsychiatry 8:64-69, 1938

Malone CA: Observations on the role of family therapy in child psychiatry training. J Am Acad Child Psychiatry 13:437, 1974

Marohn RC, Dalle-Molle D, McCarter E, et al: Juvenile Delinquents: Psychodynamic Assessment and Hospital Treatment. New York, Brunner/Mazel, 1980

Masterson J: Treatment of the Borderline Adolescent: A Developmental Approach. New York, Wiley-Interscience, 1972

McDermott JF, Char WF: The undeclared war between child and family therapy. J Am Acad Child Psychiatry 13:422-436, 1974

Montalvo B, Haley J: In defense of child therapy. Fam Process 12:227, 1973

Mowrer OH: Learning Theory and Personality Dynamics. New York, Ronald Press, 1950

Noshpitz JD: The psychotherapist in residential treatment, in Healing Through Living: Symposium on Residential Care. Edited by Mayer MF, Blum A. Springfield, Ill, Charles C Thomas, 1971

Parad LG, Parad HJ: A study of crisis-oriented planned short-term treatment. Social Casework 49:418-426, 1968

Piaget S: The stages of the intellectual development in the child, in Childhood Psychopathology. Edited by Harrison SI, McDermott JF. New York, International Universities Press, 1972

Proskauer S: Focused time-limited psychotherapy with children. J Am Acad Child Psychiatry 10:619-639, 1971

Proskauer S: Some technical issues in time-limited psychotherapy with children. J Am Acad Child Psychiatry 8:154-169, 1969

Rapaport D: The theory of ego autonomy, in The Collected Papers of David Rapaport. Edited by Gill MM. New York, Basic Books, 1967

Rosenthal AJ, Levine SV: Brief psychotherapy with children: a preliminary report. Am J Psychiatry 127:646-651, 1970

Rosenthal AJ, Levine SV: Brief psychotherapy with children: process of therapy. Am J Psychiatry 128:141-146, 1971

Thomas A, Chess S, Birch H: Temperament and Behavior Disorders in Children. New York, New York University Press, 1968

von Hug-Hellmuth H: On the technique of child analysis. Int J Psychoanal 2:287, 19

Watson JB, Raynot R: Conditioned emotional reactions. J Exp Psychol 3:1, 19

Werner H: Comparative Psychology of Mental Development. New York, International Universities Press, 1957

Williams F: Family therapy: its role in adolescent psychiatry. Adolesc Psychiatry 2:324-339, 1973

Winnicott DW: The squiggle technique, in Psychiatric Treatment of the Child. Edited by McDermott JF, Harrison SI. New York, Jason Aronson, 1977

Witmer HL: Psychiatric Interviews with Children. New York, Commonwealth, 1946

Zinner J, Shapiro R: Projective identification as a mode of perception and behavior in families of adolescents. Int J Psychoanal 53:523-530, 1972

Disorder Specific and
Manual Based Psychotherapies

The next two psychotherapies described—interpersonal psychotherapy (IPT) and cognitive therapy—have several features in common. Both treatments are short-term, were developed specifically for depressed patients, are explicit about the relationship between theory and clinical practice, and are specified in treatment manuals for efficacy research. Both have been tested in at least two randomized clinical trials against a pharmacotherapy and a no-treatment control group and have been included in the NIMH Treatment of Depression Collaborative Research Program taking place at the University of Pittsburgh, the University of Oklahoma, and George Washington University (Waskow et al., 1980).

Efficacy studies of pharmacotherapy have a long history of using well defined protocols; multiple outcome criteria; independent treatment evaluators; and randomized, controlled clinical trials as crucial elements of the research design. These methods have been incorporated into the NIMH study, which is the first multi-site collaborative study of psychotherapy. Two additional features, which have enhanced the ability of researchers to test the efficacy of psychotherapy, also have been incorporated into the study. These are:

A. The use of treatment manuals that specify the main techniques and procedures for the psychotherapy and guide the therapists during training; and

B. The use of standardized training programs on manual-specified procedures of the psychotherapy, which increases consistency among therapists in the psychotherapy being tested.

The treatment manuals developed for psychotherapy outcome studies specify identifying characteristics of the psychotherapy, including the tasks and their sequence. The tasks are explicitly described through both definition and case example. Training programs are used to transmit and further explain the information in the manual and to provide supervised clinical practicum experiences for participating psychotherapists. The training programs developed for psychotherapy outcome studies are not designed to teach the inexperienced therapist how to become a therapist. Training to become a psychotherapist involves the learning of fundamental skills such as empathy, handling of transference, etc. and is extensive in time (a minimum of two years) and intensive in depth. Training experienced psychotherapists to participate in outcome studies, on the other hand, is a brief process designed to modify the practices of fully trained and competent psychotherapists to conduct the psychotherapy under study as specified in the manual. The development of a shared language and specified procedures in an agreed-upon sequence is a major focus.

The certification criteria used in these training programs are based on the goals and tasks outlined in the treatment manual. Through the viewing of videotapes of the trainees' psychotherapy sessions, several independent evaluators determine whether the therapists have met competence criteria and can be certified to participate in the clinical trial.

Treatment manuals have a long history. As reviewed by Luborsky et al. (1982), the first manuals were designed by behavior therapists. It was their ability to specify interventions (such as implosion, desensitization, etc.) with great precision which gave impetus to the field. The first nonbehaviorally-oriented treatment manual (supportive-expressive psychoanalytically-oriented psychotherapy) was developed by Luborsky.*

The development of treatment manuals and training programs for outcome studies is a burgeoning field. Several other psychotherapies, both for depression and for other disorders, have been developed and specified in manuals (Luborsky et al., 1982). In fact, treatment manuals are applicable not just to psychotherapy. Fawcett and Epstein have developed comparable manuals and training programs for pharmacotherapy as it is being used in the NIMH Collaborative Study as a standard reference condition against which to compare interpersonal therapy and cognitive therapy (Waskow et al., 1980).

Many psychotherapies would be amenable to both specification and testing. The availability of treatment manuals and standardized training programs does not necessarily mean that the treatment is efficacious or that it should be endorsed. Treatment manuals and training procedures are a

---

* Luborsky L: A general manual for supportive-expressive psychoanalytically oriented psychotherapy, unpublished manuscript, 1976 (Available from Piersol Building, Room 203, Hospital of University of Pennsylvania, 36th and Spruce Streets, Philadelphia, PA 19104)

necessary requirement for enhancing the consistency and reliability of the treatment procedure under study; they do not ensure its validity.

The field of psychotherapy research has made major advances in testing efficacy. Regardless of the final results of the collaborative study, the specification of psychotherapy in manuals, as a basis for training, will have an impact on clinical training and practice.

REFERENCES

Luborsky L, Woody GE, McLellan AT, et al: Can independent judges recognize different psychotherapies? An experience with manual-guided therapies. J Consult Clin Psychol 50:49-62, 1982

Waskow IE, Hadley SW, Autry JH, et al: NIMH Treatment of Depression Research Program (Pilot Phase), Revised Research Plan. Rockville, Md, Psychosocial Treatment Research Branch, National Institute of Mental Health, Jan 1980

Interpersonal Therapy

INTRODUCTION

The history of attempts to understand depression in an interpersonal context is a long one, and some clinical descriptions of interpersonal psychotherapeutic approaches have been excellent. Arieti and Bemporad (1979) have contributed the most recent description of an interpersonal understanding of depression. Their therapy, as well as that of others, has usually been long-term and aimed at personality as well as symptom change.

Interpersonal psychotherapy (IPT) differs from previous treatment approaches in four ways:

A. It is short-term (12 to 16 weeks).

B. It is oriented toward symptom relief and resolution of the immediate interpersonal difficulties and not toward personality change.

C. Its efficacy is being tested in controlled clinical trials.

D. Its techniques and methods have been specified in a manual.

Short-term interpersonal psychotherapy (IPT) is a brief (12 to 16 week) psychological treatment that focuses on current social and interpersonal difficulties in ambulatory, non-bipolar, nonpsychotic, depressed patients. IPT is based on the assumption that depression, regardless of symptom patterns, severity, biological vulnerability, or personality traits, occurs in an interpersonal context and that clarifying and renegotiating the context associated with the onset of symptoms is important to the person's recovery and possibly to the prevention of further episodes.

IPT is designed so that it may be used alone or in conjunction with pharmacologic agents. IPT has evolved over nearly 15 years from the experience of the New Haven-Boston Collaborative Depression Project. Variants of IPT have been tested by this group as it has evolved in two clinical trials of depressed patients, one of maintenance therapy (Klerman et al., 1974; Weissman et al., 1974) and one of acute treatment (Weissman et al., 1979; DiMascio et al., 1979a; Weissman et al., 1981). IPT has been tested with and without the addition of a tricyclic antidepressant. In 1980 a further testing of IPT in comparison with cognitive therapy and a tricyclic antidepressant was begun in a collaborative clinical trial sponsored by the National Institute of Mental Health (NIMH, 1980).

The concepts, techniques, and strategies of IPT have been specified in a procedural manual (Klerman et al., 1984), which was developed as a training tool so that further refinement of the procedures and replication of the efficacy studies could be undertaken. A program for the training of experienced therapists of differing disciplines has been developed at Yale (Weissman et al., 1982; Chevron et al., 1983).

IPT was designed to fill a gap in the field, in which the only therapies that have been sufficiently specified in procedural manuals to enable serious replication trials have been those based on cognitive (Lewinsohn et al., 1976) and behavioral approaches (Weissman and Paykel, 1974). In contrast, IPT is based on interpersonal approaches, as will be described.

A variety of treatments may be suitable for depression. The depressed patient's interests are best served by the availability and scientific testing of different psychological as well as pharmacologic treatments, which can be used alone or in combination. The ultimate aim of these studies is to determine which treatments are best for particular subgroups of depressed patients. This chapter will briefly describe the conceptual framework and goals of IPT and will summarize the efficacy data available thus far.

THEORETICAL AND EMPIRICAL ISSUES

IPT derives from a number of theoretical and empirical sources. (The full details and references are outlined in the IPT book [Klerman et al., 1984]). The most prominent source is Adolph Meyer, whose psychobiological approach to understanding psychiatric disorders placed great emphasis on the patient's psychosocial environment. Meyer viewed psychiatric disorders as an expression of the patient's attempt to adapt to that environment. An individual's response to environmental change and stress is determined by prior experiences, particularly early experiences in the family and the individual's affiliation with various social groups. Among Meyer's associates, Harry Stack Sullivan stands out for his theory on interpersonal relationships and for his writings linking clinical psychiatry to the emerging social sciences.

The empirical basis for understanding and treating depression with IPT includes studies associating stress and life events with the onset of depression; longitudinal studies demonstrating the social impairment of depressed women during the acute depressive phase and following symptomatic recovery; recent studies by Brown et al. (1975) which demonstrate the role of intimacy and social supports as protections against depression in the face of life stress; the studies of Pearlin and Lieberman (1977) and Ilfield (1977), which show the impact of chronic social and interpersonal stress, particularly marital stress, on the onset of depression; and finally, the works of Bowlby (1969) and, more recently, Henderson et al. (1978), which emphasize the importance of attachment bonds or, alternately, show that loss of social attachments can be associated with the onset of depression.

Goals and Focus of IPT for Depression

Depression may be seen as involving three components:

Symptom formation, involving the development of depressive affect and vegetative signs and symptoms, which may derive from psychobiological and/or psychodynamic mechanisms;

Social adjustment and interpersonal relations, involving social interactions with other persons which derive from learning based on childhood experiences, concurrent social reinforcement, and/or current personal mastery and competence;

Personality, involving more enduring traits and behaviors, i.e., the handling of anger and guilt and overall self-esteem, which constitute the person's unique reactions and patterns of functioning and which also may contribute to a predisposition to manifest symptom episodes.

IPT attempts to intervene in the first two processes. Because of the brevity of the treatment, the low level of psychotherapeutic intensity, and the focus on the context of the current depressive episode, no claim is made that IPT will have an impact on the enduring aspects of personality, although personality functioning is assessed.

IPT focuses on:
- The patient's immediate "here and now" problems,
- The patient's current important social and interpersonal relations,
- Engagement of the patient in an evaluation of himself and his current situation, and
- Assistance for the patient in mastering the current situation by clarify-

ing and modifying the current interpersonal relationships and/or by changing maladaptive perceptions.

These goals are achieved by finding solutions to existing interpersonal disputes. Little attention is given to uncovering deeply unconscious, conflicted areas; developing a transference; relating current problems to early childhood developmental antecedents; and reconstructing the patient's personality.

IPT strategies were developed to deal specifically with the acute depressive syndrome and four interpersonal problem areas often associated with the onset of depression—grief, role disputes, role transitions, and interpersonal deficits (Klerman et al., 1984).

EFFICACY DATA

IPT has evolved and become increasingly more specified on the basis of two trials that have been completed by the New Haven-Boston Collaborative Depression Project.

IPT as Maintenance Treatment

Description of Study. The first study, begun in 1967, was an eight-month maintenance trial of 150 women who were treated for six to eight weeks with a tricyclic antidepressant (amitriptyline) and were recovering from an acute depressive episode. Criteria for entrance into the study of acute treatment were definite depression of at least two weeks' duration and of sufficient intensity to reach a total score of seven or more on the Raskin Depression Scale (range 3-15). Most of the patients (88 percent) were diagnosed as having a neurotic depression according to *DSM-II*.

This study tested the efficacy of IPT (administered weekly by experienced psychiatric social workers) in comparison with low therapist contact (brief monthly visits for assessment) with either amitriptyline, placebo, or no pill, using random assignment in a 2 x 3 factorial design. The full design, methodology, and results have been reported elsewhere (Klerman et al., 1974; Weissman et al., 1974).

Results. The findings showed that maintenance IPT as compared with low contact had no significant differential impact on prevention of relapse or symptom return. However, IPT significantly enhanced social and interpersonal functioning for patients who did not relapse. IPT's effects on social functioning, assessed by the Social Adjustment Scale (Weissman et al., 1974; Spitzer et al., 1978), took six to eight months to become statistically apparent. Patients receiving IPT as compared to low contact were significantly less impaired in work performance, with the extended family, and in marriage. The overall mean of the assessed social adjustment items reflected

Table 1. IPT Effects on Social Adjustment After 8 Months of Maintenance Treatment in Depressed Patients who did not Relapse

Social Adjustment Means[1]	Low Contact	IPT	F-Value
Work	1.7	1.5	5.3*
Social and Leisure	2.3	2.1	1.6
Extended Family	1.7	1.5	5.2*
Marital	2.3	2.0	2.9[+]
Parental	1.8	1.7	0.5
Family Unit	1.8	1.7	1.1
OVERALL ADJUSTMENT	2.0	1.8	7.2**
RATER'S GLOBAL ASSESSMENT	3.4	2.9	5.0*

[1]All means are adjusted for initial level. The scale for all roles is 1-5, except for the global evaluation which is 1-7. In all cases, higher score means more impairment.
[+]$p = < .10$
*$p = < .05$
**$p = < .01$

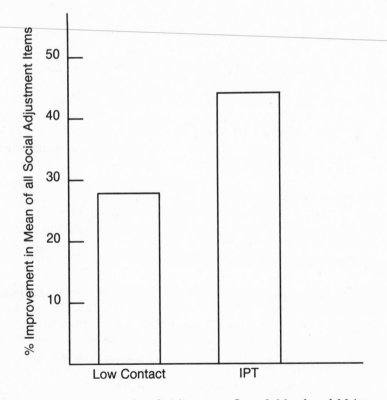

Figure 1. Improvement in Social Adjustment Over 8 Months of Maintenance Treatment

these differences between groups, as did the rater's overall evaluation of the patient (Table 1). The percentage of improvement on social adjustment was substantially greater in the IPT group (44 percent) as contrasted with the low-contact group (28 percent) (Figure 1).

The maintenance study had several problems. First, the sample of depressed patients, while all women, was not diagnostically homogeneous. In 1967, the new research diagnostic approaches, which included operationalized diagnostic criteria and systematic methods for collecting information on signs and symptoms to make these diagnoses, were not available (DiMascio et al., 1979a). The diagnostic criteria most often used for depressed patients were *DSM-II* accompanied by a symptom severity measure.

The psychotherapy was described in terms of conceptual framework, goals, frequency of contact, and criteria for therapists' suitability (Weissman et al., 1974). However, the IPT techniques and strategies had not been set out in a procedural manual. Finally, the maintenance study was not the best design for testing the efficacy of a psychological treatment. Patients who entered maintenance treatment were all drug responders, and the IPT did not begin until the patient had had at least four weeks of drug treatment. Having already established a therapeutic relationship with the psychiatrist who was not administering IPT, the patients were not acutely depressed at the point of randomization to the social worker for IPT treatment.

IPT as Acute Treatment

Description of Study. In 1973, a 16-week study of the acute treatment of ambulatory depressed patients, both men and women, was initiated using IPT and amitriptyline, each alone and in combination against a nonscheduled psychotherapy treatment. IPT was administered weekly by experienced psychiatrists. Eighty-one patients entered the study and accepted the randomized treatment assignment. On the basis of the experience in the maintenance study, changes were incorporated into this acute treatment study which resulted in a better design for testing psychotherapy in a clinical trial.

By 1973, the SADS-RDC were available for making more precise diagnostic judgments, thereby allowing the inclusion of a more homogeneous sample of depressed patients. Based on the SADS-RDC approach, the inclusion criteria were non-bipolar, nonpsychotic, ambulatory patients who were experiencing an acute primary, major depression of sufficient intensity to reach a score of at least 7 on the Raskin Depression Scale.

A procedural manual for IPT was developed (Klerman et al., 1984). Patients were assigned randomly to IPT or the control treatment at the beginning of treatment, which was limited to 16 weeks since this was an acute and not a maintenance treatment trial. Patients were followed up one year after treatment had ended to determine any long-term treatment effects. The assessment of outcome was made by a clinical evaluator who was independent of and blind to the treatment the patient was receiving. The full details of this study have been described elsewhere (Weissman et al., 1979; DiMascio et al., 1979b; Weissman et al., 1981).

The control treatment for IPT was nonscheduled psychotherapy in which patients were assigned to a psychiatrist whom they were told to contact whenever they felt a need for treatment. No active treatment was scheduled for these patients; but they could call for an appointment if their needs were of sufficient intensity, and a 50-minute session (a maximum of one a month) would then be scheduled. Patients who were still symptomatic and required further treatment (Raskin 9 or over) after eight weeks or whose clinical condition worsened sufficiently to require other treatment were considered failures of this treatment and were withdrawn from the study. This procedure served as an ethically feasible control for psychotherapy in that it allowed a patient to receive periodic supportive help "on demand."

Results. Figure 2 summarizes the results of the study using lifetime calculations and demonstrates that the probability of symptomatic failure over 16 weeks was significantly lower with IPT as compared with nonscheduled treatment. The results were upheld using other symptom outcome measures, including both self-report and clinical ratings (DiMascio et al., 1979b).

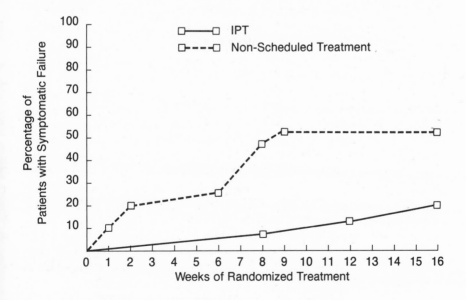

Figure 2. Life Table Calculations of the Product-Limit Estimate of Symptomatic Failure Time

Table 2. IPT Effects on Social Adjustment One Year After Acute Treatment for Depression

Social Adjustment Means[1]	Non-Scheduled Treatment	IPT	F-Value
Work	1.5	1.5	.1
Social and Leisure	1.9	1.7	3.6*
Extended Family	1.7	1.6	.6
Marital	1.3	1.4	.09
Parental	1.5	0.9	3.1*
Family Unit	2.1	1.4	9.0**
OVERALL ADJUSTMENT	1.7	1.5	2.6
RATER'S GLOBAL EVALUATIONS	2.9	2.5	3.1+

[1]All means are adjusted for initial level. The scale for all roles is 1-5, except for the global evaluation which is 1-7. In all cases, higher score means more impairment.
+$p = < .10$
*$p = < .05$
**$p = < .01$

As noted earlier, differential effects of IPT on patients' social functioning were not found at the end of four months of maintenance treatment but took six to eight months to develop. Similarly, in the acute treatment study, which ended at four months, no differential effects of IPT on social functioning were found. However, at one-year follow-up, patients who had received IPT, in comparison to those who had not, were functioning at a less impaired level in social activities, as parents, and in the family unit; and this difference was reflected in the rater's global assessment (Weissman et al., 1981) (Table 2).

CONCLUSION

In addition to the use of randomized treatment assignment and independent blind clinical assessments of outcome, the work described here has attempted to incorporate two important methodologic advances for clinical trials of psychotherapy: operationalized and defined diagnostic criteria to allow for relatively homogeneous patient groups and operationalized and defined psychotherapeutic procedures to facilitate comparability of goals and focus between therapists and to allow replication. IPT has now been further refined based on new experience since these studies were completed; the IPT approach is now ready for replication studies outside of the New Haven-Boston centers.

Substantively, two collaborative clinical trials demonstrated (a) the efficacy of maintenance IPT in enhancing social functioning in recovering depressed patients and (b) the efficacy of IPT in reducing symptoms and improving social functioning in acute depressives. The effects on social functioning take at least six to eight months to become apparent. These findings are consistent with the general concept of IPT.

As yet, the studies of IPT, as well as of cognitive therapy, i.e., therapies developed specifically for depressed patients, are based on relatively small samples. Moreover, the therapeutic trials have been conducted at the centers where the therapies were developed. The results must be replicated elsewhere before definitive conclusions can be drawn. The National Institute of Mental Health, Clinical Research Branch, has initiated a multi-site collaborative study of cognitive therapy, IPT, and imipramine in nonpsychotic, non-bipolar, ambulatory depressed patients (Waskow, 1980). This study will be critical in providing answers about the short- and long-term differential effects of the various treatments for some types of depression. The study has other important features: First, it includes large samples pooled from three research sites; second, the therapists from each site have received uniform training in the psychotherapy method by its developers; finally, the therapies are being tested in sites other than those where the methods were originally developed. An 18-month follow-up of patients is included.

Pending the results of this important study, there are now some general guidelines as to the treatment of acutely depressed patients which suggest the value of both tricyclic antidepressants and psychotherapy because of the differential effects that each of these treatments seems to have on both the type and the timing of response.

REFERENCES

Arieti S, Bemporad J: Severe-Mild Depression: The Psychotherapeutic Approach. New York, Basic Books, 1979

Bowlby J: Attachment and Loss. London, Hogarth Press, 1969

Brown G, Bhrokhain M, Harris T: Social class and psychiatric disturbance among women in an urban population. Sociology 9:225-254, 1975

Chevron E, Rounsaville B, Prusoff B, et al: Selecting psychotherapists to participate in psychotherapy outcome studies: a pilot training program. J Nerv Ment Dis 171:348-353, 1983

DiMascio A, Klerman GL, Weissman MM, et al: A control group for psychotherapy research in acute depression: one solution to ethical and methodological issues. J Psychiatr Res 15:189-197, 1979a

DiMascio A, Weissman MM, Prusoff BA, et al: Differential symptom reduction by drugs and psychotherapy in acute depression. Arch Gen Psychiatry 36:1450-1456, 1979b

Henderson S, Byrne DG, Duncan-Jones P, et al: Social bonds in the epidemiology of neurosis. Br J Psychiatry 132:463-466, 1978

Ilfeld FW: Current social stressors and symptoms of depression. Am J Psychiatry 134:161-166, 1977

Klerman GL, DiMascio A, Weissman M, et al: Treatment of depression by drugs and psychotherapy. Am J Psychiatry 131:186-191, 1974

Klerman GL, Weissman MM, Rounsaville BJ, et al: Interpersonal Psychotherapy of Depression. New York, Basic Books, 1984

Lewinsohn P, Biglan A, Zeiss A: Behavioral treatment of depression, in The Behavioral Management of Anxiety, Depression and Pain. Edited by Davidson P. New York, Brunner/Mazel, 1976

Pearlin LI, Lieberman MA: Social sources of emotional distress, in Research in Community and Mental Health. Edited by Simmons R. Greenwich, Ct, JAI Press, 1977

Spitzer RL, Endicott J, Robins E: Research diagnostic criteria: rationale and reliability. Arch Gen Psychiatry 35:773-785, 1978

Waskow IE: NIMH Treatment of Depression Collaborative Research Program (Pilot Phase) Revised Research Plan. Rockville, Md, Psychosocial Treatments Research Branch, NIMH 1980

Weissman MM, Klerman GL, Paykel ES, et al: Treatment effects on the social adjustment of depressed patients. Arch Gen Psychiatry 30:771-778, 1974

Weissman MM, Klerman GL, Prusoff BA, et al: Depressed outpatients: results one year after treatment with drugs and/or interpersonal psychotherapy. Arch Gen Psychiatry 38:51-55, 1981

Weissman MM, Prusoff BA, DiMascio A, et al: The efficacy of drugs and psychotherapy in the treatment of acute depressive episodes. Am J Psychiatry 136 (4B):555-558, 1979

Weissman MM, Rounsaville BJ, Chevron ES: Training psychotherapists to participate in psychotherapy outcome studies: identifying and dealing with the research requirements. Am J Psychiatry 139:1442-1446, 1982

Weissman MM, Paykel ES: The Depressed Woman: A Study of Social Relationships. Chicago, University of Chicago Press, 1974

Cognitive Therapy

INTRODUCTION

Cognitive therapy as it applies to various psychiatric disorders has been the subject of several reviews in recent years (Beck, 1976; Rush, 1982). Cognitive therapy is usually defined as a short-term psychotherapy aimed at specific target conditions or symptoms. These symptoms are used as clues by which to define specific cognitions (verbal thoughts or pictorial images) and assumptions or schemata that, according to the theory, account for both the symptomatic state and the psychological vulnerability to that state. According to cognitive theory, negative cognitions play a pivotal role in the development and/or maintenance of the psychopathological state. Thus, the initial objectives of this treatment are to teach the patient to recognize and record these cognitions; thereafter, the patient learns to evaluate objectively and modify such thinking patterns. This initial phase of treatment aims at symptom reduction.

The second half of therapy focuses on the identification and subsequent modification of specific assumptions or dysfunctional attitudes that are inferred from the patient's stereotyped thinking and behavioral patterns. These schemata are values or notions that derive from early life experiences and that support the cognitions or moment-to-moment thinking patterns. These schemata are viewed as highly related to vulnerability to future recurrence. Thus, this psychotherapeutic approach aims at symptom reduction, prophylaxis, and treatment of the underlying problem.

Discussion will focus on the cognitive approach to the affective disorders in order to illustrate basic points. However, this treatment has been used clinically with a variety of nonpsychotic psychiatric conditions. Research to document indications, limitations, and acute and prophylactic effects is ongoing.

HISTORICAL BACKGROUND

Cognitive therapy derives from the so-called "phenomenological" approach to psychology. The philosophical basis for this approach has been described in detail (Spiegelberg, 1971, 1972). The phenomenological emphasis assigns a central role to an individual's view of himself and the world as determinants of behavior—a notion initially proposed by Greek Stoic philosophers. Alfred Adler emphasized the idea that each person lives in a personal conceptualization or representation of the objective world (Ansbacher and Ansbacher, 1956). The profusion of stimuli that bombard us is immediately organized, conceptualized, and given meaning based on our individual and very personal prior experiences. Adler termed this constructed representation of objective reality the "phenomenal field." The phenomenal field is a construct that is used to explain why different people respond differently to the same event or series of events. For example, moving to a new city may be seen as a loss by some and as an adventure by others. Thus, it is not things in themselves but the views that we take of things which upset or please us.

In the twentieth century, the phenomenological emphasis apparently arose in part from dissatisfaction with unconscious motivation as a system sufficient to explain and predict various behaviors. Generally speaking, unconscious motivation is inferred from a behavior or series of behaviors by examining the results of the behavioral sequence. The clinician assumes that the consequences of the behavior express or make apparent the individual's unconscious wishes and desires. Thus, if the person denies that he actually desires the end products of a behavioral sequence, the testimony may be discounted.

If the consequences of a behavior constitute the *sole* basis for inferring unconscious motivations, diagnostic errors may result. For instance, one may erroneously infer an unconscious desire from a behavioral consequence that the individual actually neither desired nor foresaw. Motivational inferences that rely *exclusively* on the consequences of a behavior assume (a) that the patient can make anything happen which he wants, (b) that nothing happens that he does not want, and (c) that he can consciously or unconsciously foresee all the consequences of any particular behavioral sequence before undertaking it. Obviously, these assumptions are rarely applicable to everyday situations.

On the other hand, the cognitive perspective assumes that a person chooses those options that are in his own best interest, based on his particular, albeit idiosyncratic, view of things. Not only are these views *rarely* objective, they are often highly biased in a stereotyped fashion. Thus, self-defeating behaviors ensue not from a desire to lose, for example, but from the patient's inability either to conceive of or to act upon and carry out more constructive alternative plans of action.

Initially, the cognitive therapist clarifies how the patient views things (that is, how he conceptualizes and gives meaning to particular events): What are the bases for these views? Are they accurate? To what behaviors and feelings do these views lead? For instance, a depressed person often fails to undertake specified measures that might relieve his depression, not because he wants to suffer (one of several possible unconscious motivational assumptions) but because he does not conceive of undertaking particular steps to reduce the depression or does not believe that any action will result in relief. On the other hand, the patient may not believe he can successfully undertake these steps. If a patient is convinced that corrective actions are unavailable or doomed to failure, this conviction logically leads to a decision not to try.

Beck (1963, 1976) has emphasized the critical role that cognitions (conscious verbal or pictorial mental activity) and assumptions or beliefs play in stereotyped repetitive "neurotic" behavior. Recently, ego psychoanalytic (Klein, 1970), neobehavioral (Mahoney, 1974; Meichenbaum, 1977), and cognitive psychological (Kelley, 1955; Ellis, 1962) movements have added impetus to this emphasis on cognition.

A cognitive explanatory system allows for a significant degree of direct empirical testing of many of the presumed determinants of behavior. If a patient's view of events leads to particular responses, and if this view is consciously available to him, then the relationship between this view and observed behaviors can be evaluated. Thus, a cognitive perspective appears to permit greater empirical testing than does a strictly unconscious motivational explanation of behavior. Indeed, cognitive theory is supported by various kinds of empirical data (for a review see Beck and Rush, 1978).

In some instances, however, this empirical attraction may be more apparent than real. People are notorious for making up explanations for what, in fact, they literally find themselves doing, as evidenced by split-brain studies (Gazzaniga and Ledoux, 1978). While they may truthfully report how they conceive of a particular event, this conceptualization may not be formulated until the person is asked to shape his view. Thus, some conceptualizations may be retrospectively and inaccurately deduced. In addition, specific conceptualizations may be influenced by the perceived "demands" in specific situations, by what has transpired since the conceptualization occurred, by the relationship between the interviewer and conceptualizer, etc. These difficulties may be overcome only with improved methods of measuring cognitions and beliefs.

THEORETICAL ISSUES

Cognitive therapy is a generic term that refers to a variety of psychotherapeutic techniques that are applied within a theoretical perspective. These techniques are designed to accomplish the following specific objectives: (a) Patients are taught to become aware of the views that they take of various events, particularly upsetting events (i.e., the therapist leads the patient to recognize and examine his "phenomenal" field). (b) Patients learn to assess, reality-test, and correct these views (i.e., patients learn to make a better match of objective reality with particular meanings attributed to specific events). Thus, stereotyped perceptions are identified and corrected. (c) Patients learn to identify specific silent assumptions or beliefs by inferring these general rules or assumptions from what they say and think in various situations. These general rules are not conscious thoughts or behaviors. Rather, they are the premises by which a person weighs, encodes, and gives meaning to specific events. (d) Patients practice various cognitive and behavioral responses to anticipated and unusual stresses. (e) Finally, new assumptions are generated and applied to actual and anticipated circumstances.

The therapist acts as a guide. The data of therapy consist of cognitions or thoughts, as well as behaviors and feelings, which the patient records or reports. Both experiences within the therapeutic relationship and data provided by the patient about his ongoing interpersonal relationships are used to teach the patient to recognize and correct stereotyped, biased thinking and self-defeating behavioral patterns.

Cognitive therapy is designed to provide both symptom reduction and prophylaxis. According to cognitive theory, the former objective is met by learning to identify and correct biased cognitive patterns, the interpretations that are given to moment to moment events. Prophylaxis is believed to follow from learning to identify and change maladaptive assumptions or beliefs.

The relationship among cognitions, schemata, and logical errors—the three critical elements in cognitive theory—deserves further comment. Cognitions are thoughts or images that are available to consciousness. They are immediate, nearly automatic ideas to which each person is subject when confronted with any stimulus condition. Their content reflects the meaning an individual gives to an event. They are not what a person thinks *about* a situation; rather, they are what a person thinks to himself *in* a situation. These cognitions are closely tied to and are said to account for both the feeling(s) raised and the behavior(s) displayed in the situation.

Depressed persons have negatively biased views of themselves, their world, and their future (Beck, 1976; Beck and Rush, 1978; Rush and Beck, 1978a,b). Empirical data support this contention (Beck and Rush, 1978; Rush et al., 1982). Schemas are assumptions or beliefs derived from early experience which direct the person to attend to certain events, ignore others, and to value or encode these events in particular ways. Thus, schemas account for cognitions. A careful logical analysis of a series of cognitions leads to a rule that can be inferred. This rule is typically an "if . . . , then . . . " statement. This statement is a premise that is not thought by the patient but that guides the patient's thinking. For example, "If I am not loved and valued by others, my life has no meaning," might constitute such a rule.

A depressed person is said to endorse a variety of such illogical notions. Thus, when an event that might often lead to transient dysphoria (e.g., breaking up with a loved one or the death of a spouse) occurs, the person who bases his happiness and self-worth on attention from a single other person will develop a depressive syndrome that exceeds normal dysphoria. When such a schema is activated, it begins to influence how the person thinks about other analogous events (e.g., a friend's forgetting to call at a specific time). Notions such as, "I am generally unlovable," or, "My life has no meaning," begin to enter consciousness. Events that are otherwise neutral in content are construed as further evidence that these negative notions are, in fact, true. For example, being ignored by a salesperson in a department store may stimulate such thoughts as, "No one cares about me," or, "I'll never get what I want." Silent assumptions both direct the content of cognitions and account for vulnerability to recurrence of depressive episodes.

Logical errors are seen when one examines the relationship between cognitions and the associated events. Consider the above case. When the

Table 1. A Synopsis of Beck's Cognitive Theory[1]

A. Cognitions
1. Consist of thoughts and images
2. Reflect unrealistically negative views of self, world, and future
3. Based on schemata
4. Reinforced by current interpretations of events
5. Explain symptoms of depressive syndrome
6. Covary with severity of depression
7. Logical errors occur in cognitions that are negatively distorted

B. Schemata (silent assumptions)
1. Consist of unspoken, inflexible assumptions or beliefs
2. Result from past (early) experience
3. Form basis for screening, discriminating, weighing, and encoding stimuli
4. Form basis for categorizing, evaluating experiences, and making judgments and distorting actual experience
5. Determine the content of cognitions formed in situations and the affective response to them
6. Increase vulnerability to relapse

[1]From Beck (1976)

friend does *not* call, although he promised to do so, the event is a non-event; that is, nothing at all actually happened. Furthermore, the patient's thought, "My life has no meaning," is unrelated to the non-event. This *arbitrary inference* is a conclusion drawn on insufficient evidence. The thought, "I'll never get what I want," is an *overgeneralization* from the current frustrating circumstance. Other errors include *personalization*, that is, giving personal meaning to a neutral event; *magnification*; and *selective attention* (specifically, ignoring the positive aspects of a situation, etc.). These logical errors are *consequences*, not causes, of negatively biased thinking (Rush and Beck, 1978a,b).

Table 1 summarizes the relationships among cognitions, assumptions, and logical errors. Table 2 provides examples of cognitions or automatic thoughts taken from the Automatic Thoughts Questionnaire (Hollon and Kendall, 1980). Table 3 provides examples of dysfunctional attitudes derived from the Dysfunctional Attitudes Scale (Weissman, 1979).

The therapist selects specific cognitive techniques, depending on the degree and type of psychopathology present (Beck et al., 1979; Rush, 1980). For example, the therapist provides greater structure, direction, and guidance to more severely depressed patients who are less able to think objectively. Typically, therapy begins with techniques that focus on behavioral monitoring and change. These techniques are often simple and are designed to provide patients with success experiences. Subsequently, task assignments are given to provide stimuli for the collection and later correction of cognitions.

Table 2. Examples of Cognitions from the Automatic Thoughts Questionnaire[1]

1. I feel like I'm up against the world.
2. I'm no good.
3. Why can't I ever succeed?
4. No one understands me.
5. I've let people down.
6. I don't think I can go on.
7. I wish I were a better person.
8. I'm so weak.
9. My life's not going the way I want it to.
10. I'm so disappointed in myself.
11. Nothing feels good any more.
12. I can't stand this any more.
13. I can't get started.

[1]Hollon and Kendall (1980)

Table 3. Sample Items from Dysfunctional Attitude Scale[1]

It is difficult to be happy unless one is good looking, intelligent, rich, and creative

Happiness is more a matter of my attitude toward myself than the way other people feel about me

People will probably think less of me if I make a mistake

If I do not do well all the time, people will not respect me

Taking even a small risk is foolish because the loss is likely to be a disaster

It is possible to gain another person's respect without being especially talented at anything

I cannot be happy unless most people I know admire me

If a person asks for help, it is a sign of weakness

[1]Weissman, AW (1979)

Table 4. Behavioral Techniques

Activity scheduling
Mastery and pleasure ratings
Graded task assignment
Cognitive rehearsal
Assertive training/role playing
Mood graph

Table 5. Cognitive Techniques

Recording automatic thoughts (cognitions)
Reattribution techniques
Responding to negative cognitions
Counting automatic thoughts
Identifying assumptions
Modifying shoulds
Pro-con refutation of assumptions
Homework to test old assumptions
Homework to test new assumptions

The homework assignments are critical to treatment. These assignments are created to help the patient (a) develop objectivity about situations that otherwise are stereotypically misconstrued, (b) identify underlying assumptions, and (c) develop and test alternative conceptualizations and guiding assumptions.

Table 4 lists some of the behaviorally-oriented techniques while Table 5 lists some of the techniques aimed at changing cognitions or beliefs. This list of techniques is not exhaustive (Beck et al., 1979). In fact, an experienced cognitive therapist will design homework assignments for each individual patient in each session depending on the cognitive and behavioral targets to be addressed.

To illustrate one technique, consider the Graded Task Assignment (Beck et al., 1979; Rush and Beck, 1978a,b). A very depressed woman might state that she is unable to do her housework. The therapist takes this general statement and converts it into a specific series of activities that are encompassed in the patient's version of the term "housework." Assume that the patient proffers that she cannot vacuum the rooms, empty the wastebaskets, do the wash, and clean the bathrooms. Each of these components is further broken down into smaller steps (e.g., plugging in the vacuum cleaner, doing the living room, the stairs, etc.). The therapist then asks the patient to supply evidence to support the notion that she "can't do" each step. The patient is urged to specify precisely what is meant by "I can't do it." Does the patient believe that she cannot find the vacuum cleaner, has insufficient energy to vacuum, will not do it as thoroughly as she would like, etc.? Next, the patient is encouraged to undertake one step at a time to determine whether the anticipated difficulties are actually encountered and to elicit the specific thoughts that occur while she tries to accomplish each step. Typically, these thoughts are either self-critical (e.g., "I'm not doing it correctly, fast enough," etc.) or anticipate failure (e.g., "I'll never do this well enough," or, "It will be dirty before I finish the house."). Using a dialogue, the therapist points out partial successes, helps the patient to realize that she is anticipating negative events before they occur, and provides reassurance for undertaking what the patient perceives as a difficult task.

Once the first task is completed, a second, more complex task is designed; and the same process is followed. The patient is asked to verbalize her anticipations about each step, her thinking during the task, and her thoughts after she has completed the task. This method provides for repeated identification and correction of negatively biased thinking. Furthermore, a carefully designed hierarchy of tasks which is successfully completed may begin to provide the patient with a series of experiences that contradict long-held notions about being personally defective, helpless, incompetent, and worthless. The therapist functions as an objective, independent, nonjudgmental source of information. This role is often essential to counteract the depressed patient's tendency to discount, neglect, or minimize successes, or otherwise misjudge herself.

The Graded Task Assignment is only one of many techniques that constitute cognitive therapy. Both behavioral and cognitive techniques can provide methods for elucidating and modifying cognitions and assumptions. As the patient reports his thinking patterns in specific situations, the therapist helps him to reappraise each situation objectively, to recognize specific logical errors in his thinking (e.g., personalization, selective attention), to identify recurrent silent assumptions, and to modify these stereotyped thinking patterns and unrealistic or rigid beliefs.

The therapeutic relationship must be carefully attended to in this form of therapy (Beck et al., 1979; Rush, 1980, 1982). In fact, cognitive therapy (at least when kept to a maximum of 20 sessions) has definite limitations for patients who have difficulty forming a working alliance within a short period of time (e.g., borderline patients). The therapist must be both empathetic and objective. He must be able to think as the patient does, to understand both the cognitive and emotional responses of the patient, and to see the world as the patient does. In addition, he must remain objective about the events reported and logical and objective about the patient's thinking.

Depressed patients are notorious for overpersonalizing interactions with others. When the therapist identifies and points out negatively biased thinking, many patients may feel as if they are being attacked. As one patient put it, "When I came here, I thought I had just a depression. Now you tell me I can't think straight either." Great tact is required in helping patients to become objective about their views.

In order to develop a collaborative alliance, a great deal of time is spent introducing the patient to the rationale for treatment. A brief pamphlet, *Coping with Depression* (Beck and Greenberg, 1974), is used as part of this introduction. In addition, patients are strongly encouraged to point out when they feel criticized or attacked during a session. Each session begins with a review of the patient's responses to the previous session, and each session is reviewed before the patient is dismissed.

Negative transference is dealt with through a cognitive framework (Beck, 1976; Beck et al., 1979; Rush, 1980). The patient's views of the therapist, the therapy, or specific transactions in the session which were associated with increased dysphoria are elicited, evaluated collaboratively, and considered objectively.

While Tables 4 and 5 suggest that the various techniques can be divided conceptually into those with a primary focus on changing behavior and those with a primary focus on changing cognitions and/or assumptions, this dichotomy is artificial. Actually, behavioral assignments are often used to elicit cognitions in specific situations. For example, by recording activities actually undertaken and by rating the senses of mastery (M) and pleasure (P) derived from each, the patient collects data that help the therapist to select particular targets for the session to follow. The therapist selects activities that sound likely to give a nondepressed person a sense of mastery and pleasure yet are not associated with such feelings by the depressed patient. An inquiry into the cognitions surrounding such an activity typically leads to recollection of negatively biased thinking. For example, a patient who applied wallpaper to a neighbor's kitchen reported absolutely no sense of either mastery or pleasure. The thoughts that surrounded this event focused on how poorly he felt he had done the job and how he had ruined the kitchen as a result. Further discussion, along with an independent report by his wife about the quality of the work and the neighbor's sense of gratitude, eventually led to the discovery of this patient's perfectionistic assumptions such as, "If I don't do the job perfectly, it doesn't count at all" (Rush et al., 1975a).

Similarly, techniques designed to elicit or change cognitions or beliefs often involve carrying out specific behaviors. For example, a shy, insecure, 26-year-old single man reported having difficulty meeting women at various singles bars. His assignment was to engage three different women in conversations that were not to exceed five minutes in length and to record his cognitions before the event as well as after it. Only by carrying out the feared behavior could the patient compare his dire predictions with the actual events and correct his cognitive distortions. In general, experiential testing of cognitions and beliefs, that is, carrying out actual assignments or behaviors, appears to be more powerful in both eliciting and changing cognitions or assumptions than is intellectual, logical discussion. The latter is more useful in preparing and persuading patients to try such experiments.

Members of the patient's social system (spouse, friend, etc.) can be especially useful in certain situations (Rush et al., 1980). Such persons can be engaged to promote compliance with homework, to provide independent views of events to which the patient is reacting, and eventually to cue the patient when he appears to be making erroneous assumptions or coloring new information with a negative bias. Finally, cognitive therapy can be used with groups, couples, or individuals (Rush and Watkins, 1981).

CLINICAL ISSUES

Indications

Cognitive therapy has been applied to a variety of psychopathological conditions (e.g., major nonpsychotic, unipolar depressions, generalized anxiety disorders, phobic disorders, obesity, alcoholism, drug dependency, chronic pain, and others). The specific techniques differ depending on the condition to be treated and on the phase of therapy. Cognitive theory (Beck, 1976) predicts the kinds of thinking patterns encountered with each disorder. For example, anxious patients frequently perceive danger in situations that are not dangerous, while depressed patients often see evidence for personal defect in situations that offer no objective reasons for self deprecation. Paranoid patients may misconstrue situations in terms of being gypped or attacked. Cognitive theory also suggests that specific beliefs are more commonly found in certain disorders. For example, the need for love, approval, and/or success is likely to underlie negatively biased thinking in depression.

With several exceptions (Khatami and Rush, 1978, 1982), there are few empirical data to document the efficacy of this approach except in depression. The available outcome studies in depression suggest that patients who are particularly suitable for cognitive therapy are mildly to moderately depressed, unipolar, nonpsychotic persons with a capacity for establishing a working alliance in a short period of time. These patients appear most likely to obtain significant symptom reduction in ten weeks of treatment. Chronic depressions are *not* more responsive and may be less responsive than more acute disorders (Rush et al., 1978c). Depressions with melancholic features (APA, 1980) have not been systematically evaluated.

It is controversial whether those patients with endogenous features according to the Research Diagnostic Criteria (Spitzer et al., 1978) will respond to cognitive therapy (Kovacs et al., 1981; Blackburn and Bishop, 1981). While the answer to this question awaits further research, the clinician is well advised *not* to use cognitive therapy alone in such patients in order to obtain symptom reduction. On the other hand, we must remember that symptom reduction is *not* the only objective of cognitive or other psychotherapies. The evidence for the prophylactic utility of cognitive therapy is reviewed below.

It is conceivable that some patients may reach a better level of interepisode recovery because of cognitive therapy even if antidepressant medications are essential for initial symptom reduction. For example, consider a patient who has endured three episodes of major depression with substantial but not total interepisode recovery. Assume further that the patient has obtained almost full symptomatic remission with amitriptyline. The patient has still been depressed a good deal of time in the recent past. Might this experience not have affected his view of himself, his sense of competence, and his view of things around him? Such a patient might profit from a short course (five to ten weeks) of cognitive therapy to help him become more objective about both himself and his illness. Thus, cognitive therapy may be indicated in a patient who requires antidepressants for symptom reduction and/or prophylaxis but who also needs to relearn or unlearn specific self-defeating views or notions that either preceded or arose in conjunction with the symptomatic manifestations of the depression.

Limitations

While Beck et al. (1979) caution that many depressed patients may require medication or may not respond to cognitive therapy, specific limitations to this treatment are yet to be identified. Clinical experience suggests that patients with impaired reality testing (e.g., hallucinations, delusions), impaired reasoning abilities or memory function (e.g., organic brain syndromes), those with borderline personality structures, and those with schizoaffective disorder will not respond to this treatment (Rush, 1980, 1982; Beck et al., 1979). Whether patients with antisocial personalities with

major depression or other forms of secondary depressions will respond to
cognitive therapy is yet to be established empirically. However, clinical
experience suggests that many secondary depressions will respond.

The clinical experience of several cognitive therapists suggests that major
depressions that accompany medical disorders, but *are not biologically
caused* by such disorders, may respond rapidly to cognitive therapy, especially with patients who do not have a history of pre-existing psychopathology. For example, patients with their first myocardial infarction, with some
forms of cancer, and/or with physical injuries that require marked psychological readjustments (e.g., blindness, loss of limb) may profit from this
approach.

One apparent limitation of cognitive therapy has been suggested based
on a subtype of depression, namely, endogenous depression with associated dexamethasone nonsuppression (Carroll et al., 1981). In one study, five
such patients with severe endogenous depressions and dexamethasone
nonsuppression all failed to respond at all to cognitive therapy alone.
Perhaps in the future specific biological measures will help to identify
responders and nonresponders to cognitive or other psychotherapies.

Most patients who ultimately respond well, in terms of acute symptom
reduction, will do so within five to seven weeks of twice-weekly treatment
with cognitive therapy alone; others may have a more gradual response. If
50 percent symptom reduction by Hamilton Rating Scale (Hamilton, 1960)
or Beck Depression Inventory (Beck et al., 1961) is *not* achieved by 14
sessions, the treatment plan should be revised.

No reports of adverse reactions to cognitive therapy have as yet been
made. Adverse reactions may be difficult to differentiate from lack of
efficacy. For instance, suicide attempts, as well as premature terminations,
may be evidence of either adverse reactions or lack of efficacy. Two studies
(McLean and Hakstian, 1979; Rush et al., 1977) found that cognitive
behavioral methods were associated with a significantly lower premature
dropout rate than antidepressant pharmacotherapy alone, while a more
recent report (Blackburn and Bishop, 1981) did not replicate these findings.
One might suspect that the structured, planned, directive nature of this
approach helps retain depressed outpatients. If so, cognitive therapy might
be particularly useful in outpatients of low socioeconomic class, whose
dropout rate from psychotherapy is particularly high (Rush and Watkins,
1980).

Few data are available to evaluate the relationship between the frequency
of treatment sessions and outcome. Only one pilot study* has found that for
moderately/severely depressed outpatients, twice-weekly treatment was
associated with a lower dropout rate and better symptom reduction than

* Rush AJ, Beck AT, Kovacs M, et al: A comparison of cognitive and pharmacotherapy in
depressed outpatients: a preliminary report. Presented at Society for Psychotherapy Research,
Boston, Mass, June 1975

was once-a-week treatment. However, treatment assignment was *not* randomized in this study. This preliminary report and clinical experience suggest that once-a-week treatment may be sufficient for mild to moderately depressed patients, whereas sessions twice a week are indicated for the more severely depressed.

Maintenance treatment may consist of "booster" sessions once or twice a month for six to 12 months after a course of more intensive once- or twice-weekly treatment is completed. The effect of maintenance treatment has not been empirically evaluated.

DEVELOPMENTAL AND AGE RELATED ISSUES

Cognitive therapy can be applied to all adults and is likely to be of value in adolescents, although empirical studies of teenagers are not available. Whether the parts of this treatment which require less capacity for abstract thought would be effective in children is unknown.

PROFESSIONAL AND ETHICAL ISSUES

While cognitive therapy appears to be "simple," great skill is required in applying the basic techniques, and supervised training is needed to learn many of its more complex aspects. In addition, medical and psychiatric diagnostic evaluations are essential before placing a patient in this form of treatment since some types of depressions, anxiety disorders, and other psychiatric syndromes may be caused by undiagnosed medical conditions or may best be treated with medication.

The nature, type, and length of training required to learn this approach are being studied through an NIMH collaborative study. At least four closely supervised cases seem to constitute the minimum clinical experience necessary to learn cognitive therapy techniques. Co-therapists can be used in a group or family format with ease. There is no experience with co-therapists for individual patients.

RESEARCH AND EVALUATION

Cognitive therapy has been most thoroughly assessed in nonpsychotic, non-bipolar depressed outpatients. While many studies have been conducted on "depressed college student volunteers," several recent trials have been carried out on psychiatric patients. Tables 6 and 7 summarize studies with patients treated individually and in a group format, respectively.

There are no predictors as to which patients are best suited for cognitive

Table 6. Individual Therapy—Clinic Patients

Study	Measures	Treatment	Sessions Number/Weeks		Results
Schmickley (1976)	BDI, MMPI (N = 11)	1. cognitive modification	4	2	Within-sub. Improvement
Rush et al. (1977)	BDI, HRSD (N = 41)	1. CT 2. Imipramine	20	11	CT>Imipramine
Beck et al. (1979)	BDI, HRSD (N = 26)	1. CT 2. CT + amitriptyline (A)	20	12	CT = CT + A
McLean and Hakstian* (1979)	BDI, DACL (N = 154)	1. amitriptyline (A) 2. relaxation tg (RT) 3. BC 4. insight (I)	10	10	BC>A = RT I
Blackburn et al. (1981)	BDI, HRSD (N = 64)	1. CT 2. medication 3. combination	16-17,	12-15	Hosp. Clinic: Comb>CT=Med Gen. Practice: CT=Comb>Med

BDI—Beck Depression Inventory
HRSD—Hamilton Rating Scale for Depression
DACL—Depression Adjective Checklist
CT—cognitive therapy
A—amitriptyline

BC—behavioral cognitive therapy
I—insight therapy
med—medication
comb—combination

*Included community volunteers and clinic patients.

therapy alone, medication alone, or the combination. Endogenous symptoms have *not* been correlated with a poor response to cognitive therapy (Kovacs et al., 1981; Blackburn and Bishop, 1981). Further studies are needed to identify the specific indications for cognitive therapy or the combined approach. Rush et al. (1982) found that cognitive therapy had a more pervasive and significant impact on self-concept than did amitriptyline by the end of treatment. In addition, cognitive therapy resulted in a greater reduction in hopelessness compared to medication. While chemotherapy did reduce hopelessness by the end of treatment, it had little effect on self-concept dimensions. While these findings require replication, they suggest that cognitive therapy more profoundly improves patients' views of themselves and their future than does chemotherapy. Furthermore, cognitive therapy differs from imipramine in the timing of its effects on particular symptoms (Rush et al., 1981). Specifically, views of self and future appear to improve *prior to* other symptom groups (e.g., motivational, vegetative) during cognitive therapy. This finding is consistent with predictions from cognitive theory.

Does cognitive therapy provide prophylaxis? Only one study has exam-

Table 7. Group Therapy—Clinic Patients

Study	Measures	Treatment	Sessions Number/Weeks		Results
Rush and Watkins (1980)	BDI, HRSD (N = 39)	1. group CT (GC) 2. ind. CT (IC) 3. ind. CT + medication	10	10-12	GC<IC=IC+meds
McDonald (1978)	BDI, DACL (N = 28)	1. cog mod + day care (CM + DC) 2. day care (DC)	12	4	Improved but CM+DC=DC
Magers (1978)	BDI, MMPI TSCS (N = 18)	1. CB 2. WLC	6	6	CB>WLC
Shaw* (1977)	BDI, HRSD (N = 32)	1. cog mod (CM) 2. behav mod (BM) 3. nondirective (ND) 4. WLC	6	3	CM>BM CM>ND BM=ND Each>WLC
Morris (1975)	BDI, HRSD (N = 51)	1. cog mod (CM) 2. insight group 3. WLC	6	3	CM>Insight Each>WLC

BDI—Beck Depression Inventory
HRSD—Hamilton Rating Scale for Depression
CT—cognitive therapy
GC—group cognitive therapy
IC—individual cognitive therapy
CM—cognitive modification

DC—day care
CB—cognitive behavioral therapy
WLC—waiting-list control
BM—behavior modification
ND—nondirective treatment

*Student Health Clinic Patients

ined this question (Kovacs et al., 1981). Subjects treated with cognitive therapy alone (n=18) or imipramine without cognitive therapy (n=17) were followed monthly for one year after active treatment was terminated. Both patient groups maintained the overall symptomatic gains made during active treatment throughout the follow-up. The imipramine treated group had twice the "risk of relapse" during follow-up, although this between-group difference did not reach statistical significance.

It is not clear which of the various techniques included in the cognitive therapy treatment program account for the treatment effects. What does the relationship itself contribute to the process over and above providing a medium for applying specific techniques? Do the homework assignments actually contribute to efficacy? Only one study (Shaw, 1977) suggests that both cognitive and behavioral components significantly contribute to a positive outcome. If further research can identify specific "active ingredients," then the treatment package itself might be revised to improve both efficiency and specificity in selected patients.

While research data provide some general guidelines about patient selection, the clinician is confronted with individualized decisions: when to attempt cognitive therapy, when to discontinue it, and when to supplement it with medication. Clinical impressions and some new research data may help in these complex decisions.

Those inpatients with the most marked cognitive distortions, as assessed by responses to a card-sorting task, appear to do better with cognitive therapy (Shaw, 1980). However, the overall effect of the treatment was less impressive than published outpatient studies. Another recent report (Rush et al., 1982) suggests that outpatients with unipolar, nonpsychotic major depressions can be subdivided into three groups based on the dexamethasone suppression test (DST) and the sleep EEG: those with neither DST nonsuppression nor reduced REM latency, those with both abnormalities, and those with only reduced REM latency. Whether these groups differ in their responsiveness to cognitive therapy has not yet been fully evaluated. However, with antidepressant pharmacotherapy, those with one or both biological derangements did significantly better with antidepressant pharmacotherapy than those with neither derangement (Rush, 1983).

While many questions remain for cognitive as well as for other psychotherapies, a growing body of data suggest that this therapy is effective for some types of depression. Additional research is needed to clarify the specific indications, limitations, active ingredients, and adverse reactions to this treatment approach.

REFERENCES

Ansbacher HL, Ansbacher RR (eds): The Individual Psychology of Alfred Adler: A Systematic Presentation in Selections from His Writing. New York, Basic Books, 1956

Beck AT, Rush AJ, Shaw BF, et al: Cognitive Therapy of Depression. New York, Guilford, 1979

Beck AT, Ward CH, Mendelson, M, et al: An inventory for measuring depression. Arch Gen Psychiatry 4:561-571, 1961

Beck AT, Greenberg RL: Coping with Depression. Philadelphia, Center for Cognitive Therapy, University of Pennsylvania, 1974

Beck AT, Rush AJ: Cognitive approaches to depression and suicide, in Cognitive Defects in Development of Mental Illness. Edited by Serban G. New York, Brunner/Mazel, 1978

Beck AT: Cognitive Therapy and the Emotional Disorders. New York, International Universities Press, 1976

Beck AT: Thinking and depression, I: idiosyncratic content and cognitive distortion. Arch Gen Psychiatry, 9:324-333, 1963

Blackburn I, Bishop S: Is there an alternative to drugs in the treatment of depressed ambulatory patients? Behavioral Psychotherapy 9:96-104, 1981

Carroll BJ, Feinberg M, Greden JF, et al: A specific laboratory test for the diagnosis of melancholia. Arch Gen Psychiatry 38:15-22, 1981

Diagnostic and Statistical Manual of Mental Disorders, Third Edition, Washington DC, American Psychiatric Association, 1980

Ellis A: Reason and Emotion in Psychotherapy, Secaucus, NJ, Lyle Steward, 1962

Gazzaniga MS, Ledoux J (eds): The Integrated Mind. New York, Plenum, 1978

Hamilton M: A rating scale for depression. Neurol Neurosurg Psychiatry 12:56-62, 1960

Hollon SD, Kendall PC: Cognitive self-statements in depression: development of an automatic thoughts questionnaire. Cognitive Therapy and Research 4:383-395, 1980

Kelley GA: The Psychology of Personal Constructs. New York, WW Norton & Co, 1955

Khatami M, Rush AJ: One year followup of multimodal treatment of chronic pain. Pain 14:45-52, 1982

Khatami M, Rush AJ: A pilot study of the treatment of outpatients with chronic pain: symptom control, stimulus control, and social system intervention. Pain 5:163-172, 1978

Klein GS: Perception, Motives and Personality. New York, Alfred A Knopf, 1970

Kovacs M, Rush AJ, Beck AT, et al: Depressed outpatients treated with cognitive therapy or pharmacotherapy: a one-year followup. Arch Gen Psychiatry 38:33-39, 1981

Mahoney JJ: Cognition and Behavior Modification. Cambridge, Mass, Ballinger, 1974

McLean PD, Hakstian AR: Clinical depression: comparative efficacy of outpatient treatments. J Consult Clin Psychol 47:818-836, 1979

Meichenbaum D: Cognitive-Behavior Modification. New York, Plenum, 1977

Rush AJ, Kovacs M, Beck AT, et al: Differential effects of cognitive therapy and pharmacotherapy on depressive symptoms. J Affective Disord 3:221-229, 1981

Rush AJ, Beck AT, Kovacs M, et al: Comparative efficacy of cognitive therapy and pharmacotherapy in the treatment of depressed outpatients. Cognitive Therapy and Research 1:17-37, 1977

Rush AJ, Giles DE, Roffwarg HP, et al: Sleep EEG and dexamethasone suppression test findings in outpatients with unipolar major depressive disorders. Biol Psychiatry 17:327-341, 1982

Rush AJ, Hollon SD, Beck AT, et al: Depression: must pharmacotherapy fail for cognitive therapy to succeed? Cognitive Therapy and Research 2:199-206, 1978c

Rush AJ, Khatami M, Beck AT: Cognitive and behavior therapy in chronic depression. Behavior Therapy 6:698-404, 1975a

Rush AJ, Shaw B, Khatami M: Cognitive therapy of depression: utilizing the couples system. Cognitive Therapy and Research 4:103-113, 1980

Rush AJ, Beck AT: Adults with affective disorders, in Behavioral Therapy in the Psychiatric Setting. Edited by Hersen M, Bellack AS. Baltimore, Williams & Wilkins Co, 1978a

Rush AJ, Beck AT: Cognitive therapy of depression and suicide. Am J Psychother 32:201-219, 1978b

Rush AJ, Watkins JT: Cognitive therapy with psychologically naive depressed outpatients, in Cognitive Therapy Casebook. Edited by Emery G, Hollon S, Bedrosian R. New York, Guilford, 1980

Rush AJ: Biological markers and treatment response in affective disorders. McLean Hospital Bulletin, 8:38-61, 1983

Rush AJ (ed): Short-Term Psychotherapies for Depression. New York, Guilford, 1982

Rush AJ: Psychotherapy of the affective psychoses. Am J Psychoanal 40:99-123, 1980

Shaw B: Predictors of successful outcome in cognitive therapy: a pilot study. Jerusalem, Israel, World Congress on Behavior Therapy, 1980

Shaw BF: Comparison of cognitive therapy and behavior therapy in the treatment of depression. J Consult Clin Psychol 45:543-551, 1977

Spiegelberg H: Phenomenology in Psychology and Psychiatry. Evanston, Ill, Northwestern University Press, 1972

Spiegelberg H: The Phenomenological Movement, vols 1,2. The Hague, Nijhoff, 1971

Spitzer RL, Endicott J, Robins E: Research diagnostic criteria: rationale and reliability. Arch Gen Psychiatry 3:773-782, 1978

Weissman AW: The Dysfunctional Attitude Scale: a validation study. Dissertation Abstracts International 40:1389-1390B, 1979 (University Microfilm No 79-19533)

8
Group Therapy

8
Group Therapy

INTRODUCTION AND HISTORICAL BACKGROUND

The origins of group psychotherapy in the United States can be traced to Joseph Pratt's (1907) work with tubercular patients. He reported that his patients were helped in coping with the effects of their illness and its subsequent problems by sharing their experiences in groups. Lazell (1921) was one of the early practitioners who described group treatment with schizophrenics, consisting mainly of lectures to patients. Burrow (1927), a student of Freud's, treated patients in groups because he felt that a patient in a group was less resistant. Schilder (1936) also conducted group psychotherapy, emphasizing such psychoanalytic phenomena as resistance and transference in groups. Wender (1940) provided the first major translation of analytic concepts to hospital group psychotherapy. Slavson (1955) designed a model for activity group therapy with children and relied on screening and the composition of his groups to correct the children's behavior problems.

Moreno (1957), who is credited with publicizing the expression "group psychotherapy," stressed that the members of a group are therapeutic agents and that their interactions are important for the therapeutic process, as is the concept of the "here and now." He also developed psychodrama and trained practitioners in this approach. Lewin (1945) introduced the "Gestalt" concept of field theory to describe the interaction between the individual and his environment; his work contributed to the theories of group dynamics. Foulkes (1948) emphasized group processes but focused on the individual patients in the group. Bion (1959) emphasized the importance of interpretations to the group as a whole and saw individual patient behaviors as manifestations of group forces. Wolf (1950) described psychoanalysis in groups, eschewing the notion of group dynamics.

By 1953 the use of group psychotherapy was widespread. Powdermaker and Frank (1953) set out to study the therapeutic process in groups and early on attempted to evaluate its efficacy. Since then, the literature on group psychotherapy has become extensive, focusing on theory, practice, technique, patient selection, research, and empirical data. Dies (1979) has highlighted the major trends in the empirical investigation of group psychotherapy in the past 30 years.

THEORETICAL ISSUES

Many types of group therapy are practiced in the United States today. Lieberman (1977) distinguished four major types of groups: (a) professionally led traditional groups; (b) peer self-help groups; (c) groups of the human potential movement, including sensitivity training and encounter groups; and (d) consciousness raising groups. The philosophy of each of these types of groups varies. This chapter will focus mainly on the more traditional types of group psychotherapy, with the other types of groups covered elsewhere in this volume.

In regard to these more traditional modalities, there are three basic types of group therapy, based on the focus of therapeutic intervention. Parloff (1968) outlines these three approaches as (a) focus on the individual, (b) focus on the interactions, and (c) focus on the group-as-a-whole. In actual practice, most group therapies make use of some combination of these approaches. In addition, the approach varies within each of these broad categories (psychodynamic, behavioral, existential, etc.).

In those groups in which the focus is on the individual, the approach is derived mainly from psychoanalysis, and a dynamic understanding of each member is sought. This approach transposes the practice and theory of individual therapy into the group setting and essentially promotes individual therapy within groups. The group is viewed as the transferential family, and the goal is to arrive at an intrapsychic analysis of each group member. Transference to the leader as well as between and among group members is of primary importance. Wolf (1974) has suggested that the group is more challenging than the dyad for psychoanalysis. The basic orientation is to the individual patient and his relationship with the therapist.

In those groups in which the focus is on interactions, interpersonal exchanges become the primary area for interventions. Here attention is focused on the subgroup or dyad. Group members are stimulated to demonstrate their unique modes of relating to others. The leader prompts and acknowledges member-to-member feedback; and emphasis is on the here-and-now experience, including here-and-now memories. Interactional group therapy makes it the task of the group to help each individual analyze, as completely as possible, his or her interactions with the therapist and with each group member. The facets of the individual's interpersonal problem areas are illuminated and worked through (the past may be used in this regard). This approach places more emphasis on the actual interactions that occur between group members than on the use of group members as observers of an individual's behavior.

The group-as-a-whole approach places the major emphasis on group dynamics. Through study of the group as an entity, the functioning of each member is revealed. The common group members' unconscious transference wishes toward the therapist make for the common group conflict. Comments in this approach are made to and about the whole group and its fantasies about the leader. This group-wide interpretation highlights commonalities among members, creates greater cohesion in the group, offers protection or support, and enhances the understanding of each member's contribution. Primary attention is not paid to member-member relationships except as they illustrate the nature of the leader-whole group fantasies on the behavior of the individual members; attention is paid, however, to the relationship of the individual member to the group as an entity and the relationship of each member to the collective whole.

Transference also seems to be a major goal in all three approaches. Grotjahn (1977) cites the tripartite nature of transference in groups: transference toward the central figure (patterned on the transference neurosis in psychoanalysis), transference toward peers in the group (patterned on that of the family neurosis), and transference toward the group as a whole (symbolizing the preoedipal mother figure and basic trust). The group setting is important because it provides a variety of character structures and personalities for transferential relationships.

Again, it is important to note that few group therapists adhere rigidly to only one theoretical position. Most use an interactional focus with aspects of the other theoretical positions. There is usually a relative balance or emphasis on group, interpersonal, and individual events.

Variations in Practice

There is much variation in the practice of group psychotherapy. Group therapy is conducted in many settings: inpatient hospital settings, outpatient clinics, private offices and homes, and other arranged locations (work setting, medical/surgical floors, etc.). Those referred to as "small groups" usually contain no fewer than four patients and no more than ten. Most practitioners regard six to eight members as the ideal number, allowing for greater participation (and therapist comfort).

The length of group treatment varies widely from short-term and crisis intervention groups (several sessions to a fixed number of sessions) to long-term groups. A distinction is made between open and closed groups. A closed group meets for a predetermined number of sessions and accepts no new members, whereas an open group maintains a consistent size by replacing members as they leave the group.

The duration of group meetings varies, depending on the setting and the diagnostic composition of the group, though most therapists agree that a period of at least 60 minutes is required for the warm-up interval and for working through the major themes of the session. Consensus is also that after two hours a point of diminishing returns is reached. The frequency of meetings varies from one to five times a week. Most outpatient groups meet once or twice a week.

The composition of therapy groups has been widely considered. A diagnosis of the individual is usually made, as well as a diagnosis of the individual's interpersonal skills. Groups vary as to whether they are homogeneous or heterogeneous. Homogeneous groups are composed of patients in the same diagnostic category or who present with the same symptoms. In group therapy for medical patients, for instance, patients with a particular organic illness are treated together. Most private practice groups are heterogeneous, as the balancing of persons with diversely structured personalities facilitates the development of therapeutic interchanges. Homogeneity of ego strength and heterogeneity of conflict areas may be ideal for the members of a therapeutic group. It is, however, sometimes helpful in groups in which symptom reduction is the major goal to have a symptomatically homogeneous group. At times homogeneous groups may be preferred when treating certain subgroups of patients (homosexuals, adolescents, etc.).

The goals of a therapy group will obviously vary depending on who is in the group and how it is structured. Some groups may have as their goal the therapeutic working through of their members' unresolved intrapsychic conflicts or the illumination of members' repetitive, maladaptive ways of relating interpersonally. Other groups may have symptomatic relief as their goal. Inpatient groups may focus more on hospital adjustment and diagnostic assessment as well as behavioral management. Other groups may be intended to be purely supportive or to provide a place for socializing and improving social skills.

The amount of preparation a patient is given before starting in a group also varies greatly. Some therapists meet only once or twice with an individual for a selection interview and then have no further contact until the group begins. Others continue individual sessions until the group begins. A number of preparatory sessions give the therapist the chance to clarify misconceptions, unrealistic expectations, and fears; to provide support; and to anticipate and thus diminish group therapy problems. Preparatory sessions provide the patients with a cognitive understanding that will enable them to participate more effectively in the group, allow an opportunity to raise the issue of confidentiality, and help the therapist to build rapport with the patients which may help to keep them in the group during periods of discouragement and anger. Such preparation also serves to decrease premature terminations from the group (Piper et al., 1979).

The Role and Tasks of the Group Therapist

Yalom (1975) sees the group therapist's role as centered around three basic tasks: (a) the construction and maintenance of a physical system, (b) the construction of a therapeutic culture (norm building), and (c) the activation and illumination of here-and-now interaction. The therapist is responsible for creating, selecting, and convening the group, and must be aware of forces that threaten group cohesiveness. Culture building refers to the establishment of a code of behavioral rules, or norms, which guide the group's interactions and are based on the group's expectations and goals. The therapist steers the group members away from discussions of certain outside material and focuses on the interactions and relationships that develop within the group. This, of course, encourages discussion of the here-and-now.

Group therapists also are often responsible for the setting of therapeutic contracts, which may involve the exclusion of certain group members for not maintaining agreed upon standards. The group therapist must have knowledge of group dynamics and theory in addition to a working knowledge or theory of personality development and dysfunction.

The group therapist must pay attention to the stages of group therapy, from its beginning (diagnosing, setting goals, planning treatment, and the early preparation of patients), to entrance into the therapy and participation in group cohesion, to movement into the primary work and exploration of issues in the group, to facing indications for termination, and finally to parting (Kanter, 1976). The group therapy situation, then, is a uniquely complicated one since the group therapist's areas of influence are more diverse than in a one-to-one context. The leader must have insight into both an individual member's personality structure and the level of his or her interpersonal skills. Interpretations need to be directed toward individual issues as well as toward group process issues. The concept of the therapist as the "leader" of the group is also unique. Direct leadership occurs through the therapist's role as technical expert; indirect leadership occurs through his role as model-setting participant, though "experts" can be nondirective, and "models" can be directive.

Therapeutic Change Agents

In general, group therapy attempts to be therapeutic by enhancing the patient's understanding of himself and his relationships with others and by effecting change in his behavior and his capacity for relatedness. It is difficult to ascertain common therapeutic factors for all group therapies. As shown by Berzon and Farson (1963) and Taylor (1961), patients perceive and experience the same group event in different ways. In addition, there are many types of group therapies for different types of patients, and treatment goals may vary widely.

Yalom (1975) classified the therapeutic factors of groups as (a) the instillation of hope, (b) universality, (c) imparting of information, (d) altruism, (e) the corrective recapitulation of the primary family group, (f) development of socializing techniques, (g) imitative behavior (benefits derived by "vicarious therapy"), (h) interpersonal learning (the gaining of insight into what a patient's behavior is, how it affects others, and what the motivation for the behavior is), (i) group cohesiveness, (j) catharsis, and (k) existential factors (the patient learns that he alone is ultimately responsible for himself and for the quality of his life).

It has been found that patients in different kinds of groups, and indeed different patients, value different therapeutic factors (Berzon and Farson, 1963; Dickoff and Lakin, 1963; Yalom, 1975; Maxmen, 1973; Rohrbaugh and Bartels, 1975).

Groups, then, give patients practice in expressing feelings to peers, and feedback on such expression fosters understanding and empathy toward others and allows for comparisons of a patient's behavior with that of his peers. This process provides an opportunity not only for the resolution of the patient's individual issues and difficulties but also for resolution of interpersonal problems through direct interaction with others in the group.

Differences Between Individual and Group Psychotherapy

There are many differences between group and individual psychotherapy, some of which underline the uniqueness of group therapies. The group provides a more genuine social experience. The presence of a number of people fosters multiple interpersonal relationships. A group of eight or nine people has a far better chance of representing a true social setting for the patient than a one-to-one, more insular situation with the therapist. More facets of the individual's interpersonal problem areas (and strengths) can, therefore, be illuminated. As a group member's characteristic ways of relating emerge and evoke reactions from others, verbal and nonverbal interventions by the other members and the therapist set the stage for the working through of problem areas. The group also allows for the development of multiple, simultaneous transferences. In addition, groups provide support because they allow for a sense of belonging and offer an increased opportunity for reality testing. Imagined hurts, fears, retaliations, and transference distortions may thus be subject to easier here-and-now exploration and correction. A group can provide more direct support from peers; the disheartened patient can be helped to see that he or she is not alone or necessarily the worst off. The group provides a setting in which a patient's dependency needs are divided and not directed solely toward the therapist. And transferences that develop can be diluted in groups, preventing certain overwhelming affects that may impede the patient's progress.

Confrontations and interpretations by peers are often more readily accepted than those from the authority figure. This may be particularly true of groups for adolescents and substance abusers. More experienced group members can also serve as role models in the acceptance of certain feelings as well as the need for self-exploration. Vicarious participation in a group may offer a unique means for the expression of hostility or other feelings. In this way, groups permit patients to self-regulate the emotional intensity of therapy since they allow for differential degrees of participation among the members. Certain unique motivational factors for change and growth may, therefore, be inherent in the group setting. Emotional change and insight in a group may be more immediately related to external conflict than to its intrapsychic representation, and dynamic movement in groups occurs to a large extent "outside inwards" instead of "inside outwards" (Ackerman, 1975). Anthony (1971) states that in a group the sense of risk is more acute than in individual treatment. Also, the patient has to share the therapist and may thus experience a loss of his sense of uniqueness.

Battegay (1977), in Switzerland, proposes an interesting differentiation of the therapeutic factors in groups as opposed to individual treatment. He suggests that the group offers the possibility of learning a more integrative manner of behavior. However, since there are always several people present, it may make it more difficult to work through individual conflicts. In the extreme, therefore, he suggests that in group therapy the patient's behavior becomes more adapted to social reality but the internal conflicts themselves may not be much affected. One solution is the combination of group and individual therapy, which will be covered more extensively later in this chapter.

CLINICAL ISSUES

Indications for Group Therapy

Not every patient is suitable for group psychotherapy. Selection criteria vary widely depending on the structure, goals, and procedure of the group. On many inpatient units, all patients (except the grossly psychotic) are assigned to groups. For groups with specialized goals, admission criteria may be simply the existence of the target symptom (alcoholism, obesity, addiction, etc.), and selection is relatively straightforward. The selection of patients for outpatient group therapy is more complicated, and contradictory impressions abound in the literature. Bednar and Lawlis (1971), Lewis and McCants (1973), and others have stressed the impact of client selection variables on outcome. Most research has also focused on exclusion criteria rather than on clear indications for group psychotherapy as the treatment of choice. The state of the art is such that it is easier to predict who will not be able to work in groups than to predict who will profit from a group.

Some variables that seem to be predictive of success are the patient's attraction to the group and his general popularity in the group (Houts et al., 1967); motivation for group therapy (Yalom, 1975); high levels of discomfort initially coupled with low levels of overt behavioral disturbance (Truax, 1971); bright, younger, moderately anxious, psychologically-minded patients with good premorbid histories (Salzberg, 1969; Sethna and Harrington, 1971); and patients with sufficient flexibility to reduce or heighten intragroup tension and to serve at times as the catalyst for the group (Leopold, 1957). In summary, then, to benefit from group psychotherapy, a patient must have at least a minimum level of interpersonal skills, motivation for treatment, psychological discomfort, and expectancy of therapeutic gain.

The types of patients who will benefit from groups depend on the goals of the group. Nondirective or insight-oriented groups may not be appropriate for psychotic individuals, who would benefit from a group that emphasizes structure, social skill development, and interaction. Also in dynamic group therapy, there is concern for therapeutic matching and group composition. A patient for whom group therapy is indicated may not be suitable for a particular treatment group but might do well in another group. Group therapy may also be useful for patients with specific medical conditions* and in the treatment of alcoholism (Hill and Blane, 1967; Brown and Yalom, 1977) and drug abuse. Approaches are modified with specific groups of patients, allowing the treatment to be useful.

Limitations of Group Therapy

There is some clinical consensus that several types of patients should be excluded from heterogeneous dynamically-oriented groups (though not necessarily excluded from group treatment per se). These include brain damaged and addicted patients (Nash et al., 1957; Johnson, 1963); paranoid patients (Graham, 1959); extremely narcissistic, hypochondriacal, suicidal, or acutely psychotic patients (Slavson, 1964); and sociopathic patients

* Peptic ulcers (Fortin and Abse, 1956), asthma (Clapham and Sclare, 1958; Groen and Pelser, 1960; Forth and Jackson, 1976), cardiac illness (Adsett and Bruhn, 1968; Rahe et al., 1979; Hackett, 1978), diabetes (Frizzell, 1968), epilepsy (Yeager et al., 1960), migraine and tension headaches (Cooper and Katz, 1956), intractable pain (Pinsky, 1978), rheumatoid arthritis (Schwartz et al., 1978), amputees (Freeman and Applegate, 1976), and paraplegics (Banik and Mendelson, 1978).

(Abrahams and McKorkle, 1947; Bach, 1954). In long-term dynamic interactional groups these patients may construct an interpersonal role that is detrimental to themselves and to the group, though they may derive benefit from a group with specialized goals and/or different techniques.

The limitations of group therapy become clearer when examining those patients who tend to terminate from the group prematurely. Premature terminators generally leave treatment unimproved and can produce negative effects for themselves and for the remaining group members. Patients terminate early because of problems of intimacy; an inability to share the leader; inadequate orientation to therapy; fears of emotional contagion (Yalom, 1966); manifest or threatening psychotic breakdown; isolation; use of the group for only crisis resolution (Grotjahn, 1972); lack of the requisite emotional, interpersonal, and intellectual resources (Woods and Melnick, 1979); lack of motivation; little perceived discomfort; excessive passivity or hostility; and somatization of problems (Kotkov, 1958; Nash, 1957; Sethna and Harrington, 1971). Mullan and Rosenbaum (1962) state that a patient is unsuitable for a dynamically-oriented group who (a) paralyzes group interaction over an extended period of time; (b) cannot be reached by other members in the group because of constant chaotic behavior; (c) is in a state of constant acute anxiety and thus becomes a burden and responsibility to the group; or (d) shows antisocial, destructive, impulse-motivated behavior that arouses fear in the other group members. Combinations of the above characteristics create a group deviant who will either terminate from the group prematurely or act to inhibit group progress.

There is evidence that among a certain small percentage of group participants, group therapy can produce adverse effects (Bednar and Lawlis, 1971; Smith, 1975; Hartley et al., 1976). The casualty rates vary and the hypothesized antecedents to these negative outcomes are not fully understood, but there is some cause for concern. Yalom and Lieberman (1971) studied the casualties of 18 encounter groups, defining a casualty as an individual who, as a result of the group experience, suffered persistent psychological distress of considerable degree (anxiety, psychosis, depression, suicidal ideation, and increased isolation). The casualty rate was 7.5 percent. It should be highlighted that these were encounter groups and not traditional therapy groups, but some of the findings are relevant to group therapy as a whole. Casualties appear to be partly related to therapist style and approach. When therapists use a more supportive, less confrontative style, the rates of patient dropouts and casualties are minimized (Malan, 1976; Galigor, 1977).

The adverse effects of some forms of group therapy can, therefore, be significantly reduced if careful attention is paid to selection and if potential group deviants are placed in other types of treatment or other types of groups. There must also be a match between group goals and member expectations.

The Use of Concurrent Group and Individual Therapy

Many therapists have considered the advantages of concurrent individual and group psychotherapy for different patient populations. In "combined" therapy the two treatments are conducted by the same therapist; "conjoint" therapy refers to treatment by two different therapists. Potential advantages of both forms of concurrent treatment are: individual treatment may help patients develop the frustration tolerance and ego strength that are often needed to benefit from intensive group therapy, the multiplicity of stimuli in a group can create a degree of fragmentation which some patients can tolerate only through the integrative work of parallel individual therapy, individual treatment can allow for a working through of group-induced frustrations and help to diminish resistance toward disclosures in the group (Fried, 1971), resistance to individual therapy can be reduced (Anthony, 1971), and the ongoing interactions of group and individual treatment can form a more integrated therapeutic experience (Bieber, 1971).

Heigl-Evans and Heigl (1974) recommend the combined approach for patients with narcissistic problems so that the group therapy can serve to avoid a countertherapeutic gratification of transference wishes raised in the individual treatment. Wong (1979) also recommends the combined approach for narcissistic patients because the group can serve as a transitional object to reduce the fears of engulfment and retaliation that are projected onto the therapist and can allow the patient greater individualization. The group can also be valuable in working through grandiose and aggressive issues and in easing the individual therapist's countertransference burden. The group provides a variety of role models and different behavioral options. Individual therapy can foster a therapeutic alliance that may protect the patient from intolerable feelings that may be raised in the group.

For patients with borderline personality disorders Grobman (1980) feels that a combination of individual and group treatment is often necessary. The group may help these patients establish adequate cognitive skills and a more coherent sense of self, which is necessary for the development of a therapeutic alliance. Without group therapy, these patients may have a more difficult time tolerating the regression and participating in the process of insight required by individual psychotherapy. A particular benefit of conjoint therapy is that undue regression may be decreased, given that during vacations and illnesses at least one therapist is always present and that the therapists themselves can support each other while working with these sometimes difficult patients (Roth and Stiglitz, 1971). Scheidlinger and Porter (1980) conclude that concurrent therapy may be the treatment of choice for patients with characterological, borderline, and narcissistic disorders, especially those with primitive preoedipal transferences and rigid character defenses. The technical issues involved in the concurrent approach include timing the introduction of group or individual therapy, the composition of the therapy group, the handling of confidentiality, the intensity of the individual sessions, and the choice of combined (one therapist) versus conjoint (different therapists) therapy.

Potential drawbacks have been raised concerning the use of concurrent therapy. Battegay (1972) suggests that the concurrent approach may interfere with the full development of the transference, that there may be severe sibling rivalry, and that there may be a draining off of clinical material from the therapy group by the individual sessions. Yalom (1975) worries that the two therapies may work at cross purposes with one another: The group may be attacked because it offers less attention and narcissistic gratification, and the individual therapy may decrease involvement and participation in the group. Scheidlinger and Porter (1980) also caution against the concurrent approach for some borderline, psychotic, and masochistic patients, whose ego structure is such that they respond to the addition of group therapy with increased anxiety, regressed behavior, or depression.

In conclusion, it seems that the concurrent group and individual psychotherapy approach can be helpful for some patients, may be the treatment of choice for others, and that its effectiveness will be increased if attention is paid to careful selection of patients who are most likely to benefit from this approach.

DEVELOPMENTAL AND AGE RELATED ISSUES

Group therapy is used for people of all ages and, when limited to a particular age group, focuses on the specific developmental issues of that group.

Therapy groups may be used in the treatment of children. Rosenbaum and Kraft (1975) state that the therapist tries to provide situations that encourage behavior that reveals information about the child. Its emotional content can then be extracted and translated intellectually. Experiential insight comes through interaction with other children in the group and through identification with others. Response to treatment can be measured in terms of each child's verbal and nonverbal behavior, activity level, and interrelationships with other children in the group.

Schamess (1976) reviewed the current group treatment modalities for children and classified them into four categories: (a) groups for preoedipal children with developmental and personality problems (activity therapy and therapeutic play groups); (b) groups for "atypical" ego-damaged children, which are modified activity groups designed to provide corrective object relationships; (c) groups for "impulse ridden," acting-out children, which provide a structured environment in which aggression can be expressed without retaliation and identification with the authority figure is fostered (mastery of specific developmental tasks can thus be achieved); and

(d) groups for neurotic children. Children's groups, therefore, should preferably be homogeneous with respect to age and overall level of dysfunction. Other groups that have been used for children include short-term diagnostic groups, school groups for maladaptive behavior, and groups in residential treatment settings.

Group therapy may be preferable to individual therapy for certain adolescents. Muroff* feels that group psychotherapy is the treatment of choice for most adolescents since it is concordant with the natural need of the adolescent to belong to groups and to work directly through the basic conflict of being dependent while wishing to be independent. Group psychotherapy with adolescents helps them to bypass both their lack of desire to evaluate themselves and their resistance to working in a one-to-one relationship with an adult toward whom they feel rebellious.

Issues addressed in adolescent groups may revolve around peer support for problems with separation, identity formation, impulse control, sexuality, and experienced interpersonal pressures. Brandes (1977), however, points out that group therapy is not suitable for every adolescent.

For the young adult, the group can be particularly helpful in dealing with issues such as leaving home, differentiating from families, selecting a career goal, and dealing with difficulties with intimacy and commitment to others. For adults with families, groups can help with problems in child-rearing, the assumption of new roles and responsibilities, and the problems associated with aging. Groups have also been found to be helpful for marital discord, sexual dysfunction, and other specific problems. As has already been mentioned, most outpatient groups for adults tend to be more heterogeneous, addressing a broad range of conflicts and problems.

Finally, group therapy for the elderly may involve treatment both in institutions and for those who remain at home. Goldfarb (1971) sees the goals of group work in institutions as increasing the discharge rate, decreasing disturbing behavior and management problems, and maximizing the patient's comfort and well-being through social integration. Outside of institutions, group goals may vary from the alteration of the elderly person's way of life through interaction with others to the provision of guidance, counsel, and information. Prophylactic groups have been used to assist in the preretirement and retirement problems of the relatively well (Ross, 1975). The Committee on Aging of the Group for the Advancement of Psychiatry (1971) has recommended that group psychotherapy be made available to the elderly both in mixed groups with patients of all ages (to increase the range of life problems presented in the group) and in groups with aged patients only (to avoid domination by younger, more verbal members and to address solely the common needs of the elderly patient). Outpatient

---

* Muroff M: Group psychotherapy with children. Presented at the ITT International Congress of Group Psychotherapy, Copenhagen, 1980

group psychotherapy has been suggested as an alternative to institutional-ization of the elderly (Deutsch and Kramer, 1977). The elderly patient's coping abilities may be strengthened by the opportunity to interact freely with peers in a supportive environment (Ingersoll and Silverman, 1978).

Group involvement for different ages may, therefore, serve either a rehabilitative, social, or more psychotherapeutic role, depending on the needs of the individual.

PROFESSIONAL AND ETHICAL ISSUES

Training Issues

Training in group psychotherapy is offered in some professional training programs, by a few specialized centers, and informally in a number of clinics and agencies. Standards have been outlined for the practice of group therapy, though there are no formal requirements. The American Group Psychotherapy Association (1979) has developed a model for post-profes-sional specialization in group psychotherapy. The suggested guidelines, however, are only for preparation to do group therapy with adults. Further training is suggested for other age groups and specialized problems.

As discussed, group therapy differs in certain important respects from other treatment modalities and, therefore, requires a complete understand-ing of these differences as well as knowledge of how to implement the unique interventions that are required.

Training and supervision in group therapy involve the didactic teaching of group theory and technique, the selection of patients and the composition of groups, and actual supervision around the treatment of individuals in the group and the group as a whole. Clinical material is either presented to a su-pervisor after the therapy session, or supervision is done "live" by having the trainee observe an ongoing group treatment or by having him be present in the group as a co-therapist. Through direct observation the trainee can obtain a better sense of group process and model his therapeutic interven-tions. Mistakes can also be corrected as they occur. In a recent survey of practitioners, Dies (1980) found that group trainers favored direct supervi-sion (conducting a group and receiving feedback) and experiential groups (being a group member) over academic and observational techniques in the training of group therapists.

It is not enough for the group therapist to have training only in individual psychodynamics and treatment, as group therapy involves an understand-ing of group dynamics and requires certain skills. Similarly, since group therapy is not effective for every type of problem, training must encompass a broad understanding of different treatment modalities and approaches to various problems. Certain patients may not be suitable for group therapy or may for one reason or another have to be terminated from a group. The group therapist must maintain a flexible approach to treatment.

The nature of group therapy also requires a different level of activity on the therapist's part. There are more people present at a given time and many more variables to be kept in mind while conducting a group. These differences can potentially be more stressful and confusing for the beginning group therapist. Beginning group therapists often seem to experience substantial difficulty with the group therapeutic model (Dies, 1980); this difficulty has been seen as arising from the trainees' insensitivity to group process or from their failure to use the resources of the group effectively.

Beginning group therapists have also frequently been seen as being intimidated by the intensity of the group process. The most difficult patients for the beginning therapist are the "problem patients"—those patients who are help-rejecting, monopolistic, or otherwise problematic. These patients demand individual management and management in the context of the entire group, thus requiring special skills on the part of the group psychotherapist.

Co-Therapist Issues

Co-therapists are frequently used in group therapy. Advantages of co-therapy include: (a) male and female co-therapists may elicit different transferences, (b) two people often understand the meaning of a particular group's interaction differently and can model the communication of differences openly, (c) co-therapists' discussions after a group meeting can help to focus on countertransference reactions, (d) more than one leader may allow for the expression of different feelings; and (e) the presence of a more senior therapist may be reassuring to a less experienced therapist (Fried, 1971).

Potential difficulties in the use of co-therapists may be intimidation of group members, unresolved issues between the therapists which interfere with treatment, and difficulties in working together which may create more stress and dissonance for the group members. The co-therapist must also pay attention to the co-therapy relationship in addition to the other variables in the group. Difficulties may arise if a therapist is not seen by the group to be of equal stature with his or her co-therapist because of experience or sex-role stereotypes. Economic factors in certain clinical settings may also prohibit co-therapy.

Overall, co-therapy is a useful, informative, and therapeutically enhancing experience for a group. If the potential difficulties cited are worked through, both the therapists and the group will benefit from co-therapy.

The Risk/Benefit Ratio in Group Therapy

Deterioration rates in group psychotherapy are probably about the same as they are for individual psychotherapy. The drop-out rate is probably no higher in groups than in other forms of therapy, provided that attention is paid to selection and preparation of patients for group therapy. The risk/benefit ratio would therefore appear to be about the same as for other effective forms of psychotherapy and may be the treatment of choice for certain types of problems, as outlined above.

Ethical Issues

In considering ethical issues pertaining to group therapy, the question of the leader's responsibility to individual members in a group is raised. What may be important and therapeutic for one member in a group may not be helpful for all members. By focusing on group cohesion and growth of the group as a whole, the needs of certain members may not be met. It may at times be better for a group member to drop out of a group for the good of the group (if the member is too disruptive, attacking, or if he blocks group progress). The therapist is, in fact, responsible for every member of a group. Potential difficulties in sacrificing an individual for the sake of the group can be diminished if extreme care is taken in the selection of group members so that obviously deviant or disruptive individuals are referred elsewhere.

Once a group has begun, the therapist has less control over how members in the group will affect each other. Certain patients may experience a negative effect from the group or fail to improve because of the interactions with the other group members. This may be particularly true when members of a group drop out. The therapist must take responsibility for those remaining members as well as for the patient who drops out (by suggesting another form of treatment, helping to clarify the reasons for termination, and not just allowing the patient to disappear). The therapist may judiciously remove a patient from the group when there is substantial evidence that the patient has little likelihood of benefiting from the therapy and an increased potential for being disturbed by the experience.

The issue of confidentiality is a particularly difficult one for group therapy. The therapist often knows things about a member's life which others in the group do not know. The premature disclosure of information may be destructive for a group member and violate his or her right to privacy. This situation may be avoided if the therapist has previously contracted with the patient that certain information they share may be relevant for the group and if the therapist gives the patient the option to reveal something or not at a particular time. In addition, confidentiality in a group may be violated by other group members. Group members are not professionally bound to keep confidential information they have learned about others in the group and may be tempted to discuss group members outside of the therapy setting. The need for confidentiality must be stressed and insisted upon. This can be accomplished in the screening interview prior to actual group involvement.

In groups there is always peer pressure for certain types of behavior as a group culture develops. A forced atmosphere of confession may result in pressure to disclose certain information and feelings prematurely. Group members will have different rates of development, comfort, and tolerance of stress within the group; and these must be respected by the leader and the other members.

The management of acute crises may be a difficult ethical problem for the therapist. In a group there are limitations as to how well the therapist knows each member and how much attention is paid to each member. If a patient becomes acutely suicidal or psychotic, the group setting makes it more difficult for the therapist to intervene directly and make a complete evaluation of the situation. This situation is less of a problem when a patient has an individual therapist in addition to the group. Some therapists deal with this potential difficulty by immediately offering to see a patient who has entered an acute crisis in an individual session or a series of individual sessions. A responsible referral for individual treatment or additional services can then be made if indicated.

Finally, the extra-therapeutic contact that occurs between group members may raise ethical issues. Group members frequently will have liaisons outside of the group which may be harmful for the group process or damaging to an individual. Therapists differ in their tolerance of such situations; some encourage them, while others make it a group rule that there be no outside contact between members. Therapists should promote the alliance of patients in the group therapeutic process and inform them about the problems that extra-group meetings pose for the group. In this way the group therapist can encourage patients to bring the important aspects of extra-group liaisons back into the group for discussion and analysis or discourage patients from potentially destructive relationships.

FINANCIAL AND SOCIAL ISSUES

Group therapy is often less expensive than individual therapy. In addition, when professional resources are limited, one therapist can treat a number of patients at the same time for a similar time investment, making the cost/benefit ratio for group therapy low. Potential problems are that patients who are not suitable for a group but cannot afford individual therapy may be inappropriately placed in a group. The lack of professional resources may also result in grouping patients inappropriately. The formation of groups can also take a great deal of time with screening, pre-group preparation, and consultations with outside agencies and individual therapists.

Group therapy may play an increasingly important role in social issues. With evolving technology and urbanization, our times have become an era of alienation. Group therapy, with its focus on interpersonal relationships and improved communication between people, may help to counter some of the effects of this alienation. The value system the group therapist employs involves the belief that people are important to one another and can share and help each other. One of the major therapeutic effects of group treatment is thought to be an understanding of the universality of certain feelings and difficulties so that each member feels less isolated and alone.

This is also an era in which the role of the family has become less important; with increasing divorce rates, families are becoming fragmented. As the family dissolves, a group may serve as a substitute for support, cohesion, and the provision of a sense of identity.

Groups may also serve as important ways of dealing with specific problems that arise out of changing social issues. Groups for women in an age of increased options and shifting roles may help deal with conflicts around these changes. Similarly, as life expectancy increases and our society contains greater numbers of elderly people, groups for the aged may help with support and problem solving for the elderly in a youth-oriented society.

Finally, as life becomes more complex, the need for teaming may become greater; different collaborative skills and approaches may become necessary to get a job done. A knowledge of small group dynamics in therapy and nontherapy settings may be an adaptive skill. Through group therapy, individuals may gain the kind of mastery of group dynamics which allows them to negotiate more effectively with families, work, and community groups.

REFERENCES

Abrahams J, McKorkle L: Group psychotherapy at an army rehabilitation center. Dis Nerv Syst 8:50-62, 1947

Ackerman N: Psychoanalysis and group psychotherapy, in Group Psychotherapy and Group Function. Edited by Rosenbaum M, Berger M. New York, Basic Books, 1975

Adsett C, Bruhn J: Short-term group psychotherapy for post-myocardial infarction patients and their wives. Can Med Assoc J 99:577-584, 1968

Anthony E: Comparison between individual and group psychotherapy, in Comprehensive Group Psychotherapy. Edited by Kaplan H, Sadock B. Baltimore, Williams & Wilkins Co, 1971

Bach G: Intensive Group Therapy. New York, Ronald Press, 1954

Banik S, Mendelson M: Group psychotherapy with a paraplegic group. Int J Group Psychother 28:123-128, 1978

Battegay R: Characteristics and new trends in group psychotherapy. Acta Psychiatr Scand 56:21-31, 1977

Battegay R: Individual psychotherapy and group psychotherapy as single treatment methods and in combination. Acta Psychiatr Scand 48:43-48, 1972

Bednar R, Lawlis G: Empirical research in group psychotherapy, in Handbook of Psychotherapy and Behavior Change. Edited by Bergin A, Garfield S. New York, John Wiley & Sons, 1971

Berzon B, Farson R: The therapeutic event in group psychotherapy: a study of subjective reports by group members. J Individ Psychol 19:204-212, 1963

Bieber T: Combined individual and group psychotherapy, in Comprehensive Group Psychotherapy. Edited by Kaplan H, Sadock B. Baltimore, Williams & Wilkins Co, 1971

Bion W: Experiences in Groups. London, Tavistock, 1959

Brandes N: Group therapy is not for every adolescent: two case illustrations. Int J Group Psychother 27:507-510, 1977

Brown S, Yalom I: Interactional group therapy with alcoholics. J Stud Alcohol 88:426-456, 1977

Burrow T: The group method of analysis. Psychoanal Rev 14:268-280, 1927

Clapham M, Sclare A: Group psychotherapy with asthmatic patients. Int J Group Psychother 8:44-54, 1958

Cooper M, Katz J: The treatment of migraine and tension headache with group psychotherapy. Int J Group Psychother 6:266, 1956

Deutsch C, Kramer M: Outpatient group psychotherapy for the elderly: an alternative to institutionalization. Hosp Community Psychiatry 28:440-442, 1977

Dickoff H, Lakin M: Patients views of group psychotherapy: retrospections and interpretations. Int J Group Psychother 13:61-73, 1963

Dies R: Current practice in the training of group psychotherapists. Int J Group Psychother 30:169-185, 1980

Dies R: Group psychotherapy: reflections on three decades of research. J Applied Behav Science, 15:361-373, 1979

Forth M, Jackson M: Group psychotherapy in management of bronchial asthma. Br J Med Psychol 49:257-260, 1976

Fortin J, Abse D: Group psychotherapy with peptic ulcer: a preliminary report. Int J Group Psychother 6:383-391, 1956

Foulkes S: Introduction to Group-Analytic Psychotherapy. London, William Heinemann, 1948

Freeman A, Applegate W: Psychiatric consultation to a rehabilitative program for amputees. Hosp Community Psychiatry 27:40-42, 1976

Fried E: Basic concepts in group psychotherapy, in Comprehensive Group Psychotherapy. Edited by Kaplan H, Sadock B. Baltimore: Williams & Wilkins Co, 1971

Frizell M: Group therapy for diabetic mental patients. Hosp Community Psychiatry 19:297-298, 1968

Galigor J: Perceptions of the group therapist and the drop-out from group, in Group Therapy 1977: An Overview. Edited by Wolberg I, Aronson M, Wolberg A. New York, Stratton Intercontinental Medical Book Corp, 1977

Goldfarb A: Group therapy with the old and aged, in Comprehensive Group Psychotherapy. Edited by Kaplan H, Sadock B. Baltimore, Williams & Wilkins Co, 1971

Graham I: Observations on analytic group therapy. Int J Group Psychother 9:150-157, 1959

Grobman J: The borderline patient in group psychotherapy: a case report. Int J Group Psychother 30:299-318, 1980

Groen S, Pelser H: Experiences with and results of group psychotherapy in patients with bronchial asthma. J Psychosom Res 4:191-205, 1960

Grotjahn M: The Art and Technique of Analytic Group Therapy. New York, Jason Aronson Inc, 1977

Grotjahn M: Learning from drop-out patients: a clinical view of patients who discontinued group psychotherapy. Int J Group Psychother 22:306-319, 1972

Guidelines for the Training of Group Psychotherapists. New York, American Group Psychotherapy Association Inc, 1979

Hackett TP: The use of groups in the rehabilitation of the postcoronary patient. Adv Cardiol 24:127-135, 1978

Hartley D, Roback H, Abramowitz S: Deterioration effects in encounter groups. Am Psychol 31:247-255, 1976

Heigl-Evans A, Heigl F: On the combination of psychoanalytic individual and group therapy. Gruppenpsychother Gruppendyn 8:97-121, 1974

Hill MJ, Blane HT: Evaluation of psychotherapy with alcoholics: a critical review. Q J Stud Alcohol 28:76-104, 1967

Houts P, Yalom I, Zimerberg S, et al: Prediction of improvement in group therapy. Arch Gen Psychiatry 17:159-168, 1967

Ingersoll B, Silverman A: Comparative group psychotherapy for the aged. Gerontology 18:201-206, 1978

Johnson J: Group Psychotherapy: A Practical Approach. New York, McGraw-Hill, 1963

Kanter S: The therapists' leadership in psychoanalytically oriented group psychotherapy. Int J Group Psychotherapy 26:139-147, 1976

Kotkov B: Favorable clinical indications for group attendance. Int J Group Psychotherapy 23:346-359, 1958

Lazell E: The group treatment of dementia praecox. Psychoanal Rev 8:168-179, 1921

Leopold H: Selection of patients for group psychotherapy. Am J Psychotherapy 11:634-637, 1957

Lewin K: The research center for group dynamics at Massachusetts Institute of Technology. Sociometry 8:126-136, 1945

Lewis P, McCants J: Some current issues in group psychotherapy research. Int J Group Psychotherapy 23:268-291, 1973

Lieberman M: Problems in integrating traditional group therapies with new forms. Int J Group Psychotherapy 27:19-32, 1977

Malan D: Group psychotherapy: long term follow-up study. Arch Gen Psychiatry 33:1303-1315, 1976

Maxmen J: Group therapy as viewed by hospitalized patients. Arch Gen Psychiatry 28:404-408, 1973

Moreno J: The First Book on Group Psychotherapy. New York, Beacon House, 1957

Mullan H, Rosenbaum W: The suitability for the group experience. Group Psychotherapy Theory and Practice. New York, Macmillan, 1962

Nash E, Frank J, Gliedman L, et al: Some factors related to patients remaining in group psychotherapy. Int J Group Psychotherapy 7:264-275, 1957

Parloff M: Analytic group psychotherapy, in Modern Psychoanalysis. Edited by Marmor J. New York, Basic Books, 1968

Pinsky J: Chronic, intractable benign pain: a syndrome and its treatment with intensive short-term group psychotherapy. J Human Stress 4:17-21, 1978

Piper W, Debbane I, Garant J, et al: Pretraining for group psychotherapy. Arch Gen Psychiatry 36:1250-1256, 1979

Powdermaker F, Frank J: Group Psychotherapy: Studies in Methodology of Research and Therapy. Cambridge, Mass, Harvard University Press, 1953

Pratt J: The class method of treating consumption in the homes of the poor. JAMA 49:755-759, 1907

Rahe R, Ward H, Hayes V: Brief group therapy in myocardial infarction rehabilitation: three-to-four-year follow-up of a controlled trial. Psychosom Med 41:229-242, 1979

Rohrbaugh M, Bartels BD: Participants' perception of curative factors in therapy and growth groups. Small Group Behavior 6:430-456, 1975

Rosenbaum M, Kraft I: Group psychotherapy for children, in Group Psychotherapy and Group Function. Edited by Rosenbaum M, Berger M. New York, Basic Books, 1975

Ross M: Community geriatric group therapies: a comprehensive review, in Group Psychotherapy and Group Function. Edited by Rosenbaum M, Berger M. New York, Basic Books, 1975

Roth M, Stiglitz M: The shared patient: separate therapists for group and individual psychotherapy. Int J Group Psychother 21:44-52, 1971

Salzberg H: Group psychotherapy screening scale: a validation study. Int J Group Psychother 19:226-228, 1969

Schamess G: Group treatment modalities for latency-age children. Int J Group Psychother 26:455-474, 1976

Scheidlinger S, Porter K: Group therapy combined with individual psychotherapy, in Special Techniques in Individual Psychotherapy. Edited by Karasu T, Bellak L. New York, Brunner/Mazel, 1980

Schilder P: The analysis of ideologies as a psychotherapeutic method, especially in group treatment. Am J Psychiatry 93:601-617, 1936

Schwartz L, Marcus R, Condon R: Multidisciplinary group therapy for rheumatoid arthritis. Psychosomatics 19:289-293, 1978

Sethna E, Harrington J: A study of patients who lapsed from group psychotherapy. Br J Psychiatry 119:59-60, 1971

Slavson S: A Textbook in Analytic Group Psychotherapy. New York, International Universities Press, 1964

Slavson S: Criteria for selection and rejection of patients for various kinds of group therapy. Int J Group Psychother 5:3-30, 1955

Smith P: Are there adverse effects of sensitivity training? Journal of Humanistic Psychology 15:29-47, 1975

Taylor F: The Analysis of Therapeutic Groups. New York, Oxford University Press, 1961

The Aged and Community Mental Health: A guide to Program Development. Publication #81. New York, Group for the Advancement of Psychiatry, 1971

Truax C: The initial status of the client and the predictability of psychotherapeutic change. Comparative Group Studies 2:3-16, 1971

Wender L: Group psychotherapy: a study of its application. Psychiatr Q 14:708-718, 1940

Wolf A: Psychoanalysis in groups, in The Challenge for Group Psychotherapy: Present and Future. Edited by Deschill S. New York, International Universities Press, 1974

Wolf A: The psychoanalysis of groups. Am J Psychother 4:16-50, 1950

Wong N: Clinical considerations in group treatment of narcissistic disorders. Int J Group Psychother 29:317-345, 1979

Woods M, Melnick J: A review of group therapy selection criteria. Small Group Behavior 10:155-171, 1979

Yalom I, Lieberman M: A study of encounter group casualties. Arch Gen Psychiatry 25:16-30, 1971

Yalom I: The Theory and Practice of Group Psychotherapy. New York, Basic Books, 1975

Yalom I: A study of group therapy dropouts. Arch Gen Psychiatry 14:393-414, 1966

Yeager C, Shaskan D, Rigney F: A study of epileptics receiving group psychotherapy. Dis Nerv Syst 21:491-498, 1960

9

Family Therapy

9

Family Therapy

INTRODUCTION

In its 30-year history, family therapy has had phenomenal growth, from an almost underground position to wide acceptance. In 1973, the field had only one professional journal, *Family Process*; today there are nearly two dozen family therapy journals, about half of them published in English, and more than 300 freestanding family institutes in the United States alone. The American Association for Marriage and Family Therapy, one of the better known professional organizations, dates from 1945; its membership has grown from just under 1,000 in 1970 to more than 11,000 in 1983. In 1977, after a long gestation period which avoided premature crystallization of the family therapy field, the American Family Therapy Association was organized.

Many patients find that it makes sense for them to participate in a kind of therapy that provides a window for direct observation of how they and their loved ones interact. Family members also appreciate a forum for airing and resolving differences in which they are actually present and able to respond, rather than remaining outside the process.

Widespread concern about fragmentation of the family, particularly in the United States, has probably been responsible for some of the increasing public acceptance of family therapy. Family therapists often focus on working out practical solutions to problems at home, frequently using a "down-to-earth," direct approach.

With family therapy's great growth and acceptance, however, misconceptions have arisen and sometimes have proliferated. These include the assumption that family therapy is always the treatment of choice and the associated notion that other treatment modalities, such as individual therapy or chemotherapy, are incompatible with family therapy. Such attitudes have been eroded: from the psychoanalytic direction by Grotjahn (1959) and from the family therapy direction by Hallowitz (1966). Pearce and L.J. Friedman (1980), Stierlin (1977), and Glick and Kessler (1980) provide bridging perspectives. A broadened view of family therapy also can be gained from books detailing case studies such as those by Haley and Hoffman (1967), Napier and Whitaker (1978), and Papp (1977).

There is a misconception that family therapy must always include the whole family. Various realities of family living make this rule impractical, however. Absent members communicate indirectly about the system. Another misconception is apparent when participants are limited to members of the immediate household or nuclear family. It may be important to include not only all household members—such as in-laws, uncles, and boarders—but it also may be important to include members of the nuclear family who do not live in the same household. Furthermore, there may be distinct advantages in including many members of the extended family, and some therapists find it helpful to work with several unrelated families. Some family therapists have also found it useful to apply "network" approaches (Speck and Attneave, 1973) involving the family's, friends, teachers, lawyers, probation officers, employers, and even business partners in the family therapy situation. The principles of human communication and systems theory have been successfully applied to business partnerships struggling with problems that proved similar in many respects to those occurring in families. The growing field of mediation is now rediscovering these similarities but is also discerning the differences.

Family therapy is not so much a technique as a viewpoint. This viewpoint is often termed *family systems orientation*. It is important to understand this way of thinking if the significance of the family therapy movement is to be appreciated.

Revolutionary strides were taken when Pinel struck the chains from "asylum inmates" and when Freud used talking treatment to understand unconscious determinants of behavior. Current mental health concepts have shifted the focus from individuals to the groups with which they interact and to the interpersonal behaviors that constitute observable events which thus influence and are influenced by their community. Thus, family therapy constitutes one aspect of what might be termed "the sociotherapeutic shift." This orientation has been defined by Strauss et al. (1964), and Langsley (Langsley and Kaplan, 1968; Langsley, 1980).

The two most salient features of the sociotherapeutic shift are its emphasis on sociological as well as psychological factors and its attention to synthesis as well as analysis. These concepts converge in those forms of therapy which emphasize the forces of building and sustaining relationships between people, such as group therapy in general and family therapy in particular.

Family therapy, through its concern with individuals and their contextual systems, extends attention beyond what goes on within the individual to *observing* what actually happens between people. Several fundamental changes in our thinking occur because the nature of our questions changes, causing us to seek different solutions with a heightened appreciation of the fact that even individual therapy and testing are misnomers since the context is at least dyadic. Some concepts of causality must also change as *interpersonal* interactions are increasingly viewed as the contexts in which *intrapersonal* phenomena emerge and are maintained.

While all forms of therapy support the goal of helping patients become more responsible, family therapy may derive some of its growing popularity from the fact that it recognizes an intermediate condition that is neither pure independence nor pure dependence, namely *interdependence*. This condition is no mere compromise: It is a richer and more complete description of each family member's situation. Moreover, it leavens the burden of responsibility with a recognition that each family member is affected by the others. This recognition of interactional impact, in turn, entails for each family a greater impetus to exercise maximum individual responsibility. Dilemmas develop with the recognition that conflicts of interest abound, but family members may derive some comfort from appreciating that the burden is shared since they are all in it together.

HISTORICAL BACKGROUND

Family therapy is both very new and very old. Only in the past three decades have family members been seen together for therapy. It was not until 1959 that the field was given a special phrase specifically describing the situation in which the *whole family works with the same therapist in the same room at the same time*: "conjoint family therapy" (Jackson, 1959). The essential features of this form of treatment had been reported six years earlier by Bell (1953), but he later credited his breakthrough to a misunderstanding of a secondhand account of Bowlby's family-focused treatment. Bell attributed his courage to his misconception that another therapist had broken the ice (Bell, 1961).

Fortunately for the field of family therapy there will probably be no polemics about who can claim priority. Don D. Jackson, while vacationing in Hawaii in the summer of 1966, verified a rumor, passed along to him by Gregory Bateson, of an ancient tribal tradition presaging even a logical but radical development in family therapy: "network therapy" of extended family social systems sometimes including dozens of related participants.* Jackson spoke with an octogenarian practitioner of the ancient art of O'Ho Puna Puna, who told him that she was the last of a line of women charged with responsibility for helping families with their problems. She brought together all family members whose presence struck her as potentially helpful. Any family member with a grievance was required to report to her, and even the more distant relatives were supposed to carry such tales to her. Family members were bound by custom to let such interventions inform their hearts as arrows of loving communication rather than as shafts of hateful tattling. The tribal tradition of O'Ho Puna Puna is many centuries old, yet refreshingly free from the weighty theoretical superstructure that sometimes stultifies the spontaneity and common sense of "modern" therapists in their work with families.

A seminal paper for the field of family therapy probably appeared in 1937 in the *Bulletin of the Kansas Mental Hygiene Society*. This lead article, by Nathan Ackerman (1937), was titled "The Family as a Social and Emotional Unit." In his opening paragraph Ackerman laid the cornerstone for the field of family therapy:

> None of us live [sic] our lives utterly alone. Those who try are doomed to a miserable existence. It can fairly be said that some aspects of life experience are more individual than societal, and others are more social than individual. Nevertheless, principally we live with others, and in early years almost exclusively with members of our own family.

Ackerman viewed his family work as stemming from roots in the child guidance movement, a fact he feared would be forgotten as a rash of reports appeared on schizophrenia. Salvador Minuchin and Dick Auerswald worked in the former tradition at the Wiltwyck School in the early 1960's, where they treated and studied the families of delinquent boys. Nevertheless, as Guerin (1976) observed,

> Family research with schizophrenia was the primary focus of the majority of pioneers in the family movement: Bateson, Jackson, Weakland, and Haley in California; Bowen in Topeka and Washington; Lidz in Baltimore and then in New Haven; Whitaker and Malone in Atlanta; Scheflen and Berkowitz in Philadelphia.

Two institutes have had a seminal role in the family field. In 1959 Don Jackson founded the Mental Research Institute (MRI) with Jules Riskin and Virginia Satir as the original staff, and with John Weakland, Jay Haley, Paul Wazlawick, and Dick Fisch joining shortly thereafter. The development of MRI's "interactional view" over two decades is described by Bodin (1981). In 1960 Nathan Ackerman founded the Family Institute, renamed the

---

*Speck RV: Psychotherapy of the social network of a schizophrenic family. Presented at American Psychological Association, New York, September, 1966.

Ackerman Institute only after his death. The *Psychodynamics of Family Life* (Ackerman, 1958) was the first book devoted to the diagnosis and treatment of family relationships. In 1961 Don Jackson and Nathan Ackerman founded the journal *Family Process*, which has proved to be an important influence in integrating the field.

The growing literature of family therapy has been compiled in bibliographies by Framo and Green (1980) and by Glick et al. (1982). They recognized a truth stated by Luther H. Evans, librarian of Congress: "Without bibliography, the records of civilization would be an uncharted chaos of miscellaneous contributions to knowledge, unorganized and inapplicable to human needs." Landmark work includes the first book detailing techniques for doing family therapy, *Conjoint Family Therapy*, by Satir (1967), a systematic overview by Goldenberg and Goldenberg (1980), a collection of commentary on major contributions selected through a survey of family therapists by Green and Framo (1981), and a handbook by Gurman and Kniskern (1981) organizing the field around ten themes central to any approach and useful in studying and teaching family and couples therapy.

FORMAT: A SPECTRUM OF STRUCTURES

Family therapy embodies an approach to thinking about people and their problems which goes beyond what Ackerman (1962) termed "a one-person phenomenon, non-social," to include what he termed "a two-or-more-person, true social phenomenon."

The developmental path of family therapy traverses a variety of possibilities. The spectrum of potential clinical situations, along with some of their antecedents, has been classified by Solomon and Greene (1963). A modified classification would be as follows: (a) consecutive therapy, (b) collaborative therapy, (c) concurrent therapy, (d) conjoint therapy, and (e) combined therapy.

Consecutive Therapy

Some family focus was advocated by Freud (1905) who wrote:

> It follows from the nature of the facts which form the material of psychoanalysis that we are obliged to pay as much attention in our case histories to purely human and social circumstances of our patients as to the somatic data and the symptoms of the disorder. Above all, our interest will be directed toward their family circumstances.

Within the framework of psychodynamic therapy there can be consecutive treatment of family members and even spouses by one therapist. This latter approach is a delicate one but has the advantage of giving one therapist a view of the major events of each spouse's therapy, putting the therapist in a relatively good position to compare, integrate, and use cognitively whatever is learned from these separate sources.

Collaborative Therapy

Collaborative treatment is the first step toward overcoming the idea that the problem is inherent in *one* individual whose therapy can proceed in isolation from communication regarding significant others, except for what the individual chooses to tell. Collaborative treatment by two or more therapists may be either consecutive or, sometimes preferably, concurrent. This arrangement, however, risks an exacerbation of family conflict through a reflection of disagreements between the therapists. Moreover, even if the therapists are in substantial agreement regarding their treatment philosophies and techniques, their understanding of the situation and their plans to manage it would still be handicapped by the incompleteness of the picture presented by their individual patients. Thus, each therapist would have only an indirect, incomplete, and biased view of the interaction.

Concurrent Therapy

Concurrent treatment by one therapist requires a high level of dexterity and experience but has the advantage of permitting the therapist to use his integrated information in the treatment of both spouses or other family members he may be seeing synchronously. According to Solomon and Greene (1963), the first psychoanalyst to do concurrent therapy was Mittelman (1948). A more recent discussion of the concurrent method of spousal therapy has been presented by Rodgers (1965). Concurrent treatment by one therapist favors a higher degree of coordination than is likely in collaborative therapy. It also answers objections to consecutive treatment which state that only the second patient can benefit from the combined knowledge available when the second spouse starts treatment after the first spouse terminates.

Conjoint Therapy

Only with the advent of conjoint family therapy, lead by such pioneers as Nathan Ackerman, John Bell, Murray Bowen, Jay Haley, Don Jackson, Salvadore Minuchin, Virginia Satir, Paul Watzlawick, John Weakland, and Carl Whitaker, were the crucial steps taken of having the *whole family work with the same therapist in the same room at the same time*. These conditions set the stage for the family to be viewed as an integral system having emergent properties transcending the characteristics of any or all of its individual members. This is not to say that there is nothing to be gained from focusing on individuals in their family context. However, to concentrate on therapeutic work in an individual frame of reference when dealing with the family unit is to leave relatively untapped the unique potential of conjoint family therapy for revealing and changing the dysfunctional rules by which the family has been governing itself as a homeostatic system. Thus, the conjoint system favors emphasis on *process* aspects of interaction, both in their own right and in relation to the kinds of *content* which initiate, maintain, and sustain dysfunctional interpersonal processes.

An alternative to emphasizing process and interpersonal interaction as joint and inextricably linked behavior sequences is to emphasize content and intrapsychic inferences about individuals. The latter approach would relegate the use of the family context mainly to overcoming inaccuracy, incompleteness, and hesitation on the part of individuals. The relationship between these two alternative types of family therapy may be clarified by pointing out that they are roughly analogous, respectively, to transactional or process-oriented group therapy and to psychoanalytically-oriented group therapy. Conjoint family therapy, however, affords many advantages and makes sense to a wide variety of people of all social strata. A restrictive consideration is whether patients have families who will attend.

Combined Therapy

Combined approaches include the simultaneous treatment of a family in conjoint family therapy and one or more of its members in individual therapy, as well as the increasing tendency toward flexibility in shifting from seeing the whole family to seeing various segments, such as parents, children, male or female members, and various individuals when it seems appropriate. MacGregor et al. (1964) described the development of multiple impact therapy (MIT), a flexible marathon treatment of a single family with shifting combinations of therapists and family members. MIT was designed partly to meet the needs of families who could not meet a regular therapy schedule and, thus, wanted help in one large dose. This form of treatment is noteworthy because of its imaginative integration of various techniques. For instance, two or more therapists may see the same individual and compare their discrepant impressions in front of the individual and even his family. Thus, the therapists may set an example about the handling of discrepant perceptions. The use of self as a model extends even to the frankly corrective comments an experienced therapist may make to a trainee in front of the family. Such open handling of unequal status communicates not only the content of the correction but also the implication to the family that it is all right for the parents to follow the therapist's example of firmness in exercising the prerogatives earned by experience.

Another dimension of combined approaches is the simultaneous treatment of more than one family system, as in couples group therapy. Some writers have described an extension of this technique called multiple family therapy in which several families are seen together in one therapy group (Laqueur et al., 1964; Blinder et al., 1965; Curry, 1965). All of the foregoing methods may be applied on either an intermittent or a marathon basis and with either one therapist or multiple therapists. The use of two or more therapists presents special difficulties in coordination and advantages in modeling and in family members' ability to find allies (Sonne and Lincoln, 1965).

Other Situations. An interesting innovation is the treatment of families in the home setting (Fisch, 1964; AS Friedman, 1965; and T Friedman et al., 1960). Extended home observation of families for research purposes has been described by Henry (1965) and by Hansen (1968), who blended the marathon feature into therapy by living in the home for as long as a week to effect specific goals with a family in crisis. For obvious practical reasons, use of this innovation remains limited.

Still other variations of family therapy are represented by such developments as the movement called Parents Without Partners, which sponsors special therapy (discussion) groups to help those contemplating or coping with divorce; Parent Effectiveness Training (PET), which focuses on parent-child communication (Gordon, 1970); programmed instructional materials for improving communication (Berlin et al., 1964); and family workshops to enhance open communication through an intensive marathon multiple family group experience lasting from two to five days.

THEORETICAL AND PHILOSOPHICAL ISSUES

Certain theoretical and philosophical themes emerge from a perusal of reviews of family therapy (Jackson and Satir, 1961; Meissner, 1964; Mottola, 1967; Bodin, 1968; GAP, 1970; Beels and Ferber, 1972; Guerin, 1976; Madanes and Haley, 1977; Ritterman, 1977; Goldenberg and Goldenberg, 1980; Olson et al., 1980; Kaslow, in press; Levant, 1980; Green, 1981).

To set the stage for his consideration of family theory, Meissner (1964) set forth ten points summarizing then extant views as a guide to consider when evaluating families. In essence these points are (a) Similarity of maturity levels and complementarity of needs both operate in mate selection. (b) An emotionally interdependent triad is formed by parents and their disturbed child. (c) Incongruent communication and contradictory demands abound in such relationships. (d) The interaction of emotionally immature parents involves and influences their children. (e) Parental maladjustment fosters child maladjustment. (f) Family interaction patterns are not specific to particular types of pathology. (g) Parental patterns of relating to disturbed children are not specific to particular forms of child pathology. (h) Immature functioning includes poor parental and marital functioning. (i) Outside influence has little impact on interdependent family triad interaction. (j) The functioning of family members is often affected by pressure from the extended family. In discussing family therapy theory, Meissner cites a central insight and premise: A missing link between theory and therapy must be provided by identifying and locating the significant etiological and pathogenic variables within the range of levels of family functioning. However, contemporary systems theorists would promote the notion of associated rather than etiological variables.

General systems and communication concepts can be added to concepts of interpersonal perception and social learning as four areas of theoretical support to which family therapy is particularly indebted.

General Systems Theory

General systems theory (von Bertanlanffy, 1968) cuts across many disciplines, culling from their common features some useful unifying generalizations. It is not a discrete discipline per se, but represents an extension of and generalization from priniciples evolved in such fields as organic biology, Gestalt psychology, and cybernetics. General systems theory formalizes some concepts anticipated by anthropologists, such as the emphasis on families as social systems with patterns rather than focusing on individual characteristics (which change over time) or on striking events. Thus, general systems theory has encouraged family therapists to remain alert for interpersonal counterparts of homeostasis which help describe tendencies to restore group or family equilibrium (Berrien, 1964; Jackson, 1959); figure-ground aspects of communication with multiple meanings as mutually exclusive logical levels, as in the "double bind" (Bateson et al., 1956); contextual influences on behavior, such as demand characteristics (Orne, 1962) and artifactual self-fulfilling or self-negating effects of experimenter bias (Rosenthal, 1964); and "disturbances in correction, feedback, and reply" (Ruesch, 1961).

Communication

Though particularly crucial to clinical work, the pragmatics of human communication has generally been slighted in courses on psycholinguistics in favor of such topics as information theory and descriptive linguistics. The neglect of this vital subject may result from its relatively recent emergence as one of the three branches of the larger domain of human communication termed semiotics. Its branches are semantics (Hayakawa, 1952), syntactics, and pragmatics. Semantics concerns the relationship between words and what they signify (roughly, their meaning). Syntactics concerns the relationship between words and other words (roughly, their grammar). Pragmatics concerns the relationship between words and human behavior (roughly, their impact). The interest of clinicians centers increasingly on pragmatics, the branch of semiotics most concerned with influence and change.

The contribution of communication to the development of dysfunction, to the maintenance of good functioning, and to the entire spectrum of interactional influence as people deal with one another has been rigorously developed in the book *Pragmatics of Human Communication* by Walztawick et al. (1967), who present in considerable detail a number of postulates about communication. Their central axioms are:

A. One cannot *not* communicate.

B. Every communication has a content and a relationship aspect such that the latter classifies the former and is therefore a meta-communication.

C. The nature of a relationship is contingent upon the punctuation of the communicational sequences between the communicants.

D. Human beings communicate both digitally and analogically. Digital language has a highly complex and powerful logical syntax but lacks adequate semantics in the field of relationship, while analogic language possesses the semantics but has no adequate syntax for the unambiguous definition of the nature of the relationships.

E. All communicational interchanges are either symmetrical or complementary, depending on whether they are based on equality or difference.

These five axioms, once grasped, have far-reaching implications for understanding normal as well as pathological communication and psychotherapy in general and family therapy in particular.

Interpersonal Perception

Development of self-concept is a recurrent theme in personality theory and psychotherapy. A particularly powerful determinant of self-concept consists of messages we receive from others which tell us how they perceive us. These messages may or may not be discrepant from what we already think of ourselves. If discrepancies of a particular kind are consistent, our self-concept may well be modified by repeated experiences of learning that others tend to see us differently from the way we see ourselves. Those who do not learn from such experiences have socially inaccurate perceptions—they cannot adequately anticipate the responses of others. Sometimes family members deny the reality of one another's perceptions, often causing other family members to question their perceptions of reality. Such interpersonal maneuvers have been referred to as "disconfirmation" (Laing, 1962).

Laing et al. (1966) distinguish three levels of interpersonal perception. The first is the "direct perspective," which is simply the view that the husband and wife, or any other two people, have of a particular person or object, such as their child. The second level is the "metaperspective," or the view that each person has of the other's direct perspective, e.g., "my notion of your perception of our child." To the extent that one person's metaperspective differs from the other person's direct perspective, the first person has misunderstood the second person's view of the object. Two people may disagree at the level of their direct perspectives but may nevertheless enjoy some empathy by understanding each other correctly; in this case they are in a position to avoid conflict by agreeing to disagree. The third level in interpersonal perception is the "meta-metaperspective," or each person's perception of the other person's metaperspective. If one *actually* agrees with another person *who thinks* one disagrees, one can correct his misimpression only if one is aware of it. Thus, correcting the other person's erroneous metaperspective requires a correct metaperspective on one's own part. In other words, the ability to provide corrective feedback requires a realization on one's own part that one has been misunderstood.

Social Learning

The systematic application of social learning principles is another approach to family therapy. A person initially presented by the family as the patient is viewed by the cautious therapist as the "identified patient" or "index patient" (IP). Some of the work of family therapy involves removing the label from this person by focusing on the interpersonal functions of the behavior that the family found unpleasant enough to justify calling one of its members a patient. The family may construe the IP's disturbing behavior as "symptoms" and as evidence of "illness." Yet it may be that the rest of the family is disturbed by the IP's behavior, perhaps because it communicates some truth the others cannot tolerate unless they disconfirm its validity by disqualifying the source. In other words, the family can dismiss the unpleasant truth by saying, "What a crazy thing to say!" or, "Why get upset about such notions; they only show how sick he is." The latter example, in addition to disqualifying the IP's sense of reality, isolates him from the family group by the use of the third person in his presence, thus powerfully ostracizing him. Such exclusion induces a sense of "patient-hood," a fate many families foist upon the tactless "truth teller" by relentless though perhaps subtle scapegoating.

The relevance of social learning principles to family interactions in general, and family therapy in particular, is by no means limited to the self-conscious application of theoretical concepts. On the contrary, some social learning will occur regardless of the presence or absence of any intention to have it occur. For this very reason, it is important to try to understand how such learning occurs spontaneously, for the existing conditions for learning are the foundations on which the therapist's efforts must be built. Such efforts may be designed to disrupt the usual dysfunctional patterns in a family or to convert them to more functional patterns by capitalizing on particular features of the existing patterns.

Whatever form the therapist's interventions take, he will have made implicit decisions about what behaviors to reinforce or to encourage the family members to reinforce. Since communication is a pervasive and influential component of interpersonal behavior, it receives continued attention from family therapists both as a behavior domain to modify and as a vehicle for creating and obtaining behavior change.

In workshop presentations, Gerald Patterson has taught that "the family is a social system whose members exercise mutual control over one another's social reinforcement schedules." Control occurs through words and actions. This statement points to the relationships between the four areas: general systems theory, communication, perception, and social learning. More explicitly, the family system comprises a complex and integrated context in which all behavior is inevitably perceived as communication containing relationship messages that also constitute sequences of mutual social reinforcement.

Behavioral analysis relies on obtaining a "functional analysis" of what maintains the behavior and perhaps a "conditioning history" of the patient as a basis for behavioral change experiments involving re-programming the contingencies and rewards comprising the family reinforcement system (Falloon and Liberman, 1973; Weathers and Liberman, 1978).

FAMILY AND THERAPIST PARAMETERS AND CLASSIFICATION

Premises about therapists and families were explored in a report from the Group for the Advancement of Psychiatry (GAP, 1970), which described two hypothetical extreme positions involving the treatment of whole families as follows:

> Position A will locate those one-to-one therapists who occasionally see families but who retain a primary focus upon the individual system, and Position Z those who use exclusively a family system orientation . . . and that, between these two positions, most therapists by far combine these two positions in differing proportions. Position N might identify those family therapists who see equal validity in an approach to the individual and to the family system, and who may elect to use either or both systems levels in conceptualizing about as well as treating illness.

This report goes on to suggest that Position A is associated with doing family therapy as a *method* of treatment, while Position Z regards it as an orientation to one's profession. The report also suggests that Position A therapists are more comfortable emphasizing the individual patient while Position N and Z therapists seek terms other than "patient" such as "identified patient." History and diagnosis are more strongly emphasized by Position A than by Position Z therapists, the latter being more likely to include themselves in the diagnostic description of a family. Position A therapists place more emphasis on the expression of affect, whether positive or negative. Position Z therapists place more emphasis on the participation of all family members in conjoint sessions. More generally, Position A therapists use joint sessions to gather more information about individuals, Position N therapists as a broadening of theory and practice, and Position Z therapists as an extension of psychiatric thinking to embrace an ecological framework for describing and dealing with individuals and families with conceptual unity.

The relation of the therapist to the family group was a central theoretical dimension considered by Beels and Ferber (1972), who stated, ". . . we begin by dividing *conductors* from *reactors.*" They describe conductors as more likely to initiate than to respond; more likely to be dominant than submissive, identifying usually with the senior side in a generation gap situation; and more likely to propound ideas vigorously, including their own values and goals. The reactors are further divided by Beels and Ferber into the *analysts* and the *system purists,* the former tending to conceptualize in recognizably psychoanalytic terms such as "transference," "counter-transference," and "acting-out," while the latter are more likely to look on the family as a rule-governed network of influences, more accessible to change through system interventions than through interpsychic interpretations.

A three-dimensional view of family therapy is presented by Guerin (1976), who discusses theoretical developments according to geography, ideology, and what might be called "penetrance." Guerin (1976) has observed that "the systems approach has moved from the periphery to the center of the field," and that "there are basically four kinds of systems orientations present: general systems; structural family therapy; strategic family therapy; and Bowenian family systems and therapy," and that another way to classify family therapists, cutting across theoretical positions, hinges on whether the therapist seeks intervention on an individual or a family level if emotional dysfunction develops in his or her personal family system. Another position, not mentioned by Guerin, is also possible: The family therapist with personal system problems might seek intervention based on the nature of the problems, possibly even addressing different aspects through some concurrent or consecutive mixture of family and individual therapy.

Dimensions of family therapy were described by Madanes and Haley (1977) as including (a) past versus present as the crucial cause of the problem; (b) interpretation versus action as vital intervention emphases; (c) growth versus presenting problem amelioration as goals of therapy; (d) method versus specific plan for each problem as preconceived versus tailored approaches to the problem at hand; (e) units of one, two, and three or more people as salient in the therapist's thinking about the problem; (f) quality versus hierarchy as attitudes toward equality, status, power, rights, and responsibilities in relation to generation lines; and (g) analogical versus digital categorization of symptoms as methaphoric communication or as discrete "bits" of behavior. Madanes' (1981) recent work underscores correctly reorganizing covertly incongruous family hierarchies.

A new paradigmatic model developed inductively through a qualitative factor and analytic method applied by Levant (1980) in preference to imposing deductively derived *a priori* categories consisted of the following: (a) a first order factor concerning time perspective or orientation as past-historical or present-historical, (b) a second order factor for the present-focused groups concerning whether the goal is to change the family's structure or process on the one hand or (c) to provide an intensive emotional experience for its members on the other hand. The three resulting paradigms of family therapy are termed respectively, "historical approaches," "structure/process approaches," and "experiential approaches." These approaches, respectively, are concerned with resolving problematic or conflict laden attachments to past figures which would otherwise be transmitted to future generations, changing the structure or current interactions of the family to remove the symptom, and enhancing the quality of life for family members regardless of any family system changes or alleviation of symptoms.

These three therapeutic paradigms were offered by Levant as broader than either schools or theories of family therapy, since each paradigm contains several schools that share certain formal characteristics, particularly pertaining to their premises about family dysfunction as the process of therapeutic change.

Fisher (1977) reviewed family classification literature from the mid-1950's to the mid-1970's and described five "schemata" for characterizing families as follows: (a) style of adaptation (approach to the world, pattern of handling stress, tendencies for dealing with crises—as displayed within the family either broadly or individually), (b) developmental stage (family developmental), (c) presenting problem or diagnosis of the identified patient (grouping of families according to the individual diagnosis or problem behavior seen as having brought the family to treatment), (d) family theme or dimension (distinctive family dimensions regarding salient features such as power allocation or family structure), and (e) type of marital relationship (included because the parents are the architects of the family and its functioning). He then presented a typology reflecting six ways families clustered according to the above schemata. Each type is followed by some of the descriptive terms or phrases it was meant to embrace, drawn from the family classification literature: (a) constricted family types (repressive, passive-negative, perfectionistic), (b) internalized family types (externally isolated, two against the world, suicidal, stable-unsatisfactory, family-centered, enmeshed, consensus-sensitive, family character neurosis), (c) object-focused family types: child-focused (children come first, child-centered), externally-focused (externally integrated, devitalized), self-focused (unintended, every man for himself, egocentric), (d) impulsive family types (delinquent, aggressive/anti-social, childish maladjustment reaction), (e) childlike family types (immature, detached, demanding, oral dependent, inadequate), and (f) chaotic family types (disintegrated, unsocial).

An integrative model of family functioning was the Circumplex Model, developed and described by Olson et al. (1980) as having a *cohesion* dimension, an *adaptability* dimension, and a *communication* dimension.

From the major contributions to family therapy they identified, Green (1981), with the collaboration of Framo, distilled 12 major concepts of family functioning and arranged them beginning with whole-family concepts and moving toward those that reflect relationships among individuals as family subsystems. These key concepts and brief explanations are summarized below.

Concept 1: The Family as an Open System. Family members function within and outside the family, influencing one another. Interdependence characterizes the family system, including disturbed behavior as an integral part of reciprocal interactions among family system members.

Concept 2: Family Stability (Homeostasis) and Change. Families act as if governed by rules, tending toward stability (homeostasis); they are able to change over time. Family members tend to restore previous equilibrium levels through a variety of behaviors that counteract the actions of other family members if these deviate beyond some implicitly permissible range. Families adjust their rules to accommodate life cycle and other changes in their members, but dysfunctional family systems lack this flexibility.

Concept 3: Family and Social Organization. The nuclear family system functions in relation to other systems such as those involving the extended family, work, school, and ethnic and religious subcultures. Just as these larger and higher systems provide the context within which the nuclear family functions, the nuclear family provides the context for its own subsystems, including (a) the spouse subsystem, (b) the parent-child subsystem, and (c) the sibling subsystem. The better the therapist's understanding of these hierarchically nested systems in relation to one another, the more therapeutic options the therapist will be able to generate.

Concept 4: Family Communication Disorder. All behavior in social situations constitutes communication, and all communication has a content and a relationship level. If incongruent, these levels create confusion and engender disturbed behavior, particularly if the family communication pattern continually contains contradictions that disqualify the communication and becloud the relationships of family members.

Concept 5: Individuality and Family Conflict. Because of the unique position occupied by each individual, relationships necessarily entail differences in respective perceptions, needs, and beliefs. Such differences are the fuel for family counseling, which may be overt or covert. Family systems typically evolve enduring patterns of conflict management. Three basic styles are collaborative conflict resolution, avoidance of open conflict through submerged individuality, and a competitive approach to conflict.

Concept 6: Marital Conflict and the Parental Alliance in Well Functioning Families. Collaboration characterizes the conflict management of a well functioning family, whose mates maintain a strong alliance through acceptance of individual differences and mutual satisfaction of needs. Though usually supporting each other in front of the children, the parents may disagree but do not permit a child to act as a judge or umpire. Thus, children are barred from some specifically marital functions such as sexuality and negotiating husband-wife conflicts, though more flexible boundaries may characterize other family functions.

Concept 7: Dysfunction and Unresolved Marital Conflict. Failure to resolve marital conflict, whether through submersion or continuing competition, may produce either alienation, symptoms in one spouse and compensatory "caretaker" behavior from the other, or involvement of third parties in the marital conflict, such as lovers, policemen, psychotherapists, or children, usually to their detriment in at least the last instance. These consequences of marital conflict can contribute new components that intensify the problem.

Concept 8: The "Triangled" Child and the Breaching of Generational Boundaries. A child may become involved in marital conflict as a referee, a decoy, an ally, or even as a surrogate spouse or parent. Such breaching of the appropriate boundary between generations leads to fusion or enmeshment of the child with one or both parents, compromising the autonomy of all. Children as well as their parents participate in the triangulation process, which can take several forms: over protection, scapegoating, inter-parent competition, and rigid cross-generational coalitions.

Concept 9: Transference and Projection. Mate selection may be guided by conscious or unconscious attempts to replicate or avoid relationship patterns experienced in childhood. In either case, the feared or wished for characteristics may materialize through the responsiveness of the spouse to projected attributions, which may be negative or positive.

Concept 10: Parent Involvement With Family of Origin. Very high or low involvement with the family of origin by either spouse can be associated with marital dysfunction. A give and take with each partner's old family, accommodating the fit of prime loyalty to the new family, can harmonize potentially conflicting loyalty claims from old and new family systems.

Concept 11: Affective Expression. Rigid family rules, through severely restricting the expression and even the experience of feelings, can produce symptomatic behavior.

Concept 12: Incomplete Mourning. Rules that block family members from showing and sharing grief about death and other losses may also block their subsequent separation and individuation, leaving them locked in "anxious attachment."

CLINICAL ISSUES

Procedures

What therapists do may depend on their orientation, particularly regarding their use of themselves. Gurman (1978) identified 13 therapist roles and functions in marital therapy which seem applicable as well in family therapy:

> All of the approaches attach major importance to four therapist activities: (1) directing and structuring the flow of therapy sessions and guiding the sequencing of treatment goals; (2) challenging the assumptions, beliefs, and attitudes of couples about the nature of marriage in general and of their difficulties in particular, and providing alternative world views; (3) clarifying communication; and (4) assigning out of therapy "homework" of various sorts.

More explicitly the 13 therapist roles and functions Gurman identified and used as a basis for the above synthesis were (a) teaches skills, imparts knowledge; (b) models new modes of interpersonal behavior; (c) directs, structures sessions, sequences goals; (d) clarifies communication; (e) gives practical advice, support; (f) provides rationale for couple's difficulties and for treatment offered; (g) encourages and supports expression of feelings; (h) manipulates environment; (i) assigns 'homework'; (j) challenges couple's assumptions, beliefs; (k) interprets patients' feelings and behavior, facilitates insight; (l) facilitates and interprets transference; and (m) shares own values, uses self, including transference feelings and behavior. The relative importance of each of these points has been detailed in tabular form by Gurman (1978).

The most far-reaching pattern of distinctions among the three therapy perspectives compared hinges on their handling of the therapeutic relationship. In the psychoanalytic approach this relationship is salient, and transference is facilitated and interpreted. In the systems approach the relationship is of intermediate importance, the Bowen therapists avoiding intense involvement and those who emphasize communications tending to view the relationship as an arena in which the successfully treated couple or family ultimately prevails. In the behavioral approach the relationship is regarded mainly as providing the rapport that allows the application of selected technical interventions. Thus, there is a continuum along which the proportion of attention devoted to relationship matters decreases as attention paid to technical interventions increases: The psychoanalytic approach emphasizes relationships, the behavioral approach emphasizes techniques, and the communications approaches have intermediate positions.

Though leading advocates of the major approaches to family therapy may suspect that therapists trained at other centers neglect their contributions, the tenor of recent consideration of this issue suggests the widespread emergence of an eclecticism that no longer reflects a lack of decisiveness but rather a thoughtful integration and tailored application of various approaches.

A summary of 23 treatment guidelines for family therapy, distilled by Green with the collaboration of Framo (1981), reflects much current clinical practice:

Assessment and Taking a Family History. Most family therapists gather historical material as it arises in the course of therapy, occasionally probing specific past areas that appear likely to illuminate current concerns. Some conceptualize the therapy within a multi-generational context, making use of systematic and multi-generational history-taking about the family's branches. Such information is gathered to (a) elucidate possible functions of symptom behavior within the family; (b) discern patterns of problem formation and attempted problem resolution, possibly spanning generations; (c) uncover the parental and marital models the spouses may be emulating; (d) appreciate how the present dysfunctional patterns may derive from past deprivations and shift from blaming parents to accepting responsibility for changing the pattern; and (e) mobilize awareness of past successes and present strengths for coping with the current crisis.

Treatment Goals. Symptom relief without symptom substitution is a widely accepted goal among family therapists. Those who work briefly believe success reflects a change in the family system's rules. Such change is regarded as structural, often directed toward the accomplishment of developmentally appropriate but blocked tasks. Goals reflect the people and problems of particular families. For growth as well as symptom relief, these goals may include (a) increasing or decreasing the contact with people beyond the immediate family; (b) communicating and acknowledging communication more clearly; (c) individuating; (d) collaborating in resolving conflicts; (e) guiding the family to rearing the children with strong husband-wife bonds as mates and parents; (f) allowing one-to-one communication without drawing in others, even if conflict and anxiety are involved; (g) increasing family members' self-direction; (h) removing parataxic and projective distortions as barriers to realistic interpersonal perception in a family; (i) decreasing inhibitions that block appropriate sharing of feeling within the family; and (j) increasing and enhancing the enjoyment of family life.

The Use of Time in Family Therapy. Most family therapists conduct weekly sessions of 50 to 90 minutes, though some meet less often for longer sessions, perhaps of marathon proportions when crisis resolution is involved. Tapering off from weekly to less frequent sessions is common, and some brief therapists set a maximum number of sessions from the start to spur responsibility for progress by accepting suggestions and setting realistic rather than utopian goals.

Orientation to the System as a Whole. The family therapist's influence and consequent ethical concern extends to all who may be affected by the problem or its resolution or who may help or hinder the process. Thus, the therapist's attention is not limited to the "symptom-bearer" or "identified patient" (IP) or to only those who attend the family sessions.

Therapist Side Taking. Family therapists generally avoid taking sides, though some depart from neutrality momentarily to assist in restoring severely compromised homeostasis or reality testing or in unbalancing a system for specific therapeutic goals. Despite such brief fluctuation, the therapist must be sensitive to each family member's need for a feeling of equity so as to further an overall sense of fairness. The "Milan Team" therapists are particularly stringent about maintaining neutrality (Palazzoli et al., 1978).

Inclusion in Sessions. Usually, all household members are included in the first session and those whose presence will help or whose absence may hinder the therapy are invited to subsequent sessions. Specific sub-systems, possibly including people outside the nuclear family, may be included for particular purposes as the therapy progresses.

Defining the Problem in Systems Terms. Disturbed behavior of the identified patient is defined as a problem involving the family interaction patterns. Members are regarded as responsible for exercising whatever personal power they possess to relate in altered ways that will help resolve the problems.

The Therapist as Intervener-Reactor-Observer. The family therapist places one foot in the turbulent stream of the family's flow of events while keeping the other foot planted firmly on the shore. Thus, the therapist can subjectively feel the pull of the family's cross-currents while retaining the ability to observe and think objectively about the people and their problems, integrating subjective and objective facets into coherent therapeutic interventions.

Countertransference, Co-Therapy, and Live Supervision. Powerful family pressures limit therapists' vision and the options they can perceive and promulgate. Some therapists work in pairs or in live supervision, allocating their attention to the complex family currents flowing before and around them. Such team efforts help in achieving objectivity, although they are replete with risks that unresolved differences between the therapists may confuse the family, as well as being more expensive and slowing the process.

Building the Therapist-Family System. The therapist's partial participation in the family system alters both the system and its rules. Mutual accommodation occurs regarding language, other interactional rules, and the structure and contract of the therapy. The therapist's partial accommodation to the family builds rapport as a basis for later leverage.

The Therapist as Model and Teacher. In relating to family members or to a co-therapist, the family therapist offers a model demonstrating options for relating (a) by showing concern for all family members, (b) by lending objectivity and involvement, (c) by presenting personal positions as his or her own and by following through, (d) by communicating clearly, (e) by sharing personal experiences pertinent to the purposes of therapy, (f) by relating warmly, (g) by relating with humor and playfulness, (h) by honest sharing of personal reactions designed to promote changes in problematic behavior, and (i) by appropriate modeling of many aspects of behavior. The family may learn about its own system through explicit as well as implicit teaching as the therapist elucidates nonlinear causality, triangulation, and the maintenance of appropriate coalitions within generational boundaries.

The Therapist as Leader of the Therapeutic System. The therapist joins the family system, transmuting it and leading the new therapist-family system. The therapist's influence derives from the active assumption of leadership and an implicit negotiation process.

The remaining guidelines outline options available for therapists to influence family systems.

Establishing the Treatment Structure. The therapist believes in determining who will attend therapy, what the fee will be, what co-therapist or consultant will be present, where and when sessions will be held, whether sessions will be audio or video taped, and what policies about telephone contacts and cancellations will be in effect.

Limit Setting and Protection of Family Members from Harmful Interactions. For the well-being of all participants during the sessions, the therapist establishes implicit limits against physical aggression, property damage, and abusive verbal attacks.

Directing the Flow of Communication in the Sessions. The therapist usually prevents one family member from speaking for another family member ("mind reading") and asks each to speak only for himself or herself, using the word "I." All family members are encouraged to participate, and to describe how they perceive one another's motives, feelings, and thoughts and how they test them. The therapist sometimes directs communication, rerouting it, keeping it on track, derailing disruptions, and using other strategies as necessary. The therapist may move people around to symbolize or even stimulate appropriate shifts in subsystem boundaries, such as by having parents sit together while discussing how to deal with a child who has literally as well as figuratively been getting between them. The therapist encourages family members to seek clarification of unclear communication and acknowledgment of what is said.

Directing the Focus of Communication in the Sessions. The therapist sets and keeps the focus on issues relevant to therapy, selecting and exploring conflict and themes judged most likely to facilitate progress toward the goals of therapy. The therapist seeks consensus or closure comprehensive to all family members, helping them learn to keep dyadic disagreements from attracting allies and thereby complicating the conflict resolution process. The therapist's restructuring of communication patterns in the sessions provides opportunities for practice and implicit or explicit encouragement for generalized application beyond the sessions.

Increasing the Family's Awareness of Interactional Patterns. The therapist points out dysfunctional interaction patterns, along with their distressing consequences and alternatives. Opportunities for change are described and/or enacted, e.g., fostering conflict or unaccustomed positive exchange. Family members may be helped to recognize their contributions to such patterns by audio or video feedback. The therapist calls attention to incongruities between verbal and nonverbal channels and encourages clear and candid communication. It should be noted, however, that many therapists believe "increasing awareness" *is not* helpful in inducing experiential change.

Fostering Insight into Multi-Generational Dynamics. When disturbed behavior occurs, most family therapists explore the involvement of extended family members living with the nuclear family or having other salient interaction with its members or the identified patient. Some examine the extended family's past and present involvement with a broadly focused multi-generational approach, using interpretation to accelerate appreciation of such dynamics. Interpretation is also used to clarify and unhook present patterns from past problems. The therapist traces distorted or displaced contributions to their sources and encourages recognition and acceptance of disowned individual characteristics.

Facilitating Operational Mourning. The therapist asks about mourning in the wake of past losses, encouraging belated grief work where appropriate. Completion of truncated mourning helps with acceptance of the loss and the resumption of progress toward necessary changes in family rules commensurate with developmentally appropriate differentiation and separation.

Conducting Family-of-Origin Sessions. Special opportunities for corrected emotional experiences are presented by sessions involving extended family members. Uncovering previously hidden information, clarifying past misunderstandings, revising inter-generational boundaries, and encouraging more realistic perceptions of parents and siblings all help to reorient internalized interaction patterns from the past, reducing residual distortions in the present.

Coaching One Family Member (Differentiation of Self in One's Family-of-Origin). A coaching method that has been developed to encourage individuation entails the following: (a) teaching family systems concepts, (b) arranging visits with extended family members between sessions, (c) promoting the establishment of dyadic relationships with each family member without drawing in any others, (d) engaging in guided practice in observing one's own family system and governing one's own emotional participation, and (e) encouraging the individuation necessary for nonpartisan involvement in emotional issues between other family members.

Reframing and Positive Connotation. Reframing prompts the family to attach new meanings or motives to behaviors that previously evoked dysfunctional attributions. Reframing usually entails replacing negative labels with positive labels, resulting in a redefinition of dysfunctional behavior in more sympathetic and optimistic terms. It may be easier for someone feeling verbally attacked to respond positively if he or she has accepted the idea that the "attack" represents "reaching out for contact." Reframing is usually but not always done in the benevolent direction. Relabeling in a negative direction is occasionally useful but must be approached with particular care. A therapist may, for example, instigate more individuation in an anxiously compliant child by redefining over-protective parental "helpfulness" as well meaning but no longer needed "restrictiveness." Such relabeling has special risks, however, in that it may undermine parental authority if done in front of the child and may unite parents in resentment and resistance, resulting in aborted therapy. Less risk results from relabeling the behavior of all family members in positive terms; "positive connotation," as this technique is called, ascribes positive intentions to all behaviors, viewing them as manifestations of such noble sentiments or motives as love, altruistic sacrifice, and the yearning for family unity. Refocusing the family's attention on such mutual benevolence supports the system's homeostatic tendency, relieving its members of any need to oppose the therapist and freeing them to consider changes in the service of maintaining overall stability. The family can be praised for cooperation and trying to preserve stability.

Prescribing Simple, Paradoxical, and Ritualistic Tasks. Family therapists often assign homework aimed at altering the system's rules, generalizing the impact of therapy beyond the sessions and strengthening family responsibility for actions leading to change. Some such tasks are simple and straightforward enactments of altered family rules. The most distressed families are the most motivated to perform tasks suggested by the therapist. Less motivated families may respond best to tasks presented through suggestion, or even just permission, rather than with authoritative direction; such families may be most readily mobilized through emphasizing the modest size and importance of the task. The ultimate modesty in asking for change is asking for no change at all. This *reductio ad absurdum* can take the form of asking the family to keep things just the same, at least for now, perhaps noting more carefully how they go about maintaining the *status quo*. Such an assignment harnesses the family's homeostatic tendency, undermining resistance to change by rendering it unnecessary through the paradoxical proscription against change. This intervention constitutes prescribing the symptom, which may be mixed with a request to alter slightly its frequency, duration, or intensity, perhaps even against the desired direction, as a means of establishing some control over the symptoms. Cautions to "go slowly" serve the same function, particularly with patients who are expressing discouragement and impatience about their lack of rapid improvement. Patients who fear a relapse may be asked to produce one so as to master the fear by establishing that symptom removal was no fluke but a repeatable act.

Dysfunctional rules may be disrupted by the prescription of a family ritual down to the last detail of timing, location, roles, and content. Such an intervention replaces old norms with new ones through action and metaphor rather than through criticism and explanation.

Additional Approaches. In summarizing his 23 guidelines, Green (1981) stated:

> There are, of course, many techniques not cited in this overview, including multi-family therapy (Laqueur, 1976); couples group therapy (Framo, 1973); family sculpture (Duhl, Kantor, and Duhl, 1973); family network intervention (Speck and Attneave, 1973); triadic-based family therapy (Zuk, 1971); fight training (Bach and Wyden, 1968); behavioral family therapy (Patterson, Reid, Jones, and Conger, 1975); family group therapy (Bell, 1975); the "Greek chorus" strategy (Papp, 1977; 1980); and many others.

INDICATIONS AND LIMITATIONS

Applications

Family therapy has been used to treat people with a tremendously wide variety of diagnoses. These have frequently included (a) diagnoses of physical problems that have profound impact on the family and that may be profoundly affected by the family reaction to the primary patient; (b) psychoses, including schizophrenia and major affective disorders, which affect and are affected by the family; (c) somatoform disorders affecting or affected by the family and psychological factors affecting physical conditions with impact on or from the family; (d) conditions not attributable to a mental disorder which are a focus of attention for treatment (marital problem, parent-child problem, other specified family circumstances); and (e) psychosocial stressors, including family changes such as a vacation, a birth, serious illness, major financial loss, marital separation or divorce, discipline problems, repeated physical or sexual abuse, death of a parent or sibling, adoption, and remarriage. Family therapy has not been limited to the conditions just mentioned since a wide variety and perhaps all of the other diagnoses in *DSM-III* may influence or be influenced by the family.

Family therapists generally try to relieve presenting symptoms and resolve presenting problems. Many family therapists also try to help the family learn how to resolve future impasses by themselves. Such therapists would say they are trying to help the family through fostering (a) clearer communication and more accurate understanding of one another's points of view and feelings; (b) skill in interpersonal processes for defusing and avoiding interpsychic conflict; (c) positive self concepts of family members through acceptance of differences without blaming or scapegoating; and (d) functional processes for appropriate balancing of competing values such as family cohesiveness and individuation, balanced separateness *and* togetherness, stability, and flexibility, to name only a few.

Recognizing and using the family's impact on and involvement in psychosomatic and somatic conditions has been termed "family somatics" by Weakland (1977), who suggests looking beyond traditional linear explanations of human events. Family approaches to psychosomatic problems have been reviewed by White (1983), with special emphasis on structural and strategic approaches. Family therapy has also been used in the treatment of alcoholism (Steinglass, 1976), drug abuse (Liberman and Weathers, 1975), schizophrenia (Falloon et al., 1981, 1982; Goldstein, 1981b; Goldstein and Doane, 1982; Liberman et al., in press; and Snyder and Liberman, 1981). Schizophrenia and the affective disorders are among the topics covered in *Family Therapy and Major Psychopathology* (Lansky, 1981). The details of aftercare for acute schizophrenia are described by Goldstein (1981a), and communication and problem-solving skills training with relapsing schizophrenics and their families are described by Falloon (1981). Treatment of married bipolar patients in conjoint couples therapy groups is described by Davenport (1981). Family therapy approaches have likewise been described for hysteria (Mumford and Liberman, 1982), adolescent delinquency (Weathers and Liberman, 1975), and work and school phobia (Pittman et al., 1968).

Family therapy is useful during "family changes" and when families are undergoing stressful situations. Family life cycles considerations are set forth in some detail in Haley's chapter on "The Family Life Cycle" in *Uncommon Therapy* (1973). The family life cycle characteristically has two types of markers: predictable and unpredictable. The predictable junctures, in turn, may also be of two types: expected and unexpected. "Expected" denotes a lack of surprise rather than a societal or family demand. Events that typically occur with expected timing include marriage, the birth of a child, a child starting school, a child's leaving school, a child's leaving home, a child's getting married, the parents' becoming grandparents, and retirement. Death is an example of an indeterminate marker, the time of which can be either expected or unexpected, though predictably inevitable. Divorce, on the other hand, is not predictably inevitable, though when it occurs, its timing may or may not be expected. Unpredictable and unexpected life cycle markers include major illnesses, serious accidents, and unusual failures or triumphs in the course of school or career. Such events would also include accidental misfortunes such as robbery, rape, and murder. Unpredictable but expected events may also occur, such as a woman's returning to work when the child(ren)'s age permits. The significance of expectability and predictability is that both permit some preparation.

Conventional family therapy and crisis intervention techniques have been applied to helping families move beyond the stresses of anticipated and unanticipated crises. For example, an approach to modifying the mental health of parental responses to premature birth was supported by Caplan (1960), who also found that home intervention is most effective when the crisis is most acute. Immediate family intervention in acute crisis was found useful in reducing hospitalization in a controlled study by Pittman et al., (1968). Bard and Berkowitz (1967) have tailored family crisis intervention for the police so that the first people on the scene can provide immediate help when violence and negative consequences may hang in the balance. Everstine and Everstine (1983) have described an emergency treatment center that combines family therapy and crisis intervention techniques in its 24-hour, seven-day-a-week mobile service, backing up police departments in dealing with family crises.

The interactional family therapy approach of MRI has been applied to counseling elders and their families, as described by Herr and Weakland (1979). Illumination of the bonds between grandparents and grandchildren has been provided by Kornhaber and Woodward (1981), and an approach to helping families move beyond past object losses through facilitation of mourning has been described by Paul and Grosser (1965).

ETHICAL AND PROFESSIONAL ISSUES

Ethical Issues

The shift from a predominantly individual focus to a wider focus on the family as a system encompassing its individual members is a conceptual step with concrete implications. This "sociotherapeutic shift" raises the question of whether the therapist's primary loyalty is to the individual identified by the family as the patient, to all family members actually being treated, to all family members regardless of whether they attend therapy sessions, to the family as a system, or to some weighted combination of these possibilities. Whatever choice the therapist may make, values are inevitably involved. Some therapists make this choice on a case by case basis; others have a relatively unchanging position. Whatever the therapist's position, however, it may have a profound impact on the family. Some therapists have no explicit position either because they have no implicit position or because they have decided to avoid making their position explicit. Other therapists disclose their position, and still others work out their position with the family members. How and whether this is done may itself have great importance to the family members, partly because there may be deep disagreements among them as to what position they would prefer the therapist to take. For example, a man who is contemplating divorcing his wife might take the position that his individual happiness is so compromised by remaining in the family system that he hopes the therapist attaches greater importance to individual well being than to the maintenance of some abstraction called "the family system." His wife, on the other hand, might prefer that the therapist emphasize maintaining the family as an entity and helping individuals adjust their expectations and actions for the sake of the collective well being.

Morrison et al. (1982) have identified four classes of ethical issues in family therapy. First, whose interests should the therapist serve? Should the therapist who begins individual therapy try to involve others in the family? If so, which others, and when are they adjuncts to the treatment of an individual or full and equal participants in the treatment of a family? Should the therapist who begins treatment of a family see one or more of the individuals separately and with what explicit understanding about the confidentiality rules? One increasingly common practice among eclectic family therapists is to allow for the whole spectrum of possibilities, sometimes seeing the whole family, sometimes one or another member, and sometimes a particular combination of family members. This "segmental" approach allows the therapist to understand how particular configurations of a family affect the functioning of the family and its individuals. Some therapists structure the attendance to create particular effects. A frequent approach to the ethical concern about confidentiality is to have such meetings known to all members of the family while preserving for each member the decision as to what, if anything, to say about the content of such visits. Some family therapists even vary the structure within a particular session, approximating what has because known as "shuttle diplomacy."

Second, what position should the family therapist take, if any, regarding whether family members should reveal to one another their secrets, and, if so, whether these should be revealed only to or between the parents or also from parents to children? How can the family therapist be sure the anxiety and loss of respect or even love will not outweigh whatever benefits are envisioned from the sharing of secrets? Mariner (1971) suggested that family members should enter into a pre-therapy agreement specifying whether information revealed to the therapist by one family member should then be shared with the rest of the family. Exceptions can be specified to allow therapists to follow their legal obligations in states that have mandatory reporting requirements about such matters as credibly expressed intentions to commit future bodily harm and about past physical, sexual, or mental child abuse. However, the discussion of such hypothetical exigencies in any prelude to the therapeutic process might cloud the beginning with ominous warnings. Moreover, such agreements leave little room for the exercise of clinical judgment *after* the therapist knows both the secrets and the family members with whom they might be shared. Parallel problems are present for the family members since, like the therapist, they can hardly be expected to anticipate what secrets might emanate from other members; thus, they have little basis for evaluating whether the sharing of such secrets would cause more harm than good.

Third, the family therapist possibly has some power to reduce conflict. Yet, the therapy format itself may imply some favoring of traditional concepts of the ideal family model, thus fostering role relationships that are not necessarily equally advantageous to all family members. However, any shift away from such traditional ideals would simply reallocate the still unequally distributed advantages.

Two of the more common dilemmas in family therapy are (a) when to have the same therapist and when to have different therapists for one or more individual family members and for the family, and (b) how to deal with confidentiality and problems posed by "secrets."

In approaching (a) above, we must be aware of the tremendous range of circumstances in which such a question can arise. More specifically, was a particular family member seen for a long time in individual therapy after which it appeared desirable to shift into family therapy? In this case, the individual therapist may have an advantage in doing the family therapy, provided, of course, that the therapist is professionally equipped to do family therapy and is accepted by the other family members, who must first be aware of that therapist's work with one of their members on an individual basis. Problems could arise, nevertheless, because of the reluctance of one or more family members to become genuinely involved in family therapy; such reluctance might take the form of agreeing overtly to an arrangement with a built-in basis for covert resistance. Another possibility is that the therapist may have worked with the family for some time and may feel that one or more members need individual therapy to progress. This need could arise from the creation of extreme tensions in joint sessions, making it difficult for the individuals to focus on their own feelings or contributions to the interaction because of their instantaneous reactivity to some other family member(s).

The patients, themselves, may have strong preferences in these matters. For example, they might prefer to have one or more separate therapists on the basis that they want to feel completely free to explore the fullest range of their feelings and alternatives, including the possibility of divorce. They may feel that the *family* therapist might have some difficulties with helping them consider such alternatives.

The choice at this point is critical since it may predict the ultimate outcome and since individual treatment by a therapist who does not know the whole family cannot be guided by a first-hand perspective on the family system, including the development of an opinion on individual changes that might improve the impact of family members on one another. Nevertheless, if one or more therapists are seeing family member(s) individually who are also being seen in family therapy, it is useful if some arrangement were made for the therapists to consult periodically to coordinate and share significant developments. The ground rules would have to be carefully worked out so as not to inhibit the free exploration of thoughts and feelings by those in individual therapy. Another circumstance in which individual therapy by a separate therapist might be warranted is with adolescents and even adults struggling with autonomy problems. It is increasingly common for family therapists to have an eclectic orientation and to use their best clinical judgment about mixing some individual and some family sessions, as well as some sessions with particular segments of the family, such as the older generation, the younger generation, the males, the females, and so forth.

Information may be provided in an individual session with one member which might help the therapist progress more rapidly with another individual in a separate session. The individual providing the information may not want the therapist to disclose the source of this information or even the fact that it has been transmitted. Yet the provider of the information may not want to tie the therapist's tongue in exploring the matter. Under such circumstances it is possible for the therapist to proceed by taking care to explore a variety of issues related in some way to the target area, leading in a natural sequence to a consideration of the area. In other words, another family member's hint has alerted the therapist to the possibility of some focused fishing, saving time by pointing out where the fishing is likely to be best.

The sharing of secrets has long been considered an important aspect of family therapy. This assumption rests on the idea that it is important to have an open system and that unshared secrets become increasingly guarded barriers to intimacy. Therefore, some therapists simply announce that there will be no secrets and that it will be assumed that any information shared with the therapist by any family member was for sharing with the entire family. Such a position presents several problems. One is that there is a hierarchical organization within families which makes it appropriate for certain information to be shared, if at all, only between the parents and not between parents and children. Secondly, family members may become sufficiently emotionally engaged in what they are discussing in an individual session, that they may not be considering whether they want to share with other family members what they are confiding to the therapist. Further, they may have an insufficient basis for predicting the consequences of sharing such information with other family members. Thus, the therapist may prefer to support privacy rights by avoiding the "no secrets" rule and hunting for another. Such rules could consist of withholding only what the patient tells the therapist is vital to withhold, disclosing only what the patient tells the therapist is vital to disclose, or not disclosing to other family members what was told the therapist in an individual session. This last rule has a great deal to recommend it. It avoids the complexity of the intermediate rules, it avoids having the therapist agree to be used as a messenger, and it encourages the therapist to be creative in getting the family members to communicate with one another. Many therapists indicate that they should be told only that which they are free to use their own judgment about discussing openly. This policy also seems to resolve the "secrets" problem.

Contemporary overviews of the hidden ethical issues can be found in articles by Hines and Hare-Mustin (1978) and Sider and Clements (1982).

Professional Issues

Training Needs. Liddle et al. (1979) have summarized in tabular form six content categories characteristically covered in the literature: (a) goals of training and supervision and skills of the supervisor, (b) training and supervision techniques, (c) the supervisor-supervisee relationship, (d) personal therapy for trainees, (e) politics of family therapy training, and (f) evaluation of training. Their recommendations include the following: (a) Evaluation research should address the selection of suitable family therapy trainees, a matching of supervisory methods to particular types of trainees, and the specification of program goals in measurable terms. (b) Conferences should be conducted and local networks of family therapists should be formed as forums for sharing training and supervision materials and methods. (c) Training programs should equip trainees to cope with the considerable professional resistance and institutional inertia likely to be encountered in connection with the interactional view of human problems inherent in family therapy, and trainees should be exposed to evaluation methods and instruments for studying their own work with families, perhaps emulating such evaluation of the training by their teachers and supervisors. (d) Sophisticated selection of supervisors, perhaps with the aid of earlier evaluations by trainees and video tape teaching samples, may enhance the quality of training. (e) While the selection of family therapy trainees should be studied and broadened to assure quality and cross-fertilization, the outreach of an interactional or ecological view of human problems and solutions is vital to prepare the public to accept and seek family therapy, particularly through the informed referrals of teachers, lawyers, probation and peace officers, and the whole range of health professionals.

Most family training programs for psychiatrists have both didactic and clinical components, including live supervision. The task is to integrate the family model into a pluralistic model that is the foundation of most programs.

According to Kniskern and Gurman (1979), family therapy training programs derive their emphases from the definition of family therapy either as a *technique* or as a new *conceptual approach* to understanding problem behavior, the former definition emphasizing the acquisition of specific interventions and the latter emphasizing the acquisition of a new conceptual framework for therapy.

Though some question whether individual therapists need to learn couples and family therapy, few question whether family therapists should learn individual therapy. This is particularly important now that flexible formats in which family members may be seen separately, all together, and in various combinations are commonplace. Research and curriculum experimentation remain to be done to ascertain the relative costs and gains of teaching individual therapy first, family and marital therapy first, or both concurrently.

Supervisory methods commonly encountered in training family therapists include individual and group supervision with and without audio and video tape, live supervision, co-therapy, and supervision in doing supervision. Some supervision focuses on formulating approaches to problems and emphasizes technique, while other supervision emphasizes the development of relationship skills in the family therapy context. The latter approach is more likely to emphasize an understanding of countertransference issues deriving from the family therapist's past or present family experience as well as the use of such personal factors in understanding the family system and empathizing with its members. Some programs suggest trainee participation in therapy with his or her family of origin or adult family. Alternative approaches to working with one's own family include charting and discussing one's family tree, role playing one's family problems, and visiting one's parents to promote further progress toward balanced identification and individuation.

Family therapists, just as individual therapists, have been intrigued by the question of whether previous personal therapy is important and, if so, in what ways. The overwhelming majority of psychiatrists and clinical psychologists have had some individual or group psychotherapy (most commonly individual), but information is lacking about the proportion of family therapists who have had family therapy.

Many significant training issues have been identified. Those remaining unresolved are questions of balance, involving optimizing the "mix" of several values so that integration may be appropriate to the particular course. Ideological issues include: the balance between interpersonal and intrapsychic points of view, action and insight-oriented interventions, the seminal viewpoint of one pioneer and an eclectic spectrum of views. Pedagogical issues include the balance between theory and practice; studying and treating families; prestructuring and evolving the course with trainee participation in decisions; lecture, and discussion; observation and doing; substantive feedback by video and audio tape, and unaided observer feedback; supervision by teacher and outside consultation; task-centered teaching and supervision, and trainee-centered teaching and supervision with personal and perhaps therapeutic elements. Training needs include more knowledge of when to see which subgroups within a family, a new interactional vocabulary, earlier and more continuous teaching of family therapy, audio and video tape libraries, co-teachers, more knowledge of therapist selection of families, and balancing brief therapy of several families and extensive therapy of one family during training.

Opportunities for training in family therapy are proliferating rapidly, and are becoming an integral part of many training programs.

Co-therapist Possibilities and Problems. Information about co-therapy for families was first reported by the Group for the Advancement of Psychiatry (1970), which stated that 90 percent of the respondents usually worked alone, 68 percent sometimes had two therapists in the room, and only six percent regularly used two therapists. Arguments advanced in support of co-therapy included having a greater capability to keep up with the rapidly unfolding complexities of family sessions, offering the family a model of male-female interaction (where the therapists were of opposite sexes), and anchoring the therapists' sanity in dealing with families of schizophrenics or providing the freedom for one therapist to move in and out of the psychotic system while the other "administered" the process of the session. Where the co-therapists were from different professions only 16 percent described the situation as being defined so that one therapist was clearly "in charge." The report continued:

> Disagreements arising between the therapists are usually acknowledged in the presence of the family, although most respondents work out such altercations outside the treatment room. In this connection an argument in favor of the single therapist should be mentioned—it is difficult enough to keep up with what is happening in the family without adding the difficulties of relationships between co-therapists.

The frequently cited advantage of male-female co-therapists modeling behavior in male-female situations including conflict resolution (Haupt, 1971) may be overshadowed by drawbacks (Bodin, 1981) such as the therapists' not sharing the same theoretical framework, activity level or tempo.

Due to the diffusion of responsibility and dilution of pressure, co-therapy might provide a relatively comfortable mode of entering into the field. A rather different advantage may be that, in the linking of a junior therapist (trainee) with a senior therapist, the latter may use the reality of their discrepant experience levels by asking directly that the junior co-therapist observe much and say little. This technique was described earlier as modeling a clear role differentiation for chaotic families whose parents are unable to make specific requests and structure appropriate generational boundaries (MacGregor et al., 1964).

FINANCIAL AND LEGAL ISSUES

Financial Issues

The meaning of who pays the bill is particularly significant in all therapy, even when third-party payment covers part of the fee. For example, if a husband and wife both have insurance coverage through separate employment, one of them may state the strong preference that the other's insurance company be billed for the sessions. Though it is possible that such a preference might rest on a desire to be officially recognized as the non-labeled spouse, it is possible that no such motive exists and/or that another reason actually underlies the request. Such a request often reflects the patient's perception that the health care billing under his or her insurance policy does not go directly to the insurance company but is processed by the personnel department at work.

Even without insurance coverage there may be issues about who pays. Some husbands and wives, particularly when separation or divorce is an issue, act as if they believe that accepting responsibility for paying the bill is tantamount to accepting responsibility for having caused the problem. Also, some partners seem caught in a stalemate over the allocation of responsibility within the marriage in general, including the areas of providing and controlling financial resources. Some couples have tightly drawn verbal or written agreements about who is responsible for what expenses to be paid from their separate bank accounts; some of these couples have no joint account and are, accordingly, particularly concerned about whether the family therapy is paid for by the husband, the wife, or both, in which case the respective proportions of payment may still be an issue.

Who pays what proportion of the bill may also prove to be a significant issue in multi-generational therapy involving parents and grown children, in therapy involving adult brothers and/or sisters, and in therapy of separated spouses, of blended families with children from previous marriages, and of couples who are simply living together.

The fee for therapy depends on such factors as the duration of sessions in particular therapeutic modalities and the rate per unit of time. In addition, the frequency of sessions and the probable duration of treatment may be factors considered by the therapist and the patients. In the survey by the Group for the Advancement of Psychiatry (1970), more than 60 percent of therapists reported having some sessions lasting between one and two hours, though 83 percent expressed a preference for the 50-minute hour. Sessions longer than two hours were reported by one-third of the respondents, as were sessions shorter than one hour. Though only about one-third of the respondents reported preferring short-term therapy, the impression left by the survey is that family treatment is typically briefer than individual treatment. Flexibility characterized the course of therapy, with 71 percent of the respondents reporting a preference for seeing families regularly until the problems are resolved, 64 percent reporting seeing some families for a short time, followed by a recess and resumption of treatment, and eight percent reporting therapy with intermittent recesses. Sixty-six percent of the respondents reported charging for family sessions at the same rate as for individual sessions, though 18 percent reported feeling that family therapy deserves a higher rate per unit of time than individual therapy.

Legal Issues

Privileged Communication. The most exhaustive treatment of confidentiality and privileged communication in psychotherapy is probably that of Slovenko (1966), who stated:

> Indeed, in recent years, the conjoint family therapy approach has commanded increasing attention in psychiatry. In such cases, the legal question arises whether or not the psychiatrist can testify on behalf of the spouse who wants him to testify. The opponent spouse can apparently claim privilege as to communications obtained from him and observations made of him by the psychitrist. Yet by seeing the opponent spouse in therapy, the psychiatrist will naturally be affected in his evaluation and testimony on behalf of the proponent spouse. No medical statute expressly covers the problem.

Ordinarily no privilege exists where the disclosure was made in the presence of any third party not necessary to the proceedings. In fact, Gumper and Sprenkle (1981) have stated:

> The third-party limitation may, however, have somewhat less impact on the privilege as applied in the context of family or marital therapy. In isolated cases, "the presence of one sustaining and intimate family relationship with the patient . . . "* has been held not to waive the physician-patient privilege. (Note that such language would not necessarily extend to the couple in premarital [or nonmarital] counseling.) In most jurisdictions, the marital or family therapy client seeking to prevent disclosure must rely on the argument that the therapy participants are the therapist's agents in the treatment process. The success of the agency argument in the context of group, marital, or family therapy is still far from certain.

Family therapists could well argue, if the need arose, that other family members, unlike virtually interchangeable strangers at the start of group therapy, are necessary for the proceedings.

Gumper and Sprenkle (1981) cited a case that went to a Tennessee Appellate Court (*Ellis v. Ellis*, 472 S.W. 2d 741 1971) which concluded that the testimony of the psychiatrist who had been seeing both spouses prior to the divorce was inadmissible under a statute extending the privilege of communications to psychiatrists. The good news for advocates of a strong psychotherapy privilege was the court's conclusion that the presence of a

---

Bassil et al. v. Ford Motor Co., 278 Mich. 173, 270 N.W. 258, 259 (1936)

spouse does not negate the confidentiality of the professional relationship and thus does not destroy psychotherapist-patient privilege. The bad news was the court's determination that one spouse could testify as to the therapy communication of the other spouse. The spouse's testimony was admissible, first, because the psychotherapist-patient privilege statute covered only communications "between" patient and therapist and did not expressly protect interpatient therapy communications and, further, because of a basic exception to the husband-wife privilege recognizing that testimony about marital communications is necessary for the determination of issues in divorce proceedings.

An exception to the Evidence Code exists in some states through statutory requirements for reporting child abuse. This may cover physical abuse, sexual abuse and molestation, neglect, and even psychological abuse, though for this last type, perhaps with authorized rather than mandated reporting.

Nonmarital, Premarital, Separation, and Divorce Counseling. Family therapists work increasingly with people living together (including homosexual couples) and increasingly with couples contemplating or going through separation or divorce. The therapist's awareness of legal considerations may be important in these areas as well as in dealing with the elderly, the dying, the grieving, and with children as witnesses; an introductory survey of these areas has been presented by Bernstein (1982). A further survey, including issues of abortion, paternity, legitimacy, adoption, abuse, neglect, delinquency, and status offenses is presented by Ruback (1982).

Family therapists wishing to function in these forensic fields would be well advised to obtain special training through course work or continuing education programs, consult with and work with attorneys, and consult such outstanding specialized background sources as those on marriage contracts by Sager (1976) and Weitzman (1981), and those on dealing with divorce and its impact, such as the survey by Kaslow (1981) and three seminal books by Gardner (1977), Ricci (1980), and Wallerstein and Kelly (1980). Those family therapists contemplating forensic involvement in child custody evaluation would do well to be familiar with the books by Goldstein et al. (1973), Goldzband (1980), the Group for the Advancement of Psychiatry (1980), and Gardner (1982). Family therapists contemplating work in the nonadversarial or alternative dispute resolution mode of dealing with divorce would benefit from familiarity with the original book in the field by Coogler (1978), another early text by Haynes (1981), recent, psychologically specific texts by Bienenfeld (1983) and Saposnek (1983), and the inspiring combination of high principles and helpful practicalities cogently summarizing the field of negotiation from the Harvard Negotiation Project by Fisher and Uri (1981).

Family therapists may encounter a number of other situations with legal ramifications beyond those already mentioned. Whether to advise an abused spouse to move out of the house is one such situation. Leaving a child behind may set up a situation that a court might subsequently interpret adversely in custody determination. A family therapist may suggest that an abused spouse seek immediate legal counsel regarding a prospective move to an independent residence or battered women's shelter, as well as to explore what other legal remedies may be available, including restraining orders. Testamentary capacity, adoption, and termination of parental rights are among the other kinds of legal issues that may arise during and after family therapy. In each case, the family therapist would do well to consult with the patient(s) and with his or her attorney before deciding how to proceed. If uncertainty remains after such consultation, it would be well for the family therapist to obtain independent legal advice from an attorney well versed in family law, mental health law, privileged communication, and experienced in working with psychotherapists as clients.

SOME TASKS AND TRENDS

The future of family therapy will probably reflect the future of families. In this country, divorce and remarriage are becoming more common, and people are living longer. Thus, divorce therapy, custody evaluation, divorce mediation, and the treatment of families formed by remarriage are of growing importance, along with the therapy of elders and their families.

Several additional areas within the family therapy field are becoming ripe for research. These include: (a) the effects of different epistemological assumptions on the process and outcome of therapy; (b) the efficacy and impact of different approaches to evaluating families; and (c) the range and variety of individual cognition, emotion, and behavior and of interpersonal interaction in "normal," "healthy," or at least nonlabeled families. Another type of research need concerns the method rather than the focus of investigation: Specifically, the family field has lacked longitudinal research, perhaps because it requires a steady stream of determined investigators as well as an exceptionally stable institutional support structure within which to organize and sustain such studies. Longitudinal research is sorely needed to answer myriad questions about family therapy approaches across the spectrum of individual and family disturbances and about the long-range development of normal families and their individual members.

It is apparent that the family field is shifting from the polarized positions of its pioneers. Many among the new generation of family therapists are able to assimilate and integrate various positions without sacrificing the coherence of their approach. Thus, as the family field matures, its new practioners seem more eclectic, reflecting the courage to appreciate and apply a broad spectrum of available theories and techniques.

REFERENCES

Ackerman NW: Family psychotherapy and psychoanalysis: implications of difference. Family Process 1:30-43, 1962

Ackerman N: The psychodynamics of family life. New York, Basic Books, 1958

Ackerman N: The family as a social and emotional unit. Bulletin of the Kansas Mental Hygiene Society 12:1-3,7-8, 1937

Bard M, Berkowitz B: Training police as specialists in family crisis intervention: a community psychology action program. Community MHJ 3:315-337, 1967

Bateson G, Jackson DD, Haley J, et al: Toward a theory of schizophrenia. Behav Sci 1:251-264, 1956

Beels C, Ferber A: What family therapists do, in The Book of Family Therapy. Edited by Ferber A, Mendelsohn M, Napler A. Boston, Houghton Mifflin, 1973

Bell JE: Family Group Therapy. Public Health Monograph 64. Washington, DC, US Government Printing Office, 1961

Bell JE: Family group therapy as a treatment method. Am Psychol 8:515, 1953

Berlin H, Wycoff LF, Mermin D: HDI: Improving Communication in Marriage. Atlanta, Human Development Institute, 1964

Berrien K: Homeostasis in groups. General Systems Yearbook 9:205-217, 1964

Bernstein BE: Ignornace of the law is no excuse, in Values, Ethics, Legalities and the Family Therapist. Edited by Hansen JC, L'Abate L. Rockville, Md, Aspen Systems, 1982

Bienenfeld F: Child Custody Mediation: techniques for counselors, attorneys, and parents. Palo Alto, Calif, Science and Behavior Books, 1983

Blinder M, Coleman A, Curry A, et al: "MCFT": simultaneous treatment of several families. Am Psychother 19:559-569, 1965

Bodin AM: The interactional view: family therapy approaches of the Mental Research Institute, in Handbook of Family Therapy. Edited by Gurman AS, Kniskern DP. New York, Brunner/Mazel, 1981

Bodin AM: Training in conjoint family therapy, in Product Summaries of Experiments in Mental Health Training. Rockville, Md, National Institute of Mental Health, 1971

Bodin AM: Conjoint family therapy, in Readings in General Psychology. Edited by Vinacke WE. New York, American Book Co, 1968

Caplan G: Patterns of parental response to the crisis of premature birth: a preliminary approach to modifying the mental health outcome. Psychiatry 23:365-374, 1960

Coogler LJ: Structured Mediation in Divorce Settlement. Lexington, Mass, Lexington Books, 1978

Curry C: Therapeutic management of multiple family groups. Int J Group Psychother 15:90-96, 1965

Davenport YB: Treatment of the married bi-polar patient in conjoint couples psychotherapy groups, in Family Therapy and major psychopathology. Edited by Lansky MR. New York, Grune & Stratton, 1981

Everstin DS, Everstine L: People in Crisis: Strategic Therapeutic Interventions. New York, Bruner/Mazel, 1983

Falloon IRH, Boyd JL, McGill CW, et al: Family management in the prevention of exacerbations of schizophrenia. N Engl J Med 306:1437-1440, 1982

Falloon IRH, Liberman RP, Lillie FJ, et al: Family therapy of schizophrenics with high risk relapse. Fam Process 20:211-221, 1981

Falloon IRH, Liberman RP: Behavioral analysis and therapy with families, in Theory and Practice in Family Therapy. Edited by Textor M. Schoningh-Verlag, West Germany, Paderborn, 1973

Falloon IRH: Communication and problem-solving schizophrenics and their families, in Family Therapy and Major Psychopathology. Edited by Lansky MR. New York, Grune & Stratton, 1981

Fisch R: Home visits in a private practice. Fam Process 3:114-126, 1964

Fisher L: On the classification of families: a progress report. Arch Gen Psychiatry 34:424-433, 1977

Fisher R, Uri W: Getting to Yes: Negotiating Agreement Without Giving In. Boston, Houghton Mifflin, 1981

Framo JL, Green RJ: Bibliography of Books Related to Family and Marital Systems Theory and Therapy. Upland, Calif, American Association for Marriage and Family Therapy, 1980 (Available from AAMFT, 1717 K Street, NW, Suite 407, Washington, DC 20006)

Friedman AS: Family therapy as conducted in the home. Fam Process 1:132-140, 1962

Friedman T, Rolfe P, Perry N: Home treatment of psychotic patients. Am J Psychiatry 116:807-809, 1960

Gardner RA: Family Evaluations in Child Custody Litigation. Cresskill, NH, Creative Therapeutics, 1982

Gardner RA: A Parents Book About Divorce. Garden City, NJ, Doubleday, 1977

Glick ID, Kessler DR: Marital and Family Therapy, 2nd ed. New York, Grune & Stratton, 1980

Glick, ID, Weber DH, Rubinstein D, et al: Family Therapy and Research: An Annotated Bibliography, 2nd ed. New York, Grune & Stratton, 1982

Goldenberg I, Goldenberg H: Family Therapy: An Overview. Monterey, Calif, Brooks/Cole, 1980

Goldstein J, Freud A, Solnit AJ: Beyond the Best Interests of the Child. New York, Free Press, 1973

Goldstein MJ, Doane JA: Family factors in the onset, course and treatment of schizophrenia spectrum disorders: Update of current research. J Nerv Ment Dis 170:692-700, 1982

Goldstein MJ: Family therapy during the after-care treatment of acute schizophrenia, in Family Therapy and Major Psychopathology. Edited by Lansky MR. New York, Grune & Stratton, 1981a

Goldstein MJ (ed): New Directions for Mental Health Services: New Developments in Interventions with Families of Schizophrenics, no 12. San Francisco, Jossey-Bass, 1981b

Goldzband MG: Custody Cases and Expert Witnesses: A Manual for Attorneys. New York, Harcourt Brace Jovanovich, 1980

Gordon T: P.E.T.: Parent Effectiveness Training: The Tested New Way to Raise Responsible Children. New York, Peter H Wyden, 1970

Green RJ, Framo JL (eds): Family Therapy: Major Contributions. New York, International Universities Press, 1981

Green RJ: An overview of major contributions to family therapy, in Family Therapy: Major Contributions. Edited by Green RJ, Framo, JL. New York, International Universities Press, 1981

Grotjahn M: Analytic family therapy: a study of trends on research and practice, in Individual and Family Dynamics. Edited by Masserman J. New York, Grune & Stratton, 1959

Group for the Advancement of Psychiatry: Divorce, Child Custody and the Family. New York, Mental Health Materials Center, 1980

Group for the Advancement of Psychiatry: The Field of Family Therapy, Vol 7, report no 78. New York, Group for the Advancement of Psychiatry, 1970

Guerin PH: Family therapy: the first twenty-five years, in Family Therapy: Theory and Practice. Edited by Guerin PJ. New York, Gardner Press, 1976

Gumper LL, Sprenkle DH: Privileged communication in therapy: special problems for the family and couples therapist. Fam Process 20:11-23, 1981

Gurman AS, Kniskern DP: Handbook of Family Therapy. New York, Brunner/Mazel, 1981

Gurman AS: Contemporary marital therapies: a critique and comparative analysis of psychoanalytic, behavioral and systems theory approches, in Marriage and Marital Therapy. Edited by Paolino TJ Jr, McCrady BS. New York, Brunner/Mazel, 1978

Haley J, Hoffman L: Techniques of Family Therapy. New York, Basic Books, 1967

Haley J: Uncommon Therapy: The Psychiatric Techniques of Milton Erikson. New York, Norton, 1973

Hallowitz D: Individual treatment of the child in the context of family therapy. Social Casework 47:82-86, 1966

Hansen C: An extended home visit with conjoint family therapy. Fam Process 7:67-87, 1968

Haupt E: A male-female co-therapy team as a model (doctoral dissertation). Berkeley, California School of Professional Psychology, 1971

Hayakawa SI: Semantics. ETC: A Review of General Semantics 9:243-257, 1952

Haynes JM: Divorce Mediation: A Practical Guide for Therapists and Counselors. New York, Springer, 1981

Henry J: My life with the families of psychotic children, in The American Family in Crisis. Des Plaines, Ill, Forest Hospital, 1965

Herr JJ, Weakland JH: Counseling Elders and Their Families: Practical Techniques for Applied Gerontology. New York, Springer, 1979

Hines PM, Hare-Mustin RT: Ethical concerns of family therapy. Professional Psychology 9:165-171, 1978

Jackson DD, Satir V: A review of psychiatric developments in family diagnosis and family therapy, in Exploring the Base of Family Therapy. Edited by Ackerman NW, Beatman FL, Sherman SN. New York, Family Service Associations of America, 1961

Jackson DD: Family interaction, family homeostasis, and some implications for conjoint family psychotherapy, in Science and Psychoanalysis, vol 5: Psychoanalytic Education. Edited by Masserman JH. New York, Grune & Stratton, 1959

Kaslow F: Marriage and family therapists, in Handbook on Marriage and the Family. Edited by Sussman M, Steinmetz S. New York, Plenum (in press)

Kaslow FW: Divorce and divorce therapy, in Handbook of Family Therapy. Edited by Gurman AS, Kniskern DP. New York, Brunner/Mazel, 1981

Kornhaber A, Woodward K (eds): Grandparents, Grandchildren, The Vital Connection. New York, Doubleday, 1981

Kniskern DP, Gurman AS: Research on training in marriage and family therapy: status, issues and directions. Journal of Marriage and Family Therapy 5:83-94, 1979

Laing RD, Phillipson H, Lee AR: Interpersonal Perception: A Theory and a Method of Research. New York, Springer, 1966

Laing RD: The Self and Others: Further Studies in Madness. Chicago, Quadrangle Books, 1962

Lansky MR: Family Therapy and Major Psychopathology. New York, Grune & Stratton, 1981

Langsley DG, Kaplan DM: The Treatment of Families in Crisis. New York, Grune & Stratton, 1968

Langsley DG: Teaching family therapy to psychiatric residents and child fellows—a department chairman's point of view, in Downstate Series of Research in Psychiatry and Psychology, vol 3: Challenge of Family Therapy. Edited by Flomenhaft K, Christ AE. New York, Plenum, 1980

Laqueur P, LaBurt HA, Morong E: Multiple family therapy, in Current Psychiatric Therapies, vol 4. Edited by Masserman J. New York, Grune & Stratton, 1964

Levant R: A classification of the field of family therapy: a review of prior attempts and a new paradigmatic model. American Journal of Family Therapy 8:3-16, 1980

Liberman RP, Falloon IRH, Aitchison RA: Multiple family therapy for schizophrenia: a behavioral problem-solving approach. Psychosocial Rehab J, in press

Liberman RP, Weathers L: Working with families of drug abusers, in Junkies and Straights. Edited by Coombs RH. Lexington, Mass, Lexington Books, 1975

Liddle H, Vance S, Pastushak R: Family therapy training opportunities in psychology and counselor education. Professional Psychology 5:760-765, 1979

MacGregor R, Ritchie A, Serrano A, et al: Multiple Impact Therapy with Families. New York, McGraw-Hill, 1964

Madanes C: Strategic Family Therapy. San Francisco, Jossey-Bass, 1981

Madanes C, Haley J: Dimensions of family therapy. J Nerv Ment Dis 165:88-98, 1977

Mariner A: Psychotherapists' communication with patients' relatives and referring professionals. Am J Psychother 25:517-529, 1971

Meissner WW: Thinking about the family: psychiatric aspects. Fam Process 3:1-40, 1964

Mittelman B: The concurrent analysis of married couples. Psychoanal Q 17:192, 1948

Morrison JK, Layton D, Newman J: Ethical conflict in decision making, in Values, Ethics, Legalities and the Family Therapist. Edited by Hansen JC, L'Abate L. Rockville, Md, Aspen Systems, 1982

Mottola WC: Family therapy: a review. Psychotherapy: Theory, Research and Practice 4:116-124, 1967

Mumford P, Liberman RP: Behavioral approaches for hysterical disorders, in Hysteria. Edited by Roy A. London, Wiley, 1982

Napier A, Whitaker C: The Family Crucible. New York, Harper and Row, 1978

Olson DH, Russell CS, Sprenkle DH: Marital and family therapy: a decade of review. Journal of Marriage and the Family 24:973-993, 1980

Orne MT: On the social psychology of the psychological experiment: with particular reference to demand characteristics and their implications. Am Psychol 17:776-783, 1962

Palazzoli MS, Cecchin G, Prata G, et al: Paradox and Counterparadox: A New Model in the Therapy of the Family in Schizophrenic Transaction. New York, Jason Aronson, 1978

Papp P: The family that had all the answers, in Family Therapy: Full Length Case Studies. Edited by Papp P. New York, Gardner Press, 1977

Paul NL, Grosser GH: Operational mourning and its role in conjoint family therapy. Community Ment Health J 1:339-345, 1965

Pearce JK, Friedman LJ: Family Therapy: Combining Psychodynamic and Family Systems Approaches. New York, Grune & Stratton, 1980

Pittman E, Langsley D, DeYoung L: Work and School phobia: a family approach to treatment. Am J Psychiatry 124:1535-1541, 1968

Ricci I: Mom's House, Dad's House. New York, Macmillan, 1980

Ritterman MK: Paradigmatic classification of family therapy theories. Fam Process 16:29-48, 1977

Rodgers TC: A specific parameter: concurrent psychotherapy of the spouse of an analyst by the same analyst. Part 2 Int J Psychoanal 46:237-243, 1965

Rosenthal R: The effects of the experimenter on the results of psychological research, in Progress in Experiential Personality Research. Edited by Maher BA. vol 1. New York, Academic Press, 1964

Ruback RB: Issues in family law: implications for therapists, in Values, Ethics, Legalities and the Family Therapist. Edited by Hansen JC, L'Abate L. Rockville, Md, Aspen Systems, 1982

Ruesch J: Therapeutic Communication. New York, WW Norton, 1961

Sager CJ: Marriage Contracts and Couple Therapy: Hidden Forces in Intimate Relationships. New York, Brunner/Mazel, 1976

Saposnek DT: Mediating Child Custody Disputes. San Francisco, Jossey-Bass, 1983

Satir V: Conjoint Family Therapy, revised ed. Palo Alto, Calif, Science and Behavior Books Inc, 1967

Sider RC, Clements C: Family or individual therapy: The ethics of modality choice. Am J Psychiatry 139: 1455-1459, 1982

Slovenko R: Psychotherapy Confidentiality and Privileged Communication. Springfield, Ill, Charles C Thomas, 1966

Solomon AP, Greene BL: Marital disharmony: concurrent therapy of the husband and wife by the same psychiatrist, III: an analysis of the therapeutic elements and action. Dis Nerv Sys 24:1-7, 1963

Sonne JC, Lincoln G: Heterosexual co-therapy team experiences during family therapy. Fam Process 4:177-197, 1965

Snyder KS, Liberman RP: Family assessment and intervention with schizophrenics at risk for relapse, in New Directions in Mental Health Services. Edited by Goldstein MJ. San Francisco, Jossey-Bass, 1981

Speck RV, Attneave CL: Family Networks. New York, Pantheon, 1973

Steinglass P: Experimenting with family treatment approaches to alcoholism 1950-1975: a review. Fam Process 15:97-123, 1976

Stierlin H: Psychoanalysis and Family Therapy. New York, Jason Aronson, 1977

von Bertanlanffy L: General System Theory. New York, Braziller, 1968

Wallerstein JB, Kelly JB: Surviving the Breakup: How Parents and Children Cope with Divorce. New York, Basic Books, 1980

Walztawick P, Beavin JH, Jackson DD: Pragmatics of Human Communication. New York, WW Norton & Co, 1967

Weakland JH: "Family somatics"—a neglected edge, in The Interactional View: Studies at the Mental Research Institute, Palo Alto, 1965-74. New York, Norton, 1977

Weathers L, Liberman RP: Modification of family behavior, in Child Behavior Therapy. Edited by Marholin D. New York, Gardiner Press, 1978

Weathers L, Liberman RP: Contingency contracting with families of delinquent adolescents. Behav Therapy 6:356–366, 1975

Weitzman LJ: The Marriage Contract: Spouses, Lovers, and the Law. New York, Free Press, 1981

White M: Psychosomatic problems, in Helping Families with Special Problems. Edited by Textor MR. New York, Jason Aronson, 1983

Zuk GH: Family Therapy: A triadic-Based Approach. New York, Behavioral Publications, 1971

10
Behavior Therapy

10

Behavior Therapy

INTRODUCTION

In 1973 an American Psychiatric Association Task Force Report entitled *Behavior Therapy in Psychiatry* (Birk et al., 1973) concluded with the following comment:

> The work of the Task Force has reaffirmed our belief that behavior therapy and behavioral principles employed in the analysis of clinical phenomena have reached the stage of development where they now unquestionably have much to offer informed clinicians in the service of modern clinical and social psychiatry.

Since that time the proliferation of experimental and clinical studies has continued, the number of textbooks on the subject has grown exponentially, and membership in behavior therapy organizations has increased dramatically. In addition, there has been a massive expansion in the types of behavioral techniques and their applications. Currently, almost the entire content of *DSM-III* can be shown to intersect to some extent with the behavioral armamentarium.

One major change since 1973 has been the growing acceptance of the idea that internal (mental) processes are suitable areas for behavioral study and intervention, and that they may play a major role in the generation and maintenance of dysphoric affects and dysfunctional behaviors (e.g., Beck, 1976; Mahoney, 1974). Another important change has been the development of behavioral medicine, now a specialty in its own right (e.g., Pomerleau and Brady, 1979; Williams and Gentry, 1977). Behavioral methodology and techniques have been applied to a variety of psychophysiological disorders and habits such as bronchial asthma, essential hypertension, cardiac arrhythmias, cigarette smoking, obesity, alcoholism, tension headaches, and enuresis (see Ferguson and Taylor, 1980).

Contemporary behavior therapy is marked by a diversity of views and continues to spawn a broad range of procedures; it is predicated on the seminal assumption that clinical practice should adhere firmly to the principles and findings of experimental psychology. This philosophy does not preclude the use of concepts and treatment methods borrowed from areas not directly connected with experimental psychology (e.g., systems theory, communications training, psychopharmacology).

Behavior therapy can no longer be defined in terms of "modern learning theory" (Eysenck, 1959). Instead, it transcends narrow stimulus-response formulations and is committed to interdisciplinary research and treatment. Behavior therapy has come a long way since the appearance of Wolpe's classic text (1958) and the development of "the conditioning therapies" (Wolpe et al., 1964).

There is no general agreement about the nature and scope of behavior therapy, and numerous definitions have been put forth. It has even been stated that the term is not definable (Erwin, 1978). The terms "behavior therapy" and "behavior modification" are used synonymously by most behavior therapists and in some major textbooks on the subject (Rimm and Masters, 1979; Wilson and O'leary, 1980). Others have chosen to make a distinction (e.g., Kalish, 1981; Redd et al., 1979). Failure to distinguish the two has created confusion, and certain luminaries have suggested eliminating one or both terms (Bandura, 1969; Goldfried and Davison, 1976).

The confusion is partly due to the fact that *behavior modification* has a public usage as well as a professional meaning. Attempts to modify the behavior of planaria, political dissidents, and deodorant consumers can scarcely be considered therapy. In addition, the public tends to equate behavior modification with aversive methods as portrayed in the film *A Clockwork Orange*, and most laymen polled on the subject have expressed negative views of behavior modification (Turkat et al., 1979; Woolfolk et al., 1977).

Whereas behavior modification may be a humanistic enterprise *or* a dehumanizing and exploitive endeavor, *therapy* is by definition a humanistic activity involving a benevolently motivated implementer and an overtly, or at least tacitly, consenting subject. The *intent* of therapy is to improve the quality of feeling and the level of functioning of an individual or group of patients.

Some behavior therapists have restricted the use of the term *behavior modification* to operant conditioning procedures and have reserved *behavior therapy* for techniques derived from classical conditioning (Eysenck, 1982). Still others have suggested that the term *behavior modification* be limited to attempts to influence or change social institutions or groups of people and that *behavior therapy* be restricted to work with individuals (Franzini and Tilker, 1972). Behavior modifiers, in contrast to behavior therapists, are more apt to confine themselves to tangible reinforcers rather than search for values, attitudes, or other conceptual or social variables. Perusal of the *Journal of Applied Behavior Analysis* reveals that a majority of papers are concerned with the control of behavior and its technological ramifications, with scarcely any space devoted to the understanding of behavior. In contrast, *Cognitive Therapy and Research*, though behaviorally-oriented, deals with such concepts as "expectancies," "encoding," "plans," "values," and "self-regulatory systems," which are operationally defined.

Wolpe (1969) defined behavior therapy as "the use of experimentally established principles of learning for the purpose of changing unadaptive behavior." The Association for Advancement of Behavior Therapy suggested the following definition: " . . . the primary application of principles derived from research in experimental and social psychology to alleviate human suffering and enhance human functioning" (July, 1974).

Ullmann and Krasner (1975) have pointed out that everyone from radical behaviorists to staunch psychoanalysts are in the business of *behavior influence*, a term that transcends therapeutic applications and includes formal school education, environmental design, advertising, and psychological experiments. More specifically, behavior therapy addresses clinical problems using (a) a testable conceptual framework, (b) treatment methods that can be objectively measured and replicated, (c) outcome criteria that can be validated, and (d) evaluative procedures for determining the effectiveness of specific methods applied to particular problems.

Behavior therapy is a set of beliefs, assumptions, and hypotheses about human beings and the nature of their problems; a methodology for assessing and evaluating these problems; and a technology for intervening. The basic assumptions are related to the role of learning and the emphasis on therapy as education. An extensive literature on behavioral assessment (see Barlow, 1981) has provided a degree of precision that has been lacking in other nonbiological orientations. Moreover, a sizable technical armamentarium has been made available to clinicians so that they can approach a large number of psychiatric problems in a highly specific and focused manner. These issues and techniques will be discussed in later sections of this chapter.

HISTORICAL BACKGROUND

Whereas behavior therapy historians have reached into antiquity to find anlagen of behavioral philosophy and examples of behavioral techniques applied to clinical, interpersonal, and social problems (Franks, 1969; Kazdin, 1978; Ullmann and Krasner, 1969; Yates, 1970), the development of an experimental approach to the study of learning and the systematic application of those findings to human concerns is a phenomenon of the twentieth century. The extension of clinical studies beyond a few isolated cases did not occur until the 1960's.

Ullmann and Krasner (1969) discuss modern behaviorism in relation to Locke's *tabula rasa* doctrine, Hartley and Hobbes' "association of ideas," and Bentham's "association principle" and "greatest happiness principle." The latter concepts contain adumbrations of the work of Pavlov and Skinner, respectively.

The twentieth century behaviorist movement is directly attributable to the Russian physiologists Sechenov, Pavlov, and Bechterev. Sechenov's position (1865) was that all motoric and psychic behavior is determined by external sensory stimulation; he rejected the concept of mentalism and explained all internal phenomena in terms of reflexology. Pavlov's (1927) experiments on conditioning and his extrapolation to human behavior provided the strongest basis for the development of behaviorism as a scientific endeavor. Bechterev (1932) was a pioneer in reflexology and attempted to apply scientific observation to individual human behavior and group interactions.

J. B. Watson, who was profoundly influenced by the Russian physiologists, proposed that all human behavior, normal and abnormal, was attributable to learning. His classical experiments, including the most dramatic case of development of fear in a young child (Watson and Rayner, 1920), are well known. In 1924, Mary Cover Jones treated a three-year-old child whose fear of a white rabbit had generalized to other furry objects. The feared stimuli were presented in the presence of food, using a graded exposure technique; during part of the treatment, other children were present and served as fearless models. Dunlap (1932) introduced the concept and technique of "negative practice" for the treatment of such undesirable habits as tics, stuttering, and nail-biting. (The dysfunctional behavior is practiced by the patient to the point of fatigue.) Mowrer and Mowrer (1938) published a classic article on conditioning therapy for enuresis. The work of Thorndike, resulting in the "law of effect," presaged Skinner's experiments on operant conditioning. Thorndike (1932) postulated that a behavior followed by "satisfying" consequences is apt to be learned, whereas a behavior followed by "annoying" consequences is likely to be attenuated. Skinner (1938) made the distinction between classical (respondent) and operant (instrumental) conditioning, the former being derived from the work of Pavlov and the latter being derived from Thorndike's studies. *Science and Human Behavior* (1953) contains the practical applications of Skinner's experimental and theoretical work. Salter (1949) was the first to attempt a general clinical presentation based mainly on the Pavlovian concepts of "inhibition" and "excitation."

It was not until the late 1950's that systematized and explicitly formulated

principles of behavior acquisition and change appeared relatively independently in England, South Africa, and America. In England, Eysenck and his
students at the University of London studied behavior in its own right
instead of viewing it as a superficial manifestation of underlying conflicts.
They emphasized the conditioning principles of Pavlov and Hull as well as
the work of learning theorists such as Mowrer (1947) and Miller (1948).
Eysenck argued that clinical problems could be more effectively handled by
formulating treatment strategies based on "modern learning theory." His
first foray into print on behalf of learning theory and behavior therapy
appeared in the *Journal of Mental Science* (Eysenck, 1959). In 1963 he
launched *Behaviour Research and Therapy*, the first scientific journal devoted
exclusively to behavioral theories and strategies.

In South Africa during the late 1940's and much of the 1950's, Wolpe, a
medical practitioner, was stimulated by the writings of Pavlov (1927)
(classical conditioning) and Hull (1943) (stimulus-response learning) to
conduct experimental research into the reduction of fear in cats. Extrapolat-
ing from animals to humans, Wolpe's (1958) classic book *Psychotherapy by
Reciprocal Inhibition* described several now well known behavior therapy
techniques (e.g., systematic desensitization, assertion training, sexual retraining, and avoidance conditioning), all predicated on the assumption that
"if a response antagonistic to anxiety can be made to occur in the presence
of anxiety-evoking stimuli so that it is accompanied by a complete or partial
suppression of the anxiety responses, the bond between these stimuli and
the anxiety responses will be weakened." This approach has been referred
to as *counter-conditioning*. After more than a decade in the United States,
Wolpe, in 1970, founded the *Journal of Behavior Therapy and Experimental
Psychiatry*.

Skinner and his associates in the U.S. were also investigating the application of behavioral principles to psychological problems. Having studied
animals in laboratories, they were interested in learning whether operant
conditioning principles might be relevant to severely disturbed adult mental
patients. Skinner's (1953) book *Science and Human Behavior* emphasized
observable behavior as the critical subject matter of therapeutic change. It is
noteworthy that the Skinnerian position is one of *radical behaviorism*—overt
behavior is regarded as the *only* acceptable subject of scientific investigation—a position not adopted by Wolpe, Eysenck, and their associates.
Skinner's view stressed that internal or subjective states (such as images or
thoughts) do not exert a causal effect on behavior but are merely correlated
with behavior as a function of external consequences. Skinner also departed
from Eysenck and Wolpe's neo-behaviorist position by arguing that statistical comparisons between groups of subjects or patients bypass significant
nuances of the actual behavior of individuals. Thus, the hallmark of his
approach is repeated objective measurements of the single subject under
highly controlled conditions (applied behavior analysis).

Bandura has made far reaching contributions to the field of clinical behavior therapy. His social learning theory (Bandura, 1969, 1977a) elegantly integrates elements of operant conditioning, classical conditioning, and cognitive processes. Unlike Eysenck, Wolpe, and Skinner, whose theories of learning were based on animal analogues, Bandura's research (devoted mainly to vicarious learning, modeling, and imitation) derived from human subjects studied in the laboratory and under ordinary living conditions. Bandura's emphasis is on reciprocal interaction among three interlocking elements: behavior, cognitions, and environmental influences. His "self-efficacy" concept (Bandura, 1977b) stresses the significance of positive self-expectations in accounting for therapeutic changes from diverse interventions.

In the 1960's, modeling techniques were added to methods derived from classical and operant conditioning paradigms, particularly for the treatment of children's phobias (Bandura, 1969b). Although observational learning had its roots in the work of Hull (1920) and Jones (1924), it was mainly the work of Bandura (1963, 1965, 1969, 1971, 1976) which seriously challenged the supremacy of operant psychology. He demonstrated that learning could occur in the absence of overt behavioral practice ("no trial learning") and differentiated between *acquisition* and *performance*.

Starting from a Wolpean framework (Wolpe and Lazarus, 1966), Lazarus' clinical orientation led to a broadening of behavior therapy (Lazarus, 1971), culminating in a multimodal approach (Lazarus, 1976, 1981). He postulated seven discrete but interactive modalities of personality: behavior, affect, sensation, imagery, cognition, interpersonal relationships, and biological factors. In keeping with broad-spectrum behavioral approaches, multimodal therapy accords full tribute to the totality of human personality and shows how humanistic values are entirely congruent with behavior therapy procedures. While some critics consider the multimodal orientation outside the boundaries of behavior therapy (Kazdin and Wilson, 1978), it has also been referred to as "the most comprehensive behavioral system in existence today" (Franks, 1976).

It is worth noting that two prominent cognitive behavioral therapists, Aaron T. Beck and Albert Ellis, had previously acquired well established reputations outside the mainstream of behavior therapy. Although Beck's (1963) "cognitive therapy" and Ellis' (1962) "rational-emotive therapy" leaned heavily on methods to assist patients in identifying and modifying irrational ideas, they subsequently added a variety of behavioral techniques to their cognitive repertoires (Beck, 1976; Ellis and Grieger, 1977). This modification was in keeping with evidence in the behavioral literature that performance-based methods are usually more effective than purely verbal or cognitive interventions (see Wilson, 1980).

Two milestones in the history of behavior therapy as a movement were the founding of the Association for Advancement of Behavior Therapy in

1967, with Franks as its first president, and the organization of the World Association of Behavior Therapy in 1980 (see Rosenbaum et al., 1983).

The history of behavior modification and therapy is vast and complex. Kazdin's (1978) 468-page volume is recommended to those who seek a comprehensive understanding of the historical and conceptual underpinnings of contemporary behavior therapy. Another useful text is by Erwin (1978), whose concerns are primarily with the scientific and philosophical foundations of behavior therapy and their implications for theory and practice.

THEORETICAL ISSUES AND PHILOSOPHY

Behavior therapy is inextricably related to learning; its main intent is the development of effective psychological treatment. The role of behavioral science in changing human behavior is a central concern. Wherever possible, clinical phenomena are operationally defined, and those variables that are amenable to experimental investigation are given priority. Thus, constructs such as "the unconscious" and inferences derived from "psychodynamics" are avoided.

Behavior, instead of being viewed as necessarily symptomatic or reflective of deeper processes within the psyche, is often regarded as significant in its own right. It is held that any psychopathological syndrome, when analyzed in terms of antecedents and consequences, may be dissected into a series of target behaviors that require augmentation or elimination. This assessment would include cognitive processes. Even behavior with major biological determinants such as occurs in schizophrenia (Curran et al., 1982) and primary affective disorders (DeRubeis and Hollon, 1981; Lewinsohn and Hoberman, 1982) may be evaluated and often modified in accordance with this formulation.

The social learning orientation to personality development underscores the importance of contiguous events, the impact of rewards and punishments, and the influential role of modeling and imitation in the acquisition and maintenance of many actions, attitudes, and beliefs. Treatment interventions are aimed directly at altering unwanted behavior, establishing its incompatible alternatives, or promoting desired behavior. Thus, behavior therapists attend to a range of specified behaviors on the assumption that behavior change often precedes rather than follows attitude and affect change.

Observation and measurement are pivotal concepts. Both process and outcome variables are closely scrutinized. The goal is to derive a body of well established knowledge whereby publicly verifiable facts replace intuitive and anecdotal formulations. The search for more specific data about the relevance of particular procedures to selected problems is a persistent one. Consequently, responsibility rests primarily with the therapist; he or she is accountable for selecting, designing, implementing, and evaluating the plan of intervention.

Another central issue in behavior therapy is the emphasis on generalization, that is, the transferring of learned behavior from the clinician's office to extramural settings. Many a therapist has been misled by the transformation of a formerly timid, reticent, withdrawn, and uncommunicative patient into an outspoken and assertive person in the individual or group therapy context. Actually, gains are often person- and situation-specific, and frequently deliberate steps must be taken to ensure that treatment benefits extend to the extratherapy environment.

Most behavior therapists are opposed to descriptive or diagnostic labels. Instead of referring to a patient as having a "passive-aggressive personality," the behavioral clinician seeks operational ingredients. What behaviors do patients demonstrate which lead others to label them as passive-aggressive? In what specific situations, as the result of which stimuli, does the patient respond maladaptively? The crucial focus is on observable behaviors and the selection of appropriate interventions (Mischel, 1968, 1973).

In summary, the basic assumptions of behavior therapy include the following:

A. Psychological disorders represent some combination of biological determinants and learning factors.

B. Abnormal behavior that is a product of learning factors is acquired and maintained according to the same principles as normal behavior.

C. Dysfunctions attributable to faulty or inadequate learning, and even many disturbances with strong biological inputs, may be alleviated by applying techniques derived from learning principles.

D. Presenting problems are viewed as real and are investigated on their own merits, rather than being regarded as symptoms of some underlying problem or process.

E. The focus is on the present rather than on remote antecedents or unconscious processes. Immediate antecedents and current factors maintaining behavior are emphasized.

F. Assessment involves investigation of all areas of behavioral, cognitive, and interpersonal functioning to discover dysfunctions or deficits that are not immediately presented.

G. Simple behavioral descriptions are preferred to diagnostic labels.

H. Although recognizing that therapy, to some extent, involves transmission of values, behavior therapists minimize value *statements*. Rather than behavior's being labeled as good or bad, its consequences are specified.

I. The therapist is active and interactive, often assuming the role of teacher and serving as a model.

J. The locus of resistance is primarily in the therapy and the therapist rather than in the patient.

K. Emphasis is on self management. Patients are taught specific self-management techniques so that the likelihood of autonomous functioning in problem areas is maximized and dependency on the therapist is reduced. Assigned homework is an essential part of the behavioral approach (e.g., Shelton and Ackerman, 1974).

L. Involvement of the identified patient's social network is desirable and often necessary. It permits the therapist to structure an optimal reinforcement environment and to resolve interpersonal conflicts through such approaches as communication training and contracting (e.g., Guerney, 1977; Patterson et al., 1975; Stuart, 1971).

The Therapist-Patient Relationship

The emphasis on precision in assessment and specificity of intervention does not imply that the therapeutic relationship in behavior therapy is less important than in other therapies. While the social learning conceptualization of relationship factors differs from the traditional psychodynamic perspective (Lazarus, 1971, 1981; Wilson and Evans, 1977), behavior therapists would agree that qualitative aspects of the patient-therapist relationship have a significant impact on the course of therapy (DeVoge and Beck, 1978; Wilson et al., 1968).

Behavioral techniques are not administered in a vacuum; the context of patient-therapist rapport is the soil that enables the techniques to take root. Thus, the respect that therapist and patient have for each other, the therapist's willingness and ability to be flexible in adjusting to different patients' (and the same patient's) varying needs, the level of trust, and appropriate expectations all provide a framework for the implementation of effective procedures. Wilson (1980) has stressed the importance of each of the foregoing factors in achieving the patient's compliance with treatment prescriptions.

Many behavior therapists have commented negatively on the application of a unitary model of therapist-patient interaction to all cases. For example, warmth, empathy, and genuineness are not universal facilitators; some patients are more responsive to distant and impersonal therapist styles. Beck et al. (1979) state that the

> therapist is well advised to exercise caution and vigilance in displaying this warm attitude. If the therapist is too active in demonstrating a warm, caring concern (or more importantly, if the patient thinks the warm attitude is too intense), the patient may react negatively. . . . The patient may construe minimal warmth as rejection, while too hearty a display of caring may be misinterpreted in either a negative or overly positive way. Thus, the therapist must carefully attend to signs that suggest that his attitudes are counterproductive.

The indiscriminately supportive therapist will, in many cases, reinforce the very behavior he or she wishes to extinguish.

In behavior therapy, the therapist's personal contributions to effective treatment are explicitly described and measured and their effects on treatment outcome evaluated (Ford, 1978; Rabavilis et al., 1979; Wilson, 1980). In the behavior therapy literature, concrete suggestions are made about how the therapist might go about promoting these conditions (e.g., Goldfried and Davison, 1976; Lazarus, 1971, 1981; Wilson and Evans, 1977).

Models of Learning

There are essentially four theoretical models of learning: the classical conditioning model, the operant model, the observational learning model, and the cognitive-behavioral model (see Wilson and Franks, 1982, for a review). Although some adherents to each of these models espouse only their own limited viewpoint, the models themselves are complementary; and most clinicians use techniques derived from several or all of them. These four formulations simply represent different mechanisms by which learning may occur, and each has its own terminology and technical armamentarium. What they have in common is an adherence to the concept that behavior can be understood and modified in accordance with learning principles. The complexity of these models precludes an extensive review in this clinically-oriented chapter, but specific techniques derived from each will be discussed in the following sections.

BASIC ISSUES AND TECHNIQUES

When behavior therapy was in its formative stages, Ullmann and Krasner (1965) emphasized "that while there are many *techniques*, there are few *concepts* or *principles* involved." London (1972) expressed the view that espousal of any theoretical model is secondary to the development and application of effective clinical techniques.

Basically, from a behavioral standpoint, problems fall into one or more of the following three categories: (a) behavioral excesses (e.g., compulsive rituals, substance abuse), (b) behavioral deficits (e.g., memory impairment, limited social skills), and (c) behavioral inappropriateness, (e.g., intimate disclosures to uninterested strangers). To effect constructive changes, behavior therapists draw primarily from the principles of extinction, positive and negative reinforcement, stimulus control, modeling, generalization, and other components of operant and respondent (classical) conditioning. (These terms are defined later in the chapter.)

Commencing with presenting complaints, a thorough functional or behavioral analysis (diagnostic process/problem identification sequence/

stimulus-response assessment) is conducted. Antecedent factors, overt behavioral responses, and maintaining consequences are rigorously evaluated.

A behavioral assessment pinpoints specific inappropriate reactions that require remediation or change. In a behavior therapy framework, one would not, for example, refer to a child's "bad attitude in school." Rather, precise behaviors would be defined (i.e., Does the child not comply in class? Does he leave his seat, swear at the teacher, disrupt the other children? Does she come late to classes or skip them entirely?). After specific behaviors have been clearly delineated, the therapist focuses on who or what appears to be eliciting and maintaining this behavior. Most behaviors are assumed to be elicited and maintained primarily by environmental events.

Walen et al. (1977) emphasize "five cardinal rules of strategy" in behavior therapy:

A. *Parsimony*. Use the simplest and least intrusive procedures that are deemed effective with a particular problem.

B. *Self-management*. Wherever possible, teach the patient the elements of behavior analysis and control to minimize dependence on the therapist and to maximize personal coping skills.

C. *Positive Procedures*. Negative or suppressive procedures are rarely indicated, whereas positive reinforcement of desirable behavior is often sufficient to effect therapeutic change.

D. *Overt Procedures*. In general, overt and external contingencies are more effective at initiating and maintaining prosocial behaviors than procedures that rely on covert or internal factors.

E. *Broad-Spectrum Approach*. Parsimony is not to be confused with oversimplification. It is necessary to determine how the "whole person" interacts with his or her environment.

In addition to their use with individuals (e.g., Cautela and Upper, 1975), behavioral methods have been employed in the therapy of couples (e.g., Jacobson and Margolin, 1979; Knox, 1972; Liberman et al., 1980; O'Leary and Turkewitz, 1978; Stuart, 1980; Weiss, 1978), families (e.g., Mash et al., 1976; Patterson et al., 1975), groups (e.g., Upper and Ross, 1979, 1980, 1981), and patients in institutional settings (e.g., Hersen and Bellack, 1978). There are literally dozens of behavioral techniques. The most frequently applied procedures will be described.

Relaxation Training

It has been postulated that muscle tension is related to anxiety and that a significant reduction in subjective anxiety tends to accompany the deliberate "letting go" of tense muscles (Jacobson, 1938; Wolpe, 1958). The most widely used procedure has been the successive contracting and relaxing of the major groups of voluntary muscles in a systematic order until a marked diminution of tension is accomplished. Researchers have differed with regard to the optimal duration of contraction and relaxation, the precise order in which the muscles are to be relaxed, and the value of incorporating hypnotic and related suggestions (Rimm and Masters, 1979).

After the therapist explains the rationale for deep muscle relaxation, the patient is asked to position him/herself in a comfortable chair or couch. A few preliminary slow, rhythmic inhalations and exhalations may be used to facilitate a positive mental set. It is customary to begin alternate tension-relaxation exercises with the dominant hand and forearm (Bernstein and Borkovec, 1973). "Make a fist, really hard, tighter and tighter. Notice the uncomfortable tension in your hand, fingers, and forearm." After about ten seconds of tensing, the patient is instructed: "Relax your hand, open your fingers, let your hand rest limply on your lap, and notice the difference in your sensations." The same tension-relaxation sequence is repeated after about 15 seconds.

Next, the biceps and triceps may be the focus of tension-relaxation contrasts. With most patients, a 30-minute session allows sufficient time to encompass most of the major muscle areas—hands, forearms, arms, shoulders, neck, jaws, mouth, tongue, eyes, forehead, chest, abdomen, buttocks, thighs, calves, and toes. The therapist may make a recording for the patient's home use or recommend commercially available relaxation tapes. Since the therapeutic goal is self-directed relaxation, patients are encouraged to phase out the use of tape recordings in favor of self-instructions. After practicing the entire relaxation procedure several times, most people are able to identify their foci of tension, whereupon they are advised to pay particular attention to relaxing those specific areas.

When deeply relaxed, patients often find it helpful to link certain words to the accompanying feelings of serenity and tranquility. Thus, they may be told to think the words, "calm," "relax," or "peace" each time they exhale during a two- to three-minute practice period. Russell and Sipich (1973) used the term *cue-controlled* relaxation to describe this procedure.

The use of differential relaxation is recommended after the patient has achieved a satisfactory level of relaxation. Here, the patient is instructed to relax ("let go of") those muscles not in use during a given activity. For example, during the act of walking, it is unnecessary to tense much of the upper body.

The use of metronome-conditioned relaxation was developed by Brady et al. (1974). Tape recorded instructions to "re-lax" and "let-go" are rhythmically cued to the click of a metronome set at 60 beats per minute. Typically, patients receive 30-minute sessions each day. One of the most widely publicized behavioral techniques for inducing relaxation is biofeedback, which is the subject of another chapter. Relaxation procedures formed the basis of most of the early work on systematic desensitization.

Systematic Densensitization

Wolpe (1954, 1958) developed the technique of "systematic desensitization based on relaxation." His patients, after being taught an abbreviated version of Jacobson's (1938) progressive muscle relaxation, were exposed in imagination to a series of anxiety-generating events. Desensitization procedures were applied to the treatment of classical phobias and various hypersensitivities such as excessive fear of criticism, rejection, failure, and disapproval.

It is often clinically sufficient to counterpose relaxation to the tension and fears that are evoked by vivid mental pictures of distressing events (Paul, 1969), but the most effective desensitization procedures appear to involve actual exposure to real-life situations (Bandura, 1977a; Dyckman and Cowan, 1978; Emmelkamp, 1982; Sherman, 1972). Wilson (1980) has underscored that "the most potent methods of therapeutic change appear to be those that are performance based." This *in vivo* desensitization is predicated on the assumption that irrational fears can be reduced by graded and progressive exposure to a hierarchy of anxiety-generating situations.

Probably no other behavioral or psychotherapeutic technique has been as thoroughly researched as systematic desensitization. For example, after a "cursory count" of five journals published during 1970-1974, Kazdin and Wilcoxon (1976) found 74 studies that involved controlled outcome research with desensitization methods. While there is little debate over the efficacy of systematic desensitization in the treatment of phobic disorders, there is lively controversy over the theoretical mechanisms that are responsible for its effects. Kazdin and Wilcoxon (1976) have argued that the results may be attributable to various placebo influences and expectations of therapeutic improvement. Wilson's (1973) well controlled study seems to disconfirm the foregoing conclusion and points up the necessity of including exposure to the feared situation "be it *in vivo*, pictorial, or imaginal." Indeed, it has repeatedly been confirmed that graduated exposure to anxiety-creating objects, people, situations, and events is a critical ingredient in the effective treatment of phobic conditions (Leitenberg, 1976; Marks, 1978).

Flooding

Flooding involves prolonged exposure to high intensity anxiety-evoking stimuli. It may be conducted in imagination or *in vivo*. Whether the feared stimuli are presented in imagination or in real life, the patient is strongly encouraged to endure the stressful effects of the intense anxiety that is usually engendered, with the expectation that relief will ensue. Lazarus (1971) referred to flooding as the "blow-up technique" and described a 22-year-old man with debilitating obsessive-compulsive symptoms, among which were repeated and irresistible urges to check men's rooms at theaters and movie houses during performances to see if he had started a fire. The therapist suggested that he remain seated while imagining that a fire had actually broken out. He was instructed to picture the fire spreading to the lobby and the entire theater, ravaging adjacent buildings, the entire neighborhood, and then engulfing the whole city. Ultimately, the planet becomes a raging inferno as a result of his actions. The patient reported that after applying this procedure, there was an initial escalation of anxiety, followed by a definite and rapid shift to calm indifference and amusement.

As illustrated in this example, imaginal flooding often has elements in common with "paradoxical intention" (Frankl, 1960). With the *in vivo* methods (e.g., driving a bridge phobic patient back and forth over a long bridge for several hours at a time), an extinction paradigm (i.e., absence of consequences leads to decrease in intensity and/or frequency of a response) appears to provide the best explanation for the results, although the process of exposure may also be construed as a form of "reality testing" (i.e., negative expectations are disconfirmed). Comparative studies between flooding and systematic desensitization indicate that flooding is generally the more effective method (Leitenberg, 1976; Marks, 1978; Marks et al., 1971).

Implosion therapy (Stampfl and Levis, 1967) is an imaginal flooding procedure that entails exposure to primary process psychodynamic themes, with an emphasis on invasion, mutilation, and bizarre transformations. The standard flooding technique, by contrast, simply uses real or imagined high intensity exposure to feared objects or situations. In the treatment of snake phobias, for example, implosive therapy would involve the conjuring up of terrifying images of snakes crawling into body orifices or strangling the patient.

In the behavioral management of severe obsessive-compulsive disorders, *in vivo* exposure is considered essential (Marks et al., 1975; Rachman and Hodgson, 1980; Steketee et al., 1982). Patients often require supervision in a psychiatric setting where trained personnel apply response prevention (i.e., they ensure that the patients refrain from carrying out their rituals). This may also be accomplished by family members or auxiliary therapists in the home setting. The flooding sessions themselves consist of the patients' engaging in their most feared activities. Thus, individuals with handwashing rituals and contamination anxieties may be urged to handle dirty laundry and other soiled objects without washing for at least eight hours thereafter. When finally permitted to wash, they would be supervised in order to preclude their engaging in the activity for more than a minute or two. Response prevention (which, in and of itself, often induces considerable anxiety) coupled with *in vivo* exposure, renders the treatment of formerly intractable cases much more feasible.

Foa, Steketee, and Turner (1980) and Foa, Steketee, and Milby (1980) have indicated that the exposure component of the treatment tends to reduce anxiety, while response prevention reduces the ritualistic behaviors. Further, they have found that imaginal exposure facilitates the maintenance of therapeutic gains. The presence of depression appears to contribute to treatment failures and relapses (Steketee et al., 1982) and constitutes the major indication for pharmacological intervention in obsessive-compulsive disorders.

Behavior therapy tends to be less effective with obsessions than compulsions (Marks, 1978, 1981a). *Thought stopping* was incorporated into the behavior therapy repertoire by Wolpe (1958) for the management of obsessions. In this technique, the patient is asked to engage in the characteristic ruminative activity, whereupon the therapist shouts the word "STOP!" or introduces any strong disruptive stimulus. After several repetitions with the therapist, the patient practices the procedure at home, shouting the word "STOP!" aloud or subvocally whenever obsessive thoughts intrude.

Techniques such as thought stopping, electrical aversion, covert sensitization, and systematic desensitization, have produced mixed results (Emmelkamp and Kwee, 1977; Stern, 1978). The total clinical management of severe obsessive-compulsive disorders often requires a multi-faceted treatment regimen that includes both behavior therapy and pharmacotherapy (Marks et al., 1980; Turner et al., 1979).

Behavior Rehearsal, Assertiveness, and Social Skills Training

The behavioral emphasis on performance results in several interlocking techniques aimed at enhancing interpersonal effectiveness. The term *behavior rehearsal* is a specific procedure that seeks to replace deficient or inadequate social or interpersonal responses with efficient and effective behavior patterns. The patient achieves this substitution by practicing the desired forms of behavior under the direction of the therapist (Lazarus, 1966). Unlike other forms of role-playing such as "psychodrama" (Moreno, 1958), behavior rehearsal aims primarily to modify currently maladaptive patterns of behavior.

In behavior rehearsal, the therapist assumes the role of significant people in the patient's life and, in a progressive stepwise fashion, more difficult encounters are enacted. Role reversal is an important component of behavior rehearsal, wherein the therapist acts the part of the patient and models the desired verbal and nonverbal behaviors, while the patient assumes the role of the person(s) with whom he/she has (or anticipates having) a problem. The use of video tapes is helpful in monitoring the patient's mode of expression, including tone of voice, inflection, hesitations, querulous undertones, posture, gait, and eye contact.

Behavior rehearsal is most frequently used within the context of assertiveness training. The main components of assertiveness include: (a) the ability to make requests of others without undue anxiety; (b) the capacity to refuse unacceptable requests or demands from others; (c) the wherewithal to identify and express feelings, opinions, and values in a frank and forthright manner; and (d) the willingness to display affection and tenderness. Training is accomplished in three basic steps: (a) instructions in how to perform a desired behavior, (b) modeling (the therapist enacts the scenes or situations as he or she considers them best executed), and (c) rehearsal with the therapist or surrogates. The combination of instruction, modeling, and rehearsal is often referred to as social skills training (see Kelly, 1982; Twentyman and Zimering, 1979).

Chaney et al., (1978) used social skills training to teach alcoholic men how to cope constructively with problematic interpersonal situations that typically had triggered excessive drinking. Several studies have shown that social skills training facilitates interpersonal contact and diminishes social anxiety (e.g., Bellack et al., 1976; Goldsmith and McFall, 1975).

A broad-based behavior therapy approach including social skills training has been used in nonpsychotic depressed outpatient populations with good results (Lewinsohn and Hoberman, 1982; McLean and Hakstian, 1979).

Graduated Sexual Prescriptions

The direct use of behavioral retraining for eliminating anxiety-associated cues attached to sexual participation has been described by Wolpe (1958) and by Wolpe and Lazarus (1966). Subsequently, Masters and Johnson (1970) provided a more elaborate sequence of sexual prescriptions for treating sexual inadequacy. However, Masters and Johnson have insisted on certain elements that many behavior therapists have found to be unnecessary (e.g., a male-female cotherapy team to work with a husband and wife unit), and they tend to omit certain procedures. For example, they do not use systematic desensitization to overcome nonsexual fears (e.g., irrational fears of assault, of control, or of blood, or hypersensitivity to rejection and disapproval).

Performance anxiety often contributes to sexual inadequacy (e.g., erectile and orgasmic dysfunctions). Anticipatory anxiety is associated with predominantly sympathetic autonomic discharges that inhibit sexual arousal and/or performance. The basic strategy for overcoming sexual anxiety is for the patient to avoid reaching the point at which sexual arousal is truncated by fear, tension, or other inhibitory sensations. Wolpe (1958) stated:

> The patient is told to inform his sexual partner (quoting the therapist if necessary) that his sexual difficulties are due to absurd but automatic fears in the sexual situation and that he will overcome them if she will help him, i.e., if she will participate on a few occasions in situations of great sexual closeness without expecting intercourse or exerting pressure toward it. He is to ask her to be patient and affectionate and not to criticize. . . . It is found that from one love session to the next there is a decrease in anxiety and an increase in sexual excitation. . . .

Wolpe and Lazarus (1966) added:

> In some cases, it is a powerful aid to remove the onus of an expected level of performance from the sufferer by informing him that there are several ways besides direct genital contact by which one's partner may attain orgasmic satisfaction and sexual fulfillment; and then to instruct him in the relevant oral, manual, and digital manipulations.

These activities serve two important functions—they provide powerful sources of sexual arousal, and they divert the patient's attention away from his own problems through focusing on pleasures bestowed on the other person.

Most of the foregoing sexual prescriptions fall under the *in vivo* desensitization rubric. Graded exposure procedures are applicable in the treatment of dyspareunia, retarded ejaculation, anorgasmia, vaginismus, and other sexual dysfunctions (Leiblum and Pervin, 1980; LoPiccolo and LoPiccolo, 1978). For example, in applying the technique of orgasmic reconditioning to a woman with vaginismus, the following sequence is recommended: While masturbating in the privacy of her home, the woman, immediately before achieving orgasm, would be told to picture penile insertion into her vagina. She would be instructed to imagine this scene as vividly as possible. Thereafter, she would repeatedly imagine the intromission scene earlier in the masturbatory sequence until the image of penile insertion generated sexual arousal. Successful completion of the imagery sequence is followed by gradual insertion into the vagina of objects (e.g., fingers, tampons, dilators) of increasing size under conditions of relaxation. Thereafter, penile-vaginal intromission may be attempted, with the male partner instructed to stop or to withdraw on request and to proceed in a graduated manner.

In premature ejaculation, the use of Semans' (1956) method of controlled partner-induced manual stimulation has proved useful.

> This consists of controlled acts of manual stimulation of the penis by the wife which lead to a progressive increase in the amount of tactile stimulation needed to bring about ejaculation.... When the husband feels a sensation which is, for him, premonitory to ejaculation, he informs his wife and removes her hand until the sensation disappears. Stimulation is begun again and interrupted by the husband when the premonitory sensation returns.

Masters and Johnson (1970) recommend a "squeeze technique" in which the woman applies pressure to the penis, just below the coronal ridge, maintaining pressure for about 20 seconds at the "moment of inevitability."

A caveat at this juncture seems opportune. While the documented effectiveness of many behavioral techniques has been replicated, a "push-button panacea outlook" would be unfortunate. The breakdown of sexual responsiveness is often one manifestation of larger interpersonal problems. Hence, as with all behavior disorders, the need for adequate, multimodal assessment cannot be overemphasized. Furthermore, while many behavioral techniques have mechanistic overtones, the actual implementation of these procedures calls for sensitivity, artistry, and a therapeutic alliance based on consideration, empathy, and caring.

Modeling

Campbell's (1981) *Psychiatric Dictionary* defines modeling as "a form of behavior therapy, based on principles of imitative learning." In a broad social context, it is well known that teenagers imitate people in the sports and entertainment fields, young children imitate other children (especially those whom they admire), sons and daughters tend to mimic the behavior of their parents, and we all learn a wide range of skills by observing competent individuals performing the necessary actions. Thus, modeling or imitation plays an important role in teaching someone how to use intricate machinery or enhance social facility. People can learn new responses merely by observing the behavior of others. One of the first systematic accounts of imitation, identification, and modeling from a social learning perspective was presented by Bandura and Walters (1963). Since then the literature on modeling has expanded and deals more extensively with characteristics of the model and the observer (Bandura, 1977a).

Participant modeling is singularly effective in eliminating phobic responses (Bandura, 1976). This procedure involves three basic steps: (a) displays of desired behaviors by a model, (b) performance by the patient, and (c) corrective feedback. In an early and well controlled study, Bandura et al. (1969) found participant modeling significantly more effective than systematic desensitization, symbolic modeling (e.g., observing a film), and a no-treatment control in overcoming intense fear of snakes. Rachman and Wilson (1980) cited several studies that document the effectiveness of modeling techniques for reducing or eliminating a variety of phobias, obsessive-compulsive habits, and anxiety-related sexual problems. Bandura (1977a) also cited evidence of the therapeutic value of modeling methods in developing new behavioral repertoires and overcoming numerous skill deficits. (Since modeling has been applied most extensively to the problems of children and adolescents, the technique is discussed more fully in the section entitled "Developmental and Age Related Issues.")

Aversion Therapy

Aversion therapy was introduced (Max, 1935; Voegtlin et al., 1941) to eliminate or control unwanted or undesirable behavior such as substance abuse or the paraphilias. In accordance with the classical conditioning paradigm, a target behavior was repeatedly paired with an aversive event such as a painful electric shock or drug-induced nausea. Aversion conditioning has always been controversial, and many beliefs about its effects are erroneous. Even with the use of powerful emetic drugs, conditioned aversions are unlikely to develop without the patient's deliberate, conscious cooperation. The patient's freely obtained prior informed consent is an ethical imperative. Since aversion conditioning is an intrusive procedure, it is recommended only after more conservative alternatives have proven futile (Wilson and O'Leary, 1980).

Electrical aversion conditioning has proved effective in treating some of the paraphilias such as transvestism and exhibitionism (Marks, 1978). Again, this method must be part of a broader treatment approach that enables the patient to cope with the psychosocial problems that frequently accompany these conditions. Given that the patient's self-directed involvement in the learning process is probably crucial (aversive reactions do not automatically result from the simple pairing of two external stimuli), *aversive imagery* is often a preferred form of treatment. The patient is instructed to picture most vividly and realistically various aversive consequences. Thus, a pedophilic patient might be asked to imagine experiencing nausea and vomiting at the thought of initiating sexual contact with children. This method is often referred to as covert sensitization (Cautela, 1967).

Several considerations recommend aversive imagery in place of electrical and chemical aversion. It is more practical and can be implemented by the patient in any setting without cumbersome apparatus. It emphasizes the type of self-activation that is considered crucial to the conditioning process, and it is more humane. Meletsky (1978) reported on the use of covert sensitization in the treatment of 186 patients with exhibitionism and found that about 90 percent improved to the point where all overt acts of exposure were eliminated. Several patients showed objective evidence of sustained efficacy over a 30-month follow-up period.

The treatment of alcoholism with broad-spectrum behavioral methods (Lazarus, 1965) in which aversive imagery is part of an all-embracing program of self-monitoring, goal setting, stress reduction, contingency management, and social reinforcement of sobriety through group support, along with several other behavior therapy procedures, has been proven useful "in producing substantial changes in abusive drinking" (Rachman and Wilson, 1980). The work of Marlatt (1978), Nathan (1976), Nathan and Goldman (1979), and Nathan and Marlatt (1978) is among the most important in the behavioral treatment of alcoholism. In treating non-ethanol substance abuse, Rachman and Wilson (1980) conclude that behavior therapy offers no advantages over alternative approaches.

Behavioral Self-Control Procedures

In its earlier phase, behavior therapy placed much emphasis on the control of behavior by environmental manipulation. The idea that the human organism might develop control over its own conditioning was foreshadowed by Skinner (1953) in a discussion of *self-control*. Kanfer (1970, 1971) described self-regulation as consisting of three processes: self-monitoring, self-evaluation, and self-reinforcement. Self-monitoring involves observing one's own behavior, especially a behavior targeted for change. This process may be accomplished by recording events in a notebook or by making a mental notation. Some experimental evidence suggests that this widely used technique may be effective by itself in modifying behavior, especially in the early stages of the change process (Kazdin, 1974) and when positive efforts (rather than undesired habits) are monitored. Self-evaluation refers to comparison of one's behavior with a standard (internal or external) to assess its adequacy. Self-reinforcement is the administration of consequences to one's self, contingent upon the performance of a particular behavior in a specific manner. The reinforcement may take the form of self-verbalization (e.g., the patient says to himself, "Well done, you're terrific.") or some behavioral or material reinforcer (patient buys herself a new pair of shoes after walking three miles a day and avoiding sweets for a week). Self-reinforcement is perhaps the most important of all the self-management techniques, and numerous studies have shown its effectiveness (Bandura and Perloff, 1967; Brownell et al., 1977; Felixbrod and O'Leary, 1973; Lovitt and Curtiss, 1969).

Self-control procedures were launched by Goldiamond's (1965) influential paper, and the concept of self-control came into its own with the publication of Thoresen and Mahoney's volume (1974). Although the term *self-control* has been widely used, its implication of self-denial in the public sense has led to the suggested use of "coping skills training" as an alternative (Goldfried, 1980). Self-management has become one of the central focuses of behavior therapy (see for example Stuart, 1977), with behavioral techniques being used by patients to modify their overt behavior as well as their thought processes.

Homme's (1965) concept of *coverant control* (coverant=covert, i.e., mental operant) stressed that operant conditioning principles are applicable to mental as well as to overt behavior. Thus emerged an array of conditioning techniques involving private events (internal processes), including covert positive reinforcement, covert negative reinforcement, covert extinction, and covert response cost (see section entitled "Developmental and Age Related Issues"). Subsequently, covert modeling was added (Cautela, 1971). As already mentioned, Cautela (1967) had used "covert sensitization" for attenuating undesired habits. The advent of Bandura's (1969) classic text spurred more interest in the role of self-regulation of behavior in the absence of immediate external supports (cf., Kanfer and Karoly, 1972). Self-monitoring, self-evaluation, and self-reinforcement are now being investigated as important behavior change methods in and of themselves.

Modification of overeating in obese subjects represented one of the first applications of self-control procedures (Stuart, 1967). Behavioral weight reduction programs teach patients to keep detailed records of food consumption and exercise habits as well as the circumstances under which these activities occur. In addition, the importance of *stimulus control* is emphasized. This technique is based on the assumption that a primary determinant of behavior is the stimulus environment in which it occurs. Thus, the patient is instructed to reduce and narrow the number of stimuli associated with the act of eating (e.g., avoid eating while reading or watching television, do not eat while standing up, eat only at specified times and in specified places). Additional procedures are used to disrupt and control the actual act of eating (e.g., all food has to be chewed slowly and completely swallowed before the next bite, eating utensils have to be placed on the table between bites). Furthermore, explicit sources of reinforcement are arranged to support behavior that delays or controls eating. Thus, if the patient has achieved a preset caloric intake of fewer than 1,500 calories for that day, he or she would apply self-reinforcement (e.g., attending a special concert, making an appointment at the beauty parlor, or whatever fits the subjective pleasures of the individual).

Self-instructional training is another self-control procedure that has been well researched (Meichenbaum, 1977). In this procedure, patients are explicitly trained to monitor irrational, self-defeating thoughts; to realize how these thoughts or self-verbalizations generate emotional turmoil; and to acquire alternative self-statements that are incompatible with anxiety. (Many behavior therapists assume that most covert processes obey the same psychological laws as do overt behaviors and can be modified by the same techniques—modeling, reinforcement, and aversitructional training distinctly ameliorates such problems as impulsivity (Bender, 1976) and low resistance to temptation (Hartig and Kanfer, 1973).

With children, self-instruction training involves five steps (Meichenbaum, 1977): (a) an adult model first performs the task while talking to himself aloud (cognitive modeling), (b) the child then performs the same task under the direction of the model's instructions (overt external guidance), (c) the child next performs the task while instructing himself aloud (overt self-guidance), (d) the child then whispers the instructions to himself as he performs the task (faded overt self-guidance), (e) the child performs the task while guiding his performance via private speech (covert self-instruction).

These and other cognitive restructuring procedures were introduced into the behavioral literature during the 1970's (Beck, 1970, 1976; Goldfried et al., 1974; Lazarus, 1971; Mahoney, 1974; Meichenbaum, 1977) and are discussed extensively in Chapter 7. As mentioned previously, behavior therapists focus primarily on conscious thought processes and seldom search for unconscious, symbolic meanings. The emphasis is on how to change cognitive distortions without necessarily examining how and why the distortions arose.

Token Economies

Ayllon and Azrin (1968) pioneered in developing token economy programs for chronically psychotic inpatients. Since then, token reinforcement programs have been applied in many correctional, rehabilitative, and educational settings (Hersen and Bellack, 1978). They have been used with an extraordinarily diverse range of populations—psychiatric inpatients and outpatients, normal and disturbed children in classroom settings, retarded and autistic children, delinquent youths, and even low-income families in a community-improvement program (Kazdin, 1977).

Many different procedures and goals are subsumed under the token economy rubric. Nevertheless, they share common characteristics. Where the goal is augmentation of self-care behaviors in psychotic patients, the following procedures are implemented:

A. The specific behaviors to be modified or developed are clearly identified and operationally defined.

B. Reinforcers available in the environment are determined. (These are desiderata that the patients are willing to work for, such as special desserts, extra television time, or private accommodations.)

C. The tokens themselves are specified. In some settings plastic chips are used; in others, numerical ratings are more suitable.

D. A set of rules is established for exchanging tokens for back-up reinforcers (a private room, extra television time, or other activities that the patients consider rewarding).

E. Personnel are trained to hand out tokens for appropriate behaviors, and a predetermined number of tokens enables the patient to purchase the back-up reinforcer.

In essence, the programs mirror economic principles governing society outside the token economy environment. An important feature of successful token economy programs is the rewarding of personnel (usually nurses, attendants, aides, or volunteers) for correctly and appropriately dispensing the tokens and back-up reinforcers (Gelfand et al., 1967; Hersen and Bellack, 1978). The most sophisticated and elegant token economy programs (e.g., Paul and Lentz, 1977) attempt to go beyond the induction of therapeutic change for a specific set of problem behaviors within a circumscribed environment. Through a progressive series of bridging procedures, they try to expand these changes to situations outside of the institution, and they address issues involving long-term maintenance of improvement.

The fact that token economies repeatedly have been successful in improving behavior within the hospital should not be seen as trivial. Greater social involvement and better self-management usually result in a happier, more dignified, and more productive life for patients, even if they remain hospitalized.

Further discussion of operant conditioning principles and techniques is presented in the section on "Developmental and Age Related Issues."

Behavioral Medicine

One of the most quoted definitions of behavioral medicine is that put forth by Schwartz and Weiss (1978), who refer to it as

> ... the interdisciplinary field concerned with the development and integration of behavioral and biomedical science, knowledge and techniques relevant to health, illness and related conditions and the application of this knowledge and these techniques to prevention, diagnosis, treatment, and rehabilitation.

The scope of behavioral medicine is so broad as to involve

> the integration of relevant parts of epidemiology, anthropology, sociology, psychology, physiology, pharmacology, nutrition, neuroanatomy, endocrinology, immunology, and the various branches of medicine and public health, as well as related professions such as dentistry, nursing, social work, and health education (Miller, 1983).

Behavioral medicine generally focuses on conditions traditionally viewed as medical rather than psychiatric and on habits with predominantly medical consequences. Thus, schizophrenia, primary affective disorders, and phobic neuroses would not come under the rubric, whereas hypertension and asthma would. On the other hand, social phobia leading to an inhibition of micturition in public bathrooms would qualify. Obesity and alcoholism would be included, whereas compulsive gambling would not. The distinction is sometimes arbitrary, and basic textbooks on the subject have differed in their selection of content (see Davidson and Davidson, 1980; Doleys et al., 1982; Ferguson and Taylor, 1980; McNamara, 1979; Melamed and Siegel, 1980; Pomerleau and Brady, 1979; Serwit et al., 1982; Weiss et al., 1981; Williams and Gentry, 1977). Melamed and Siegel (1980) include a chapter on "Management of Psychiatric Disorders Associated with Medical Problems" and list anorexia nervosa, headaches, spasmodic torticollis, insomnia, and sexual dysfunction, as well as phobias and obsessions concerned with illness or bodily injury. An even broader conceptualization would encompass the entire bio-psycho-social domain (West and Stein, 1982).

The specific area of biofeedback, an integral part of behavioral medicine (Birk, 1973), has become a domain unto itself; although it is based on learning principles, it is fundamentally distinct in that physiological parameters rather than overt behavior are the focus of attention. Therefore, behavioral procedures have sometimes been divided into biofeedback and non-biofeedback areas (Epstein and Parker, 1977). The subject of biofeedback is covered in another chapter; this section will review other behavioral approaches.

Behavioral medicine may be divided as well according to medical specialties—there are fields of pediatric and adolescent behavioral medicine (e.g., McGrath and Firestone, 1983) and behavioral gerontology (Patterson, 1982), as well as areas of behavioral cardiology (e.g., Matarazzo et al., 1982), behavioral ophthalmology (Collins, 1981), and behavioral urology (Doleys and Meredith, 1982) among others. As early as 1976, a national conference on "behavioral dentistry" was convened (Ingersoll et al., 1977). The practice of creating subspecialties in behavioral medicine has been deplored in some quarters as premature and presumptuous (Brownell, 1982).

Blanchard (1977) regards behavioral medicine as having several subdomains: (a) direct psychological intervention in problems that have traditionally been considered medical, such as hypertension and obesity. Here, behavioral medicine provides an alternative or adjunct to traditional pharmacological or surgical intervention, (b) the use of psychological intervention to facilitate or enhance standard medical care. The major focus is patient compliance or adherence to the prescribed medical regimen, (c) psychological intervention at the physiological level through biofeedback training, and (d) primary prevention.

Despite substantial gains in the fields of epidemiology, medical diagnosis, and clinical pharmacology, the health of individuals in technologically advanced countries has not improved *pari passu*. One major reason is the traditional focus on illness rather than "wellness." Another crucial problem centers around the issue of compliance (Davidson, 1982; Epstein and Cluss, 1982; Haynes, 1981), which has been defined as "the extent to which a person's behavior coincides with medical or health advice" (Haynes, 1979). Clearly, health care providers' medical knowledge is not a sufficient condition for clinical effectiveness; implementation is critical, and it is here that behavioral methods may be particularly useful (Zifferblat, 1975).

Before discussing the behavioral management of specific medical entities, it is important to point out that behavioral medicine is a relatively new field; a large number of conditions have been studied, and numerous techniques applied. Many of the studies suffer from significant design limitations, are anecdotal rather than scientific, and/or lack long-term follow-ups. Many data are contradictory and conclusions are unclear. Miller (1979) has sounded a note of caution about claims in this area which do not rest on an adequate experimental base. Because the field is so vast as to preclude a review of all topics that have been studied, a few representative problems that have received a great deal of attention will be discussed.

Among the medical areas most thoroughly investigated are cardiovascular disease, asthma, pain, and insomnia.

Cardiovascular Disorders. Most of the work on cardiovascular disorders has centered on hypertension, arrhythmias, Raynaud's disease, and the mitigation of risk for coronary artery disease, including modification of smoking, diet, activity patterns, and Type A behavior.

Relaxation procedures have been shown to be useful in essential hypertension. These techniques have been studied alone, in comparison with biofeedback, and in conjunction with biofeedback. While the comparison data are contradictory, various relaxation techniques have been successfully used (Agras and Jacob, 1979) since Jacobson's initial report (1939).

Whereas most of the work on arrhythmias and Raynaud's phenomenon has used biofeedback, one study showed a significant reduction in the frequency of premature ventricular contractions in eight of 11 patients treated with the "relaxation response," essentially a meditation procedure (Benson et al., 1975).

There is an extensive literature on the modification of smoking (e.g., Lichtenstein and Brown, 1982), obesity (e.g., Stunkard, 1982), and Type A behavior (e.g., Suinn, 1982).

Asthma. Several authors (e.g., Dekker et al., 1957; Turnball, 1962) have formulated explanations for the phenomenon of bronchial asthma which invoke classical and operant conditioning. An asthma attack may become associated with a variety of conditioned stimuli (e.g., the sight of a cat or mention of the word "dust"). Operant explanations focus on the increased attention that often accompanies an episode, as well as on the avoidance of work, school, unwelcome chores, or social or sexual encounters. Desensitization to emotionally disturbing stimuli has been reported in several studies (e.g., Philander et al., 1979; Yorkston et al., 1974). Alexander (1981, 1983) and Creer and Kotses (1983) have reviewed a variety of behavioral techniques in the management of bronchial asthma, including positive reinforcement, punishment, satiation, response cost, and systematic desensitization. This area is still highly controversial, and much of the research has been called into question (e.g., King, 1980; Richter and Dahme, 1982).

Pain. The behavioral approach to the alleviation of pain has been reported most extensively by Fordyce and associates (Fordyce, 1976, 1982; Fordyce et al., 1968, 1982; Steger and Fordyce, 1982). This group's basic approach to pain control rests on several fundamental assumptions:

A. Pain may be conceptualized in terms of "pain behavior," which includes complaints, characteristic facial expressions and posture, use of health care facilities, taking of analgesics, and refusal to work.

B. Pain (pain behavior) may become chronic for reasons other than the original etiology.

C. Chronic pain may be understood in terms of learning or conditioning factors that exist in the interactions between patient and social environment.

D. Since chronic pain behaviors may be linked to conditioning effects, strategies for treatment can be based on counterconditioning or behavior change principles.

E. Behavioral methods can help patients alter their pain behavior. They share the basic premise that treatment, in appropriately selected cases, can focus on altering pain behavior directly.

Fordyce emphasizes the positive reinforcement that strengthens pain behaviors: "When I hurt (i.e., emit pain behaviors), 'good' things happen which otherwise would not." He cites the p.r.n. scheduling of analgesic medication as an illustration. He also stresses the importance of avoidance learning, which he paraphrases as, "When I hurt (emit pain behaviors), 'bad' things don't happen which otherwise would" (Fordyce et al., 1982). Numerous studies have documented the effectiveness of reducing pain behavior, without focusing on organic etiology, in producing significant and lasting improvement (Cairns et al., 1980; Fordyce et al., 1973; Gottlieb et al., 1977; Greenhoot and Sternbach, 1974; Newman et al., 1978; Roberts and Reinhardt, 1980; Swanson et al., 1979).

In summary, the approach includes: (a) nonreinforcement of pain behavior, (b) encouragement of physical activity to the limit of tolerance, (c) positive reinforcement of non-pain behaviors, and (d) instructing families in operant procedures to facilitate generalization. While this orientation is intriguing and the results encouraging, methodological limitations preclude unqualified acceptance (Latimer, 1982).

The specific problem of headache has received a great deal of attention from behavioral researchers and therapists. Tension headache and migraine have been most extensively studied. The main techniques include progressive relaxation, biofeedback, hypnosis, operant conditioning, and cognitive restructuring. (See Blanchard et al., 1979; Turner and Chapman, 1982a, 1982b, for a review.) In addition the subject of pain management has been reviewed from a broad cognitive-behavioral perspective by Sanders (1979).

Insomnia. The behavioral treatment of persistent insomnia (more than three weeks' duration) has its greatest usefulness and appropriateness in those problems without specific medical referents (e.g., congestive heart failure, duodenal ulcer pain) or psychiatric determinants (e.g., affective disorder). According to the "Diagnostic Classification of Sleep and Arousal Disorders" (1979), persistent psychophysiological DIMS (Disorders of Initiating and Maintaining Sleep) is "a sleep onset and intermediary sleep maintenance insomnia that develops as a result of the mutually reinforcing factors of chronic, somatized tension-anxiety and negative conditioning to sleep."

Relaxation training (Bernstein and Borkovec, 1973) is probably the intervention of choice for the tension-anxiety component (e.g., Borkovec and Fowles, 1973; Jacobson, 1938), while stimulus control procedures (Bootzin, 1972, 1977) have been widely used to recondition patients whose bedtime habits are incompatible with normal sleep patterns.

Bootzin developed stimulus control procedures for insomnia, on the assumption that insomnia is often a function of conditioned associations between the bed and sleep-incompatible behaviors (e.g., worrying about problems). The objective is to strengthen the association between bed cues and sleep and weaken the connection between bed cues and non-sleep (or sleep-incompatible) cues. Patients are given the following instructions:

A. Lie down only when you feel sleepy.

B. Set an alarm clock for the same time every morning regardless of the amount of sleep obtained the previous night.

C. Avoid daytime naps.

D. Use the bed and bedroom only for sleeping. No other activities (e.g., eating, reading, watching television) with the exception of sex are allowed.

E. If you are in bed and unable to fall asleep within ten minutes, leave the bedroom immediately. Return to bed only when you again feel sleepy. This step is to be repeated as often as necessary throughout the night until rapid sleep onset occurs.

Hauri (1979) has emphasized that among the major factors in heightening arousal and interfering with sleep are "trying too hard" and the expectation and fear of insomnia. Such patterns are disrupted in some patients by the paradoxical instruction to remain awake as long as possible rather than try to fall asleep (Ascher and Efran, 1978; Borkovec and Boudewyns, 1976). Finally, most behavioral work with patients involves self-monitoring procedures, and there is evidence that this technique itself may be effective in the treatment of insomnia (Jason, 1975).

CLINICAL ISSUES

Indications

Perusal of major textbooks of behavior therapy (Bellack and Hersen, 1977; Leitenberg, 1976; O'Leary and Wilson, 1975; Rimm and Masters, 1979; Walen et al., 1977; Wilson and O'Leary, 1980), the 14 volumes of *Progress in Behavior Modification*, and the nine volumes of the *Annual Review of Behavior Therapy* attests to the development and application of a variety of behavior therapy approaches to almost every clinical problem confronting the psychiatric practitioner. Sometimes a behavioral orientation is used adjunctively with primary biological interventions, but there is scarcely a clinical entity for which a behavioral intervention strategy cannot be proposed and implemented. Current assessment methods encompass a broad range of symptoms, dysfunctions, deficits, and relationship problems.

Although behavior therapists tend to eschew traditional nosology, a recent series of volumes on behavior therapy is precisely organized around *DSM-II* and *DSM-III* (Daitzman, 1980). While the "pathology" model (in the sense of searching for underlying causes) is disavowed by behavior therapists, simplistic relief strategies are also considered inadequate for the resolution of most clinical problems. Comprehensive behavioral assessment and intervention are generally considered *de rigeur*.

The range of problems addressed by behavior therapy includes depression, obsessive-compulsive disorders, anxiety states, phobias, alcohol abuse, obesity, cigarette smoking, delinquent behavior, sexual dysfunctions, shyness, insomnia, stuttering, enuresis and encopresis, marital discord, headache, pain, and hyperactivity in children. In addition, the principles and techniques of behavior therapy cut across distinctions of schools and settings, so that behavioral methods are relevant to family therapy, sex therapy, group therapy, and therapies that are primarily cognitive and affective.

It has been shown that patients with identical psychiatric diagnoses fare better when treatment is tailored to individual response patterns. For example, phobic patients who were divided into behavioral and physiological reactors responded better to social skills training (social phobia) and exposure (claustrophobia) on the one hand and applied relaxation on the other (Öst et al., 1981, 1982).

Limitations

Clinically, it would seem that the major contraindication to behavior therapy would be a strong mismatch between patient and therapist in terms of expectations. It is clear that significant discrepancies between the patient's expectations and the nature of the therapy predispose to unfavorable outcomes or premature termination of treatment (Garfield, 1980). Some patients, for example, clearly want answers to "why" questions and expect exploration of early anamnestic material and interpretations of their rich dream life as a part of the process. Some patients find the term *behavior therapy* odious and will not work with someone they feel is behaviorally oriented. In terms of specific problems, diagnoses, symptoms, or psychological dysfunctions, there probably are no real contraindications. There are certain caveats to be issued, however, in terms of the use of any psychological technique by itself in the face of major biological disturbances that are amenable to somatic interventions.

While offering no specific contraindications, Foa and Emmelkamp's (1983) book, *Failures in Behavior Therapy*, contains 22 chapters detailing two basic kinds of nonsuccess: (a) absence of change, or limited responses to the techniques administered; and (b) initial gains that were shortlived (i.e., relapses). Thus, examples are provided in which token economies failed to achieve desired ends, where self-control procedures were unsuccessful, desensitization techniques proved futile, and other standard behavioral interventions were of little value. The contributors to this book have emphasized how one may deduce constructive clues from examining failures in therapy so that one emerges with a clearer understanding of the mechanisms that appear to underlie behavior change.

Hersen (1979, 1981) has underscored various limitations and problems in the simplistic application of behavioral techniques. He has addressed problems of nonresponse to specific treatment strategies as well as failures to effect generalization outside of the treatment setting and to achieve long-term maintenance of initial behavioral changes.

DEVELOPMENTAL AND AGE RELATED ISSUES

The focus of developmental psychology has been on behavior changes in normal subjects in normal environments as a function of age. The principles and techniques of behavior therapy have been shown to be applicable not only to a wide spectrum of diagnostic categories but also across the full range of developmental stages. While the basic learning principles are identical for children, adolescents, and adults of all ages, and many problems such as anxiety, phobias, obsessions, depression, and social isolation may occur at any age, some clinical phenomena are more characteristic of one developmental period than another. In addition, certain techniques are more relevant to problems at specific stages of life. Traditionally, operant procedures have been used most frequently to modify the behavior of persons who are not highly motivated, particularly where parents, teachers, and custodians have substantial control over reinforcers. Within the past decade, however, self-control procedures have also been used successfully, even in young children (Kanfer and Karoly, 1972).

Children acquire an array of skills and habits in the course of development. Behavior modification techniques have been used successfully to facilitate the development of normal children at home and in the classroom as well as in the management of behavior problems and psychiatric disorders. Normal behavior, "normal" problems, and unusual problems (O'Leary and Wilson, 1975) have been areas of interest to behavioral researchers and therapists alike. Conditioning techniques have been used to modify the sucking reflex in three-day-old infants, and the smiling response has been modified in slightly older subjects (Brackbill, 1958). The latter studies showed that the smiling of three- to four-month-old infants can be significantly increased or decreased in response to reinforcement or nonreinforcement by adults. Such "normal" problems as toilet training, crying, and tantrums are generally easily modified by behavioral techniques (See O'Leary and Wilson, 1975; Ross, 1981). It is sometimes difficult to draw the line between normal behavior, "normal" problems, and problem behaviors. The issue is often resolved on the basis of the environment's capacity to tolerate the behavior in question.

Children's disorders have been among the most amenable to behavioral interventions, in part because children have greater elasticity, and in part because of their dependent status. The range of problems that have been addressed extends from such relatively minor disturbances as a messy room and nail biting to total social withdrawal and life threatening self-mutilation. A recent bibliography of child behavior modification covering the period 1956 to 1977 lists more than 2,300 references dealing with the treatment of dozens of childhood disorders (Benson, 1979). A 400-page textbook devoted to child behavior therapy (Ross, 1981) has chapters on social isolation and withdrawal, inappropriate gender behavior, academic deficits, language deficits, attention deficits, hyperactivity, urinary and fecal incontinence, delinquency, aggressive behavior, disruptive behavior, fears and phobias, somatic disorders, and self-stimulation and self-injury.

Drabman et al. (1978) have outlined three basic principles for the treatment of disturbed children: (a) eliminate behaviors that cause children to appear bizarre or that interfere with their ability to learn more appropriate behaviors through social interactions, (b) teach basic skills for adaptive functioning in the community, and (c) train parents in the use of effective behavior management procedures.

The behavior therapist tries to maximize therapeutic effects by deliberately combining several strategies and techniques. For example, Lazarus (1959) combined operant and respondent strategies in treating a child who feared traveling in moving vehicles. The child was given chocolate as a reinforcer for the operant behavior of talking about cars, then for sitting in cars, and finally for riding in cars. In the same manner, various stimuli such as toy cars and proximity to actual vehicles were paired with the pleasant and unconditioned stimulus of eating chocolate. Similarly, Lazarus et al. (1965) applied classical and operant strategies in overcoming a school phobia in a nine-year-old boy. Lazarus and Abramovitz (1962) used emotive imagery in overcoming children's fears: While vividly imaging the fear-producing situations, the children were told a story that aroused feelings of pride, mirth, serenity, or a sense of adventure. Stronger and stronger phobic images were woven into more powerful, positive, and enjoyable fantasies.

The instruction of parents in operant strategies has been essential for generalization and maintenance of changes obtained in residential settings and is critical for success with outpatients as well (Graziano, 1977). Several books specifically addressed to parents have been widely used in conjunction with parent training programs (e.g., Becker, 1970; Patterson, 1975; Patterson and Gullion, 1976). One program (Pelham, 1978) recommends five basic procedures to parents: (a) offering praise and other social reinforcements for appropriate behavior, (b) ignoring minor annoying behaviors, (c) using mild punishment procedures for behaviors that cannot be ignored, (d) employing simple environmental restructuring, and (e) establishing an incentive or token reward program. The importance of siblings (Lavigueur, 1976) and peers (Israel et al., 1980; Strain, 1981) in the behavior modification process has also been stressed.

It has been a matter of common observation and formal study (Gelfand et al., 1967) that disruptive, deviant, and dysfunctional behavior gets much more attention than socially adaptive responses. A great deal of the behavior of children is operant (controlled by consequences) and therefore potentially modifiable by altering consequences. The possible consequences of a behavior may be expressed as follows: (a) reinforcement, which strengthens a response; (b) punishment, which weakens a response; and (c) no consequence, which also weakens a response. Reinforcement is defined as the presentation of a reward (positive reinforcement) or removal of an aversive stimulus (negative reinforcement) following a behavior such that the probability of that behavior's occurring is increased. Punishment refers to the application of an aversive stimulus or the removal of a positive stimulus such that the probability of future responses is decreased. The process by which the absence of consequences decreases a behavior is called extinction. The term contingency management refers to the presentation or withdrawal of rewards and punishments contingent on the occurrence of a particular behavior. A contingency contract is a negotiated agreement (usually in writing) between two or more individuals specifying a behavior that is to occur in one or more of the individuals and the positive and negative consequences that will result if the agreement is or is not honored.

There are four basic types of reinforcers: (a) primary reinforcers (e.g., food), (b) social reinforcers (e.g., attention and approval), (c) material reinforcers (e.g., money, toys), and (d) activity reinforcers (e.g., watching T.V.). In order for reinforcement to occur, several conditions are essential: (a) There must be temporal contiguity between the reinforcer and the desired behavior, (b) the proposed reinforcement must be appropriate and meaningful to the individual, (c) the reinforcer should be available only for the particular behavior in question, and (d) the reinforcer should not be available noncontingently from other sources. Furthermore, the reinforcer should be administered initially at a high rate of frequency and then gradually decreased. There is a substantial literature dealing with the effectiveness of different schedules of reinforcement (e.g., Ferster and Skinner, 1957; Morse and Kelleher, 1970; Skinner, 1969).

When reinforcers are made available beyond the rate at which optimal responding occurs, satiation may result. This principle has been used clinically in the elimination of certain habits. For example, some studies have shown that if smokers deliberately increase their amount of smoking, the habit may become attenuated (e.g., Resnick, 1968).

Positive reinforcement is obviously dependent on the patient's performing the desired behavior to some extent. A nonoccurring behavior cannot be reinforced. When the behavior is not in the patient's repertoire, shaping, or reinforcement of approximations of the desired behavior, is often necessary. For example, if a child is mute, any mouth movements or vocalizations might be reinforced until the sounds begin to take some form. Instead of waiting for a fully formed word, the therapist reinforces successive approximations.

If the response is in the child's repertoire but insufficiently expressed, prompting may be used. There are verbal prompts (the child may be asked to do something), gestural prompts (pointing or beckoning), environmental prompts (posting a sign as a reminder), or physical prompts (touching or physically guiding the child). If the desired response is reinforced, usually the prompts can be gradually withdrawn (fading).

Punishment, as already mentioned, involves the presentation of an aversive stimulus or the removal of a positive stimulus. Aversive stimuli may be electrical shocks, spanking, or shouting, among others. Procedures that involve removal of positive reinforcement are response cost and time-out (Kazdin, 1972). Response cost involves the removal of a positive reinforcer contingent on the occurrence of an undesired behavior. Forfeit of allowance and having to stay after school for disruptive behavior are examples. In time-out-from-positive-reinforcement, the child is removed for several minutes from a reinforcing environment to a room without reinforcers. Positive-practice-overcorrection (Foxx and Azrin, 1972; Foxx and Bechtel, 1982) is a third type of punishment procedure. A child who has disrupted his surroundings is required not simply to restore the environment to its former state but to improve it markedly over its previous condition. For example, a child who scattered his toys all over the floor would be required to put the toys away, hang up his clothing, and make his bed. Thus, not only is the environment left in a better condition, but the child has the opportunity to practice relevant socially adaptive behavior. Positive practice overcorrection has been used successfully to control a number of destructive habits such as hair pulling and nail biting. This technique has been made widely available to the public (Azrin and Nunn, 1977).

Active punishment procedures are disavowed by most behavior therapists, except under the most drastic conditions when no alternatives are available. An exception would be the use of punishment as a self-management technique. For example, an obese child might be advised to wear a rubber band around his or her wrist and snap it every time he/she has the impulse to eat between meals.

Another widely used approach to children's problems uses modeling or observational learning. This involves a subject (observer) watching a model engage in some behavior. Bandura (1969) outlines four requirements for observational learning to occur: (a) attention to the model's response, (b) retention of what was attended to, (c) the motor and intellectual capacity to reproduce the model's behavior, and (d) the motivation to perform the behavior.

Modeling procedures can lead to three possible effects: (a) acquisition of new responses, (b) facilitation of already learned responses, and (c) strengthening or weakening of inhibitory responses. The three types of modeling experiences most commonly used are: (a) vicarious modeling, in which the child observes a live model but is not actually involved in the activity; (b) symbolic modeling, in which fearful children may be shown a film that depicts one or more models engaging the feared object; and (c) participant modeling, in which the fearful child joins the model in approaching the feared object or situation. A variant of participant modeling, guided participation, involves the patient's holding the hand of the therapist model, who is engaging in the behavior.

Studies by Bandura and his associates on dog phobic children (Bandura and Menlove, 1968; Bandura et al., 1967) are landmarks in the development of these techniques. Their work indicates that live models tend to be more effective than filmed models. In addition, similarity between model and subject is desirable, and identification is facilitated if the model is liked and respected by the subject. (A film for use with children who fear dentists has been developed by a team of psychologists and dentists [Adelson et al., 1972].) Meichenbaum (1977) makes the distinction between mastery models and coping models; he suggests that models who are initially unsure of themselves but who ultimately succeed in performing the task are more useful than highly competent models who perform the task with complete assurance.

Behavior Therapy in the Elderly

Lindsley's (1964) work provides one of the earliest references to the use of behavior therapy in elderly populations. The operant model of aging suggests that most of the decline in cognitive and behavioral repertoires is a function of environmental factors rather than the expression of an ineluctable biological process. An impoverished stimulus environment and a paucity of reinforcers seem to have a major effect on performance levels in older individuals. Lindsley distinguished a prosthetic environment from a therapeutic environment, the former being one in which deficits are made less debilitating by a physically supportive environment in which prosthetic devices are continually applied, whereas in the latter, behavioral changes can be induced, maintained, and generalized to extramural environments. More recently, these concepts have been amplified and refined (Baltes and Barton, 1977; McClannahan and Risley, 1974; Patterson, 1982; Patterson and Jackson, 1980).

Societal expectations of mental incompetence, physical debility, sexual incapacity, and unsuitability for employment have a profound influence on functioning in this population. At the same time, separation from children and grandchildren, as well as the loss of peers and spouses through death, contribute to social isolation.

In the elderly, cognitive deficits (Labouvie-Vief et al., 1974), deficiencies in ambulation (MacDonald and Butler, 1974), urinary and fecal incontinence (Sanavio, 1981), and social isolation (Berger and Rose, 1977) are major issues addressed by behavior therapists. Improvement in self-care and personal hygiene, physical activity, social interaction, and performance on cognitive tests has resulted from the use of differential reinforcement, assertiveness training, modeling, and self-instruction. Hussian (1981) concluded that the geriatric individual takes longer to develop conditioned responses (they require stronger and more persistent reinforcements). Moreover, in the elderly, conditioned emotional responses are easily disrupted.

The new area of behavioral thanatology (Sobel, 1981) brings behavioral principles to dying patients and their families so that this difficult experience may be handled in a less painful and more dignified manner.

PROFESSIONAL AND ETHICAL ISSUES

Ethical considerations in behavior therapy are essentially similar to those in any other form of treatment. The issues of involuntary status, confidentiality, informed consent, patient determination of goals, adequate training or supervision of the therapist, as well as the relevance and efficacy of the therapy offered are among the most important. A major question is whether there is anything distinctive about behavioral methods that would call for greater caution and whether special guidelines should be established. Positive (Griffith, 1980) and negative (Stolz, 1977a; 1980) conclusions have been drawn.

Ethical Issues for Human Services

The Association for Advancement of Behavior Therapy has spelled out basic ethical issues for its members:

A. Have the goals of treatment been adequately considered?

B. Has the choice of treatment methods been adequately considered?

C. Is the client's participation voluntary?

D. When another person or an agency is empowered to arrange for therapy, have the interests of the subordinated client been sufficiently considered?

E. Has the adequacy of treatment been evaluated?

F. Has the confidentiality of the treatment relationship been protected?

G. Does the therapist refer the clients to other therapists when necessary?

H. Is the therapist qualified to provide treatment?

Davison and Stuart (1975) have emphasized that human rights must explicitly be protected; they stress that the patient's consent is necessary prior to any coercive measures such as "the removal of privileges that would ordinarily have been granted" and other "institutional pressures." There are many occasions in the practice of therapy when difficult ethical questions arise. Sometimes one may refer to existing laws and ethical guidelines, but in many instances the information may be incomplete or not entirely relevant. Peer review can be most helpful; and when there is doubt, seeking the opinion of respected colleagues is strongly recommended. The Association for Advancement of Behavior Therapy has made available without fee, through its Professional Consultation and Peer Review Committee (Risley and Sheldon-Wildgen, 1980), consultations with experts in particular clinical areas and with authorities on specific techniques.

With regard to ethics, what seems to distinguish behavior therapy from many other orientations is its directness, specificity, definability, and simplicity. These characteristics make behavior therapy highly teachable to professionals and nonprofessionals alike, thereby rendering it capable of being used for various nontherapeutic and even nefarious purposes. Individuals particularly susceptible to abuse in any kind of therapy are the involuntarily institutionalized, the naive, the severely handicapped, the enfeebled, and any other highly dependent persons.

In a sense, there may be fewer ethical difficulties with behavioral methods precisely because it is easier to define problems, prescribe procedures, and evaluate outcomes. As many problems may arise from passive therapy as from vigorous, active, even intrusive measures. Failure to alleviate symptoms as rapidly as possible can create problems as well. Schwitzgebel and Schwitzgebel (1980) have offered the observation that "...it is no advance to trade authoritarian treatment for authoritarian nontreatment." In addition, therapy that takes less time is less costly and, therefore, becomes economically more feasible for larger numbers of individuals than therapy of longer duration.

Rarely is a technique intrinsically harmful; more likely a practitioner is applying it incorrectly or inappropriately. Certain behavioral techniques may be more susceptible to abuse than others, and the consequences of such abuse may be more apparent than with nonbehavioral techniques. Among the behavioral methods that have caused particular concern and have received the most notoriety, aversion techniques are most prominent. A case that received considerable attention in this connection involved the use of succinyl choline in the treatment of alcoholism (Sanderson et al., 1963). The use of such aversive stimuli as physical slaps, loud sounds, and electric shocks in controlling self-mutilating behavior in children has been severely criticized and banned in many institutions, although it is unlikely that these measures cause lasting adverse consequences (Lichstein and Schreibman, 1976). One of the milestones in the history of behavior therapy, but one of its sadder chapters in terms of ethical considerations, was Watson's induction of conditioned fear in a normal nine-month-old boy whose family unfortunately moved before Watson was able to de-condition his subject (Watson and Rayner, 1920).

Dramatic examples of the successful use of aversion are provided by Lang and Melamed's (1969) use of intense electrical shocks in a nine-month-old infant dying from chronic ruminative vomiting and by Lovaas' use of electric shocks and slapping in the treatment of autistic, schizophrenic, and self-mutilating children (Lovaas et al., 1965; Lovaas and Simmons, 1969). Therapists called upon to eliminate behavior such as head-banging, tongue-biting, eye-gouging, and other such self-injurious behaviors will find that a brief application of an aversive stimulus can be effective in many instances.

The dispensing of positive reinforcement on a contingent basis instead of a noncontingent basis (i.e., the withholding of positive reinforcement contingent upon a desired behavioral response), the withdrawal of re-inforcement to eliminate unwanted behaviors (to bring about extinction), the use of sensitization and flooding techniques, as well as the use of paradoxical communications and assignments to circumvent resistance and effect rapid changes in behavior have been widely criticized. The main objections are that contingent reinforcements are "manipulative," paradoxi-cal interventions are "insincere," and that "manipulation" is not only bad but can be avoided. The problem is not how influence and manipulation can be avoided but how they can best be used in the interest of the patient (cf., Watzlawick et al., 1974).

The technique of paradoxical intention, developed by Frankl (1960), is actually a self-management behavioral procedure in which the patient not only knows the rationale for the absurd assignment but practices it on his own. With regard to paradoxical instructions and communications to pa-tients, some behavior therapists (e.g., Fay, 1976) have spoken out in favor of patients' being made aware of the procedure. A recent study using paradoxical intention with insomniac subjects showed superior results in a group that had prior knowledge that the instructions were intended to be paradoxical compared to a group that had been given no such information (Ascher and Turner, 1980), although subsequently these authors questioned the effectiveness of paradoxical intention in the management of insomnia (Turner and Ascher, 1982).

While training programs in behavior therapy are proliferating at all professional levels, the most thoroughly conceptualized teaching proce-dures are found mainly in clinical psychology graduate programs. Cer-tainly, the interested professional will find no paucity of workshops, seminars, and lectures, especially if he or she has access to urban centers. Ethical issues are intimately tied to professional training. The skills of a therapist, his/her accountability, and concern with patient follow-ups all relate to professional competence and the ethics of practice. In behavior therapy it is often useful to train nonprofessional staff to become competent "behavioral engineers," thus posing further dilemmas.

ECONOMIC, LEGAL, AND SOCIAL/POLITICAL ISSUES

While the previous section touched on several economic, legal, and social/political issues, the present discussion will deal with these matters more specifically. Money, per se, is an important source of reinforcement, and many organizational psychologists have instituted cash bonuses, profit-sharing plans, merit increases, and similar programs (schedules of reinforcement) for increased effort and productivity. Private practitioners and public institutions are becoming more and more accountable for their fees. Third-party payment agencies have become more stringent about treatment outcomes and cost-effectiveness. The application of cost-effectiveness and cost-benefit analyses to behavior therapy (Yates and Newman, 1980a, 1980b) is a new and important development. Meaningful accountability cannot be achieved without some form of cost-benefit analysis. Apart from the time that therapist and patient spend in treatment, weightings have to be given to other costs such as office space, equipment, and materials.

The final criterion whereby all costs can be meaningfully calculated pertains to effectiveness. Cost-effectiveness pertains to the set of relationships between the value of resources consumed and the value of the treatment outcomes produced. Cost-benefit analyses are less ambitious and pertain to dollars spent versus dollars produced or nonmonetary benefits derived.

Among the issues to which cost-effectiveness and cost-benefit analyses may be addressed are the following:

A. The relative utility of professional and paraprofessional therapy, as well as the feasibility of self-directed therapy and its financial expediency,

B. Financial comparisons of community-based versus institutional therapy, and

C. The relative costs of residential versus institutional therapy.

At a broader societal level, organizations and committees have explored a variety of issues such as the use of behavioral control by the media, the medical profession, and the prison systems. *The Arizona Law Review*, 1975, Issue 1, published the proceedings of a conference devoted to the ethics of behavior modification in closed institutions.

Closely related to the growing awareness of the rights of patients in general is the particular right of the patient to refuse treatment. The law can ensure people the right to treatment and at the same time protect them from intrusive and hazardous procedures (see Kalish, 1981).

Schwitzgebel (1978a, 1978b), who is both a lawyer and psychologist, has provided a detailed account of psychological devices, their legal regulation, and various implications for behavior therapists. All therapists should be aware of patients' rights in three specific areas: the right to have treatment, the right to refuse treatment, and the right to informed consent. Kalish (1981) has discussed the impact of various court rulings on the practice of behavior therapy and behavior modification. He cites court decisions that establish minimal conditions of institutional living as rights rather than privileges. This mandate places severe restraints on the use of token economies and other contingency management methods. In some states it is now illegal to remove comfortable beds, chairs, or other furniture; to deny free access to television in the day room; or to make social interaction, religious services, or laundry facilities contingent on prosocial behaviors. Since privileges and rights cannot be used as rewards for behavioral goals, therapists must find different yet effective reinforcers.

Other sections of this chapter have indicated that because behavior therapists intervene more actively and more directly into the lives of their patients, they may be more open to criticism than therapists who eschew directive interventions. Certain critics have concluded that directive strategies are *ipso facto* anti-humanistic (see Krasner, 1976; Thoresen, 1973). Issues of control are often invoked, and allegations are made that behavioral procedures truncate patients' freedom. London (1969) stressed that most therapeutic problems involve some aspect of a patient's behavior that is *out* of control, from the patient's viewpoint and/or from the perspective of those who interact with him/her. The goal of behavior therapy is to restore this control.

It is often erroneously assumed that behavior therapy techniques are simple and can be applied by almost anyone. Thus, ward administrators have asked untrained and unsophisticated personnel to use "behavior modification," to design a token economy, or to draw up a behavioral contract. We have encountered school settings where the random and noncontingent use of candy, gum, and trinkets is referred to as "behavior modification." Abuses are generally perpetrated by persons who are inadequately trained in behavioral approaches.

In the treatment of autistic children, the work of Harris and her associates (e.g., Harris, 1982; Harris and Milch, 1981; Harris and Wolchik, 1982) has emphasized the value of involving parents in the treatment process but has included several significant caveats. Teaching speech to nonverbal autistic children is one area where self-help manuals, for instance, may do more harm than good.

Behavioral applications have broad-based social relevance. Stress reduction programs; smoking cessation; control of teenage pregnancy; vocational enhancement; traffic safety; population control; classroom learning; delinquency; fuel conservation; installation of smoke alarms; efficient allocation of resources to alleviate hunger, poverty, and unemployment; and promotion of harmonious relationships between peoples and among nations are all within the purview of behavioral programs.

CONCLUSION

Behavior therapy was initially portrayed as a set of treatment procedures based on learning theory—a conceptual alternative to intrapsychic orientations. It has subsequently evolved into a diverse and multifaceted approach that offers useful interventions for a variety of psychological, medical, and social problems.

As is the case with any rapidly expanding field, behavior therapy is beset with at least two major problems: (a) Quantity has outstripped quality. The literature continues to proliferate exponentially, but enthusiasm outpaces the generation of hard data. (b) The large body of information and the array of techniques currently available have not been incorporated into the therapeutic armamentarium of psychiatric practitioners. The times call for a medical education that would foster "many more well rounded experienced clinicians and teachers who are able to use a behavioral approach and behavioral techniques as part of their practice" (Birk et al., 1973).

Economic and political pressures are such that while the need for psychological services is increasing rapidly, available financial resources are diminishing. The emphasis on accountability has become ever greater and more compelling. Behavioral approaches are particularly geared to ease of implementation, accuracy of evaluation, and determination of cost-effectiveness.

Behavior therapy, once viewed as a passing fad, has already had a significant impact on research in psychotherapy and has great potential for augmenting the therapeutic repertoire of psychiatric clinicians. In addition, the application of behavioral methods to social problems is an area that holds great promise for the future.

REFERENCES

Adelson R, Liebert RM, Poulos RW, et al: A modeling film to reduce children's fear of dental treatment. International Association for Dental Research Abstracts, p 114, March 1972

Agras S, Jacob R: Hypertension, in Behavioral Medicine. Edited by Pomerleau OF, Brady JP. Baltimore, Williams & Wilkins Co, 1979

Alexander AB: The nature of asthma, in Pediatric and Adolescent Behavioral Medicine: Issues in Treatment. Edited by McGrain PJ, Firestone P. New York, Springer, 1983

Alexander AB: Asthma, in Psychosomatic Disorders: A Psychophysiological Approach to Etiology and Treatment. Edited by Haynes SN, Gannon L. New York, Praeger, 1981

Ascher LM, Efran JS: Use of paradoxical intention in a behavioral program for sleep onset insomnia. J Consult Clin Psychol 46:547-550, 1978

Ascher LM, Turner FM: A comparison of two methods for the administration of paradoxical intention. Behav Res Ther 18:121-126, 1980

Ayllon T, Azrin NH: Token Economy. New York, Appleton-Century-Crofts, 1968

Azrin NH, Nunn RG: Habit Control in a Day. New York, Simon and Schuster, 1977

Baltes MM, Barton EM: New approaches toward aging: a case for the operant model. Educational Gerontology 2:383-405, 1977

Bandura A, Blanchard EB, Ritter B: The relative efficacy of desensitization and modeling approaches for inducing behavioral, affective, and cognitive changes. J Pers Soc Psychol 13:173-199, 1969

Bandura A, Grusec JE, Menlove FL: Vicarious extinction of avoidance behavior. J Pers Soc Psychol 5:16-23, 1967

Bandura A, Menlove FL: Factors determining vicarious extinction of avoidance behavior through symbolic modeling. J Pers Soc Psychol 8:99-108, 1968

Bandura A, Perloff B: Relative efficacy of self-monitored and externally imposed reinforcement systems. J Pers Soc Psychol 7:111-116, 1967

Bandura A, Walters RH: Social Learning and Personality Development. New York, Holt, Rinehart & Winston, 1963

Bandura A: Social Learning Theory. Englewood Cliffs, NJ, Prentice-Hall, 1977a

Bandura A: Self-efficacy: toward a unifying theory of behavioral change. Psychol Rev 84:191-215, 1977b

Bandura A: Effecting change through participant modeling, in Counseling Methods. Edited by Krumboltz JD, Thoresen CE. New York, Holt, Rinehart & Winston, 1976

Bandura A: Vicarious and self-reinforcement processes, in The Nature of Reinforcement. Edited by Glaser R. New York, Academic Press, 1971

Bandura A: Principles of Behavior Modification. New York, Holt, Rinehart & Winston, 1969

Bandura A: Influence of models' reinforcement contingencies on the acquisition of imitative responses. J Pers Soc Psychol 1:589-595, 1965

Bandura A: Behavior theory and identificatory learning. Am J Orthopsychiatry 33:591-601, 1963

Barlow, DH (ed): Behavioral Assessment of Adult Disorders. New York, Guilford, 1981

Bechterev VM: General Principles of Human Reflexology: An Introduction to the Objective Study of Personality. Translated by Murphy E, Murphy W. New York, International Publishers, 1932

Beck AT, Rush AJ, Shaw BF, et al: Cognitive Therapy of Depression. New York, Guilford, 1979

Beck AT: Cognitive Therapy and the Emotional Disorders. New York, International Universities Press, 1976

Beck AT: Cognitive therapy: nature and relation to behavior therapy. Behavior Therapy 1:184-200, 1970

Beck AT: Thinking and depression, I: idiosyncratic content and cognitive distortions. Arch Gen Psychiatry 9:324-333, 1963

Becker WC: Parents Are Teachers: A Child Management Program. Champaign, Ill, Research Press, 1970

Bellack AS, Hersen M, Turner SM: Generalization effects of social skills training in chronic schizophrenics: an experimental analysis. Behav Res Ther 14:391-398, 1976

Bellack AS, Hersen M: Behavior Modification: An Introductory Textbook. Baltimore, Williams & Wilkins Co, 1977

Bender N: Self-verbalization versus tutor verbalization in modifying impulsivity. J Educ Psychol 68:347-354, 1976

Benson H, Alexander S, Feldman CL: Decreased premature ventricular contractions through use of the relaxation response in patients with stable ischaemic heart-disease. Lancet 2:380-382, 1975

Benson HB: Behavior Modification and the Child: An Annotated Bibliography. Westport, Conn, Greewood Press, 1979

Berger RM, Rose SD: Interpersonal skill training with institutionalized elderly patients. J Gerontol 32:346-353, 1977

Bernstein DA, Borkovec TD: Progressive Relaxation Training: A Manual for the Helping Professions. Champaign, Ill, Research Press, 1973

Birk L, Stolz SB, Brady JP, et al: Task Force Report 5: Behavior Therapy in Psychiatry. Washington, DC, American Psychiatric Association, 1973

Birk L (ed): Biofeedback: Behavioral Medicine. New York, Grune & Stratton, 1973

Blanchard EB, Ahles TA, Shaw WER: Behavioral treatment of headache, in Progress in Behavior Modification, vol 8. Edited by Hersen M, Eisler RM, Miller PM. New York, Academic Press, 1979

Blanchard EB: Behavioral medicine: a perspective, in Behavioral Approaches to Medical Treatment. Edited by Williams RB Jr, Gentry WD. Cambridge, Mass, Ballinger, 1977

Bootzin RR: Effects of self-control procedures for insomnia, in Behavioral Self-Management: Strategies and Outcomes. Edited by Stuart RB. New York, Brunner/Mazel, 1977

Bootzin RR: Stimulus control treatment for insomnia, in Proceedings of the American Psychological Association. Washington, DC, American Psychological Association, 1972

Borkovec TD, Boudewyns PA: Treatment of insomnia by stimulus control and progressive relaxation procedures, in Behavioral Counseling Methods. Edited by Krumboltz J, Thoresen CE. New York, Holt, Rinehart & Winston, 1976

Borkovec TD, Fowles D: Controlled investigation of the effects of progressive relaxation and hypnotic relaxation on insomnia. J Abnorm Psychol 82:153-158, 1973

Brackbill Y: Extinction of the smiling response in infants as a function of reinforcement schedule. Child Dev 29:115-124, 1958

Brady JP, Luborsky L, Kron RE: Blood pressure reduction in patients with essential hypertension through metronome-conditioned relaxation: a preliminary report. Behavior Therapy 5:203-209, 1974

Brownell KD, Colletti G, Ersner-Hershfield R, et al: Self-control in school children: stringency and leniency in self-determined and externally imposed performance standards. Behavior Therapy 8:442-455, 1977

Brownell KD: Behavioral medicine, in Annual Review of Behavior Therapy, vol 8. Edited by Franks CM, Wilson GT, Kendall KC, et al. New York, Guilford Press, 1982

Cairns D, Thomas L, Mooney V, et al: A comprehensive treatment approach to chronic low back pain: the spouse as a discriminative cue for pain behavior. Pain 6:243-252, 1980

Campbell RJ: Psychiatric Dictionary, 5th ed. New York, Oxford University Press, 1981

Cautela JR, Upper D: The process of individual behavior therapy. Progress in Behavior Modification, vol 1. Edited by Hersen IM, Eisler RM, Miller PM. New York, Academic, 1975

Cautela JR: Covert conditioning, in The Psychology of Private Events. Edited by Jacobs A, Sachs LB. New York, Academic Press, 1971

Cautela JR: Covert sensitization. Psychol Rep 20:459-468, 1967

Chaney EF, O'Leary MR, Marlatt GA: Skill training with alcoholics. J Consult Clin Psychol 46:1092-1104, 1978

Collins FL Jr: Behavioral medicine, in Future Perspectives in Behavior Therapy. Edited by Michelson L, Hersen E, Turner SM. New York, Plenum, 1981

Creer TL, Kotses H: Asthma: psychologic aspects and management, in Allergy: Principles and Practice, 2nd ed. Edited by Middleton E Jr, Reed CE, Ellis EF. St. Louis, Mosby, 1983

Curran JP, Monti PM, Corriveau DP: Treatment of schizophrenia, in International Handbook of Behavior Modification and Therapy. Edited by Bellack AS, Hersen M, Kazdin AE. New York, Plenum, 1982

Daitzman RJ (ed): Clinical Behavior Therapy and Behavior Modification, vol 1. New York, Garland STPM Press, 1980

Davidson PO, Davidson SM (eds): Behavioral Medicine: Changing Health Lifestyles. New York, Brunner/Mazel, 1980

Davidson PO: Issues in patient compliance, in Handbook of Clinical Health Psychology. Edited by Millon T, Green C, Meagher R. New York, Plenum, 1982

Davison GC, Stuart RB: Behavior therapy and civil liberties. Am Psychol 30:755-763, 1975

DeRubeis RJ, Hollon SD: Behavioral treatment of affective disorders, in Future Perspectives in Behavior Therapy. Edited by Michelson L, Hersen M, Turner SM. New York, Plenum, 1981

DeVoge JT, Beck S: The therapist-client relationship in behavior therapy, in Progress in Behavior Modification, vol 6. Edited by Hersen M, Eisler RM, Miller PM. New York, Academic Press, 1978

Dekker E, Pelser HE, Groen J: Conditioning as a cause of asthmatic attacks: a laboratory study. J Psychosom Res 2:97-108, 1957

Doleys DM, Meredith RL, Ciminero AR (eds): Behavioral Medicine: Assessment and Treatment Strategies. New York, Plenum, 1982

Doleys DM, Meredith KL: Urological disorders, in Behavioral Medicine: Assessment and Treatment Strategies. Edited by Doleys DM, Meredith RL, Ciminero AR. New York, Plenum, 1982

Drabman RD, Jarvie GJ, Hammer D: Residential child treatment, in Behavior Therapy in the Psychiatric Setting. Edited by Hersen M, Bellack AS. Baltimore, Williams & Wilkins Co, 1978

Dunlap K: Habits: Their Making and Unmaking. New York, Liveright, 1932

Dyckman JM, Cowan PA: Imaging vividness and the outcome of in vivo and imagined scene desensitization. J Consult Clin Psychol 48:1155-1156, 1978

Ellis A, Grieger R (eds): Handbook of Rational-Emotive Therapy. New York, Springer, 1977

Ellis A: Reason and Emotion in Psychotherapy. New York, Lyle Stuart, 1962

Emmelkamp PMG, Kwee KG: Obsessional ruminations: a comparison between thought-stopping and prolonged exposure in imagination. Behav Res Ther 15:441-444, 1977

Emmelkamp PMG: Anxiety and fear, in International Handbook of Behavior Modification and Therapy. Edited by Bellack AS, Hersen M, Kazdin AE. New York, Plenum, 1982

Epstein LH, Cluss PA: A behavioral medicine perspective on adherence to long term medical regimens. J Consult Clin Psychol 50:950-971, 1982

Epstein LH, Parker LH: Behavioral medicine, II: treatment. Association for Advancement of Behavior Therapy Newsletter 4:9-10, 1977

Erwin E: Behavior Therapy: Scientific Philosophical and Moral Foundations. New York, Cambridge University Press, 1978

Eysenck HJ: Neobehavioristic (S-R) theory, in Contemporary Behavior Therapy: Conceptual and Empirical Foundations. Edited by Wilson GT, Franks CM. New York, Guilford, 1982

Eysenck HJ: Learning theory and behavior therapy. J Ment Sci 105:61-75, 1959

Fay A: Clinical notes on paradoxical therapy. Psychotherapy: Theory, Research, and Practice 13:118-122, 1976

Felixbrod JJ, O'Leary KD: Effects of reinforcement on children's academic behavior as a function of self-determined and externally imposed contingencies. J Appl Behav Anal 6:241-250, 1973

Ferguson JM, Taylor CB (eds): The Comprehensive Handbook of Behavioral Medicine (vols 1-3). New York, Spectrum, 1980

Ferster CB, Skinner BF: Schedules of Reinforcement. New York, Appleton-Century-Crofts, 1957

Foa EB, Steketee G, Milby JB: Differential effects of exposure and response prevention in obsessive-compulsive washers. J Consult Clin Psychol 48:71-79, 1980

Foa EB, Steketee G, Turner RM, et al: Effects of imaginal exposure to feared disasters in obsessive-compulsive checkers. Behav Res Ther 18:449-455, 1980

Foa EB, Emmelkamp PMG (eds): Failures in Behavior Therapy. New York, John Wiley & Sons, 1983

Ford JD: Therapeutic relationship in behavior therapy: an empirical analysis. J Consult Clin Psychol 46:1302-1314, 1978

Fordyce W, Shelton J, Dundore D: The modification of avoidance learning in pain behaviors. J Behav Med 5:405-414, 1982

Fordyce WE, Fowler RS, Lehmann JF, et al: Operant conditioning in the treatment of chronic pain. Arch Phys Med Rehabil 54:399-408, 1973

Fordyce WE, Fowler RS, deLateur B: An application of behavior modification techniques to a problem of chronic pain. Behav Res Ther 6:105-107, 1968

Fordyce WE: Behavioral analysis of chronic pain, in Behavioral Treatment of Disease. Edited by Surwit RS, Williams RD Jr, Steptoe A, et al. New York, Plenum, 1982

Fordyce WE: Behavioral Methods for Chronic Pain and Illness. St Louis, Mosby, 1976

Foxx RM, Azrin NH: Restitution: a method of eliminating aggressive-disruptive behavior of retarded and brain-damaged patients. Behav Res Ther 10:15-27, 1972

Foxx RM, Bechtel DR: Overcorrection, in Progress in Behavior Modification, vol 13. Edited by Hersen M, Eisler RM, Miller PM. New York, Academic Press, 1982

Frankl VE: Paradoxical intention: a logotherapeutic technique. Am J Psychother 14:520-535, 1960

Franks CM: Foreword, in Multimodal Behavior Therapy. Edited by Lazarus AA. New York, Springer, 1976

Franks CM (ed): Behavior Therapy: Appraisal and Status. New York, McGraw-Hill, 1969

Franzini LR, Tilker HA: On the terminological confusion between behavior therapy and behavior modification. Behavior Therapy 3:279-282, 1972

Garfield SL: Psychotherapy: An Eclectic Approach. New York, John Wiley & Sons, 1980

Gelfand DM, Gelfand S, Dobson WR: Unprogrammed reinforcement of patients' behavior in a mental hospital. Behav Res Ther 5:201-207, 1967

Goldfried MR, Decenteceo ET, Weinberg L: Systematic rational restructuring as a self-control technique. Behavior Therapy 5:247-254, 1974

Goldfried MR, Davison GC: Clinical Behavior Therapy. New York, Holt, Rinehart & Winston, 1976

Goldfried MR: Psychotherapy as coping skills training, in Psychotherapy Process. Edited by Mahoney MJ. New York, Plenum, 1980

Goldiamond I: Self-control procedures in personal behavior problems. Psychol Rep 17:851-868, 1965

Goldsmith JB, McFall RM: Development and evaluation of an interpersonal skill training program for psychiatric inpatients. J Abnorm Psychol 84:51-58, 1975

Gottlieb H, Strite LC, Koller R, et al: Comprehensive rehabilitation of patients having chronic low back pain. Arch Phys Med Rehabil 58:101-108, 1977

Graziano AM: Parents as behavior therapists, in Progress in Behavior Modification, vol 4. Edited by Hersen M, Eisler RM, Miller PM. New York, Academic Press, 1977

Greenhoot JH, Sternbach RA: Conjoint treatment of chronic pain. Adv Neurol 4:595-603, 1974

Griffith RG: An administrative perspective on guidelines for behavior modification: the creation of a legally safe environment. Behavior Therapist 3:5-7, 1980

Guerney B: Relationship Enhancement. San Francisco, Jossey-Bass, 1977

Harris SL, Milch RE: Training parents as behavior therapists for their autistic children. Clinical Psychology Review 1:49-63, 1981

Harris SL, Wolchik SA: Teaching speech skills to nonverbal children and their parents, in Autism and Severe Psychopathology: Advances in Child Behavioral Analysis and Therapy, vol 2. Edited by Steffen JJ, Karoly P. Lexington, Mass, Lexington Books, 1982

Harris SL: A family systems approach to behavioral training with parents of autistic children. Child and Family Behavior Therapy 4:21-35, 1982

Hartig M, Kanfer FH: The role of verbal self-instructions in children's resistance to temptation. J Pers Soc Psychol 25:259-267, 1973

Hauri P: Behavioral treatment of insomnia. Med Times 107:36-47, 1979

Haynes RB: Improving patient compliance: an empirical view, in Compliance Generalization and Maintenance in Behavioral Medicine. Edited by Stuart RB, Davidson PO. New York, Brunner/Mazel, 1981

Haynes RB: Strategies to improve compliance with referrals, appointments, and prescribed medical regimens, in Compliance in Health Care. Edited by Haynes RB, Taylor DW, Sackett DL. Baltimore, Johns Hopkins Press, 1979

Hersen M, Bellack AS: Staff training and consultation, in Behavior Therapy in the Psychiatric Setting. Edited by Hersen M, Bellack AS. Baltimore, Williams & Wilkins Co, 1978

Hersen M: Complex problems require complex solutions. Behavior Therapy 12:15-29, 1981

Hersen M: Limitations and problems in the clinical application of behavioral techniques in psychiatric settings. Behavior Therapy 10:65-80, 1979

Homme LE: Perspectives in psychology, 24: control of coverants, the operants of the mind. Psychological Record 15:501-511, 1965

Hull CL: Principles of Behavior. New York, Appleton-Century-Crofts, 1943

Hull CL: Quantitative aspects of the evolution of concepts, and experimental study. Psychological Monographs 28, 1920

Hussian RA: Geriatric Psychology: A Behavioral Perspective. New York, Van Nostrand Reinhold, 1981

Ingersoll BD, Seime RJ, McCutcheon WR (eds): Behavioral Dentistry: Proceedings of the First National Conference. Morgantown, West Virginia University Press, 1977

Israel AC, Pravder MD, Knights SA: A peer-administered program for changing the classroom behavior of disruptive children. Behavioural Analysis and Modification 4:224-236, 1980

Jacobson E: Variation of blood pressure with skeletal muscle tension and relaxation. Ann Intern Med 12:1194-1212, 1939

Jacobson E: Progressive Relaxation, 2nd ed. Chicago, University of Chicago Press, 1938

Jacobson NS, Margolin G: Marital Therapy. New York, Brunner/Mazel, 1979

Jason L: Rapid improvement in insomnia following self-monitoring. J Behav Ther Exp Psychiatry 6:349-350, 1975

Jones MC: The elimination of children's fears. J Exp Psychol 7:382-390, 1924

Kalish HI: From Behavioral Science to Behavior Modification. New York, McGraw-Hill, 1981

Kanfer FH, Karoly P: Self-control: a behavioristic excursion into the lion's den. Behavior Therapy, 3:398-416, 1972

Kanfer FH: The maintenance of behavior by self-generated stimuli and reinforcement, in Psychology of Private Events. Edited by Jacobs A, Sachs LB. New York, Academic Press, 1971

Kanfer FH: Self-regulation: research, issues, and speculations, in Behavior Modification in Clinical Psychology. Edited by Neuringer C, Michael JL. New York, Appleton-Century-Crofts, 1970

Kazdin AE, Wilcoxon LA: Systematic desensitization and nonspecific treatment effects: a methodological evaluation. Psychol Bull 83:729-758, 1976

Kazdin AE, Wilson GT: Evaluation of Behavior Therapy. Cambridge, Mass, Ballinger, 1978

Kazdin AE: History of Behavior Modification. Baltimore, University Park Press, 1978

Kazdin AE: The Token Economy. New York, Plenum, 1977

Kazdin AE: Self-monitoring and behavior change, in Self-Control: Power to the Person. Edited by Mahoney MJ, Thoresen CE. Monterey, Brooks/Cole, 1974

Kazdin AE: Response cost: the removal of conditioned reinforcers for therapeutic change. Behavior Therapy 3:533-546, 1972

Kelly JA: Social Skills Training. New York, Springer, 1982

King NJ: The behavioral management of asthma and asthma-related problems in children: a critical review of the literature. J Behav Med 3:169-189, 1980

Knox D: Marriage Happiness: A Behavioral Approach to Counseling. Champaign, Ill, Research Press, 1972

Krasner L: Behavior modification: ethical issues and future trends, in Handbook of Behavior Modification and Behavior Therapy. Edited by Leitenberg H. Englewood Cliffs, NJ, Prentice-Hall, 1976

Labouvie-Vief G, Hoyer WJ, Baltes MM, et al: Operant analysis of intellectual behavior in old age. Hum Dev 17:259-272, 1974

Lang PJ, Melamed BG: Avoidance conditioning therapy of an infant with chronic ruminative vomiting: case report. J Abnorm Psychol 74:1-8, 1969

Latimer PR: External contingency management for chronic pain: critical review of the evidence. Am J Psychiatry 139:1308-1312, 1982

Lavigueur H: The use of siblings as an adjunct to the behavioral treatment of children in the home with parents as therapists. Behavior Therapy 7:602-613, 1976

Lazarus AA, Abramovitz A: The use of "emotive imagery" in the treatment of children's phobias. J Ment Sci 108:191-195, 1962

Lazarus AA, Davison GC, Polefka DA: Classical and operant factors in the treatment of a school phobia. J Abnorm Psychol 70:225-229, 1965

Lazarus AA: The Practice of Multimodal Therapy. New York, McGraw-Hill, 1981

Lazarus AA: Multimodal Behavior Therapy. New York, Springer, 1976

Lazarus AA: Behavior Therapy and Beyond. New York, McGraw-Hill, 1971

Lazarus AA: Behavior rehearsal vs nondirective therapy vs advice in effecting behavior change. Behav Res Ther 4:209-212, 1966

Lazarus AA: Towards the understanding and effective treatment of alcoholism. S Afr Med J 39:736-741, 1965

Lazarus AA: The elimination of children's phobias by deconditioning. Medical Proceedings (South Africa) 5:261-265, 1959

Leiblum SR, Pervin LA (eds): Principles and Practice of Sex Therapy. New York, Guilford Press, 1980

Leitenberg H (ed): Handbook of Behavior Modification and Behavior Therapy. Englewood Cliffs, NJ, Prentice-Hall, 1976

Lewinsohn PM, Hoberman HM: Depression, in International Handbook of Behavior Modification and Therapy. Edited by Bellack AS, Hersen M, Kazdin AE. New York, Plenum, 1982

Liberman RP, Wheeler EG, de Visser LAJM, et al: Handbook of Marital Therapy. New York, Plenum, 1980

Lichstein AL, Schreibman L: Employing electric shock with autistic children. Journal of Autism and Childhood Schizophrenia 6:163-173, 1976

Lichtenstein E, Brown RA: Current trends in the modification of cigarette dependence, in International Handbook of Behavior Modification and Therapy. Edited by Bellack AS, Hersen M, Kazdin AE. New York, Plenum, 1982

Lindsley OR: Geriatric behavior prosthetics, in New Thoughts on Old Age. Edited by Kastenblaum R. New York, Springer, 1964

London P: The end of ideology in behavior modification. Am Psychol 27:913-920, 1972

London P: Behavior Control. New York, Harper and Row, 1969

LoPiccolo J, LoPiccolo L (eds): Handbook of Sex Therapy. New York, Plenum, 1978

Lovaas OI, Freitag G, Gold VJ, et al: Experimental studies in childhood schizophrenia: analysis of self-destructive behavior. J Exp Child Psychol 2:67-84, 1965

Lovaas, OI, Simmons JQ: Manipulation of self-destruction in three retarded children. J Appl Behav Anal 2:143-157, 1969

Lovitt TC, Curtiss KA: Academic response rate as a function of teacher and self-imposed contingencies. J Appl Behav Anal 2:49-53, 1969

MacDonald ML, Butler AK; Reversal of helplessness: producing walking behavior in nursing home wheelchair residents using behavior modification procedures. J Gerontol 29:97-101, 1974

Mahoney MJ: Cognition and Behavior Modification. Cambridge, Mass, Ballinger, 1974

Marks IM, Boulougouris J, Marset P: Flooding versus desensitization in the treatment of phobic patients: a cross-over study. Br J Psychiatry 119:353-375, 1971

Marks IM, Hodgson R, Rachman S: Treatment of chronic obsessive-compulsive neurosis by in vivo exposure: a two-year follow-up and issues in treatment. Br J Psychiatry 127:349-364, 1975

Marks IM, Stern RS, Mawson D: Clomipramine and exposure for obsessive-compulsive rituals, I, II. Br J Psychiatry 136:1-25, 161-166, 1980

Marks IM: Review of behavioral psychotherapy, I: obsessive-compulsive disorders. Am J Psychiatry 138:584-592, 1981

Marks IM: Behavioral psychotherapy of adult neuroses, in Handbook of Psychotherapy and Behavior Change, 2nd ed. Edited by Garfield SL, Bergin AE. New York, John Wiley & Sons, 1978

Marlatt GA: Alcohol, stress and cognitive control, in Experimental and Behavioral Approaches to Alcoholism. New York, Plenum, 1978

Mash EJ, Hamerlynck LA, Handy LC (eds): Behavior Modification and Families. New York, Brunner/Mazel, 1976

Masters WH, Johnson VE: Human Sexual Inadequacy. Boston, Little, Brown, 1970

Matarazzo JD, Connor WE, Fey SG, et al: Behavioral cardiology with emphasis on the family heart study: fertile ground for psychological and biomedical research, in Handbook of Clinical Health Psychology. Edited by Millon T, Green C, Meagher R. New York,, Plenum, 1982

Max L: Breaking up a homosexual fixation by the conditioned reaction technique. Psychol Bull 32:734, 1935

McClannahan LE, Risley TR: Design of living environments for nursing home residents. Gerontologist 14:236-240, 1974

McGrath PJ, Firestone P (eds): Pediatric and Adolescent Behavioral Medicine: Issues in Treatment. New York, Springer, 1983

McLean PD, Hakstian AR: Clinical depression: comparative efficacy of outpatient treatments. J Consult Clin Psychol 47:818-836, 1979

McNamara JR (ed): Behavioral Approaches to Medicine: Application and Analysis. New York, Plenum, 1979

Meichenbaum D: Cognitive Behavior Modification. New York, Plenum, 1977

Melamed BG, Siegel LJ: Behavioral Medicine: Practical Applications in Health Care. New York, Springer, 1980

Meletzky BM, Self-referred versus court-referred sexually deviant patients: success with assisted covert sensitization. Behavior Therapy 11:306-314, 1980

Miller NE: Behavioral medicine: symbiosis between laboratory and clinic. Annual Review of Psychology 34:1-31, 1983

Miller NE: Behavioral medicine: new opportunities but serious dangers. Behavioral Medicine Update 1:5-8, 1979

Miller NE: Studies of fear as an acquired drive, I: fear as motivation and fear-reduction as reinforcement in the learning of new responses. J Exp Psychol 38:89-101, 1948

Mischel W: Toward a cognitive social learning reconceptualization of personality. Psychol Rev 80:252-283, 1973

Mischel W: Personality and Assessment. New York, John Wiley & Sons, 1968

Moreno JL: Psychodrama. New York, Beacon House, 1958

Morse WH, Kelleher RT: Schedules as fundamental determinants of behavior, in The Theory of Reinforcement Schedules. Edited by Schoenfeld WN. Englewood Cliffs, NJ, Prentice-Hall, 1970

Mowrer OH, Mowrer WM: Enuresis: a method for its study and treatment. Am J Orthopsychiatry 8:436-459, 1938

Mowrer OH: On the dual nature of learning: a reinterpretation of "conditioning" and "problem-solving." Harvard Educational Review 17:102-148, 1947

Nathan PE, Goldman MS: Problem drinking and alcoholism, in Behavioral Medicine: Theory and Practice. Edited by Pomerleau OF, Brady JP. Baltimore, Williams & Wilkins Co, 1979

Nathan PE, Marlatt GA (eds): Experimental and Behavioral Approaches to Alcoholism. New York, Plenum, 1978

Nathan PE: Alcoholism, in Handbook of Behavioral Modification and Behavior Therapy. Englewood Cliffs, NJ, Prentice-Hall, 1976

Newman R, Seres J, Yospe L, et al: Multidisciplinary treatment of chronic pain: long-term follow up of low back pain patients. Pain 4:283-292, 1978

Nicassio PM, Bootzin RR: A comparison of progressive relaxation and autogenic training as treatments of insomnia. J Abnorm Psychol 83:253-260, 1974

O'Leary KD, Turkewitz H: Marital therapy from a behavioral perspective, in Marriage and Marital Therapy. Edited by Paolino TJ, McCrady BS. New York, Brunner/Mazel, 1978

O'Leary KD, Wilson GT: Behavior Therapy: Application and Outcome. Englewood Cliffs, NJ, Prentice Hall, 1975

Öst L-G, Jerrelmalm A, Johansson J: Individual response patterns and the effects of different behavioral methods in the treatment of social phobia. Behav Res Ther 19:1-16, 1981

Öst L-G, Johansson J, Jerrelmalm A: Individual response patterns and the effects of different behavioral methods in the treatment of claustrophobia. Behav Res Ther 20:445-460, 1982

Patterson GR, Reid JB, Jones RR, et al: A Social Learning Approach to Family Intervention. Eugene, Ore, Castalia Publishing, 1975

Patterson GR, Gullion ME: Living with Children: New Methods for Parents and Teachers. Champaign, Ill, Research Press, 1976

Patterson GR: Families: Applications of Social Learning to Family Life. Champaign, Ill, Research Press, 1975

Patterson RL, Jackson GM: Behavior modification with the elderly, in Progress in Behavior Modification, vol 9. Edited by Hersen J, Eisler R, Miller P. New York, Academic Press, 1980

Patterson RL: Overcoming Deficits of Aging. New York, Plenum, 1982

Paul GL, Lentz FJ: Psychological Treatment of Chronic Mental Patients. Cambridge, Mass, Harvard University Press, 1977

Paul GL: Outcome of systematic desensitization, II: controlled investigations of individual treatment technique variations and current status, in Behavior Therapy: Appraisal and Status. Edited by Franks CM. New York, McGraw-Hill, 1969

Pavlov IP: Conditioned Reflexes; An Investigation of the Physiological Activity of the Cerebral Cortex. New York, Oxford University Press, 1927

Pelham WE: Hyperactive children. Psychiatr Clin North Am 1:227-245, 1978

Philander DA, Yorkston NJ, Eckert E, et al: Bronchial asthma: improved lung function after behavior modification. Psychosomatics 20:325-327, 330-331, 1979

Pomerleau OF, Brady JP (eds): Behavioral Medicine: Theory and Practice. Baltimore, Williams & Wilkins Co, 1979

Rabavilis A, Boulougouris JC, Perissaki C: Therapist qualities related to outcome with exposure *in vivo* in neurotic patients. J Behavior Ther Exp Psychiatry 10:293-294, 1979

Rachman SJ, Hodgson R: Obsessions and Compulsions. Englewood Cliffs, NJ, Prentice-Hall, 1980

Rachman SJ, Wilson GT: The Effects of Psychological Therapy, 2nd ed. New York, Pergamon Press, 1980

Redd WH, Porterfield AL, Andersen BL: Behavior Modification: Behavioral Approaches to Human Problems. New York, Random House, 1979

Resnick JH: The control of smoking behavior by stimulus satiation. Behav Res Ther 6:113-114, 1968

Richter R, Dahme B: Bronchial asthma in adults: there is little evidence for the effectiveness of behavioral therapy and relaxation. J Psychosom Res 26:533-540, 1982

Rimm DC, Masters JC: Behavior Therapy: Techniques and Empirical Findings, 2nd ed. New York, Academic Press, 1979

Risley TR, Sheldon-Wildgen J: Invited peer review: the AABT experience. Behavior Therapist 3:5-8, 1980

Roberts A, Reinhardt L: The behavioral management of chronic pain: long term follow up with comparison groups. Pain 8:151-162, 1980

Rosenbaum M, Franks CM, Jaffe YJ: Perspectives on Behavior Therapy in the Eighties. New York, Springer, 1983

Ross AO: Child Behavior Therapy: Principles, Procedures, and Empirical Basis. New York, John Wiley & Sons, 1981

Russell RK, Sipich JF: Cue-controlled relaxation in the treatment of test anxiety. J Behav Ther Exp Psychiatry 4:47-49, 1973

Salter A: Conditioned Reflex Therapy. New York, Creative Age Press, 1949

Sanavio E: Toilet retraining in psychogeriatric residents. Behavior Modification 5:417-427, 1981

Sanders SH: Behavioral assessment and treatment of clinical pain: appraisal of current status, in Progress in Behavior Modification, vol 8. Edited by Hersen M, Eisler RM, Miller PM. New York, Academic Press, 1979

Sanderson RE, Campbell D, Laverty SG: An investigation of a new aversive conditioning treatment for alcoholism. Q J Stud Alcohol 24:261-275, 1963

Schwartz GE, Weiss SM: Behavioral medicine revisited: an amended definition. J Behav Med 1:249-252, 1978

Schwitzgebel RK: Regulation of psychological devices. Behavior Therapist 1(3):5, July 5, 1978a

Schwitzgebel RK: Regulation of research employing psychological devices and the use of self-help material in therapy. Behavior Therapist 1(5):9-10, November 9-10, 1978b

Schwitzgebel RL, Schwitzgebel RK: Law and Psychological Practice. New York, John Wiley & Sons, 1980

Sechenov IM: Reflexes of the Brain: An Attempt to Establish the Physiological Bases of Psychological Processes (1865). Translated by Belsky S. Cambridge, Mass, MIT Press, 1965

Semans JH: Premature ejaculation: a new approach. South Med J 49:353-361, 1956

Shelton JL, Ackerman JM: Homework in Counselling and Psychotherapy. Springfield, Ill, Charles C Thomas, 1974

Sherman AR: Real-life exposure as a primary therapeutic factor in the desensitization treatment of fear. J Abnorm Psychol 79: 19-28, 1972

Skinner BF: Contingencies of Reinforcement: A Theoretical Analysis. New York, Appleton-Century-Crofts,, 1969

Skinner BF: Science and Human Behavior. New York, Macmillan, 1953

Skinner BF: The Behavior of Organisms: An Experimental Analysis. New York, Appleton-Century-Crofts,, 1938

Sleep Disorders Classification Committee: Diagnostic classification of sleep and arousal disorders. Sleep 2:137, 1979

Sobel HJ (ed): Behavior Therapy in Terminal Care: A Humanistic Approach. Cambridge, Mass, Ballinger, 1981

Stampfl TG, Levis DJ: Essentials of implosive therapy: a learning-theory-based psychodynamic behavioral therapy. J Abnorm Psychol 72:496-503, 1967

Steger J, Fordyce W: Behavioral health care in the management of chronic pain, in Handbook of Clinical Health Psychology. New York, Plenum, 1982

Steketee G, Foa EB, Grayson JB: Recent advances in the behavioral treatment of obsessive-compulsives. Arch Gen Psychiatry 39:1365-1371, 1982

Stolz SB: Who do guidelines protect? A rejoinder to Griffith and Coval. Behavior Therapist 3:24, 1980

Stolz SB: (ed): Report of the American Psychological Association Commission on Behavior Modification. Washington DC, American Psychological Association, 1977a

Stolz SB: Why no guidelines for behavior modification? J Appl Behav Anal 10:541-547, 1977b

Strain PS: The Utilization of Classroom Peers as Behavior Change Agents. New York, Plenum Press, 1981

Stuart RB: Helping Couples Change: A Social Learning Approach to Marital Therapy. New York, Guilford Press, 1980

Stuart RB: Behavioral Self-Management. New York, Brunner/Mazel, 1977

Stuart RB: Behavioral contracting within the families of delinquents. J Behav Ther Exp Psychiatry 2:1-11, 1971

Stuart RB: Behavioural control of overeating. Behav Res Ther 5:357-365, 1967

Stunkard AJ: Obesity, in International Handbook of Behavior Modification and Therapy. Edited by Bellack AS, Hersen M, Kazdin AE. New York, Plenum, 1982

Suinn RM: Intervention with Type A behaviors. J Consult Clin Psychol 50:933-949, 1982

Surwit AS, Williams RB Jr, Steptoe A, et al (eds): Behavioral Treatment of Disease. New York, Plenum, 1982

Swanson DW, Maruta T, Swenson W: Results of behavior modification in the treatment of chronic pain. Psychosom Med 41:55-61, 1979

Thoresen CE, Mahoney MJ: Behavioral Self Control. New York, Holt, Rinehart and Winston, 1974

Thoresen CE: Behavioral humanism, in Behavior Modification in Education. Edited by Thoresen CE. Chicago, University of Chicago Press, 1973

Thorndike EL: The Fundamentals of Learning. New York, Teachers College, Columbia University, 1932

Turkat ID, Harris FR, Forehand R: An assessment of the public reaction to behavior modification: a preliminary report. J Behav Ther Exp Psychiatry 10:101-103, 1979

Turnball JW: Asthma conceived of as a learned experience. J Psychosom Res 6:59-70, 1962

Turner JA, Chapman CR: Psychological interventions for chronic pain: a critical review, I: relaxation training and biofeedback. Pain 12:1-12, 1982a

Turner JA, Chapman CR: Psychological interventions for chronic pain: a critical review, II: operant conditioning, hypnosis, and cognitive-behavioral therapy. Pain 12:22-46, 1982b

Turner RM, Ascher LM: Therapist factors in the treatment of insomnia. Behav Res Ther 20:33-40, 1982

Twentyman CT, Zimering RT: Behavioral training of social skills: a critical review, in Progress in Behavior Modification, vol 7. Edited by Hersen M, Eisler RM, Miller PM. New York, Academic Press, 1979

Ullmann LP, Krasner L: A Psychological Approach to Abnormal Behavior (2nd ed). Englewood Cliffs, NJ, Prentice-Hall, 1975

Ullmann LP, Krasner L (eds): Case studies in Behavior Modification. New York, Holt, Rinehart & Winston, 1965

Ullmann LP, Krasner L: A Psychological Approach to Abnormal Behavior. Englewood Cliffs, NJ, Prentice-Hall, 1969

Upper D, Ross SM (eds): Behavioral Group Therapy. Champaign, Ill, Research Press, 1979, 1980, 1981

Voegtlin WL, Lemere F, Broz WR, et al: Conditioned reflex therapy of chronic alcoholism. Q J Stud Alcohol 2:505-511, 1941

Walen SR, Hauserman NM, Lavin PJ: Clinical Guide to Behavior Therapy. Baltimore, Williams & Wilkins Co, 1977

Watson JB, Rayner R: Conditioned emotional reactions. J Exp Psychol 3:1-14, 1920

Watzlawick P, Weakland J, Fisch R: Change: Principles of Problem Formation and Problem Resolution. New York, WW Norton, 1974

Weiss RL: The conceptualization of marriage from a behavioral perspective, in Marriage and Marital Therapy. Edited by Paolino TJ, McCrady BS. New York, Brunner/Mazel, 1978

Weiss SM, Herd JA, Fox BH: Perspectives on Behavioral Medicine. New York, Academic Press, 1981

West LJ, Stein M (eds): Critical Issues in Behavioral Medicine. Philadelphia, JB Lippincott, 1982

Williams RB Jr, Gentry WD: Behavioral Approaches to Medical Treatment. Cambridge, Mass, Ballinger, 1977

Wilson GT, Evans IM: The therapist-client relationship in behavior therapy, in Effective Psychotherapy: A Handbook of Research. Edited by Gurman AS, Razin AM. New York, Pergamon Press, 1977

Wilson GT, Franks CM: Contemporary Behavior Therapy: Conceptual and Empirical Foundations. New York, Guilford, 1982

Wilson GT, Hannon AE, Evans IM: Behavior therapy and the therapist-patient relationship. J Consult Clin Psychol 32:103-109, 1968

Wilson GT, O'Leary KD: Principles of Behavior Therapy. Englewood Cliffs, NJ, Prentice-Hall, 1980

Wilson GT: Toward specifying the "nonspecific" factors in behavior therapy: a social learning analysis, in Psychotherapy Process. Edited by Mahoney MJ. New York, Plenum, 1980

Wilson GT: Effects of false feedback on avoidance behavior: "cognitive" desensitization revisited. J Pers Soc Res 28:115-122, 1973

Wolpe J, Lazarus AA: Behavior Therapy Techniques. Oxford, Pergamon Press, 1966

Wolpe J, Salter A, Reyna LJ: The Conditioning Therapies. New York, Holt, Rinehart & Winston, 1964

Wolpe J: The Practice of Behavior Therapy. New York, Pergamon Press, 1969

Wolpe J: Psychotherapy by Reciprocal Inhibition. Stanford, Calif, Stanford University Press, 1958

Wolpe J: Reciprocal inhibition as the main basis of psychotherapeutic effects. Arch Neurol Psychiatry 72:205-226, 1954

Woolfolk A, Woolfolk RL, Wilson GT: A rose by any other name . . . labeling bias and attitude toward behavior modification. J Consult Clin Psychol 45:184-191, 1977

Yates AJ: Behavior Therapy. New York, John Wiley & Sons, 1970

Yates BT, Newman FL: Approaches to cost-effectiveness analysis and cost-benefit analysis of psychotherapy, in Psychotherapy: Practice, Research, Policy. Edited by Vandenbos GR. Beverly Hills, Calif, Sage Publications, 1980a

Yates BT, Newman FL: Findings of cost-effectiveness and cost-benefit analyses of psychotherapy, in Psychotherapy: Practice, Research, Policy. Edited by Vandenbos GR. Beverly Hills, Sage Publications, 1980b

Yorkston NJ, McHugh RB, Brady R, et al: Verbal desensitization in bronchial asthma. J Psychosom Res 18:371-376, 1974

Zifferblatt SM: Increasing patient compliance through applied analysis of behavior. Prev Med 4:173-182, 1975

11

Experiential, Inspirational, Cognitive/Emotive, and Other Therapies

11

Experiential, Inspirational, Cognitive/Emotive, and Other Therapies

INTRODUCTION

The past 30 years have witnessed an extraordinary efflorescence of a wide array of "experiential" therapies, to the extent that these developments have been spoken of as constituting a "third revolution" in psychotherapy (psychoanalysis and behavioral therapy, respectively, constitute the first two revolutions) (Karasu, 1977). Literally hundreds of approaches have been developed, all directed in one way or another toward liberating emotions, expanding consciousness, and facilitating self-realization (Appelbaum, 1979; Corsini, 1981; Herink, 1980).

The emergence of this trend in the latter half of the twentieth century is considered by some to be related to a conscious or unconscious reaction against scientific technology, which has been alleged not only to have failed to fulfill its promise of a better world but to have fostered the dangers of nuclear annihilation; pollution of our food, water, and air supply; and the depletion of our natural resources. Thus, the experiential movement, to some extent, is built on a foundation of distrust of science together with a loss of faith in material values and conventional institutions. The experiential therapies lean on the importance of controlled or released emotion or "spiritual" experiences and power of conscious cognition and responsibility as the primary vehicles for inner growth and self-actualization.

Some of these therapies operate within the framework of a one-to-one relationship, but most of them involve group settings. They can arbitrarily be divided into five major categories:

A. Emotional release therapies (see Table 1),

B. Emotional release therapies with a primary focus on body manipulation (see Table 2),

C. Emotional control therapies (see Table 3),

D. Religious and/or inspirational therapies,

E. Cognitive-emotional therapies.

These five categories are not sharply demarcated, and there is considerable overlap among them.

THE EMOTIONAL RELEASE THERAPIES

The emotional release therapies operate on the premise of abreaction originally advanced by Freud. However, when, in the course of his experience, Freud discovered that emotional release in and of itself usually resulted only in transitory improvement, he gave up the pursuit of abreaction for the more painstaking process of trying to "work through" the patient's defenses and resistances. Nevertheless, the theory that the emotional recovery of a traumatic memory leads to a sudden cure of mental illness has never lost its popular appeal and has had a remarkable renaissance in recent years. Literally scores of therapies fall into this category, and it would be beyond the scope of this document to attempt to describe them all. However, some representative examples follow.

Encounter Group Therapy

The encounter groups originated from a 1946 summer workshop in Bethel, Maine, designed to explore small groups as a vehicle for personal and social change. Major participants included Kurt Lewin, Kenneth Benne, Leland Bradford, and Ronald Lippitt. Within the context of this workshop it was discovered that mutual confrontation, evaluation ("feedback"), and focusing on the group process resulted in strong emotional experiences. The approach that grew out of this conference was marked by concentration on the immediate group process plus an emphasis on personal relations and the resultant subjective experiences (Back, 1972).

An encounter group consists of ten to 18 people and one or two trainers. Several meetings are usually held over a relatively short period of time; if the group meets continuously over a weekend, the session is called a marathon. Within a session, structured exercises are

> designed to stimulate open, intense, honest, and highly personal give-and-take among group members; [they] include not only verbal interchanges but also various nonverbal devices such as touching, massaging, holding, hugging, dancing, exercising, playing games, eyeball-to-eyeballing, acting out dreams and fantasies, etc. The purpose of these activities is to loosen people up emotionally, help them get rid of their inhibitions and resistances, and "peel off their hang-ups." (Harper, 1975)

In all of this, the emphasis is on the here-and-now.

Criticisms of encounter groups have been made on the basis of this here-and-now orientation, which not only rejects the past but the future as well. The responsibility of the leader ends when the group disbands, potentially leaving an individual stranded if he acts on something that he learned in the group and then encounters problems. Other criticisms center on the inadequate training of leaders and their failure to screen out severely disturbed individuals from the groups. Although the figures vary, encounter groups potentially can be harmful. Proponents of the movement propose that individuals are depersonalized by society and frustrated in their desire for love, intimate relationships, and self-actualization, and that these feelings can be alleviated, in part, by the encounter group experience. On the other hand, Kirschenbaum (1979) has sharply criticized the counterculture as helping "to undermine initiative, competence, and self-reliance, and thus make individuals increasingly dependent on the therapeutic state."

Therapeutic Factors. Back (1972) describes encounter groups as a social movement because they respond to the needs of the larger society by providing relief from alienation. People coming to these groups are seeking an intense emotional experience, usually aimed at personal growth. Meetings are held in a variety of settings; many of the personal growth centers are weekend facilities. Sessions are led by a trainer, and the emphasis is on group process. The popularity of sensitivity training grew rapidly in the 1960's through personal testimony, books, and the media (e.g., the film, *Bob & Carol & Ted & Alice*). In more recent years, its popularity appears to have declined. As Back (1972) notes,

> One of the difficulties in assessing sensitivity training in relation to psychotherapy is the lack of clarity regarding the aims of encounter group techniques. Sensitivity training and encounter groups do not talk about patients or about cure. They talk about group members and self-realization. Thus, even if the techniques are used in a generalized psychotherapeutic program, one is almost forced to use a criterion of "change" that amounts to any undefined effect at all. . . . In the encounter movement practically everybody is a potential participant; thus, everybody or nobody is a patient, and specific needs for therapy are little considered.

The trainers do not view themselves as therapists. Trainers work to keep the group going and to see that everyone has a chance to become involved. Lieberman et al. (1973) described the leaders in their study as carrying out the following functions, albeit to different degrees: (a) emotional stimulation, (b) caring, (c) meaning-attribution (interpreting what is going on), and (d) executive functions (management of the group as a social system). They also presented evidence about the differential effects of various leadership styles. In particular, group leaders whose pursuit of group goals was most aggressive tended to have the largest number of casualties.

As for *patient-therapist congruence*, on the surface it would seem important that there be a congruence between the participant's expectations and

Table 1. Emotional Release Therapies Without Body Manipulation

DIMENSIONS	Encounter	Gestalt	Lifespring	Primal Therapy	est
Prime concern	Emotional restriction	Alienation	Self-acceptance and enhancement	"Primal pool" of pain	Self-acceptance
Concept of pathology	Alienation, emotional inhibition, impairment of identity, inability to communicate	Existential despair: human loss of possibilities, fragmentation of self, lack of congruence with one's experiences	Failure to achieve full human potential	All psychopathology result of accumulation of pain, due to failure to satisfy needs of infants for love & gratification	Human loss of possibilities, alienation, impaired sense of identity
Concept of health	Spontaneity, authenticity	Actualization of potential: self-growth, authenticity, and spontaneity	Self-actualization, self-growth, spontaneity	Freedom from primal pain.	Self-acceptance, emotional freedom, authenticity
Mode of change	Communication of spontaneous feelings to others in a group situation with group feedback	Immediate experiencing: sensing or feeling in the immediate moment, i.e., spontaneous expression of experience	Cognitive learning & spontaneous experiencing in small groups	Discharge of accumulated pain via primal scream experiences	Immediate experiencing with group feedback
Time approach and focus	Ahistorical	Ahistorical: phenomenological moment	Ahistorical, here-and-now experiencing	Historical; recovery of painful experiences in infancy, birth, and even intrauterine	Ahistorical, existential
Type of treatment	Short-term and intense	Short-term and intense	Short-term and intense	Intensive individual sessions supplemented by group sessions. Duration ca. 8 mos.	Short-term and intense
Therapist's task	To create an atmosphere in which feelings in the group can be spontaneously and honestly communicated	To interact in a mutually accepting atmosphere for arousal of self-expression (from somatic to spiritual)	To give didactic lectures & also to interact in mutually accepting & empathic manner to encourage self-expression	To encourage release of early painful memories & associated feelings	To give didactic lectures and to create an atmosphere of emotional tension in order to facilitate abreaction
Primary tools, techniques	Encounter, exercises to reduce feelings of distance or alienation	Encounter: shared dialogue, experiments or games, dramatization or playing out of feelings	Didactic lectures, meditation, role-playing, guided fantasies, games, small group discussions	Abreaction	Marathon encounter with authoritarian group leader
Treatment model	Existential, egalitarian	Existential: egalitarian	Existential, egalitarian	Adult (therapist)—Child (patient)	Mixed, existential

DIMENSIONS	Encounter	Gestalt	Lifespring	Primal Therapy	est
Nature of therapist/patient relationship to therapeutic change	Significant	Significant & primary for change	Significant	No direct relationship. Cure presumably depends on pt's ability to release early feelings	Significant
Therapist's role and stance	Interactor-acceptor: non-authoritarian monitor	Interactor-acceptor: mutually permissive or gratifying	Interactor-acceptor: non-authoritarian facilitator of abreaction & spontaneity	Authoritarian facilitator of abreaction	Authoritarian, alternatively restrictive & permissive
Setting	Small groups—informal settings	Individual and/or group workshop	Small groups—informal settings	Individual plus groups (10-30 people)	Large group workshops
Patient variables	No serious disorders; Search for meaning	Exhibitionistic, narcissistic, no serious disorders	No serious disorders; Search for self-actualization	Exhibitionistic, all forms of functional psychopathology, repressed anger & hurt, espec. at parents	No serious disorders; Search for meaning
Therapist variables	Empathic, non-authoritarian	Creative, playful, sensitive to others' needs	Warm, spontaneous, empathic, charismatic	Powerfully suggestive & belief in uniqueness of treatment-method	Authoritarian, charismatic, persuasive
Shared belief system	Importance of emotional communication and authenticity in human growth	Awareness of body and its integration with self	Capacity for personal growth & fulfillment through increased self awareness & acceptance	All problems due to parental mishandling. Therapeutic value of strong emotional abreaction	Rapid change possible through abreaction & self-revelation
Cognitive learning	De-emphasized	De-emphasized	Included	De-emphasized—secondary	Included
Behavior modification	Group reinforcement, rehearsal of behavior	Group reinforcement, rehearsal of behavior	Group reinforcement, role-playing	Powerful suggestion, group reinforcement	Group rehearsal
Affective experience	Explosive catharsis	Explosive catharsis & feeling in touch	Affective experiencing in permissive group setting	Explosive catharsis	Explosive catharsis
Length of treatment	Usually long weekends. Sessions range from several hrs. to all day	One weekend—6 months	5 consecutive days with post-training sessions. May be repeated as often as client wishes	6-8 months	9 days, including 2 consecutive marathon weekends (60-70 hrs)
Frequency of treatment	Either episodic or may be once a week	Individual & groups once/week	3 consecutive evenings plus entire weekend	Daily indiv. session at outset; later weekly group sessions	Daily for 9 days
Method of payment	Advance payment for workshop	Advance payment for workshop	Advance payment for workshop	Advance payment for initial treatment. Supplementary charges for longer—	Advance payment for workshop

the experience provided. Lieberman et al. (1973) related the participants' values to outcome and found that

> the value structure of [dropouts] was most discrepant from the values inherent in the general characteristics of encounter group culture, particularly their low investment in growth and relationship values. In contrast, the high learners were individuals whose values mirrored some aspects of the encounter group culture, the emphasis on changing, and on hedonism; their devaluation of experiencing, however, places them in opposition to a dominant motif of the encounter group. Perhaps the closest match of the dominant encounter group values can be found among the negative changers. More than any other group, they fit the value stereotype associated with encounter groups.

The issue of *therapeutic alliance* is not applicable in the traditional sense. The group works together as a whole and provides support for individual members as well. Lieberman et al. found that those who "could not or would not sufficiently identify with the group as a collective unity and experience a feeling of identity" tended to experience a negative outcome. A feeling of belongingness in the group is important, and it also seems important that the participant be able to identify with the therapist and other participants in order to learn from experiences within the group. Principles of group process are stressed rather than transference or countertransference.

The main technique of the encounter group for fostering cognitive learning is "feedback." Lieberman et al. (1973) found evidence that feedback was negatively related to change, whereas greater positive change was related to self-disclosure. On this basis, they concluded that it was better to arrive at one's own insights than to be told by others through feedback.

The training does have the potential for providing a certain corrective *emotional experience*. Some modeling appears to occur (for example, the way the trainer and other group members freely express their feelings). Groups also exert a powerful suggestive and persuasive influence on their members. The time-limited character of encounter groups and the fact that participants remain largely anonymous as individuals (e.g., in terms of their social status and current lives) probably heighten the intensity of the experience. Group pressure is largely directed at the expression of positive and negative feelings, the rapid creation of "intimacy," and the breaking down of barriers to open and direct communication. A common feature of encounter groups is an intense emotional experience the effects of which, however, appear to be largely transient and tend to dissipate once the individual returns to his or her former social environment with its usual restraints.

Intense emotional experiencing is a major goal of sensitivity training. Interestingly, those participants in the Lieberman study who deliberately sought an intense or novel experience received less benefit from the group. These investigators concluded, "Not only must individuals experience deep emotion, but they must be helped to objectify the experience in such a way as to provide meaning for the future."

Gestalt Therapy

Gestalt therapy has been practiced in this country since the 1940's but did not gain great popularity until the early 1960's. A number of individuals have played a significant role in developing the theory and practice of Gestalt therapy, but its leader was Fritz Perls, a former psychoanalyst. Perls also received training as an actor, and apparently his gifts at this craft contributed to the development of Gestalt therapy.

Gestalt therapy has had a profound impact on the entire encounter group movement. In his later years, Perls lived at Esalen and was a leader to younger experiential therapists. There is probably not a workshop taking place in this country which does not use some Gestalt techniques.

The relationship of Gestalt therapy to Gestalt psychology is far from clear. Perls was certainly influenced by Gestalt psychology, but neither he nor other writers have been able to present a coherent picture of how Gestalt therapy derives from Gestalt psychology. The most proximate relationship is in the focus on perception and on how the mind seeks to achieve "closure," cognitively, affectively, and interpersonally. The impeding or blocking of such closure leads to frustration and psychopathology. In Gestalt therapy, health is regarded as an awareness of needs, feelings, and perceptions. The focus is always on the body and what the body is telling the patient. If the patient says, "I am feeling more and more terrified," the therapist will say, "Stay with that feeling, how is it affecting your body; what is your body telling you?" If the patient says, "I feel dead," the therapist will say, "Concentrate on being dead; what does it feel like?"

Gestalt therapists believe in focusing entirely on the "here-and-now." This does not mean that patients do not talk about past events. But since they are experiencing the past problem at the present moment, the Gestaltists argue that the therapeutic resolution of the problem must take place in the present. If a patient talks about a problem with an angry feeling toward a parent, the patient is encouraged to "bring the parent into the hour" and talk to him as if he were there. Then the patient is asked to role play the parent and report the patient's perception of what the parent may be feeling. A dialogue then follows.

Another key concept in Gestalt therapy is "responsibility." Patients are put under heavy pressure to be accountable for their behavior and are actively rewarded when they talk about being responsible. If the patient states, "I don't want to work in therapy today," he is left alone because he is not "playing games" but is taking responsibility for his action. Another frequent term is "integration." It is assumed that, in response to the stresses and child rearing practices of our society, the organism develops ways of preventing itself from achieving full awareness by splitting off various parts of itself. By focusing on maximum awareness, the organism is viewed as more likely to achieve integration.

Another common expression is "unfinished business." Gestalt therapists talk about patients still hanging on to past constructs or "unfinished Gestalts." They argue that the healthy person is constantly destroying old Gestalts and creating new ones. In effect, the argument is that one cannot linger in the past but must constantly be focusing on the experience of the present.

Throughout all of the Gestalt writing, disdain is expressed for the cognitive aspect of the mind, which is viewed as a trap or resistance and often referred to as the "computer." Some Gestaltists appear to derive great joy from making statements that would be viewed as provocative by most schools of psychotherapy. There are many catch phrases such as "lose your mind and come to your senses," "you must abandon all hope before you can begin to grow," or "the worst thing you can do for people is to help them; helping is not helpful." These paradoxes are used at times to break down resistances to treatment.

Therapeutic Factors. Gestalt therapy's focus on the "here-and-now" fits in neatly with the existential school of philosophy, and in the 1950's and 1960's a number of existential therapists were attracted to the movement. It is probably appropriate to call Gestalt therapy a movement. At various times it is described simply as a therapy or a philosophy; at others, it seems to be advocated as a "blue-print" for effective living. Although Gestalt therapy can be conducted in practically any setting, it is most commonly employed in the workshop format. The shared belief system is that awareness of the body's needs, feelings, and perceptions will lead to more effective mental and interpersonal integration. Gestalt therapy can be conducted in an individual or group context. Individual therapy is more common on the east coast. The west coast, dominated by Perls, favors groups. Usually only one patient at a time "works." The rest of the group observes, reinforces, and sometimes role plays for the patient who is in the "hot seat." In the workshop setting, the therapy may take place over a long weekend rather than on a week-to-week basis. The group can be anywhere from ten to 200 in number. Perls assumed that all were gaining help as they observed. Patients pay in advance for workshops; payment for individual psychotherapy is at a level similar to that of conventional therapies.

The media have boosted the encounter movement in general and the use of Gestalt techniques in particular. Their therapeutic methods are often caricatured on television and in films. There are, however, many serious books that extol the virtues of Gestalt therapy (Fagan and Shepherd, 1970; Marcus, 1970; Perls, 1969; Perls et al., 1965).

Patients volunteer for Gestalt therapy because they are attracted by its precepts and believe it will help them. It takes a certain amount of courage to be in a Gestalt group. The techniques are powerful and threatening; it is easy to get upset in such a setting. On the other hand, the fringe benefits for being courageous are not inconsiderable. There is a lot of love from the therapist and other group members. A great deal of touching takes place within the therapy, which not infrequently leads to sexual contacts between participants outside of the therapy. The Gestalt group is no place for a psychotic or severe "borderline" individual. It is also possible that people attracted to Gestalt groups are receiving reinforcement and justification for life styles that in past years might have been viewed as selfish.

Gestalt therapists come from all mental health professions. There are also a number of lay people—writers, poets, and theologians—who have become prominent therapists. Many are charismatic and have superb acting ability. As a group, they tend to be playful, extremely sensitive to others' needs, and highly creative. However, according to Thomas Munson (1978), a prominent West Coast Gestalt practitioner, one of the major problems facing the Gestalt school of therapy is the general lack of consistent training requirements for would-be practitioners. He attributes this problem to

> Perls' original reluctance to set qualifications, so that his seminars were a mixture of a few qualified professionals and a large group of unqualified persons, bound to become Gestalt therapists by fusion or fission. Some centers offered training programs varying from one week to three years, and many of the practitioners considered themselves trained after a year, though they had no previous psychiatric training.

Patients and therapists in Gestalt therapy tend to share common values and interests. It is a therapy for the "now" society, for people who are concerned with life in the present, with self-actualization, and with growth. In some settings there is a tendency to use Gestalt and other techniques almost as a substitute for religion.

The therapeutic alliance does not take on major significance in Gestalt therapy. The therapist is merely a facilitator. He seeks only enough trust to get the patient to take a chance and try. In the course of focusing on the present, the patient will, of course, do much relating to the therapist, so if it is to be useful there must be some positive aspect to the relationship. Mutual liking is not viewed as critical in Gestalt therapy. It is assumed that to the extent that all participants reach a state of awareness and integration, they will get along well with each other.

Gestalt therapists recognize that a certain amount of identification with the therapist is inevitable. They deplore this, however. Since each individual is unique and must find his own way, reliance on the therapist is seen as a "sick game," and identification is viewed as a factor that might foster such reliance.

Gestalt therapies recognize the occurrence of transference but view it as a phenomenon that gets in the way of the patient-therapist encounter. The patient is encouraged to relate to the therapist as therapist and not to confuse him with someone else. Most of the responses the patient has to the therapist are not viewed as an expression of transference but as real happenings in the here-and-now. When a therapist suspects that a patient is relating to him as though he were someone else, the therapist tries to clarify what is happening and prevent such interaction. Gestalt therapists believe that therapists themselves should be highly aware, responsible, and integrated. This enables them to avoid the need to give advice, to be helpers, or to interfere in their patients' lives. Countertransference would simply be viewed as the therapist's avoidance of the encounter because of his own lack of mental health.

While the Gestalt therapists eschew emphasis on cognitive learning, they recognize that their system is complex and that the patient needs to hear it explained, sometimes repeatedly. There is some emphasis on helping the patient identify behavior patterns, but there is no emphasis on explaining them. The key words in Gestalt therapy are "what" and "how." "Why" is never considered to be an important question and is actually viewed as a cognitive trap that hinders the patient.

A good deal of behavior modification takes place within Gestalt therapy. The Gestalt group functions something like a "Greek chorus," providing powerful reinforcement for the patient when he is behaving correctly and withdrawing it when he is not. Also, when an individual publicly enunciates a message he has been containing internally for a long period of time, his presentation is followed by a different response, both on his part and on the part of the therapist and the group. The contingencies of internal and external reinforcement have been changed.

There is also a great deal of *exposure* in the Gestalt method. Patients are constantly looking at things they fear. Gestalt therapy encourages counterphobic behavior. Relaxation techniques are also used and considerable attention paid to deep breathing exercises.

Although Gestalt therapists would argue that they stay out of people's lives and never advise them what to do, they are certainly quite directive within the therapeutic hour. Patients are given a clear message that salvation depends on their ability to concentrate on their bodies and to expand their awareness of their own existence.

Much of the process of holding dialogue with various parts of one's self, with figures in one's past or current life, or with the therapist and other group members can be viewed as training and rehearsal for situations the patient may encounter outside the group. Although a Gestalt therapist would insist that each subsequent encounter would be a unique situation, it appears that the therapy does train the patient to deal with future encounters in a different way. Catharsis and abreaction are a critical part of Gestalt therapy. Perls often talks about "the explosion," whether it be of anger or of grief, as an important part of therapeutic change. Gestalt therapists are preoccupied with distinguishing real expression of feelings from "phony" expression.

Gestalt therapy has played a major role in all of the experiential therapies and probably provides the best theoretical justification for the importance of focusing on the here-and-now in psychotherapy. Its techniques can power-fully influence clients. Gestalt therapy's primary contribution seems, how-ever, to have been its potential for integration into a variety of other therapies.

Lifespring

Lifespring is the name of an organization that specializes in "personal growth training." It was founded in January 1974 by a group of people with extensive experience in educational and business training. Headquartered in San Rafael, California, Lifespring also has centers in Oregon, California, Pennsylvania, Washington, D.C., and Vancouver.

Lifespring offers three kinds of programs, one called Basic Training (BT); the second, Interpersonal Experience (IPE); and the third, a Training Coordinator program (TC). Recently it has added a fourth program called Family Training.

The Lifespring Foundation publishes a monthly magazine, which, in addition to announcements about forthcoming programs and "in-house" news, is packed with testimonials of satisfied clients. In California, Lifespring has formed an association with California State University at Fullerton in which its three main courses—Basic Training, Interpersonal Experience, and the Training Coordinator program—are offered for aca-demic credits. The foundation is trying to institute similar college credit programs with local state universities wherever it has a training center.

The Lifespring perspective has been influenced by such people as Abra-ham Maslow, Fritz Perls, and Carl Rogers. Its basic assumption is that all people have "an infinite capacity to experience more joy, fulfillment, and have life work better for them." The training brochure (Lifespring, 1978) states specifically that

> while the training is supportive and safe, it is not recommended for those with a history of emotional disorder or those currently experiencing severe emotional difficulties. Lifespring is not therapy and should not be artificially injected into an established therapeutic relationship. Those who have been in therapy within the last six months must obtain their therapist's signed agreement to take the training.

The Basic Training is a 50-hour program "designed to stimulate personal growth by increasing self-awareness and acceptance." The program takes place on five consecutive days, including all day Saturday and Sunday. A post-training session is held ten days later. No drugs are allowed. Each day's program has three parts:

A. A didactic part in which the trainer discusses concepts on which the program is based;

B. An experiential part, in which the trainees participate in individual, one-to-one, or group processes. These include individual meditation, guided fantasies, games, role-playing exercises, and small group discussions. The emphasis in this part of the program is on a here-and-now experience;

C. "Sharing," wherein each participant recounts his or her experiences with the process to another trainee or to the whole group. Lifespring claims that by the end of the training on Sunday most graduates report experiencing "an overwhelming sense of self-acceptance, appreciation and personal power" (Lifespring, 1978).

Lifespring also asserts that the value of its Basic Training program has been objectively demonstrated by the results of a Personal Orientation Inventory (POI) developed earlier by one of its subsequent trainers, Everett Shostrom, Ph.D. The POI is said to measure such factors as levels of self-worth, self-reliance, independence, flexibility, and sensitivity to the needs of others.

The methods used in the Interpersonal Experience program are similar to those used in Basic Training except that they proceed in greater depth and are more personalized. Participation in the IPE program requires completion of the Basic Training course.

The Training Coordinator program (TC) is an advanced leadership training course offered to IPE graduates. The Family Training course is a four-day experience for parents who have graduated from Basic Training and for their children, ages six through 17.

According to Lifespring, about half of the graduates of Basic Training continue on to the IPE training. A smaller number also complete the TC program. Graduates are permitted to retake the Basic Training as many times as they wish at no charge. As the Lifespring manual puts it, "The Basic Training can always provide a safe environment for examining where our lives are at that moment." Lifespring also sponsors ongoing social events for its graduates.

Therapeutic Factors. Lifespring is part of the sociocultural context of the "human potential" movement and is closely related to "T groups" and sensitivity training programs. Its courses generally are given in classrooms. Like many movements of this kind the followers are proselytized by members who have taken the program previously and feel that they have benefited from it. The basic structure of the Lifespring training program involves a group context but, as in other sensitivity training groups, many of its exercises are on a one-to-one basis. People who reach out for this kind of therapy are seeking an emotional experience that promises them some benefit within a brief period of time. Judging from people who enter the human potential movement and sensitivity training programs in general, it can be assumed that some of them have emotional problems that they do not wish to deal with in standard psychotherapeutic ways while others are seeking some kind of extended support system. No specific professional training is necessary to become a trainer in the Lifespring movement.

These groups work best when there is a mutual liking between patient and therapist, and identification with the therapist plays a part in the therapeutic experience. Although not specifically recognized as such, transference and countertransference factors undoubtedly play an important part in the relationships that develop in these training sessions. And while the Lifespring program claims to be primarily an experiential type of program, it is clear that some cognitive learning takes place in the sessions, particularly when the trainers lecture and present the concepts that they consider central to the Lifespring training program. It is evident that suggestion, persuasion, reassurance, rehearsal, and approval for "good reactions" occur in the training sessions, not only from trainers to individual participants, but also within the group context from the group to the individuals. It is, therefore, reasonable to infer that a certain amount of operant conditioning and trial and error learning takes place in the training sessions.

The major emphasis in the Lifespring program is on here-and-now experiencing. As in many sensitivity training programs, the "exercises" are designed to intensify aspects of affective experience.

In summary, Lifespring's techniques involve a potpourri of processes including meditation, guided fantasies, games, role-playing exercises, and small group discussions. Its therapeutic efficacy is based on all of the factors that play a part in this type of group process—group support, catharsis, suggestion and persuasion, identification with the trainers, mutual identification, rehearsal, and some degree of cognitive training. Its primary emphasis, however, is on affective experience in a group context. Although Lifespring specifically denies that it is a therapeutic program, it clearly offers therapeutic experiences to its participants as well as an ongoing group identification. The group becomes a kind of extended family for graduates and provides them with considerable emotional support.

Primal Therapy

Primal therapy was developed around 1970 by Arthur Janov, a clinical psychologist. Janov assumes that all neurosis is the result of failure to satisfy the basic needs of infants for love and gratification. All efforts at training the child are considered to be potential interferences with these needs and to result in the accumulation of a "primal pool" of pain. Janov regards all apparently normal or well adjusted individuals as really neurotic because they have "accommodated" to this repressed pain. In the course of primal scream therapy patients are persuaded to recall and re-enact their early infantile traumata, including the presumptively painful experience of moving through the birth canal. Even intrauterine "memories" are sometimes elicited. As the pain of these events is recalled, the patients are encouraged to emit screams, which are called primals. Janov claims that a patient who has completed primal therapy thereafter has a low body temperature, a slower pulse rate, a lower blood pressure, and is less likely to develop physical illness.

Prior to instituting therapy, the patient is isolated in a hotel room for 48 hours. The aim is to "soften up" his defenses. Thus, the patient comes to the initial session in a state of heightened frustration and with his defenses more vulnerable. Therapy consists of intensive individual sessions, each session lasting until the patient is exhausted and asks for a halt. During primal experiences the patient is encouraged to regress, to assume the fetal position, to use baby-talk, and to suck on giant-sized nursing bottles. When the period of individual therapy is completed, patients then enter group therapy on an outpatient basis. These sessions can involve anywhere from ten to 30 or more people and do not focus on content. Rather, they serve as means of encouraging the individuals to continue to engage in their respective primal experiences. At the end of the group session patients are encouraged to describe their feelings during their primals. Therapy lasts about eight months.

Janov asserts that his treatment is the only true cure for neurosis as well as for severe character disorders, homosexuality, and psychosis. He overtly derogates all other forms of treatment as being inadequate. The extraordinary claims concerning the therapeutic effectiveness of primal therapy have never been substantiated by outside scientific observers.

Therapeutic Factors. Primal therapy is based on an oversimplified adaptation of the early psychoanalytic theory of abreaction. The physical setting is an office and/or clinic adapted for "primal screaming" (see above for other arrangements, especially pretherapy). The shared belief is that neurosis results from the frustration of basic infantile needs. The therapeutic context is that of intensive individual therapy, followed by group sessions. Primal therapy has been highly popularized by the media but seems to have lost some of its appeal in recent years.

Primal therapy seems to lend itself best to the treatment of neurotic patients, especially those with hysterical features. The therapist is highly directive, confrontative, and intrusive; and presumably both patient and therapist must have a flair for dramatic enactment. There is no therapeutic alliance as it is commonly understood, but the patient's full cooperation is required for reaching the "pool" of primal pain. The impression is created that the patient's dependency wishes are "utilized" rather than worked through in the traditional sense.

The patient learns to identify with Janov's theoretical position and may be selected on the basis of evidence that he/she has been "primed" (e.g., through Janov's popular books [Janov, 1970, 1971, 1972]). Insight into "primal" pain and its developmental significance is fostered.

Behavior modification probably occurs through desensitization to "primal pain" as a function of the therapeutic experience. There are strong indications that "primals" are suggested to patients who are ready to experience them, which may form a basis for their selection as suitable candidates. There also appears to be some systematic training in abandoning "neurotic goals," as defined by Janov. Intense abreaction is the major emphasis of the therapy.

Erhard Seminars Training (est)

Erhard Seminars Training was founded in 1971 by Werner Erhard, a former trainer of salesmen in the door-to-door encyclopedia sales business. In the years preceding the founding of *est*, Erhard himself had participated in a rather broad variety of therapy groups, including Dale Carnegie, Scientology, encounter groups, Gestalt therapy, yoga, zen, and Mind Dynamics. Much of *est* is said to have been patterned after Mind Dynamics, a technique of self-hypnosis which is claimed to improve personal effectiveness and mind control. The *est* program consists of a standard training period comprising a nine-day, 60- to 70-hour course that includes marathon group sessions lasting 15 to 17 hours on both days of two consecutive weekends. The group generally involves about 250 people at a time. The long hours and the physical and emotional frustration involved in the didactic sessions combine to build up a great deal of tension, thus facilitating emotional release. The training also includes self-disclosure before the entire group along with sessions of relaxation and meditation. In addition, certain cognitive concepts such as "what is, is," "you are responsible for everything about yourself, including your problems," and "accept yourself as you are" are emphasized (Rhinehart, 1976).

Part of the success of the training program lies in its remarkable merchandising program. It is organized in more than 15 cities and has almost 200 paid employees. More important, however, Erhard has found a way of enlisting ex-trainees as volunteers, working for him and trying to recruit others into the program.

In many ways *est* is closely related to the encounter group movement. Erhard himself specifically asserts that the training is not intended to be psychotherapeutic, and the official *est* policy is to discourage applicants who are currently in therapy or who have had previous psychiatric hospitalization.

Participants in *est* training often report beneficial effects after completing the seminars, but no long-term follow-up studies are available. Simon (1978) has reported good therapeutic results in some post-*est* patients with good ego strength, particularly when "motivation and readiness for change are present," but has observed severe regressions in others. There have also been other reports of psychotic episodes in *est* participants with no history of previous psychiatric disorder (Glass et al., 1977; Kirsch and Glass, 1977).

Therapeutic Factors. *est* combines Gestalt, yoga, zen, hypnosis, behavior modification, Scientology, sensory awareness, marathon sessions, and the power of positive thinking in one skillfully merchandised package. Its appeal seems to be largely to upper middle-class individuals, and its context involves large group sessions generally taking place in sizable auditoriums or hotel ballrooms. The trainers are intensively coached by Erhard himself to deliver a performance almost exactly imitating his delivery of training material, closely resembling participatory theatre. No comprehensive written explication of the theory or techniques of *est* has ever been published by *est* itself. Manuals and techniques are generally kept secret except as revealed by former trainees. The trainers' style and the group process tend to foster submission and dependence. The training seems to capitalize on the individual's infantile dependence on parental authority.

EMOTIONAL RELEASE THREAPIES WITH PRIMARY EMPHASIS ON BODY CONTACT

The recent upsurge of therapies focusing on bodily contact of various kinds as the primary road toward emotional abreaction and emotional health had its origin with techniques developed at the Esalen Institute in northern California in the mid-1960's. At Esalen a variety of massage therapies and other body contacts, often in warm pools in group situations, were found to have broad mass appeal. A variety of body massage techniques, ranging from gently titillating to harshly painful ones, have since been offered to the public for their supposed psychotherapeutic value as well as for their ability to promote relaxation and reduce tension.

The concept that psychopathology is rooted in body tension is not a new one. One such theory, that of Wilhelm Reich, was an offshoot of psychoanalytic libido theory. Reich believed that the repressed libido of neurotic individuals as expressed in their "character armor" was reflected in muscular tension that could be released by body massage and manipulation. His technique involved having the patient disrobe and lie on a couch so that the therapist could observe the patient's body behavior and manipulate presumptive areas of tension. Genital excitation during a Reichian analysis was considered a desideratum, and orgastic release was considered to be the most effective and significant discharge of repressed libido. Although Reichian therapy has lost some of its popularity in recent years, there is still a school of Reichian analysis whose followers carry on this form of therapy. It is not necessary to belabor the potential for abuse of this kind of technique, even though Reich himself specifically abjured any actual sexual relationship between patient and therapist. Three recent examples of release therapies involving bodily contact are bio-energetic psychotherapy, Rolfing, and Z-therapy.

Bio-Energetic Psychotherapy

Bio-energetic psychotherapy was developed by Alexander Lowen about 20 years ago (Lowen, 1967) and is an offshoot of the expressive, active psychotherapies developed within the psychoanalytic movement. The most important precursor to the work of Lowen was Wilhelm Reich, and Lowen's bio-energetic psychotherapy might be described as Reich without mysticism.

Lowen accepts the idea of a muscular armor as a reflection of frustrating life experiences. He also assumes that the armor reflects the presence of inhibited emotions and that there is a fairly explicit correspondence between the particular emotion that is inhibited and the particular pattern of muscular tension that develops.

Implicit in Lowen's theory is the idea that each emotion is associated with an action or an action impulse of a fairly specific kind. When overt punishment or guilt lends to the inhibition of the emotional impulse, the process of inhibition produces muscle tensions. In other words, we use one set of muscles to inhibit the action of another set. Thus, an impulse to attack or hit, if inhibited, will be associated with muscular tensions in the shoulders, arms, and neck. Inhibited sexual impulses will be associated with muscular tension in the region of the abdomen and thighs. Inhibited sadness or crying will be associated with muscular tension in the region of the lips or mouth and will often be recognized as a "stiff upper lip."

Lowen's bio-energetic analysis is an attempt to delimit these muscular tension patterns in detail and to develop methods for reducing the tensions. The assumption made by Lowen and practitioners of bio-energetic analysis is that the reduction of muscular tension and abreaction of the inhibited emotions will produce a tension-free individual capable of realizing his maximum potential.

One of the most important potentials, according to Lowen, is the capacity for pleasure. He asserts that any muscular tension or "armoring" inhibits to some extent the capacity for feeling or expressing pleasure. Therefore, a central focus of Lowen's work is the expression of pleasure, particularly the expression of sexuality. This is regarded as an indicator of the development of the individual toward an armor-free state, or toward what had earlier been called the genital character. With regard to Lowen's specific techniques, he relies heavily on the use of deep breathing, muscle palpations, and special body exercises to induce abreaction and to reduce muscle tensions. In practice, the patient is asked to disrobe partially or fully during the bio-energy session so that his patterns of muscular tension will be more evident to the therapist. The therapist then proceeds to encourage deep breathing, changes of posture, and certain forced movements (for example, pelvic thrusts) in order to elicit the expression of emotion and abreactions. This approach is uniquely oriented to one-to-one individual interactions

Table 2. Emotional Release Therapies With Body Manipulation

DIMENSIONS	Bioenergetic Psychotherapy	Rolfing	Z-Therapy	Arica
Prime concern	Reduction of muscular tension	Elimination of tensions that are "locked into" muscle, fascia, & tendons	Rage reduction	"Total self-realization"
Concept of pathology	Emotions locked in muscle tensions	Psychological disturbances result from misalignments in body structure	Sensori-motor & cognitive resistances	Failure to achieve full human potential
Concept of health	Freedom from emotional & muscular tension	Perfect symmetry between the 2 sides of the body, so that "mind & body can move through space in harmony with gravity."	Freedom from above resistances	Self-realization, "clarification of consciousness." "Freedom from muscular tension
Mode of change	Discharge of repressed emotions via postural and muscular movements	Deep, painful massage	Immediate experiencing of repressed rage	Cognitive learning, deep body massage, meditation, guided fantasy, breathing exercise, Taro cards, and Eastern mystic philosophy
Time approach and focus	Ahistorical even though pathology is traced to childhood experience	Ahistorial	Ahistorical even though pathology is traced to childhood experience	Ahistorical, mystical, phenomenological
Type of treatment	Short-term and intense	Short-term and intense	Short-term and intense	Moderate-term & intense
Therapist's task	To diagnose & release patterns of muscular tension in order to promote emotional abreaction	To diagnose & release areas of myofascial tension	To provoke & elicit violent rage reaction	Didactic, to teach & communicate complex series of ritual tasks
Primary tools, techniques	One-to-one sessions, pt. disrobed, communication of feelings, abreaction	One-to-one sessions	Painful body stimulation with patient in restraint	Didactic lectures, meditation, massage, guided fantasy, breathing exercises, Taro cards, mystic philosophy
Treatment model	Medical—therapist diagnoses, palpates, manipulates muscle groups	Medical—therapist diagnoses & eliminates areas of misalignment by deep massage	Medical—elimination of tension via provoked rage reduction	Transcendental, authoritarian

DIMENSIONS	Bioenergetic Psychotherapy	Rolfing	Z-Therapy	Arica
Nature of therapist/patient relationship to therapeutic	Significant	Indirect	None	Indirect
Therapist's role and stance	Medical model Authoritative	Authoritative	Authoritative, restrictive, but encouraging expression of rage	Teacher, guru
Setting	Individual	Individual & small groups	Individual therapy with small group as restrainers	Small groups
Patient variables	Denial of psychol. causality. Search for answers in somatic changes	Denial of psychol. causality. Search for answers in somatic changes	Depressed, masochistic. Search for quick magical cure	No serious disorders. Search for transcendental experiences and meaning
Therapist variables	Belief in dependence of psychopathology on muscular tensions. Charismatic, persuasive, suggestive	Belief in dependence of psychopathology on muscular tensions. Charismatic, persuasive, suggestive	Authoritarian. Unconscious sadism?	Charismatic, mysterious, other-worldly
Shared belief system	Muscular tensions as source of psychopathology	Muscular tensions as source of psychopathology	Rapid change through explosive expression of rage	Faith in the healing power of transcendental experience & unity with the cosmos
Cognitive learning	De-emphasized	De-emphasized	De-emphasized	Emphasized—part of total program
Behavior modification	Rel. slight	Rel. slight	Encouragement of rage expression	Group reinforcement
Affective experience	Strong catharsis in response to body manipulation	Strong catharsis in response to body manipulation	Explosive catharsis	Affective experiencing in group setting & atmosphere of mysticism
Length of treatment	Usually 6 mos.-1 year?	Usually brief	Several (2-3) sessions of 4-8 hours each	40 days, + addn'l sessions for advanced "training"
Frequency of treatment	1-2 times per week as a rule	1-2 times per week	Twice a week?	Daily for 40 days, then intermittent
Method of payment	Fee per session	Fee per session	Advance single payments	Advance payment for workshop

between patient and therapist; however, the group may look on and interact with the therapist and the patient about the experience afterward.

Lowen, like Reich before him, takes the position that human destructiveness, depression, morbidity, sadism, and the like are direct reflections of inhibitions imposed on children from the earliest years. He assumes that humans are inherently "good, cooperative, social beings" who need only freedom and joy in order to express these aspects of their nature.

Therapeutic Factors. The therapeutic setting is usually one-to-one, but group sessions are also used. Treatment is generally completed in about 15 sessions. Obvious psychiatric patients are excluded, but there is no formal diagnostic screening. The focus is said to be on life problems rather than on overt psychopathology.

Therapy is directed totally toward release of muscular and emotional tensions. No attention is paid to modifying the life situation. The shared belief is that both psychopathology and muscular tensions are due to childhood frustrations and that release of muscular tension will alleviate the psychological difficulties. Therapists are often "counter-culture," "hanging-loose" persons but are also warm and accepting. Touching tends to be gentle (although one technique is the deliberate creation of pain in order to elicit anger); the potential for mutual sexual arousal is great. Therapists are not required to have any formal schooling but do attend institutes conducted by "masters," with seminars and treatment sessions. Therapists are often former clients. Although discussions occur, they are mostly directed toward bringing out feelings rather than cognitive awareness. Major emphasis is on emotional abreaction.

Rolfing or Structural Integration

Ida Rolf, Ph.D., earned her doctoral degree in 1920 in biochemistry and physiology. She founded the Rolf Institute in the early 1960's in Boulder, Colorado, where she taught until her death in 1980.

The rationale for Rolfing rests on the thesis that human psychological disturbances result from misalignments in the body structure. In the ideal state there is perfect symmetry between the two sides of the body; the pelvis, spine, and head are centered around a vertical axis to permit a proper equilibrium between the force of gravity, on the one hand, and the electromagnetic field of force set up between an inferior electrical pole in the pelvis and a superior pole in the head, on the other. The ideal of this perfect balance, or "stacking," of the various segments of the body is rarely achieved spontaneously, however, and the average person is subject to a host of postural distortions (splayed feet, tipped pelvises, sagging bellies, winged scapulas, unhealthy curvatures of the spine, and drooping heads) that bring about myriad somatic and emotional ailments. The leading actor in this drama is the fascia, and indeed the mesoderm is elevated by the followers of Structural Integration to the highest place in the pantheon of human tissues. It is the fascia that binds muscles and bones together into units that, when they function properly, keep the body correctly aligned. If, on the other hand, the fascia becomes stretched and distorted, the various body segments fall out of alignment and illness follows.

How distortions in body structure lead to emotional illness is not entirely clear from Rolf's writings (Rolf, 1973). She clearly places physiology at the center of her scheme, emotion being merely the result of adverse bodily changes and structural imbalance. She writes,

> First is the surprising discovery that so-called emotion reflects physical material balance and unbalance. . . . An observer becomes aware that any man in an emotional crisis, responding to the emotion he thinks is driving him, is really reacting to chemical and physiological changes inside his skin. At this level, psychology is not the primal force; its place has been taken by physiology. . . . All too often . . . emotional pain— . . . depression . . . grief, even . . . anger—is a perception of physiological unbalance, an awareness of chemical lacks or overloads in blood and tissue. This may be at macro- or micro-levels, down to and including the cellular. (Rolf, 1973)

There are, furthermore, external as well as internal forces that work on the individual to produce illness or health.

> The potent, all too influential energy envelope of the earth—its gravitational field, although subliminal to man's cerebral consciousness, controls and directs him in its effect on his fascial component (derived from mesoderm). In turn, through controlling and directing his use of this derivative of mesoderm, his fascial system, man is able to use gravitational energy to his advantage. . . . His vertical extension relates a man to two separate energies, the energy of the sun and that of gravity, supplying two separate body needs. Bodies "feed" on energy; there are many and varied sources of this basic "food." Exposure to the energy of sunlight demonstrably changes chemical constituents of blood and cells; exposure to the positive effects of gravity (when the vertical is freed and unblocked) changes fluid flow (and thus chemistry) in myofascia and in mesodermal tissue throughout the body. (Rolf, 1973)

Finally, she asserts, structural balance enhances internal energies, since

> a body whose components are symmetrically distributed around a vertical line dissipates less of its energy in meaningless movements and meaningless tensions. Therefore, the electromagnetic energy field that such a body generates around itself remains of necessity greater and more consistent. In such bodies the reservoirs of available energy must stand at a higher level. (Rolf, 1973)

Rolfing as a therapy is based on the precepts and generalizations outlined above and aims to restore the distorted body to a proper structural integration. According to Rolf (1973),

> At the level of everyday problems, balancing and stabilizing emotions can be immeasurably furthered by any system able to create or restore vital physiological response. Although psychological hang-ups occur, they are maintained only to the extent that free physiological response is impaired at the glandular, visceral, myofascial and other levels. Restoration of function can be initiated from many levels, but establishment of myofascial equipoise is one of the most obvious, one of the speediest, one of the most powerful of these. To the extent (and at the speed) that restoration of physiological flow occurs, the individual is less hung-up.

Beyond these generalizations about the aims and rationale of treatment, little can be said concerning the details of the therapeutic techniques, since, as mentioned earlier, a discussion of these is specifically eschewed. Deep massage is the primary therapeutic maneuver. It is aimed at affecting the myofascial tissues, and it is often painful. Ten sessions constitute a course, although some individuals apparently undergo repeated series of treatments. Many photographs show before and after views indicating that postural changes occur, and individuals are quoted as saying that they feel emotionally better and more alive.

In summary, Rolfing seems to be a potpourri of anatomical and physiological disquisitions admixed with high-sounding concepts of gravitational and electromagnetic forces. The theoretical formulations are reminiscent, in part, of Mesmer's cosmic magnetic fluid and, in part, of the basic assumptions of the James-Lange theory of emotions. No doubt some individuals feel physically and emotionally better after being "structurally integrated" (or Rolfed), but the reasons why, the nature of the therapist-client relationship, the number of successful results, and the duration of the possible beneficial effects remain obscure.

Z-Therapy

Z-Therapy is a variety of abreaction therapy named for its developer Robert Zaslow, Ph.D. He initially developed it in 1966-1968 for the treatment of autistic children and called it "rage reduction therapy" (Zaslow, 1969). The underlying theory is a complex concept that rage reduction is essential to the progressive elimination of sensorimotor and cognitive resistances. Therapy consists of holding the autistic child down (i.e., using physical restraint) and, in addition, tickling the child so as to produce violent rage reactions. Once the rage is produced, the therapist will release the child and be loving and affectionate to him. Zaslow claimed that after only a few sessions this treatment produced dramatic changes in the autistic children with whom he worked.

He then went on to apply this method, which he now called "Z-Therapy," to the treatment of adults. Historical data are first obtained in several pre-treatment interview sessions. The patient is then instructed to lie across the laps of six or eight people seated in two rows, facing each other, with his head resting on the lap of the therapist. The six or eight "co-therapists" are usually, but not necessarily, either friends or relatives of the patient. The patient is then physically restrained while the therapist asks sharp questions designed to evoke traumatic experiences from the past. At the same time the questions are asked, or afterward, the therapist tickles or painfully prods the patient's rib cage to stimulate a rage reaction. No matter how vigorously the patient struggles or cries, the restraints are firmly maintained until the patient is literally wild with rage and expressing it in the most direct and violent fashion. Sessions may go on for several hours at a time (the typical session lasts four to eight hours) until the patient is totally exhausted and has stopped struggling. At that point the patient is released and affectionately embraced by all.

Z-Therapy is clearly a form of abreactive therapy based on the assumption that the release of primitive rage reactions helps to cure emotional disorders.

Therapeutic Factors. Z-Therapy is an outgrowth of the abreaction hypothesis originally advanced by Freud and later abandoned by him. Its physical setting is a private office. Therapy takes place in a group context but with the therapist as the sole applier of the treatment procedure. It must be assumed that patients who come for Z-Therapy, or who bring their children for it, have read about it and share the expectation that an abreaction experience will be dramatically curative.

Z-Therapy places no emphasis on cognitive learning, other than the presumption that releasing rage will remove resistances that stand in the way of emotional growth and development. It is possible that some operant conditioning occurs in Z-Therapy in that after the patient has expressed all the violent hostility and rage that the therapy has produced, he/she is nonetheless embraced affectionately and treated warmly by the therapist at the end of each session. For some patients, this might function as a corrective emotional experience. The experience involves no training for more effective coping with life.

In summary, Z-Therapy is primarily a form of abreactive treatment designed to produce the experience of rage; to enable patients to feel rage intensely; and then, when the painful treatment is completed, to experience the relief of an affectionate response from an authoritative figure. It may have a limited application for some autistic children and some depressed patients.

EMOTIONAL CONTROL THERAPIES

The techniques designated as emotional control therapies differ from the emotional release therapies in that their primary emphasis is on acquiring greater control over the body through training. Such control is expected to lead to favorable psychotherapeutic results. One of the most popular of these techniques is yoga training, which involves an organized program of stylized positions and exercises. Another is that of Silva Mind Control, a packaged program that relies mainly on meditation, self-hypnosis, and guided fantasy, which are expected to expand consciousness and help the clients to rid themselves of "negative thoughts." In more advanced sessions clients learn "effective sensory perception," which presumably enables them to sense the essence of rocks, metals, and even living things. Silva

Mind Controllers claim that they can even diagnose and heal ailments by "visualizing" patients and imagining them in good health.

One of the more popular emotional control techniques that has emerged in recent years, however, is transcendental meditation.

Transcendental Meditation

Transcendental meditation or TM is a standardized form of meditation technique adapted for Western use from an ancient Indian yoga technique (Hemingway, 1975). Its leader and founder is called Maharishi Mahesh Yogi, who, after graduating from Allahabad University in India as a physics major, studied for many years with a leading Indian swami. It is said that he began teaching the principles and practices of TM in 1955 in India, but in 1958 he launched a "world movement" to bring TM to everyone. For this purpose he created an organization of instructors which he calls the International Meditation Society (IMS). There are TM centers in and around most major cities of the United States and Europe. The technique is relatively easy to learn; it can be mastered in four lessons taught over a period of four days. In addition, clients are taught a set of beliefs based on Hindu metaphysical assumptions about the cosmos which includes exposure to certain Eastern beliefs encompassing the Hindu concept of *prana* (universal energy) and of *brahman* (the irreducible essence of all creation).

After several preliminary lectures the student is "initiated" and given a *mantra* to repeat silently in meditation. The initiation ceremony is similar to that used in ancient yoga practices with fruit and flowers, chanting, and incense to link the technique with the ancient Hindu tradition from which it comes. TM teachers claim that this mantra has special qualities and is individually chosen for each student. Students are pledged not to reveal their personal mantra to anyone else. Actually, there are only about 16 TM mantras that are regularly used and assigned to TM trainees, usually on the basis of their age. The mantra is said to possess soothing properties, and students are asked to repeat it silently to themselves for 20 minutes, twice daily, sitting quietly with their eyes closed. This technique is said to have unique properties in such diverse areas as the reduction of anxiety, the reduction of oxygen consumption, metabolic rate, the lowering of blood pressure, etc., as well as the achievement of peak experiences and transcendental states.

It is worth noting that the term "transcendental meditation" and the letters TM have been trademarked and are considered the exclusive property of the U.S. World Plan Executive Council. Its superiority over all other forms of meditation is aggressively proclaimed, and the technique is vigorously promoted throughout the country by a series of extraordinary claims. Thus it is confidently asserted that whenever one percent of an area's population begins to practice TM, taxes will go down, crime will

Table 3. Emotional Control Therapies

DIMENSIONS	**Transcendental Meditation**
Prime concern	Self-enhancement
Concept of pathology	Lack of self-fulfillment
Concept of health	Self-actualization
Mode of change	Meditation, achievement of transcendental states
Time approach and focus	Ahistorical
Type of treatment	Ongoing for life
Therapist's task	Teaching of technique, deciding of mantra
Primary tools, techniques	Meditation, mantra
Nature of t/p rel. to change	Indirect
Therapist's role and stance	Teacher
Setting	Individual alone, after training
Patient variables	Search for self-fulfillment, and transcendental experience
Therapist variables	Mystical, charismatic, persuasive
Shared belief system	Value of meditation
Cognitive learning	Minimal
Behavior modification	Training in relaxation
Affective experience	Variable—may be considerable
Length of treatment	Indeterminate
Frequency of treatment	Twice daily
Method of payment	Advanced lump sum for program

decline, illness will decline, traffic accidents will go down, and people will become happier. In addition, even the weather will improve because more people will be in tune with natural laws, and nature will respond accordingly. Another claim often made by proselytizers for TM is that when five percent of the world's population begins to practice TM, it will bring an end to war, poverty, hunger, and injustice throughout the world. Testimonials by successful athletes, businessmen, lawyers, and entertainers are widely disseminated, assuring readers that the practice of TM will result in better athletic functioning, business success, heightened legal acumen, and the bringing out of latent show business talent. Although these claims appear extravagant, they are apparently effective in selling the TM program.

In actuality, despite TM's claims of uniqueness, literally scores of practices can be listed under the heading of meditation. All of them have in common the ability to bring about a special kind of free-floating attention and to get the person completely absorbed by his/her particular object of meditation. The devices used to bring this about may be as diverse as gazing quietly at a candle flame, focusing on the repetition of a sound or mantra, following one's own breathing, concentrating on the imagined sound of rainfall, focusing on certain body sensations, or whirling about in a stereotyped dance. Patricia Carrington, a clinical psychologist, has developed her own form of meditation, which she calls Clinically Standardized Meditation (CSM) (Carrington, 1977), and a cardiologist, Herbert Benson, has developed a variation of his own called the Benson Technique (Benson, 1975). Zen instruction that may involve concentrating on an unanswerable riddle also falls into the category of meditation techniques, although the latter has the additional dimension of creating an impasse or crisis experience.

There is considerable agreement among researchers of the meditation process that meditation tends to reduce anxiety in many individuals. What has not been proven, however, is that meditation, as a special technique, has any clear advantage over other relaxation techniques in achieving this anxiety reduction. Apparently, if deep relaxation can be achieved by whatever technique, anxiety is likely to be reduced. This response to relaxation was first described in 1926 by Schultz and Luthe, two Berlin psychiatrists who developed a technique combining Western methods of autosuggestion with ancient yoga practices which they called autogenic training (Schultz and Luthe, 1969). In the mid-1930's a Chicago psychophysiologist, Edmund Jacobson, developed a method that he named progressive relaxation (Jacobson, 1938). This consisted of training patients to relax their muscles progressively with concomitant reduction in anxiety, according to Jacobson. In more recent years Joseph Wolpe (1958) has used a modification of Jacobson's approach in his technique of reciprocal inhibition for reducing anxiety in phobic patients.

Considerable research indicates that these relaxation techniques do indeed cause certain physiological changes such as slowing of the pulse rate, lowering of skin resistance, lowering of metabolic rate, and transitory lowering of blood pressure. Some physiologists assert that meditation increases the blood flow to the central nervous system and suggest that this may account for the increased mental prowess and clarity of mind that is sometimes claimed by practitioners of meditation. Although some of the results of meditation appear to be general responses to relaxation, others seem to be analogous to those described in various sensory deprivation experiments. In a sense, all meditation techniques close out the distractions of the outer world. It is possible that experienced meditators may thus achieve a kind of loosening of ego-boundaries that carries with it a transcendental feeling.

Transcendental meditation is not ordinarily promoted as a form of psychotherapy for mental illness but rather as a technique for achieving greater self-fulfillment. Thus, it may not fall appropriately into the category of specific psychotherapeutic techniques. Nevertheless, because of the extravagant claims that are made for it, emotionally disturbed individuals may turn to it hoping to find a magical solution for their problems. The heightened expectation that is generated by the special qualities claimed for TM may have a powerful suggestive effect and thus achieve a psychotherapeutic impact. However, it is not without danger and may lead to depression, agitation, and suicide attempts in some individuals. Although such negative reactions are probably few compared to the total number of individuals engaging in meditation, they reflect the dangers that exist when a program is sold indiscriminately without psychiatric screening.

Therapeutic Factors. TM belongs to an Eastern philosophical tradition rather than a Western one. It is, however, promoted as offering scientifically demonstrable physiological benefits and, to that extent, it also has roots in Western scientific tradition. Its physical setting is initially in a group seminar, later the privacy of one's own surroundings. TM has not only received wide media coverage but is aggressively promoted and, thus, has become the most popular of the meditation techniques.

TM appeals to those who seek either self-improvement or quick relief from symptoms via a method that appears to be brief, relatively inexpensive, and under the patient's own control. There are no therapists in TM in the conventional sense of the word. TM instructors, however, do surround themselves and their method with an aura of mysticism and authoritarian conviction about the value of their technique. Patient-therapist congruence is usually high, but the concept of therapeutic alliance is not applicable in the conventional sense. Identification with the therapist may be a significant factor. There is cognitive learning of the technique and of the presumptive factors behind its efficacy.

Suggestion, persuasion, training, and rehearsal all play a part in the TM process. Presumably some operant conditioning also exists in the sense that any positive results tend to reinforce the practice. There is a paradoxical response to TM in the sense that the initial goal is a blocking out of all feelings with a focus upon the mantra; the ultimate goal, however, is an experience of transcendence which may have certain abreactive elements.

In summary, TM is but one of many forms of meditative practice but one that is aggressively promoted as the "only true" form. It probably does have some beneficial effects attributable to the practice of deep relaxation for 20 minutes twice a day. Interspersed in the midst of a frenetic and tense existence such intervals may well be experienced as beneficial. In addition, for some individuals the sensory deprivation involved may produce a transcendental experience. This can have a powerful suggestive impact as well as a strong seductive and even addictive quality; but, it is not without danger for certain susceptible individuals. It must be concluded that meditation can be beneficial for many individuals but is of dubious value for persons with severe or significant psychiatric disorders. Even in the latter instances, however, it may have adjunctive value when combined with more conventional therapies.

RELIGIOUS AND INSPIRATIONAL THERAPIES

This group of therapies goes back to the prescientific and prehistoric roots of psychotherapy. In the past two decades there has been a strong resurgent interest in America in various Eastern philosophies, particularly in yoga and Zen Buddhism. The practices associated with these belief systems aim at achieving transcendental states, merging with the cosmos, and attaining a sense of ultimate release that Zen practitioners call *satori*. A wide variety of gurus, masters, babas, and maharishis are involved in the leadership of some of these groups. In contrast, Western religious healers tend to be less esoteric and more emotional. Indigenous to the American scene are revival meetings, faith healing, and the laying-on-of-hands. Particularly striking in recent years has been the emergence of numerous cults that offer their members a haven, the support of an extended family group, and the reflected power of a charismatic leader.

Religious Therapies

It is hard to make any rational and consistent classification of "religious therapies" since these comprise a wide variety of disparate categories, including nonreligious therapies. Modern religious teaching sees all healing, whether specifically medical or not, as essentially divine. Nevertheless, for centuries the major formal religions have viewed religious healing with considerable skepticism. Especially when evaluating "miracle" cures, religious investigating bodies apply extremely stringent criteria. Consequently, such cures are rarely judged to be the result of other than natural physical and psychological forces. With these caveats in mind, we shall consider the various forms of religious healing under two major headings: (a) sacramental, ritual healing and (b) faith and miracle healing.

   Sacramental, Ritual Healing. Many religions consider healing by prayer, anointing, and the laying-on-of-hands by the priest as one of their many functions. The procedures are formalized in specifically designated rituals. This function, it should be pointed out, is not a prominent part of the formal activities of the major religions. In Catholicism, for example, the anointing with oil, once aimed at curing the living, has become a sacrament performed primarily for the dying, designed to ensure their spiritual well-being in the world hereafter. From time to time, however, there has been a revival of sacramental, ritual healing by groups within the churches—a phenomenon exemplified by the attention paid by members of the clergy of the Anglican and Episcopal communions to the use of prayer as a specific aid toward curing the sick.

Faith and Miracle Healing. Ritual healing is generally unattended by any publicity or notoriety. In contrast, the activities included under faith healing are dramatic and often widely publicized. They generally center on a person or a place. A charismatic individual, either one of the ministry or an ordinary communicant of a religious sect, claims a "gift" for healing, performs a few "cures," and bursts into prominence as a healer to whom a swelling crowd of sufferers turn for relief. Oral Roberts, his fame enhanced by modern techniques of communication and advertising, is a good example. Equally commonly, a simple person has a vision of a holy figure (e.g., the Virgin Mary); the site of the vision then becomes a shrine that develops a reputation for miraculous cures. Lourdes, following St. Bernadette's visions more than a century ago, became the center of a large ecclesiastical organization devoted to healing and remains the most popular and well known of such shrines.

Faith healing is not restricted to those with specific religious affiliations. Indeed, from Mesmer to the present, a number of charismatic healers have worked outside religious organizations and concepts, often basing their theoretical schemes on materialistic, nonspiritual assumptions and constructs. The nineteenth century was marked by the rise of spiritual healing by individuals and groups whose conceptual bases lay somewhere between the realms of material agnosticism and orthodox, organized religion. The "spiritists" believed that an occasional gifted person was able to get in touch with the spirits of the dead and, under the guidance of one or more specific spirits, could diagnose and heal illness. Around such individuals there often arose a quasi-religious group of believers, which served to enhance the reputation and fame of the founding healer. Finally, it should be noted, the emergence of a nonreligious healer can occasionally lead to the development of a body of doctrine and an organizational structure that flowers into a formally recognized religious sect.

Therapeutic Factors. Faith healing appears to occur in all cultures and, in general, is associated with religious, or at least spiritual, ideas and practices. Its physical setting is usually a place that can accommodate groups of believers: a shrine, a church, a "clinic" associated with a religious organization, or a meeting room for spiritualistic seances. The shared belief system varies in doctrinal details but appears to be based on the belief that specific, gifted individuals can control universal forces (usually viewed as spiritual) in a way that enables them to diagnose and heal illness. The context is generally in groups. Cures have been claimed in individuals far removed from the locus of the healing procedures, even when the sick person was not aware that he was the focus of therapeutic attention. It is noteworthy that many of the charismatic religious healers do not accept fees, believing that they are the vehicle for God's work on earth. In terms of media effect, however, miracles make good copy; and the emergence of a healer or the discovery of a holy shrine has had a good press that has widely influenced the hopeful faithful.

Patients are often those with chronic symptoms, either neurotic or psychosomatic in nature, who have failed to find lasting help or relief from traditional medical practitioners. The "cure" may require a period of time, but most often is instantaneous and dramatic. Most investigators of faith healing (religious and agnostic) stress the centrality of psychogenic factors in the illnesses of those cured. Occasional accounts of "miraculous" cures (e.g., instant regeneration of tissue or disappearance of cancer in a fashion unexplainable on known biological grounds) have cropped up repeatedly in the literature, but solid evidence for any of these occurrences is thus far nonexistent.

Faith healers tend to be optimistic, persuasive, charismatic, highly directive individuals, often imbued with a belief that they have been given supernatural powers. Congruence between therapist and patient is generally high, taking place between a self-assured, if not authoritarian, therapist and a needy individual inspired with a faith that he will be cured. Mutual liking is presumably also high, especially when an altruistic, charitable, compassionate healer meets a believing, not to say worshipful, patient. Identification with the therapist is probably not of major importance, except for the fact that the patient may feel he shares in the divine or natural power over which the therapist putatively has control. Transference/countertransference is not dealt with therapeutically but is certainly an important factor in view of the patient's faith and childlike, often magical, trust in the therapist and the latter's self-confident, if not grandiose, conviction of his special gifts.

Compared to the affective components of faith healing, cognitive elements are minor; however, they certainly play a role in some forms of religious therapy (Christian Science, Coueism, e.g.) where specific attention is paid to changing and incorporating attitudes and ideas about the nature of health and illness.

The basic elements in religious therapy appear to be the patient's faith and hope for cure and intense suggestion and persuasion, both in the healer's approach and as part of the setting in which he or she works. In the course of healing rituals patients may experience intense feelings of worship or adoration for the healer and may undergo an emotional sense of "conversion" and of achieving contact with the Divine. These feelings may be expressed in wild outbursts of behavior with a consequent cathartic effect. The group context in which these feelings generally take place plays a very significant role in facilitating and heightening the affective experiences.

Christian Science

As a form of therapy, Christian Science falls within the province of religious healing, although, as suggested, it has at least two points of difference with the general run of such therapies: (a) Instead of being the practical application of the principles of an already established religion, Christian Science evolved as a religion from the teachings and practices of a charismatic healer, Mary Baker Eddy (Eddy, 1875). (b) In the theory and technique of Christian Science therapy, a central place is occupied by attention to cognitive processes. Mrs. Eddy and the religion she founded have both been the subject of a number of violently partisan polemics pro and con, and it is hard to get an unbiased view of either their teachings or practices.

Therapeutic Factors. It should be recognized that Christian Science views itself first and foremost as a religion with a message. Its teaching is aimed at bringing to mankind a fundamental truth about the nature of human life and the universe. Its role in the healing of human illness is only incidental; technically speaking, one should not even speak of healing, since Christian Science doctrine views "disease," like death, as merely an error in thinking and therefore nonexistent. It is a small sect, but it exercises power and influence far beyond its size since many of its members are extremely wealthy and ultraconservative in their political and social views.

Practitioners may visit their clients in their homes or, on being retained by the sick individual, may "heal" from a distance. Occasionally wealthy Christian Scientists may retain a practitioner in their personal retinue as a companion or, when incapacitated, as a kind of nurse. The Christian Science Church also maintains nursing homes for members with serious and debilitating illnesses.

Christian Science belief asserts the primacy of mind and denies the essential importance of matter. Illness is, therefore, the result of false beliefs and ideas about matter, and the "cure" of disease is achieved by recognizing this error and adopting the Truth. To illustrate, Mrs. Eddy (1875) wrote in *Science and Health,*

> Palsy is a belief that matter governs mortals, and can paralyze the body, making certain portions of it motionless. Destroy the belief, show mortal mind that muscles have no power to be lost, for Mind is supreme, and you cure the palsy.

In addition to the settings mentioned above, Christian Scientists attend regular church services where basic doctrine is expounded and carry out regular individual study of Mrs. Eddy's *Science and Health* (1875).

Science and Health is the basic Christian Science text, and every serious Christian Scientist knows its teachings intimately. In addition, the church puts out a number of publications, including a newspaper, the *Christian Science Monitor,* which promote its message and contain testimonials of those who have been healed.

Because of the lack of careful documentation in the report of cures published in the official Christian Science media, it is hard to know what kinds of disorders are treated. Despite claims for the cure of cancer and other serious medical conditions, one suspects that most of the disorders are psychogenic in origin.

Some practitioners have been described as strong, steady individuals relying heavily on the defenses of denial and reaction-formation, but one suspects that the seriously ill person experiences a good deal of dependence on his practitioner. Theoretically this should be central to the therapeutic encounter since the essence of Christian Science teaching is the thinking of proper and true thoughts. In this regard, Christian Science bears some affinity to the approach of the cognitive therapies, although its cognitive base, of course, is quite different.

Presumably suggestion and persuasion play a central role in the successful therapeutic results claimed by Christian Science. In addition, training and rehearsal are embodied in the systematic reading by practitioner and patient of relevant passages from *Science and Mind*. The element of profound faith embodied in Christian Science teaching must encompass a strong affective component.

Logotherapy

Logotherapy, a type of existential analysis, was developed by Victor Frankl, M.D., Ph.D., of Vienna, Austria. According to Frankl, logotherapy deals with a phenomenological assumption, namely, that humans are basically striving to find and fulfill meaning and purpose in life. He considers all other therapies as being "psychologistic," meaning that they represent "psychology without soul or spirit."

> Their basic mistake is to treat a person as if he were an object. A person is a spiritual entity, a subjective spirit which does not lend itself to any form of objectivization or materialization. (Frankl, 1953)

It is Frankl's belief that the human being is not driven by urges and instincts but is attracted by values and goals. Every drive, or at least every normal drive, tends toward a dynamism that is based on such value-determined goals.

To overcome psychologistic theories, Frankl introduced a psychotherapeutic method that he labeled "logotherapy." He considers this approach to be a heuristic opposite to psychotherapy in its narrow, psychologistic sense. To him, logotherapy is to be understood as a therapy that derives from spiritual sources and aims at a spiritual goal. Logotherapy has a spiritual aim, when, in the form of an existential analysis, it makes the individual reflect upon himself as a spiritual subject.

Frankl states that there is great danger that psychotherapy may commit serious misjudgments as long as it does not recognize a spiritual factor as an autonomous right. One of the goals of logotherapy is to counteract "metaphysical irresponsibility" in the individual. In some cases, in which a great spiritual need is camouflaged as emotional suffering, logotherapy has the obligation to go so far as to drive the patient into an existential crisis in order to pilot him through his spiritual need. In this instance, the therapist's approach to the patient would be, "I shall not leave you until you have found the true meaning of your existence, until you have become truly yourself" (Frankl, 1953).

Frankl feels that logotherapy and every existential-analytic endeavor goes beyond the mere treatment of illness. The individual is led not so much out of a disease as toward a truth. For the sake of truth, the patient often has to be dragged through the entire range of his existential problems in full realization of the possibility that a rude awakening from metaphysical irresponsibility and the uncovering of spiritual conflicts may lead him into a temporary increase of tension. Frankl refutes the concept that the restoration of a patient's capacity for work and enjoyment is the sole aim of psychotherapy. He asserts that psychotherapy also has the task of making the individual capable of enduring pain. He states that

> frequently, it is the aim of existential analysis to clarify the difference between meaningful and meaningless suffering and to analyze suffering in the life of an individual regarding his capacity for experiencing meaningful suffering. (Frankl, 1953)

Logotherapy disputes the pleasure principle as a functional directive. Frankl states,

> Pleasure, as a rule, ensues automatically and simultaneously with the reaching of a goal. Pleasure is a sequel, not an aim in itself, it must occur, but cannot be endeavored. It is effect, but not intention. The total human endeavor is not subject to any pleasure principle, but is oriented toward a higher meaning. (Frankl, 1953)

Frankl's focus on the spiritual aspect of man has made his therapies popular with various ecclesiastic groups. His invitations to the United States are often sponsored by church organizations, and his followers include many ministers. It may well be that logotherapy has its greatest application among theologians.

Frankl contends that logotherapy is the only school of existential psychiatry which has evolved psychotherapeutic techniques. He states that in existential analysis there are two specifically human phenomena, the "capacity for self-transcendence" and the "capacity for self-detachment." He considers these to be mobilized by two logotherapeutic techniques, namely, "paradoxical intention" and "de-reflection" (Frankl, 1960).

Paradoxical intention is a technique that Frankl uses in the short-term treatment of phobias and obsessive-compulsive disorders. He states that in order to understand this technique one has to appreciate the concept of "anticipatory anxiety." By this is meant the response and reaction to an event in terms of a fearful expectation of the recurrence of that event.

> However, fear tends to make true precisely that which one is afraid of, and in the same vein, anticipatory anxiety triggers off what the patient so frequently expects to happen. . . . A symptom evokes a phobia and the phobia provokes the symptom. The recurrence of the symptom then reinforces the phobia. (Frankl, 1960)

In paradoxical intention, when a phobic or obsessive patient is afraid that something will happen to him, the logotherapist encourages him to intend or wish for that which he fears, even if only for a second. Frankl contends that this technique brings about a change of attitude which enables the patient to place himself at a distance from the symptom, to detach himself from his neurosis. Paradoxical intention is used to enable the patient to develop a sense of detachment toward his neurosis by laughing at it.

A second logotherapeutic device is known as "de-reflection." Just as paradoxical intention is designed to counteract anticipatory anxiety, de-reflection is intended to counteract the compulsive inclination to self-observation. In these situations the patient is taught to ignore his problem to some degree. The de-reflection, however, can be achieved only to the extent to which the patient's awareness is directed toward positive aspects. Through de-reflection the patient is enabled to ignore his neurosis by focusing his attention away from himself. "He will be directed toward a life full of potential meanings and values with a specific appeal to his personal potentialities" (Frankl, 1966). Frankl recommends de-reflection as being of significant benefit in the treatment of sexual difficulties. Frankl does not believe that paradoxical intention is indicated in all patients. For example, he feels that this technique is contraindicated in psychotic depressions.

Therapeutic Factors. From a philosophic standpoint, logotherapy appeals to highly intellectual individuals who anticipate a philosophic relationship with the therapist. From a pragmatic standpoint, however, the techniques of paradoxical intention and de-reflection can be applied to individuals of all walks of life. These methods work particularly well with people who have a high degree of magical expectation; they do not involve any discussion of past events, nor do they depend on an understanding of the transference-countertransference mechanism. Apart from these strategies, logotherapy is closely related to other existential, here-and-now, analytic techniques; and elements of transference-countertransference inevitably are involved.

While the term *logos* is incorporated into the title of the therapy, the cognitive aspects of logotherapy deal more with high philosophic conceptualizations of the self and of action. Phenomenologic behavior is accentuated over cognition.

A degree of suggestion and persuasion is involved in paradoxical intention and in de-reflection. However, Frankl is quick to stress that persuasion is only a small part of his therapeutic method. Paradoxical intention includes the use of hypersensitization as a technique of desensitization. It usually is not of the degree involved in implosion techniques.

Logotherapy involves a type of gestalt learning in that there often is a "eureka" type of reaction when symptoms quickly disappear as a result of the paradoxical intention technique. There is also a substantial spiritual and inspirational element in its philosophical message.

The International Society for Krishna Consciousness (ISKOON—Hare Krishnas)

The ISKOON organization sees itself as a chain of centers (ashrams) for the study of Vedic (Hindu scriptural) lore and practice (Judah, 1974; Streiker, 1978; Edward, 1979; Ellwood, 1973; Peterson, 1975). The lifestyle of the Hare Krishna movement came out of the intent of the society's spiritual founder, the late A.C. Bhaktivedanta Bhapupadha, who came to the United States in 1965 to spread Vedanta and the particular yogic life-style called *bhakti*. Unlike some of the more abstract yogic practices that see god as totally eminent, *bhakti* yoga seeks to serve a personal deity. The strength of *bhakti*, which is the devotional style of most of lower- and middle-class India, is in its intensity of devotional practice. This devotional ardor is seen in the chanting and dancing of the street groups of Hare Krishna disciples, the saffron-costumed and bald-headed young men and the gaily saried young women. The groups distribute literature to people on the street for a small donation. Their chief publication is the ISKOON magazine, *Back to Godhead*. It is the position of ISKOON, as was that of Bhaktivedanta, that merely hearing about or reading about Krishna is a guarantee of a better birth in the next incarnation and thus a better chance for the goal of all Hindus, liberation from birth and death.

Membership in the society comes from acceptance of some beliefs and a highly structured lifestyle. The basic beliefs are that one is an external spirit soul; that there is a Supreme Person, Krishna, who is eternal; and that every believer is His servant, whose main purpose in life is to render loving service to Him. The key principle and binding force of ISKOON is the idea that the true religion is loving service to one's Lord and obedience to the transcendent teaching of the guru, Bhaktivedanta.

The life-style is based on Vedic principles, including *ahimsa*, the positive abstention of doing harm to any aware being. This means strict vegetarianism (no meat, fish, or eggs). No food is eaten before it is offered up to the image of Krishna in the temple. It then becomes a *prasadam*, a gift back to the devotee from God. There is also no illicit sex, which means strict premarital abstention and, save for procreative purposes, strict post-marital chastity as well. No intoxication is permitted and no gambling. One is expected to recite the names of God 27,000 times a day and to recite the Hare Krishna mantra constantly, whatever else one is doing. Every devotee carries a bag with *japa*, or prayer beads, and is frequently seen reciting prayers.

Obviously some people who are initially attracted to ISKOON are in some form of distress. And while there are strong cognitive and emotional pressures to stay, the demands of ISKOON are tough. Classes are held twice a day in Sanskrit, Vedantic literature, the ashramic lifestyle, Vedic hygiene, specific skills, etc. The curious drop out quickly, probably lacking the resolve to cope with this high level of demand. For the 30 percent who do remain beyond a year, there is a gradual movement into the kind of devotee they intend to become. This is a process of abandoning prior life-styles that involved a search for sex, money, and power.

Therapeutic Factors. The intense structure of ISKOON may work for people who require total commitment to a belief. The Vedic teachings it espouses are rooted solidly in an ancient philosophical tradition. Hare Krishna schools have been severely criticized about their educational styles and the conditions under which the students live, but ISKOON attorneys have won a major case involving brainwashing, kidnapping, and deprogramming. The life-style is not offered as any kind of "help." It is a rigorous and difficult way to live which is probably right only for a select few. Full members contribute 100 percent of their income to the temple and in return receive what they need to live. Thus, there is no set contribution.

One of the roots of prejudice is the extent to which people who look or act quite differently from oneself are perceived to have values and beliefs that are inferior and/or antagonistic to one's own. Such incongruence may in itself be sufficient to invalidate all or part of the other's communication. It is this illusion of incongruity, this *maya*, that the dress and manner of Hare Krishna may perpetuate. Thus, in adopting an exotic way of being in the world, the devotee may be holding in place that very secularity he wishes to influence.

Arica

The Arica Institute was founded in 1971 by a Bolivian, Oscar Ichazo. Arica means "open-door" in the language of the Bolivian Indians. In the catalogue of the Arica Institute (1980) its method is described as follows:

> Ultimately, Arica is concerned with health but recognizes that . . . mental illness falls within the realm of psychiatrists, psychologists, analysts, and sociologists. The Arica method of self-realization is presented as practical training, courses, workshops that follow the nine stages for total clarification of consciousness. . . .

The Nine Stages of Arica Training

First Stage (40-day training, temple, Arica Institute, the nine ways of Zhikr). The 40-day training is based on the study of the nine systems of mind and body.

The temple ceremony, in which the student begins a ritualized meditation for discovering the internal self, the nine ways of Zhikr, a modern form of a classical method for attaining a state of liberated consciousness, are also introduced at this stage.

Second Stage (the Domains of Consciousness, Chua K'a, Vortex Points, the 24 Lights).

In the Domains of Consciousness training the student learns that the psyche is composed of nine domains, and that every human construct and social concept falls within one of these domains.

Also at this stage begins the process of deep body massage called K'a. . . . By releasing muscle tension, Chua K'a massage also releases mental stress. Another form of body work is the Vortex Points course. Here the student learns a method of massaging certain precise points to increase the feeling of vitality in the body.

The 24 Lights meditation technique is also introduced at this stage. By picturing the various parts of the body in their corresponding colors, one awakens those parts and enhances their functioning.

Third Stage (Protoanalysis, the Outlets of Psychic Compensation, Mentations).

This stage . . . includes study of the Outlets of Psychic Compensation. When external pressures produce internal conflicts, the psyche automatically seeks ways to compensate for this stress by releasing energy through certain involuntary outlets, which are cruelty, overeating, neurosis, psychic panic, crime, over-exertion, psychosomatic illness, drug abuse, and sex.

In the study of the Mentations, the participant learns how various body parts act as receptors that supply the entire organism with specific types of information . . .

Fourth Stage (The Scarab, Psychoalchemy, Kinerhythm, Pneumorhythm).

In the fourth stage the student learns the game of the Scarab, which employs the Arica Tarot, a deck of 78 cards in which the elements of the traditional Tarot have been refined.

By studying Psychoalchemy, the movement through the body of the mystical golden serpent known as the uroboros, the student learns to transform physical energy into psychic energy.

Another method used at this stage is Kinerhythm, in which extremely slow movements are used to observe the psyche and to evoke a state of ecstasy and yantras. . . .

This stage also includes the practice of Pneumorhythm, a sequence that combines breathing with rhythmic counting regulated by the heartbeat in order to expand consciousness throughout the body.

Fifth Stage (Opening the Rainbow Eye).

The fifth stage is Opening the Rainbow Eye. . . . After opening the Rainbow Eye, the student acquires the basic satori state, which permits the clear and orderly observation of all internal and external experiences and provides the resolution of any contradictions with society's values.

Sixth Stage (Alpha Heat Ritual, Trialectics).

In the sixth stage the participant learns the ritual of the Alpha Heat, in which the mind is represented as the Tadyatha, a warrior maiden who battles the enemies of the mind until consciousness becomes free of regret, rivalry, worry, hatred, envy, pretense, fear, jealousy and prejudice.

This stage also includes a detailed study of the laws of Trialectics, the logic of unity, a form of reasoning that permits analysis of reality as it is. . . .

Seventh Stage (Cutting the Diamond, Hypergnostic Analysis).

In the seventh stage the student practices the ritual of Cutting the Diamond. Here consciousness is represented as a diamond pyramid. . . . The ritual includes techniques for completing the mystical union, known in Indian tradition as samadhi and in Zen tradition as satori.

Also included . . . is the study of Hypergnostic analysis, which uses the symbols called eidotropes (salt, fire, iron, earth, water, wood, air, alpha, and ether) to make practical analysis of the internal meanings and connections of things.

Eighth Stage (The Golden Eye Ritual, Bejewelling the Kingdom).

In the eighth stage, the participant learns the ritual of the Golden Eye, the voyage of consciousness inside the body. Also studied are techniques for the transference of consciousness.

Ninth Stage (The Universal Psyche).

The ninth stage is the ritual of Psychic Shapes, which develops the universal psyche and the internal recognition of the Unity of God. What follows is beyond words.

Arica Centers are listed in the United States, Canada, Europe, and Latin America. Membership is open to anyone. After going through the courses one is considered able to give courses on one's own. "The only requirement is that you purchase or rent the necessary materials from the Institute." A price list of equipment is offered together with an order form. There is also a monthly newspaper and a society directory. Arica is big business. Approximately 200,000 persons have been involved in its programs. An individual literally can spend many thousands of dollars in taking courses, attending special retreats, and buying an extremely broad assortment of equipment. Advantages are offered for buying the various materials in quantity.

Therapeutic Factors. Arica establishes a total sociocultural system. It has elements of a commune that is attended periodically. Local groups are extensions of the commune. It proposes a totally separate method of living one's life, with a number of hours each day being spent in specifically designed programs.

A "magical aura" is cast. The leader of the Arica system is elevated to the position of an oracle. The subject is encouraged to be totally dependent and to have magical expectations. Under the guise of preparing one to have total awareness, Arica's techniques tend to reduce the individual to a state of total dependence on a "grand therapist" with supernatural qualities. Considerable emphasis is placed on the cognitive learning of Arica's complex mystical assumptions.

The techniques, in general, depend on suggestion. In addition, there are methodologies, including meditation and physical activities, reminiscent of those used in yoga. Other phenomena suggesting autohypnosis are also used. A ritualistic method is taught, interrelating body sensations with thought processes, which are, in turn, associated with certain emotional experiences.

COGNITIVE-EMOTIONAL THERAPIES

Rational-Emotive Psychotherapy

Rational-emotive psychotherapy (RET) was developed in the 1960's by Albert Ellis, a clinical psychologist (Appelbaum, 1979; Marmor, 1980). It is based on the rationale that "human emotions are largely derived from human thinking processes" Its methodology belongs in the realm of the cognitive therapies, and its historical roots can be traced back to the popular nineteenth century Swiss psychiatrist, Paul Dubois, who achieved considerable prominence and success with a method he called rational psychotherapy. Dubois believed in "curing the will through self-education," and his therapeutic method was based on "modifying the erroneous ideas that the patient has allowed to creep into his mind" (Dubois, 1905).

Ellis (1962, 1977) states that he developed his system of psychotherapy because of his conviction that the therapeutic approaches founded upon both the psychoanalytic and existential views of man were ineffective and inadequate. He considers the Freudian view of man to be false because, in his opinion, man is not simply a biological organism deterministically driven by instincts and infantile experiences. In Ellis' view, man has the capacity to reassess early teachings and to reindoctrinate himself with different beliefs, ideas, and values; thus, he is capable of behaving quite differently in the present as compared to the past. On the other hand, Ellis asserts that the existential view of man's self-actualization tendencies also must be modified because once a man is conditioned to think or feel in certain ways, he does tend to continue behaving in that manner even though his behavior is self-defeating. Thus, it is unrealistic to assume that an existential encounter with an accepting and permissive therapist will in itself root out an individual's deeply ingrained, self-defeating behavioral patterns; persistent and consistent efforts at cognitive reorientation are essential for change to take place.

Ellis considers emotional disturbances to be the end-product of irrational or illogical ideas with which the patient has become indoctrinated. Examples of such ideas are (a) that it is necessary to be loved or approved of by everyone; (b) that one must be thoroughly competent, adequate, and achieving in all respects in order to consider oneself worthwhile; (c) that human unhappiness is caused by external circumstances over which one has no control; (d) that it is easier to avoid life's difficulties than to face them; (e) that one needs to be dependent on others and have someone stronger than oneself on whom to rely; and (f) that there is a correct, precise, and perfect solution to all human problems and that it is catastrophic not to have found it.

The task of therapy, according to Ellis, is to make the patient aware of these irrational "phrases and sentences" and to induce the patient to abandon them. RET is an active-directive method; the therapist tries to assist the individual to examine and modify his philosophy of life by confronting, persuading, lecturing, cajoling, and pressuring him to think and perform in ways that will counteract the self-defeating and incorrect beliefs to which he has been clinging.

RET therapists place great importance on emotional independence, autonomy, and self-direction as major factors in rational living, and outline specific steps to enable the patient to achieve these objectives. RET also focuses on reducing self-blame and self-condemnatory attitudes in the patient. Ellis recognizes that a few encounters are not sufficient to reverse a lifetime of false beliefs and convictions. He, therefore, emphasizes the importance of continuing effort in order to reverse the behavior and attitudes of the past.

Therapeutic Factors. Rational-emotive therapy belongs to the tradition of the cognitive therapies. It shares the psychoanalytic belief in the therapeutic power of insight, but RET differs sharply from psychoanalytic theory in its de-emphasis of unconscious factors and in its strong belief in the power of conscious cognition and rationality to modify behavior. RET may be practiced either on a one-to-one basis or in groups but takes place more often in the latter setting.

The RET therapist takes an authoritarian approach and presents himself as knowing the correct answers, which he impresses on the patient. Patients who respond to such an approach are clearly looking for direction and a strong authority figure upon whom to lean. Although not specifically dealt with in the therapy, it is clear that both transference and counter-transference elements are strongly involved in the patient-therapist interactions. RET places its major emphasis in this area on developing a cognitive awareness of the false beliefs that have been dominating one's life and on learning new cognitive attitudes to be used as guideposts for the future.

The therapist presents himself as a model whose beliefs and values are to be used as examples for the patient to copy. Repetitive practice of new ways of thinking and behaving is strongly emphasized. This involves a good deal of trial and error learning. Operant conditioning also takes place in the responses of the therapist and other members of the group to the patient's efforts.

Ellis does not discount the importance of emotions but considers them to be secondary to and derived from thinking processes. Hence, changing the patient's deeply held beliefs will, of necessity, also change his most intensely and deeply held emotions. Thus, although affective expression does take place in the course of RET, there is no emphasis on abreaction as a therapeutic goal in itself.

In summary, rational-emotive therapy belongs in the sphere of the cognitive therapies. It is an authoritative, directive approach to the patient's problems which emphasizes rationality and logic. Although Ellis insists that it is applicable to a wide range of psychiatric disorders, it is probably most suitable for patients who, although dependently seeking authoritative directions, are not too severely disturbed and who have good intellectual capacity and sufficient ego strength to take active steps in changing and modifying their behavior.

Reality Therapy

Reality therapy is a treatment technique developed by William Glasser, M.D., the emphasis of which rests on the key concepts of morality and responsibility. Glasser's objections to conventional dynamic psychotherapy may be summarized as follows: (a) Conventional categories of mental illness and efforts to treat patients in accordance with them are useless. (b) Probing the past for insights into present behavior is futile. (c) Reliving the past in the context of the transference has scant therapeutic value. (d) Insight and understanding of unconscious conflicts do not lead to behavior change. (e) Conventional psychotherapy avoids the problem of morality and fails to teach the patient better behavior.

Glasser's book, *Reality Therapy*, was published in 1965. In 1969, he organized the Institute for Reality Therapy for training teachers, psychologists, psychiatrists, court personnel, and individuals associated with various churches. An offshoot of this institute is the Educator Training Center, which has programs in the United States and Canada labeled "schools without failure."

Glasser asserts that the foremost need for human beings is to love and to be loved. Every patient requires someone about whom he deeply cares and who deeply cares for him or her in return. The patient is taught to develop a sense of caring, beginning with the therapist and expanding to involve others. The assumption is that as the patient becomes involved and begins to fulfill various needs, the presenting problem and secondary symptoms will disappear.

An essential initiating aspect in reality therapy is helping patients to understand and clarify their immediate long-range life goals. They are next helped to become aware of the ways in which they block their own progress toward their goals. The lack of alternatives is one blocking mechanism that occurs with people with emotional problems.

Responsibility is another central concept of reality therapy. It is defined as the ability to fulfill one's needs and to do so in a way that does not deprive others of the ability to fulfill their needs. According to this concept, patients with psychologic problems have either not learned or have lost the ability to lead responsible lives. Therefore, "responsible" equals "mental health," and "irresponsible" equals "mental illness."

Glasser views patients' problems as being primarily the result of an inability to comprehend and apply moral concepts and ethical values in everyday life. Change cannot occur until the patient faces the responsibility of his own acts, and Glasser has stated that "people do not act irresponsibly because they are ill, but rather they are ill because they act irresponsibly" (Glasser, 1965).

Reality therapy focuses on the here and now. It stipulates that it is possible and even desirable to ignore the past, no matter how bad it has been. Glasser feels that the past becomes of little importance when the patient learns to satisfy needs in the present. Any focus on transference relationships is negated. Reality therapy focuses on patient behavior rather than emotions. An attempt is made in all instances to relate feelings to resultant behavior. The behavior is the central problem, not the feelings evoked from the behavior. Happiness is not a central focus of therapy.

> Happiness occurs most often when we are willing to take responsibility for our behavior. Irresponsible people, always seeking to gain happiness without assuming responsibility, find only brief periods of joy but not the deep-seated satisfaction that accompanies responsible behavior. (Glasser, 1965)

Reality therapy focuses on the question of morality. The therapist weighs questions of right and wrong with patients. Reality therapy frequently involves confrontation focused against "irresponsible behavior." At all times, a patient must accept responsibility for his own behavior.

Therapeutic Factors. Reality therapy was originally developed and used in treating adolescent delinquents in a controlled environment, where it proved useful. Since then, it has had a broad acceptance by many different types of institutions, particularly educational ones. It may be defined as a "blood and guts," "Dutch uncle" type of psychotherapeutic procedure. It is a belief in "right thinking" which tends to be simplistic but which has a broad appeal to many individuals who come with the concept that they want to be directed along the "right path." Reality therapy can be practiced on an individual, group, or family basis in an office, clinic, or institution.

The discussion of any transference relationships is discouraged or even deprecated. The therapy appears to be most effective in patients who wish or need to be directed. The therapist is in reality a strong parental surrogate who guides or directs the patient into "right" thinking. The patient learns to identify behavior patterns and is taught to recognize that he is responsible for them. Conscious awareness of behavior patterns is a central focus of therapy.

In some ways, one can consider reality therapy to be in the realm of classical reconditioning. The patient is exposed to an awareness of "irresponsible behavior" on a repetitive basis. The affect associated with this behavior gradually is decreased, and a desensitization is accomplished. "Responsible behavior" is gradually inculcated through repetitive focus in an atmosphere of positive expectation and positive moral implications. Operant conditioning also takes place via therapist approval-disapproval responses.

Reality therapy includes cathartic techniques. There is a highly verbal relationship between the reality therapist and the patient. A great deal of "give and take" is incorporated. The process is reminiscent in many ways of "getting religion." It is the struggle for right thinking over wrong thinking. It focuses on the here-and-now, negating the past and implying, without stating so specifically, that correct behavior in the present will prepare one for the future.

REFERENCES

Appelbaum SA: Out in Inner Space. New York, Anchor Press/Doubleday, 1979

Arica Institute Catalogue, 1980

Back KW: Beyond Words. New York, Russell Sage Foundation, 1972

Benson H: The Relaxation Response. New York, William Morrow and Co, 1975

Carrington P: Freedom in Meditation. New York, Doubleday, 1977

Corsini RJ: Handbook of Innovative Psychotherapies. New York, John Wiley & Sons, 1981

Dubois P: Psychic Treatment of Nervous Disorders. Translated by Jelliffe SE, White WA. New York, Funk and Wagnalls, 1905

Eddy MB: Science and Health, with Key to the Scriptures (1875). Boston, The First Church of Christ, Scientist, 1971

Edward C: Crazy for God. Englewood Cliffs, NJ, Prentice-Hall, 1979

Ellis A, Grieger R: Handbook of Rational-Emotive Therapy. New York, Springer, 1977

Ellis A: Reason and Emotion in Psychotherapy. New York, Lyle Stuart, 1962

Ellwood RS: Religious and Spiritual Groups in Modern America. Englewood Cliffs, NJ, Prentice-Hall, 1973

Fagan J, Shepherd LL (eds): Gestalt Therapy Now. Palo Alto, Calif, Science and Behavior Books, 1970

Frankl V: Logotherapy and existential analysis: a review. Am J Psychother 20:252-260, 1966

Frankl V: Paradoxical intention: a logotherapeutic technique. Am J Psychother 14:520-535, 1960

Frankl V: Logos and existence in psychotherapy. Am J Psychother 7:8-15, 1953

Glass LL, Kirsch MA, Parris FN, et al: Psychiatric disturbances associated with Erhard Seminars Training, I: a report of cases. Am J Psychiatry 134:245-247, 1977

Glasser W: Reality Therapy: A New Approach to Psychiatry. New York, Harper and Row, 1965

Harper RA: The New Psychotherapies. Englewood Cliffs, NJ, Prentice-Hall, 1975

Hemingway PD: The Transcendental Mediation Primer. New York, McKay, 1975

Herink R (ed): The Psychotherapy Handbook: The A to Z Guide to More than 250 Different Therapies in Use Today. New York, New American Library, 1980

Jacobson E: Progressive Relaxation. Chicago, University of Chicago Press, 1938

Janov A: The Primal Revolution: Toward a Real World. New York, Simon and Schuster, 1972

Janov A: The Anatomy of Mental Illness: The Scientific Basis of Primal Therapy. New York, Putnam, 1971

Janov A: The Primal Scream: Primal Therapy, the Cure for Neurosis. New York, Putnam, 1970

Judah JS: Hare Krishna and the Counterculture. New York, John Wiley & Sons, 1974

Karasu TB: Psychotherapies: an overview. Am J Psychiatry 134:851-863, 1977

Kirsch MA, Glass LL: Psychiatric disturbances associated with Erhard Seminars Training, II: additional cases and theoretical considerations. Am J Psychiatry 134:1254-1258, 1977

Kirschenbaum H: On becoming Carl Rogers. New Republic 180:30-31, 1979

Lieberman MA, Yalom ID, Miles MB: Encounter Groups: First Facts. New York, Basic Books, 1973

Lowen A: The Betrayal of the Body. New York, Macmillan, 1967

Marcus E: Gestalt Therapy and Beyond. Palo Alto, Calif, Meta Press, 1970

Marmor J: Recent trends in psychotherapy. Am J Psychiatry 137:409-416, 1980

Munson TA: Gestalt on the West Coast. Toronto, Canada, Gestalt Institute of Toronto, December 1978

Perls F, Hefferline RF, Goodman P: Gestalt Therapy. New York, Dell, 1965

Perls F: Gestalt Therapy Verbatim. Moab, Utah, Real People Press, 1969

Peterson WJ: Those Curious New Cults. New Canaan, Conn, Keats Publishers, 1975

Questions and Answers about Lifespring. San Rafael, Calif, Lifespring, Inc, 1978

Rhinehart L: The Book of est. New York, Holt, Rinehart & Winston, 1976

Rolf I: Rolfing: The Integration of Human Structures. New York, Harper and Row, 1973

Schultz JH, Luthe W: Autogenic Therapy. New York, Grune & Stratton, 1969

Simon J: Observations on 67 patients who took Erhard Seminars Training. Am J Psychiatry 135:686-691, 1978

Streiker JD: The Cults are Coming! Nashville, Abingdon Press, 1978

Wolpe J: Psychotherapy by Reciprocal Inhibition. Stanford, Stanford University Press, 1958

Zaslow R: A theory and treatment of autism. In Clinical Cognitive Psychology: Models and Integrations. Edited by Berger L. New York, Irvington Pub Co, 1969

12
Biofeedback

12
Biofeedback

INTRODUCTION

The practical application of Norbert Weiner's assertion that feedback occurs when a system controls and corrects itself by reviewing results of its past performance (Kroger, 1977) has long aided the tennis coach, the piano tuner, and the first grade teacher. Its systematic and scientific application to disordered biological systems was a reasonable and even inevitable occurrence.

In psychiatry, biofeedback uses instruments to show the physiological aspects of disordered functioning side by side with the patient's stream of consciousness and unambiguously demonstrates their synchronization in a way that facilitates introspection. This capability is timely as psychiatry increasingly recognizes the large number of disorders, including those with primarily psychiatric presentations, to which a modern psychosomatic approach can be validly applied. In short, biofeedback sits astride the interaction between the physical and the mental, connecting thought, emotion, and physiology in a single therapeutic context.

Biofeedback refers to the human capacity to augment the proprioceptive or interoceptive apparatus mechanically. It uses an electronic instrument to confront a patient with a continuous stream of information about how a part of his physiology is changing in order to allow him to find out how what he thinks, feels, or does will influence it. In its most common application, the patient tries to alter that physiology in a predetermined and presumably more adaptive direction. He will see that certain mental initiatives move him in that direction and will expand upon them; others will not and he will discard them. By continuing this process, known to behaviorists as "shaping," he increasingly refines his technique over time, much as the tennis player learns to perfect the aim of his swing. In time, much of the process, as with the tennis player, becomes preconscious or even automatic.

As can be seen, the paradigm for biofeedback is straightforward; the young woman straightening her posture before the mirror is using biofeedback; so is the jogger checking his pulse as he runs. Clinically, however, biofeedback uses a sophisticated electronic instrument to feed back information about a function with little (peripheral temperature) or no (galvanic skin response) natural proprioception or for which the perceptual apparatus itself is weakened (post-stroke) or overridden (tension headache). The primary types of biofeedback used in psychiatry are: electromyogram (EMG) for striated muscles, peripheral temperature ("thermal") for sympathetic vascular tone, electroencephalogram (EEG), galvanic skin response (GSR) and its variants, and cardiotachometry.

The feedback augments proprioception/interoception in three ways:

A. By changing the perception to a more familiar or more usable form, such as a visual display in place of a dull visceral sensation;

B. By making the signal more intense (such as a clear sound of varying pitch in place of a weak signal); and

C. By pairing the sensations with a continuously changing numerical "score."

What is the experience of the patient using biofeedback? The patient settles back into a comfortable chair in a room free of distractions, and recording leads from the machine are attached to the appropriate part of the body. At this point baseline measurements are sometimes noted for use in assessing the patient's progress. Next, one of the standard methods of general relaxation is frequently used.* The patient is encouraged to make mental contact with his body by focusing on particular sensations coming from it; but he is to do this in a passive or neutral, rather than an active, striving way which may be counterproductive. He is the juror as well as the plaintiff. While tracking the shifting feedback, he makes mental notes of what works to trigger change. The ultimate arbiter of his success is the direction the feedback takes. A patient often finds that serious distortions in concept of how the body functions are rapidly revealed in this way.† In

---

*This paradigm may vary in such specialized areas as neuromuscular retraining.

†The patient finds that control of his inner world follows a curiously different pattern from his interactions with the outside world. In the outside world the fact comes first and the observation of the fact follows (i.e., only after the door is open does one think, "the door is open"). In the inner world, however, the observation, "my right arm is warm," may come first and the fact of its being warm follow in a causal manner. This is perplexing to many patients during their early experiences with biofeedback.

addition to the feedback signals and the proprioceptive or visceroceptive sensations themselves, a patient using biofeedback must keep in mind a mental representation of a "target sensation"—what he expects he will feel if he has succeeded. In the initial stages of treatment he will often conjure up images to achieve that end, such as an image of himself floating to relax his muscles or of the sun warming his hands. Other seemingly irrelevant images, thoughts, and sensations will drift into the patient's stream of consciousness and may affect the feedback. On closer analysis these associations are frequently not random but have direct or symbolic relevance to an area of conflict. If the instrument shows that the physiology regularly responds with tension to one of these images, this observation can become a bridge to discussing the reason for that reaction.

The patient is typically seen once or twice a week and is instructed to practice at home daily and whenever symptoms appear. Duration of therapy varies with the patient, the illness, and the goals; but basic biofeedback-assisted relaxation can often be taught in 20 to 40 45-minute sessions. The intent in almost all biofeedback applications is to help the patient prophylactically as well as with individual symptom episodes, to teach him to attune himself to early cues of impending difficulty, and to enable him to apply his skills without need for further feedback.*

Biofeedback can be considered a specialized branch of the self-regulatory therapies. The term is often used as a catchword to refer to those therapies collectively. Its uses are primarily in the treatment of nonstructural dysfunction in organs or systems regulated by the nervous system (i.e., psychosomatic medicine). It has been used to investigate and to educate as well as to treat. Although some have contended that all biofeedback should be considered only an educational process, if the participants are suffering emotional or medical distress and one aim of the biofeedback is to reduce that distress, then whether in the clinic or the classroom, it is treatment (Figure 1).

Much of this controversy becomes moot when it is recognized that biofeedback itself is nothing more than a tool, in the way that the stethoscope is a tool. Like the stethoscope, it can be valuable and can be used in many ways but can only produce results as good as the skill and judgment of the individual who uses it.

Although one of its major applications is as an aid in teaching relaxation, biofeedback does not function best as a primary independent relaxation therapy. Because biofeedback is an intrinsically advanced technique, it yields uneven and confusing results when divorced from more basic

---

*Further details on applications, techniques, and other specifics, because of their diversity, cannot be condensed into this document; however, they are obtainable from one of the many textbooks cited in the bibliography such as *Biofeedback: Principles and Practice for Clinicians* (Basmajian, 1983).

instructions in relaxation. Like the high power setting on a microscope, it can zero in on a specific anatomic area or physiologic function with accuracy; but, like that high power setting, it may miss the critical surrounding context if it is used first or alone. Each part of a patient's physiology is in equilibrium with the other parts, and the whole must function in equilibrium with a complex psychosocial milieu. To use biofeedback effectively, this context must be accounted for in the treatment plan. In summary, it might be most accurate to say that *biofeedback in itself is never a treatment; it is something that is used in a treatment.*

For the most part, biofeedback acts at the level of the "final common pathway" to the symptoms through which psychodynamic and personality features, current stresses, and genetic predispositions all eventually exert their influence. Some medications act in this fashion, while others, such as analgesics, act to blunt perception of symptoms. If biofeedback is continued for a sufficient time, it may lead to a permanent revision of the physiopathology, probably due to central restructuring. Thus, while biofeedback often serves a palliative function, it may also lead to more fundamental improvement.

Figure 1. The Biofeedback Star: Foundations of Biofeedback

Source: Adler CS and Adler SM, 1977. Reprinted with permission.

Biofeedback has been touted as a means to return to the patient some responsibility for his own care. It is not the only therapy to try; most psychotherapies include this as one of their several goals. Nevertheless, the readings on the feedback instrument are helpful when trying to convince a patient that he is the only one in charge of the physiology that leads to those tension headaches. He may learn directly and even "see" the association between his contracted cephalic muscles and his thoughts and emotions. This capacity has intrigued many of our general medical colleagues to learn more about the relationship between psyche and soma, an attitude psychiatry has sought to inculcate for many years.

HISTORY

As is frequent in the history of ideas, that which seems to have appeared as if by parthenogenesis can be seen to have been conceived from the union of separate germ lines, each with a long historical record. Indeed, Narcissus foreshadowed biofeedback when he caught his reflection in the lake. In the case of biofeedback, one can identify two such lines.

The "subjective" line is that of introspection/self-regulation. Attempts to intensify self-awareness were highly developed in the Orient through the use of meditation techniques, often infused with religious connotations. With prolonged periods of study and practice, impressive degrees of self-control could be achieved. In the West these tendencies also sprang from a base of religion: the meditations and prayers of early Judeo-Christian tradition. Modern analogues in the West have been (a) hypnosis (Rossi, 1980); (b) progressive relaxation (Jacobson, 1938), a means of accentuating attention on the sensations accompanying deep muscle relaxation; (c) autogenic therapy (Luthe, 1969), in which specific phrases are made the center of focus in a passive-attentive fashion; (d) autoanalysis (Bezzola, 1918), a technique described at the turn of the century in which a relaxed, detailed description of physical symptoms was used to reduce their intensity; and (e) psychoanalysis (Adler and Adler, 1972), which encourages undistracted, inner-directed attention and during which sensations and spontaneous motor phenomena are observed and experienced more intently.

The second (or "objective") line of development was a technical and theoretical one and included advances in physiological instrumentation and in the theories of cybernetics, of Pavlov (1927), and of Skinner (1938). Since the first requirement of biofeedback is a signal to feed back, one can trace this developmental line to the invention and refinement of instruments for making contact with the physiology, starting with the stethoscope of Lannec in the eighteenth century and continuing with the EMG, EKG, EEG, cardiotachometer, sphygmomanometer, galvanometer, polygraph, and finally, the computer to analyze them all. These instruments were used to explore functioning in health and disease, necessary to learn the direction of physiological change commensurate with health. For example, Mittleman and Wolff (1939) plotted the change in skin temperature over arthritic joints in response to quiet and to specific emotionally conflictual topics. The understanding of visceral responses to external stimuli was also pioneered by Beaumont (1833), Cannon (1932), Alexander (1950), Dunbar (1954), and Pavlov (1927); the theory of operant learning by Skinner (1938); and the concepts of counterconditioning by Wolpe (1958).

An integral part of what was taking shape in this technical realm was that the average person was growing more comfortable with increasingly sophisticated machines: the automobile, the television, and the computer. Machines became knowing, trustworthy, and even authoritative.* In short, the emergence of biofeedback can be seen as a cohesion of forces unfolding in society, not all of them scientific.

In the early 1950's an internist named George Whatmore (Whatmore and Kohli, 1974) decided to show his patients their EMG recordings to teach them to eliminate musculoskeletal symptoms. In 1963 Basmajian (1963) showed that with feedback, patients could learn to activate single motor units differentially and even to fire off gallop rhythms and fancy drum rolls. Kamiya (1969), at the University of California, created a popular stir in the late 1960's when he showed that subjects could learn to increase production of alpha EEG rhythm with feedback. The greatest interest in scientific circles at this time, however, came from the work of Miller et al. (for example, see Miller and Bunuazizi [1968]) at the Rockefeller Institute, which challenged the long-held belief that the human autonomic system could not be brought under direct volitional control. Autonomic activity was thought to be regulated by biology and classical conditioning and to vary secondarily as an epiphenomenon of muscular activity. Miller's laboratory rats cast the first doubt on these beliefs by varying their pulses, blood pressures, and intestinal contractions while paralyzed with curare in order to obtain a reward. Such specificity was possible that a rabbit could be trained to blush with one ear but not the other.

By the early 1970's, many of the classic studies had been completed, including those by Sterman (1973) in seizure disorders, Sargent et al. (1973) on migraine headache, Budzynski et al. (1973) on tension headache; Weiss and Engel (1971) on arrhythmias, and Shapiro et al. (1970) on hypertension. These became the platform upon which later studies would be built.

As with many scientific advances, a number of important insights about

---

*The fantasy of merging with an idealized machine is an old one well represented in mythology (Adler, 1976); and it is not surprising that in modern times, too, there can be an unconscious wish to join with our currently idealized tools, computers (Bionic Man). This extravagant wish can cause problems when it is a hidden motivation in biofeedback.

the use of biofeedback owe their existence to serendipity. The Menninger group (Sargent et al., 1973), for example, was experimentally training subjects to raise their hand temperature when one of them reported that a beginning migraine vanished as soon as she had finished raising her hand temperature 10°F. Sterman (1973) was studying cats to see whether they could learn to produce selectively a specific 11-16 Hz (sensorimotor rhythm) EEG. They could. The next part of the experiment involved inducing seizures in the animals using a standard dose of a convulsant. He was startled when many of them failed to have seizures even at greater than usual dosages. Could this unexpected reaction be a result of their training? He investigated further and found that it was. To their credit, none of these researchers dismissed the unusual observation but instead recognized that what was unexpected was their most valuable finding.

THEORETICAL ISSUES AND PHILOSOPHY

An axiom of biofeedback (the psychophysiological principle) is that any change in mental-emotional functioning, conscious or unconscious, greater or smaller, will result in a corresponding change in physiological functioning; and, conversely, any change in physiological functioning will have some effect on a person's mental/emotional life (Green et al., 1970). This axiom implies that a person's mental functioning has a nonverbal segment and that it may have an unconscious component as well.

Another fundamental belief in biofeedback is that man has more potential influence over his body than he uses. Most people are able to learn some simple form of relaxation, which, with regular use, has been found to maximize the ability of the body and the mind to protect themselves against stress-induced illness. Psychiatrists are familiar with the evidence for the detrimental effects of unremitting stress. The same control mechanisms responsible for these pathogenic effects are presumed to be capable of exerting a salutary influence instead.

The volitional (often behavioral) view can be contrasted with the naturalist ("wisdom of the body") view (Cannon, 1932). The naturalist view holds that the mind/body is a homeostasis-seeking entity that tends to efficient self-repair of its dysfunctions and that this process is facilitated if one provides the proper circumstances. Those "proper circumstances" include a regularly occurring state of lowered arousal with reduced sympathetic nervous system activity, which has been termed the trophotrophic state. The naturalists hold that automatic and often unseen corrections occur in a body at rest just as a fracture quieted in a cast will heal itself. Sub-cortical mechanisms are thought to be responsible.

The volitional view holds that natural functioning of the body is not always wise and is at times in fact archaic (otherwise, why would the body be misfunctioning?) and that it needs help from specific external corrective interventions. Its errors are genetic or due to mislearning. In the tradition of medical science, holders of this view insist that help comes only from a specific treatment for the specifically analyzed excess or deficiency that defines each disease state.

This underlying tension about the theoretical underpinnings of biofeedback is often expressed as a debate between the importance of specific, as opposed to nonspecific, treatment factors. One group emphasizes the powerful effects of relaxation and even placebo; the other holds fast to precisely validated change-to-criterion ways of thinking.

The experienced clinician recognizes that neither side in this debate can prevail exclusively. The art and science of medicine can only be separated theoretically; if they come apart in the examining room, the patient is in trouble. Higher organisms function in integrated patterns, and specific change in one area elicits accompanying or compensatory changes in another. Even when biofeedback is being used to teach a specific change, the attitude, thoughts, and expectations of the patient are also inevitably being altered and the direction of those changes will be important to the clinical outcome. Although the unique advantage of biofeedback over general relaxation is its ability to focus on the specific, those specifics are often best presented in the context of general relaxation, psychotherapy, or medical care. Within those contexts the need for specific intervention is evaluated in an illness-by-illness and even a case-by-case fashion. Just as some infections will clear with bed rest while others require penicillin, some psychophysiological problems will yield to relaxation and some only to specific retraining with feedback.

Since placebo effects are particularly enhanced in biofeedback, it is desirable to know what factors make the placebo effect accompanying biofeedback more effective, just as research seeks to discover what makes the "active ingredient" of biofeedback more effective. It is also important to know theoretically when each is operative. There has been considerable discussion among biofeedback investigators about placebo effects, which they have generally considered important and undervalued. Nevertheless, biofeedback is *not only* placebo. In many ways, placebos act automatically over pathways that biofeedback recruits intentionally. The placebo response can be seen as a powerful innate biological reflex: Sixty percent of an analgesic's effect—morphine or aspirin—is thought to be due to placebo (Evans, 1974). It is chemical: Its effect can be blocked with naloxone, an opiate antagonist (Levine et al., 1977). It is normal: Patients with a willingness to rely on others for help showed it more strongly than those who were mistrustful and isolated (Lasagna et al., 1954). It is universal: Ninety percent of patients in severe organic pain (from bone metastases) responded to a placebo to some degree (Houde et al., 1960). And it can be specific.

How do these data bear on biofeedback? Because all homeostasis-enhancing relaxation procedures facilitate the same innate capacities that are automatically activated in placebo responses, it becomes impossible to delineate distinctly the border between general relaxation and placebo effects (Frank, 1982). Indeed, it has been suggested (Stroebel and Glueck, 1973) that biofeedback-assisted relaxation can be used to ensure that these "placebo" effects do not die out but gradually shift from an epiphenomenon of hope to a more stable, learned resource. If, on the other hand, a specific physiological feedback is provided without the proper general relaxation context in order to "eliminate" placebo, it is not being used correctly and, therefore, cannot be evaluated correctly or be expected to perform correctly. Hine (1982) has documented the theoretical pitfalls and logical fallacies in trying to use experimental design to isolate single factors in complex bio-psycho-social systems.

Some authors have considered biofeedback an instrument-aided form of psychotherapy (Frank, 1982; Lazarus, 1975). The extent to which a patient perceives it as psychotherapy largely depends on the extent to which the helping professional considers it "therapy" rather than "training." Nevertheless, psychological issues will be present and relevant in most cases, whether or not this is the theoretical outlook.

Biofeedback theory, with its focus on pathways between conscious thought and sensation, pays little attention to problems that spring from the unconscious. It often equates anxiety with its measurable physical manifestations; and the literature often implies that if one alters these physical manifestations, anxiety has been dealt with adequately. Unfortunately, recommendations on how to integrate an awareness of the unconscious into biofeedback treatments have only been elaborated by a few workers in the field (Adler and Adler, 1972, 1975, 1977a; Rickles, 1976; Glucksman, 1982; Toomin and Toomin, 1975; Werbach, 1977).

When unconscious conflict is present, biofeedback can prove useful in the following ways: (a) by increasing the height of the threshold over which dynamically generated affects must cross in order to trigger physiological disturbance; (b) by encouraging a calmed state in which there is greater capacity to work through these conflicts in dynamic therapy; and (c) by signaling sources of anxiety and other affects when these are hit upon during trial and error attempts to alter the feedback, thereby yielding clues to the origins of the conflict.

In conclusion, the most important point is that the use of biofeedback must be integrated into a sensible treatment plan.

BASIC SCIENCE ISSUES

Basic science issues relevant to biofeedback include both objective (technical) and subjective (experimental) ones.

Objective issues involve problems such as developing the right instrument to reflect the physiology in the most usable form, screening out artifacts, calculating desired physiological levels, determining proper duration, and spacing training to avoid frustration or fatigue. These are technical issues in a technological age, and an entire industry has sprung up to provide answers and equipment. To the extent that "the patient" is considered in this sphere, he is generally viewed as an element of a biomedical engineering system. When biofeedback is an adjunct to general relaxation, the type of feedback is tailored to the patient's dominant pattern of psychophysiological reactivity.

Several biofeedback instruments are important for psychiatry:

Electromyographic (EMG) Biofeedback. The electrical activity generated by a muscle is an indirect but reliable measure of its contraction. For general relaxation training, surface electrodes are positioned over the frontal region or other muscle areas in the face, head, shoulders, and arms as these are often the most sensitive indicators of overall relaxation. But any distressed muscle group can be selectively targeted.

Peripheral Skin Temperature (Thermal Feedback). Temperature is recorded with thermisters, usually taped to the fingers, toes, or forehead. The most common goal is to learn to warm the extremities. The patient must discover how to decrease his sympathetic tone in order to relax the muscular walls of the arterioles and so allow for greater blood flow to the skin of the arms and legs. In other words, these temperature changes are simply surface reflections of a pattern of decreased sympathetic activity.* Given time and practice, most people can learn to increase their peripheral temperature significantly, often 10-15° F and sometimes as much as 25° F.

Electroencephalograph (EEG). Used in psychiatry, the EEG tends to be specialized; the important applications in epilepsy, hyperkinesis, and sleep disorders focus on specific frequencies. It was found, however, that one need not be relaxed to produce alpha, so this technique is currently in search of an application. Presence, amplitude, and laterality of each specific frequency range can be fed back.

Electrodermal (Galvanic) Skin Response. This measures the skin's ability to conduct or resist conduction of electricity, with one of its components (e.g., skin resistance, skin conductance) as the source of the feedback. Because skin response changes rapidly according to emotional variables, this measure has been used as an adjunct to psychotherapy where it functions to announce points of increased dysphoria or even (by fluctuating in the opposite direction) points of increased psychological resistance (Toomin and Toomin, 1975).

As with psychotherapy and certain medications, sufficient treatment

---

*A common misperception is that temperature feedback has a beneficial effect on migraine by a hydraulic repooling of blood, but this is not its actual mechanism.

time, persistence, and flexibility are necessary for effective biofeedback results. Many patients have failed to reap benefits from a lack of knowledge that more consistent practice yielded an entirely different effect than when the technique was used "as needed."

The second group of issues is subjective: discovering what the patient feels, expects, and experiences—questions of mind rather than of brain. These subjective and personality differences can affect treatment outcome. The compulsive patient, for example, often dutifully consigns his "relaxation practice" to a separate time niche emotionally isolated from his other experiences.

Since clinical practice must be a flexible, empirical, even at times intuitive business, studies that do not allow treatment to proceed in that way do not necessarily tell us how much use we can extract from a technique. Such studies are best reviewed with the aim of developing a sense of the principles underlying the use of biofeedback rather than of extracting a rigid list of indications for clinical use. Steiner and Dince (1981) note that with biofeedback, the most relevant question for clinicians is simply, "Is there a better and a safer treatment for the condition?" and, if so, "Would it be significantly better if biofeedback were added to it?"

Two other questions that often need to be answered are, "Will a patient be able to use these skills in the presence of organic disease (i.e., handwarming in scleroderma)?" and, "Will he be able to use it during acute functional disease or decompensation (i.e., such as during a panic attack)?"

As stated before, biofeedback inherently belongs to no theoretical camp. Each user transmits his personal stamp. The galvanic skin response, for example, has been called a "lie detector," a "truth detector" (Green and Green, 1977), and a "divining rod to the unconscious."* Because dynamic therapists have been slow to be recruited into biofeedback's ranks, they have made less of an impression on its public "identity," and most of the theorizing to date has been done by behaviorists, who consider biofeedback a form of conditioning. They define it as such because a patient using biofeedback gets rewarded (reinforced) when one of his spontaneous initiatives moves the feedback in the right direction and he therefore repeats and refines ("shapes") that same "behavior." There has been some debate about whether immediate reinforcement is needed to ensure adequate motivation and performance. Some have believed that the reinforcement is provided by movement of the feedback in the right direction or praise from the therapist. More important to durable motivation are internal ideals to which these situational reinforcers signal approximation, such as the sense of active mastery, of self-control, or of the long-term goal of symptom relief.

If a general relaxation response has been learned well, it can be called up

*Adler CS, Adler SM: Interface with the Unconscious in Biofeedback. Presented at the annual meeting of the American Academy of Psychoanalysis, Toronto, 1977

in the presence of previously upsetting situations as a response that is incompatible with and that can inactivate anxiety. This technique is called "reciprocal inhibition" or "counterconditioning" and is also the basis for systematic desensitization procedures. An interesting view taken by Gaarder and Montgomery (1977) is that operant conditioning may actually be one variety of feedback, which is seen as the more embracing concept. Operant conditioning is only one example of feedback; homeostasis is another.*

It has been shown that humans can learn to modify their autonomic nervous systems independently of muscular activity and in a specific rather than an all or nothing fashion. Patients paralyzed from spinal lesions or polio, for example (Pickering et al., 1977), could be taught to raise their blood pressures without increases in heart rate. The precise mechanism underlying these types of control is still being investigated.

A finding from another perspective may also be of interest (Adler and Adler, 1977b). This is the transference-like distortion of the biofeedback instrument itself. It is fostered in part by the unique relationship between patient and instrument: symbolically symbiotic. Like an idealized mother, the instrument immediately responds to every change in the patient with a change in feedback. The patient expects a soothing encounter but it often "frustrates" him by setting up its own "squall" at the very moment he is most upset, and so on. Patients will say such things as, "It seems as if it's teasing (ridiculing/invading/exposing/deceiving) me." For the therapist trained to understand them, these idiosyncratic perceptions can reveal a good deal about the earliest relationships of the patient in treatment with biofeedback.

INDICATIONS

While no longer a brand new field, biofeedback is still a young discipline and should be evaluated in comparison with other fields at a similar age. Many of the applications are still awaiting definitive studies or long-term clinical experience.

What, broadly speaking, are the conditions in psychiatry to which either biofeedback or biofeedback-assisted relaxation can be applied? Among them are: (a) teaching long-term control of the manifestations of anxiety and in disorders in which anxiety plays a prominent role; (b) treating certain psychophysiological disorders, not through general anxiety reduction but by inhibiting the access of anxiety to that patient's specifically vulnerable

---

*The starting and stopping of chemical reactions in solution is also governed by feedback mechanisms. Evolution itself, for that matter, can be thought of as the long-term consequences of feedback mechanisms in the universe.

route of discharge (final common pathway); (c) treating medical conditions that may be accompanied by emotional problems; (d) improving systematic desensitization in behavior therapy; (e) reflecting underlying psychodynamic issues that give rise to anxiety or other painful affects, and (f) investigating psychosomatic interactions and alexithymia.

General Benefits

Exploring the possibility of a simple way to return patients to a state of normal arousal seems to be a natural issue for clinicians to address. Because the need for this ability is as basic as the need for adequate sleep, nutrition, and exercise, it is surprising how few patientenefits of regularly practiced relaxation have been observed in clinical practice and can supplement more specific psychiatric therapies. They are:

A. If a patient has misconceptions about psychiatrists and other therapists, ambivalence about trusting one, confusion about whether his problem is in part psychological, and if it is, about whether "talking" can help it, the time required to learn relaxation allows patient and therapist to get to know one another. In the meantime, his perception of biofeedback as a "medical procedure" may allow the patient to save face. For this same reason, some physicians often feel more comfortable referring patients for biofeedback than for psychotherapy. This has opened the doorway to psychological treatment for many alexithymic patients.

B. Biofeedback teaches the patient an active way to fight his problems. Patients frequently lack the insight to reduce symptoms during the earliest stages of treatment and are left with the helpless/hopeless feeling that comes from not knowing anything they can do to modulate their discomfort. Being able to focus actively on combating the *experience* of anxiety in addition to its causes can cut through long-standing feelings of defeat and passivity. Patients are frequently relieved to know that even though they may not be able to change all the factors about their life which seem overwhelming, they can do *something* about their *reactions*, and in that way gain a certain autonomy from the stresses that surround them. Animals given electrical shocks differed in the subsequent level of brain norepinephrine according to whether or not they were able to combat the situation actively (Weiss, 1970).

C. In order to learn biofeedback the patient must therapeutically dissociate his observing ego from the part of him that experiences sensation and initiates changes (executive functions of the ego). By becoming both the observer (with a passive and even curious attitude toward his symptomatic self) and the observee, he can learn to gain emotional distance from his symptoms. Not only is this distance of benefit in terms of its defensive capacities, but it also may be the seed from which can grow the self-observing attitude needed in psychotherapy if this later becomes necessary.

D. As a result of focusing on his body, the patient may become more aware of its needs, such as for rest, crying, etc., and may sometimes recognize ways in which he may have ignored those needs in the past. If the migraine sufferer, for example, becomes more sensitive to internal cues, he has a head start in identifying impending difficulty before symptoms become full-blown.

E. Biofeedback may also yield diagnostic information. For example, as his physical activity diminishes, a patient may become aware of an underlying depression. Also, there are times when the physiology does not concur with the presumed diagnosis, or the patient learns to change his physiology but symptoms remain unchanged and it becomes necessary to rethink the diagnosis.

As in all psychiatric treatments, there are patient-oriented as well as disease-oriented criteria for the use of biofeedback. For example, the organic patient with eroded memory, the schizophrenic with loose body boundaries, the overly suspicious paranoid, and the sociopath who fears that his impulsively asocial behavior might be getting him into trouble are all patients whose very real anxiety would *not* be best treated with biofeedback. Other types of patients are more likely to respond to biofeedback. The patient who can intellectualize, rationalize, and resist recognition of his true feelings may find his verbal Maginot line strategically bypassed. The patient who doesn't believe his worries have anything to do with his symptoms finds that, with the feedback, seeing is believing. The patient who is more trusting of mechanical devices than of people may have a greater affinity for this form of symptom control. Biofeedback's concreteness and immediacy make it less frustrating than verbal therapy for those inarticulate or action-oriented patients who somatize and need to reinterpret their bodily sensations into feelings. Finally, the patient who needs some experience of success with a body that has frightened, discouraged, and failed him may find it this way.

Clinicians will find that the same personality traits and neurotic styles with which they are familiar from psychotherapy will wend their way into the interaction with the feedback. For example, patients with hysterical personalities tend to become restless and neglect practice between sessions, while obsessive-compulsive patients are less able to experiment comfortably with what might affect the feedback and are intolerant of their perceived failures with it. When these traits are pronounced, they cause one to question the value of biofeedback.

While biofeedback can be used with inpatients and has a number of advantages such as more frequent sessions, time away from family stresses, time in which to practice, etc., it is generally inappropriate to admit a patient for biofeedback alone. It is reasonable, however, for psychiatric inpatient facilities to consider whether a relaxation training program would be a feasible addition to their unit routine for less seriously ill patients.

Psychiatric medication may be used concomitantly with relaxation, and its effect can be synergistic. In one trial, diazepam plus EMG feedback was more useful for reducing anxiety in psychiatric patients than was either one used alone (LaVallee et al., 1977), and EEG training potentiated the effects of Ritalin on hyperkinetic children (Shouse and Lubar, 1979). On the other hand, nonpharmacologic sedation is needed in many circumstances; it may be used for the patient allergic to available compounds, the chronically suicidal patient, the ex-addict, the patient with religious beliefs precluding drug use, the patient who thinks of medication as a "crutch" that he refuses to use, and so on.

Uses of Biofeedback-Assisted Relaxation to Reduce Anxiety

Although the reduction of anxiety is biofeedback's most well known application in psychiatry, its use for this purpose should always be in conjunction with more fundamental relaxation and homeostasis-enhancing treatments. It is axiomatic that biofeedback alone is insufficient as the total treatment for clinically significant anxiety or an anxiety-induced disorder.

Finding the most appropriate general relaxation therapy (or combination) for an individual patient is not always simple; fortunately, however, there is a great deal of overlap and a person can learn to relax well in a number of ways. It is important that the technique have characteristics with which the patient feels comfortable. Progressive relaxation (Jacobson, 1938) involves the sequential contraction and relaxation of muscle groups, "progressing" to an ability to recognize and release muscle tension without prior contraction; it is, therefore, particularly useful for patients whose symptoms are primarily caused or aggravated by excess muscle tension. Autogenic training (Luthe, 1969) is an excellent technique, readily learned by most, and is often combined with progressive relaxation. Patients who strongly resist disciplined routines or who have difficulty with passivity may find this technique difficult. Quieting reflex training (Stroebel, 1982) places an emphasis on integrating relaxation practice into everyday activities. Other popular general techniques include the relaxation response (Benson, 1975), yoga, and self-hypnosis.

Other Clinical Applications

Drug and Alcohol Abuse. The aim in substance abuse is to teach the patient a means by which he can attempt to calm himself, thereby partially replacing the relief afforded by the addictive substance. To compete effectively with the immediate relief afforded by drugs and alcohol, the relaxation response must be learned well enough to become a dependable and reliable asset. A few sessions tacked onto the end of a rehabilitation program will not suffice (Bowman and Faust, 1977). Although not a panacea, relaxation skills have been found to benefit the patient who can commit himself to a full spectrum of treatment for his disorder (Graham et al., 1976).

Insomnia. Chronic insomnia is a symptom with many etiologies, only some of which may be amenable to help with biofeedback. In a well controlled study, Hauri (1981) found that insomniacs with initially elevated muscular or psychological tension were helped by EMG feedback; however, he also found many "relaxed insomniacs," who often show poorly formed sleep spindles, an EEG phenomenon seen during stage II of normal sleep, and who were not helped by relaxation. Such patients only obtained benefits from learning the sensorimotor EEG rhythm.* This waking rhythm is characterized by the appearance of 13 Hz bursts that resemble sleep spindles. He emphasizes that no one type of feedback can be uncritically applied to all patients with sleep problems.

Attention Deficit Disorder (Hyperkinesis). Significant work with hyperkinetic children has been done by Lubar et al. (1981), who found that the majority of them produced insufficient high frequency beta EEG rhythms along with an excess of slow waves (4-8 Hz) while engaged in cognitive activity. Most such children have insufficient cortical stimulation (i.e., low arousal) and, in an isolated situation, will fall asleep more readily than their peers. The hyperactive behavior is presumed to be a homeostatic attempt to correct for that insufficiency. Other patterns of hyperactivity are psychogenic, with the children simply venting emotional distress. Biofeedback treatment for the first group consists of individualized feedback training to teach them to increase 16-20 Hz beta activity and decrease 4-8 Hz slow-wave activity simultaneously, with training carried out while the child is engaged in the type of cognitive behaviors that have caused him difficulty, such as reading or drawing. EMG feedback or relaxation training is also used to reduce excess restless activity and has been shown to improve performance both in the classroom and on formal cognitive testing (Russel and Carter, 1979). Although facilities for this type of treatment are currently limited, the results have been impressive enough to consider hyperkinesis with EEG abnormalities an indication for biofeedback as an alternative treatment when pharmacotherapy is unsuccessful or inapplicable.

Phobias. Although Kiev (1983) has recently reported good success in using biofeedback with these illnesses, both panic disorder and agoraphobia require both psychotherapy and pharmacotherapy in addition to relaxation therapy. For isolated phobias, systematic desensitization has proven to be a generally effective treatment. Biofeedback can facilitate systematic desensitization: (a) by confirming that the patient has learned to relax before starting, (b) by corroborating the correct anxiogenic rank order of items in

---

*The sensorimotor rhythm feedback is the same as that used for treatment of seizure disorders.

the desensitization hierarchy, (c) by monitoring the physiologic variable most sensitive to anxiety in each patient, and (d) by continuously and silently monitoring that variable during the desensitization procedure to know exactly when to initiate and terminate visualization of scenes in the hierarchy. It has been shown that EMG and other physiological readings tend to rise before a patient will verbally report an increase in anxiety (Adler and Adler, 1977c); this early signal of rising anxiety allows the therapist to stay one step ahead of the patient throughout the desensitization.

Somatoform (Psychophysiologic) Disorders

Work in this area is one of biofeedback's strong suits and provides an entree for psychiatrists to see these frequently under-referred patients.

Tension and Migraine Headaches. Tension headache has been one of the more thoroughly studied and widely applied uses of EMG biofeedback. Electrodes are positioned over the symptomatic muscle groups, generally frontal or paracervical. The rationale for treatment is simple: Specific muscles are causing pain because they are in spasm; the patient should be able to learn how to relax them with biofeedback and, thereby, reverse the pathologic process. It is not always quite that simple, of course, as the muscles may be contracted for a covert reason—frequently anxious rage, sometimes depression. Nevertheless, since the symptom is not helping the patient solve his problems, a straightforward lesson in learning to ameliorate it should be part of the treatment. Budzynski et al. (1970) first reported the usefulness of biofeedback for tension headache in 1970. In a subsequent matched controlled study Budzynski et al. (1973), using both a false feedback control group and patients as their own controls, found that biofeedback made a statistically significant difference in the treatment of tension headaches.

Since migraine is a vascular headache, thermal biofeedback is used to treat it. Patients can learn to abort migraine headaches and to diminish their frequency (Diamond et al., 1978). Patients with classical as opposed to common migraine seem to have greater success; because they are fore-warned by a prodromal aura, they are able to interpose timely relaxation that can prevent the unfolding of the attack.

When training is thorough to begin with, psychological issues are dealt with, and relaxation practice is continued in some rudimentary fashion over the ensuing years, the treatment for headaches with biofeedback can be a durable one (Adler and Adler, 1976, in press). Sargent et al. (1973) and Diamond and Franklin (1977) have both reported positive results treating large numbers of migraine patients with biofeedback, and treatment of migraine in children was particularly successful. A sophisticated study by Mathew et al. (1980) showed that cerebrovascular flow rates as measured by xenon inhalation changed when thermal biofeedback was used and that headache ceased with these changes. The American Association for the Study of Headache (1978) has formally endorsed biofeedback for selected tension and migraine headache patients. Although generalized relaxation procedures may also be helpful for these conditions, specific biofeedback will be necessary for some and more rapid for many patients. EMG biofeedback is indicated for chronic tension headaches. Thermal biofeedback is indicated for adults with migraine occurring more than once a month and for children with migraine. At present there is no consistent evidence that biofeedback helps cluster headaches.

Bruxism, Torticollis, and Low Back Pain. The theoretical basis for treating these conditions is similar to that for tension headache. The need to deal with the attitudes frequently underlying these symptoms (such as biting anger in bruxism) also pertains, as does the need to rule out any localized pathologic processes to which the muscular bracing is a reaction.

Cardiovascular Applications. Although patients can learn to lower their blood pressure with biofeedback, most studies have not shown that the degree of decrease is dramatic or is larger than that obtained with more basic relaxation procedures. Early work by Weiss and Engel (1971) on the treatment of cardiac arrhythmias with cardiotachometry feedback showed that patients with damaged hearts could learn to reduce premature ventricular contractions significantly and could maintain these changes for years.

Thermal feedback has been successfully used by Taub and Stroebel (1978) and others to treat Raynaud's disease in the absence of active depression or collagen disease.

Bronchial Asthma. Treatment of bronchial asthma has been studied using both biofeedback-assisted relaxation training and specific feedback of respiratory resistance. As it is important to break up the mutually reinforcing interaction between panic and dyspnea which characterizes an acute attack, the application of general relaxation training or thermal biofeedback makes good sense for patients whose attacks are susceptible to psychological triggers.

Gastrointestinal Uses. Patients with irritable colon syndromes are able to decrease their peristaltic rate by paying attention to the level of amplified bowel sounds. One of the most impressive uses of biofeedback to date has been in the treatment of fecal incontinence; in the absence of denervation it is the current treatment of choice (Schuster, 1979).

Chronic Pain. Biofeedback has been incorporated into treatment programs for chronic pain but only to improve a patient's capacity to modulate that part of the suffering caused by accentuated attention to painful stimuli or by the feelings of helplessness which accompany that perception. It has been suggested that by learning to relax, patients are able to attend to the pain in a different manner, which may include some elements of self-hypnosis (Melzack and Perry, 1975).

Uses with Medical Disorders Where Psychological Factors May Play a Role

Seizure Disorders. The innovative neuropsychiatric application of biofeedback in treating seizure disorders was pioneered by Sterman (1973) and by Lubar and colleagues (Lubar et al., 1981; Lubar and Deering, 1981). Patients were taught to increase production of the 12-15 Hz sensorimotor rhythm (recorded over the sensorimotor cortex) and simultaneously to suppress paroxysmal 4-8 Hz slow activity. Sterman initially found that four out of five severe, drug-resistant epileptics improved their clinical picture dramatically with training, relapsed to previous levels of seizure activity when training was terminated, and regained their initial improvements when feedback was re-initiated (Sterman, 1973). A subsequent single-blind and well controlled study of a larger group yielded a similar success rate. This time it was found that if training were gradually tapered off rather than stopped abruptly, most patients could maintain their improvements without further instrument training, although a few required monthly "booster" sessions (Sterman and MacDonald, 1978). Lubar et al. (1981) have recently concluded a double-blind study that supported the use of this feedback paradigm even with brain-damaged or retarded epileptics. Patients appropriate for this treatment are refractory to conventional anticonvulsant medication, have adequate motivation, and have clearly defined motor components to their seizures. Use with seizure disorders offers a graphic example of how biofeedback can teach patients to modify physiology in a way unattainable without the specific information the feedback provides.

Neuro-Muscular Rehabilitation. EMG biofeedback has proven particularly valuable in re-establishing disrupted and functionally atrophied naturally occurring sensori-motor feedback systems in patients following both upper and lower motor neuron injury. Because a paralyzed muscle may provide inadequate sensory feedback, the patient may become disoriented about the new set of contingencies for activating any motor units that remain functional. EMG (using needle electrodes) can help patients to become aware of these still functional but unused motor units, although it naturally cannot revise the inherent pathology. These techniques were pioneered by Basmajian (1983) and have been successfully applied with spinal cord and peripheral nerve injuries, cerebral palsy, and hemiplegia following cerebro-vascular accidents.

Use an Aid to Dynamic Psychotherapy

Like ataraxics, biofeedback-assisted relaxation can be used in a straightforward way to reduce the anxiety symptoms of patients working through their problems in a more durable way in psychodynamic psychotherapy (Rickles et al., 1982). It can also be used to facilitate the psychotherapeutic uncovering process; this happens, in part, as a result of the deep relaxation itself. The quiet, stillness, and neutrality of deep relaxation catalyze the release of unresolved and troublesome memories, sensations, and affects. Reduction of afferent stimuli through any one of the relaxation techniques can trigger images related to recollected events or fantasy fragments in susceptible patients; remaining alert with the eyes closed facilitates visual recall of traumatic events that are less accessible with the eyes open.* In psychotherapy such rememberings, which are automatically released by homeostatic control mechanisms in the brain, can be a positive sign of reduced resistance, allowing for greater contact with repressed material. Such a technique may be particularly beneficial in treating the post-traumatic stress syndrome (Adler and Adler, 1982b).

Another route to repressed material is through what has been termed biofeedback-psychotherapy (Adler and Adler, 1972, 1975, 1977a, 1977b; Sargent et al., 1973; Glucksman, 1981, 1982). It was noted that when a patient using biofeedback permitted his mind to drift freely, the biofeedback instrument acted as a psychological barometer. Whenever his train of thought led him to a particular theme or image, the feedback might signal a rapid increase in the direction of anxiety, even if the patient had not previously associated this topic with his state of tension. The recognition that this material was anxiogenic and relevant was reinforced each time this increase was again triggered by the same or related themes. The patient was encouraged to discuss his observations of such reactions with the therapist in order to discover what unrecognized element lay at the root of them. Patients eventually learned to pay attention to cognitive antecedents of unexpected feedback shifts. Thermal and electrodermal responses reveal such reactions most dramatically. During therapy the feedback can be left running at low volume or adjusted to chime in only when undergoing rapid change; in this way it will frequently confirm the emotional valence of a discussion. This technique is useful for patients whose psychological problems present with somatoform manifestations. Glucksman (1981, 1982) has detailed experimentally some of the relationships between thematic content, therapeutic interpretations, affect, symptom occurrence, and electrodermal feedback during psychoanalytically-oriented psychotherapy. Others have also recognized the insight-producing capacity of biofeedback (Toomin and Toomin, 1975; Werbach, 1977).

Biofeedback treatment has offered hope of successful psychological treatment of those alexithymic patients who were previously thought to be psychotherapy-resistant. These patients' rigid personality structures make them highly vulnerable to a breach of their defenses, which, since they often have little capacity for self-soothing behavior, would be difficult to

---

*This process is intentionally encouraged in narcoanalysis, in hypnosis, and in autogenic neutralization. It also occurs under conditions of sensory deprivation.

repair. Biofeedback can often teach these patients how to exercise self-soothing functions similar to those they initially experienced in infancy.

Use as an Exploratory Research Tool

Biofeedback can be used to study the correlation between particular states of consciousness and the corresponding states of physiology. For example, Green (1970, 1977) found that subjects reported vivid imagery and "integrative" experiences while producing theta EEG rhythm. Whether this is specific to theta or is no different from similarly beneficial primary process experiences that occur during hypnosis and abreactive therapies remains to be determined. But biofeedback can be used to induce and study those states further.

Applications to other diseases remain experimental. Miller and Landis (Landis, 1983), among others, have found that biofeedback may eventually benefit certain subtypes of diabetics. A number of other illnesses adversely affected by stress are also being researched actively.

In conclusion, it might noted that biofeedback has been widely applied and reported to be helpful with a number of patients and disorders, has "done no harm," and has as much research support as a great many routine clinical procedures. For most conditions, it is currently advisable to allow the experienced clinician to evaluate the use of biofeedback on a case-by-case basis, taking into account tangible and intangible factors. In deferring to the clinician's judgment, we should remember that the arrow is no more accurate than its archer and the biofeedback tool no more effective than its user.

LIMITATIONS

The greatest danger of biofeedback comes not from what it is but from the risk of viewing it as what it is not: a comprehensive treatment. The patient in an acute state of agitation, depression, or situational crisis will usually require the therapist to start other treatments before initiating biofeedback; and the patient with acute medical decompensation may likewise require the initiation of other treatments first. In perspective, however, we see that biofeedback has few serious limitations or side effects because no chemical is being added to the patient's body and no invasive procedure is being performed.

The question can be raised as to whether one of the body's well chosen homeostatic coping mechanisms can be interferred with by, for example, volitionally rerouting blood away from where it is needed. Most treatments with the power to help will also have enough power, if used incorrectly, to harm. However, with biofeedback, as opposed to drugs or surgery, all changes, at some level, have to be cleared through various checkpoints in the brain; and here they are regulated by self-protective mechanisms and defenses that will usually adjust for or automatically disallow attempts to change which are incompatible with biological or unconscious needs. Biology tends to compensate for the mistakes of biofeedback professionals.

Most adverse reactions that occur during biofeedback with psychiatric patients result from its capacity to catalyze the release of repressed or suppressed psychological material if the therapist is not anticipating or prepared for it. Such reactions are not frequent, and it is uncommon for them to be of such intensity as to preclude further use of biofeedback. When a patient's psychological defenses have a physical manifestation (Adler and Adler, 1982b), such as tightening abdominal muscles to prevent crying, one may (sometimes inadvertently) allow the patient to reduce those defenses by helping him to change the accompanying physiology. Many types of repressed material may be observed in such reactions; particularly noteworthy, however, are feelings of physical vulnerability and memories of physical trauma. When focusing on the body, the site of all physical trauma, the sensations coming from it may mix with memory to recall those specific episodes to consciousness, even to the extent of occasionally re-experiencing pain, sensations of falling, etc. In susceptible individuals these reactions can be diminished by limiting the time and depth of the relaxation.

For patients with poor body boundaries, the temporary distortions of body image which are normal consequences of the decreased proprioception accompanying stillness can stimulate anxiety. In fragile schizophrenics they have even stimulated increased hallucinatory activity (Adler and Adler, 1977b; APA, 1979). Biofeedback is not recommended in acute schizophrenia; and it is generally not used with chronic varieties, for which there appear to be no safe, effective, and well researched treatment programs. Similar caution should apply to any patients who use psychotic defenses, particularly when there is a threat that those defenses will be overwhelmed. Biofeedback is virtually never recommended in patients with (a) delusions of influence, (b) severe depression, (c) mania, (d) paranoia, (e) severe obsessional states, and (f) delirium or acute psychotic disorganization.

There are also other precautions. Biofeedback treatment can reduce the dosage requirement of certain medications. The most prominent example is diabetes mellitus in which the need for insulin may be reduced after successful relaxation therapy. Blood glucose must be monitored and insulin intake adjusted to avoid the potential for insulin shock. Elderly patients receiving anti-hypertensive medications might lower their blood pressures enough to have problems with hypotension. In a less critical way it has been found that medications for hypothyroidism, glaucoma, epilepsy, and asthma may need to be readjusted after successful treatment. On the other hand, patients who have had their medication adjusted downward may simultaneously become over-confident and neglectful of their practice. The patient with angina may ignore the biological limits imposed by his coronary arteries and decide to tangle with a big mountain he has always wanted to climb. When treating such patients, the prescribing physician should be advised that dosages may need to be adjusted.

When a psychophysiological symptom is not merely a functional vestige of past conflict but is actively tied to current unconscious needs, the use of biofeedback to remove the symptom will not remove the needs. Sometimes the equilibrium has been restored through symptom substitution (Szajnberg and Diamond, 1980); on other occasions, the balance may not be restored and the symptomatic affect being defended against, such as anxiety or depression, may emerge directly (Rickles, 1976). These are not typical occurrences but show the need for psychological training of the people trying to revise psychosomatic symptoms. When using biofeedback and biofeedback-assisted relaxation, however, the likelihood of inadvertently helping some undiagnosed or preventing some potential condition is far greater than the likelihood of inadvertently causing harm.

AGE RELATED ISSUES

Age is not a barrier to learning with biofeedback. Children generally see biofeedback as a game and learn autonomic self-regulation as much as five times faster than adults (Diamond and Franklin, 1977). Since the psychiatric technique for children is "play therapy," when a young patient presents with psychosomatic difficulties, it seems reasonable to consider playing a "game" that not only elucidates the child's way of relating to others but also his way of relating to himself. An excellent child-oriented relaxation technique, called Kiddie QR (Quieting Reflex), has been developed and is used in various educational and clinical settings (Stroebel et al., 1980).

Biofeedback often appeals to adolescents for several reasons: (a) Adolescents are curious and often see biofeedback as a challenge or an adventure. (b) Early adolescents are often too "grown up" for play therapy, yet too constricted for a gratifying verbal exchange; the feedback is a compromise around which one part of treatment can be structured. (c) They can safely rebel by doing poorly on the instrument; their autonomy is assured because they know that they are the only ones in control of the feedback. (d) The image of being "coached" in learning a physical skill is an acceptable way to gratify dependency needs while, at the same time, saving face. (e) At a time when the adolescent feels that his or her body is growing too gangly, too sexual, and too fast, the feedback offers a chance to experience control over it and to rein in the sense of physiological anarchy (Adler and Adler, 1977b).

Treatment with self-regulatory methods should not be withheld because of age. Nevertheless, older patients may need more time to master the techniques and to resolve problems related to the valued existential meanings frequently acquired by long-standing symptoms (Adler and Adler, 1982c).

Because of its focus on manipulation of modes of experience and learning similar to those that dominated the earliest years of life, biofeedback may revive memories and feelings related to the period of first becoming familiar with and developing control over the body. As a result, the patient using biofeedback has a chance to make contact with some of the earliest anlage of his psychosomatic functioning, much of which has never been translated into words (Adler and Adler, 1977a).

PROFESSIONAL AND ETHICAL ISSUES

Since biofeedback is not confined to a single profession or defined by a single set of comprehensively treated illnesses, the most conspicuous ethical/professional issue in biofeedback is related to who is qualified to do what. The question lacks an easy answer. Often, it clearly has to do with fundamental questions of competence, as many of the conditions being treated are medical conditions and the interventions used are aimed at a complex physiology and even more complex psyche. Although questions about the competence of biofeedback professionals to deal with psychological issues is highlighted less often, it is no less important, as many treatment variables and adverse reactions during biofeedback are psychological. Psychiatric sophistication is more important when biofeedback is used medically or intensively than when it is used to teach a skill to presumably healthy individuals. When the patient anticipates that his experience will be limited and goal-oriented, his psychological defenses will be more effective at limiting the tendency of unconscious material to break through and cause difficulty.

Like many techniques with broad applications, the initial stages in the evolution of biofeedback have been characterized by many "therapeutic models" trying themselves out, so to speak, as natural experiments. This proliferation has included attempts to use biofeedback in the most expeditious way possible, including the use of the least extensively trained and therefore the most economic individuals to "run" the patients on biofeedback.

The best current guideline is this: Every patient should be treated with biofeedback by a professional with the appropriate credentials who is qualified to understand and treat both the illness and the patient without biofeedback, or by someone under the direct and personal supervision of a professional so qualified. For the treatment of psychiatric disorders, the therapist should have a professional level education in the diagnosis and treatment of psychological disturbances by traditional means. Supervision has not worked adequately unless such a professional has had regular contact with the facility and has taken an active part in following and making relevant decisions about the case. Because the skills required in biofeedback cover several disciplines, optimal treatment may require close collaboration among a number of professionals. Basmajian (1976) points out that in order to use EMG feedback for rehabilitation, one needs to know not only the electronics of the instrument but also the anatomy and physiology of the muscles and nerves, and, in some cases, the psychology of physical disability.

Another problem about qualifications has to do with knowledge about biofeedback instruments. While obviously important, it is not as important as understanding the disease being treated, and again, as the medical adage states, not nearly as important as understanding the patient who has the disease. If only the instrument fails, the result is usually annoyance rather than serious harm.

The ethical guidelines worked out by the professional societies whose members comprise the various biofeedback-related professions should be followed. For example, one issue about which those guidelines are already clear involves unethical advertising of biofeedback services. Because of popular appeal, it is easy to sensationalize or commercialize the benefits of biofeedback. State and national biofeedback societies have ethics committees that try to regulate this misbehavior but have found, as have most other disciplines, that many of the offenders are not members of these societies and that the societies themselves have limited legal power.

More subtle forms of commercialization are more important and less easy to define. The professional who does an evaluation designed only to find out which form of biofeedback the potential patient needs rather than whether biofeedback is even indicated may be guilty of this violation.

Training in the use of biofeedback and self-regulatory therapies is available through courses sponsored by national and state biofeedback societies and through university medical centers. Many books and several journals are available which cover all aspects of required knowledge in the field, though they tend to give insufficient attention to psychological aspects.

There is also a formal certification and peer review process. The Biofeedback Certification Institute of America has evolved to consolidate testing and certification of candidates on a national basis.

FINANCIAL, LEGAL, AND SOCIAL/POLITICAL ISSUES

In general, instrumentation should be kept as simple as possible so as not to distract patient and therapist from recognizing that the biofeedback equipment is merely an adjunctive tool being used in the treatment. Whereas substandard equipment often gives false and thereby frustrating feedback, too much sophistication often intimidates the patient (or the therapist), adds needless expense, and puts too much reliance on "tricks" and gimmicks. Moderately priced units about the size and shape of a radio are best suited for general psychiatric use. Small, portable units are unsuitable for initial office use.

Another issue is the question of third-party reimbursement. In a recent unpublished study, Middaugh reported that biofeedback was extremely cost-effective with neuromuscular rehabilitation patients who received a specific appropriate treatment for their condition. In fact, for chronic physical or psychiatric conditions—and biofeedback is basically used to treat chronic conditions—the cost of biofeedback has not been prohibitive if it goes a reasonable way toward improving the condition for which it is being used. Where allied health professionals have been trained to assist with the biofeedback (under close supervision), the charge to the patients should clearly reflect their level and their salary.

The legal issues are similar to those encountered whenever medical or psychological procedures are being used. Biofeedback instrumentation is considered to be a medical device and comes under regulation by the Food and Drug Administration (FDA).

The social and political issues surrounding biofeedback are serious. Biofeedback is a stage upon which many societal dramas are being enacted: The wish of nonphysicians to become involved in treating medically ill patients, physicians' orientation toward treating illness rather than promoting health, and the escalating cost of medical care are major examples. Also evident in this drama is the battle between the mechanistic and humanistic views of human functioning held by professionals of different theoretical persuasions. Unfortunately, the effort to bring psychological expertise to medically ill patients seems to be splintering, and some expect biofeedback to join as a feudal ally. In that context, the field called "behavioral medicine" has assumed prominence and often attempts to fill the gap left by insufficient attention by physicians to the concerns of patients mentioned earlier. The significant momentum contributed to the evolution of biofeedback theory and practice by the behavioral therapies will gain in breadth and be enriched if its future input is complemented by greater contributions from eclectic, psychoanalytically, or biologically trained psychiatrists.

It is hoped that the future will see more psychiatrists adding their special knowledge and perspective to a field the nature of which cries out for their participation. To be a significant evolutionary step, a technique does not need to be, indeed cannot be, a panacea. It may be that biofeedback will prove to be such a step by adding an enduring and innovative tool to the evolved body of scientific knowledge and technique.

REFERENCES

Adler CS, Adler SM: Physiological feedback and psychotherapeutic intervention for migraine: a ten-year follow-up, in Selected Papers from the First International Headache Society Meeting, Munich. Edited by Sjastaad O, Lundberg PO. New York, Springer, in press

Adler CS, Adler SM: Psychiatric treatment of the headache patient. Panminerva Med 24:145-149, 1982a

Adler CS, Adler SM: The importance of physical memories in the pathogenesis of psychosomatic symptoms. Presented at the American Academy of Psychoanalysis meeting, Coronado, Calif, 1982b

Adler CS, Adler SM: Existential deterrents to headache relief past midlife, in Advances in Neurology, vol 33: Headache, Pathophysiological, and Clinical Concepts. Edited by Critchley M, Friedman A, Gorini A, et al. New York, Raven Press, 1982c

Adler CS, Adler SM: Biofeedback and psychosomatic disorders, in Biofeedback—Principles and Practice for Clinicians. Edited by Basmajian JV. Baltimore, Williams & Wilkins Co, 1977a

Adler CS, Adler SM: Strategies in general psychiatry, in Biofeedback—Principles and Practice for Clinicians. Edited by Basmajian JV. Baltimore, Williams & Wilkins Co, 1977b

Adler CS, Adler SM: Biofeedback psychotherapy for the treatment of headaches: a five-year followup. Headache 16:189-191, 1976

Adler CS, Adler SM: Biofeedback in Psychotherapy (cassette tape). New York, Biomonitoring Applications, 1975

Adler CS, Adler SM: Biofeedback: Interface with the Unconscious. Boston, Proceedings of the Biofeedback Research Society, November 1972

Adler CS: Biofeedback, Evolution, and the Tools of Man. Colorado Springs, Proceedings of the Biofeedback Research Society, February 1976

Alexander F: Psychosomatic Medicine: Its Principles and Applications. New York, WW Norton, 1950

Basmajian JV (ed): Biofeedback, Principles and Practice for Clinicians, 2nd ed. Baltimore, Williams & Wilkins Co, 1983

Basmajian JV: Facts vs myths in EMG biofeedback (editorial). Biofeedback Self-Regul 1:369-371, 1976

Basmajian JV: Conscious control of individual motor units. Science 141:440-441, 1963

Beaumont W: Experiments and Observations on the Gastric Juice, and the Physiology of Digestion. Plattsburgh, NY, FP Allen, 1833

Benson H: The Relaxation Response. New York, William Morrow, 1975

Bezzola D: Elementar-autanalyse. Zeitschrift fur die gesamte Neurologie und Psychiatrie 43:27-33, 1918

Board of Directors, American Association for the Study of Headache: Biofeedback therapy. Headache 18:107, 1978

Bowman B, Faust D: EMG-autogenic training and cognitive-behavior modification: a multi-modal strategy for tension reduction for alcoholics. Biofeedback Self Regul 1:352, 1977

Budzynski H, Stoyva JM, Adler CS, et al: EMG biofeedback and tension headache: a controlled outcome study. Psychosom Med 35:484-496, 1973

Budzynski T, Stoyva J, Adler CS: Feedback-induced muscle relaxation: application to tension headache. J Behav Ther Exp Psychiatry 1:205-211, 1970

Cannon WB: The Wisdom of the Body. New York, WW Norton & Co, 1932

Diamond S, Diamond-Falk J, DeVeno T: Biofeedback in the treatment of vascular headache. Biofeedback Self Regul 3:385-408, 1978

Diamond S, Franklin M: Biofeedback—choice of treatment in childhood migraine, in Therapy in Psychosomatic Medicine, vol 4, Autogenic Therapy. Edited by Luthew, Antonelli F. Rome, Edizioni L Pozzi 1977

Dunbar F: Emotions and Bodily Changes. New York, Columbia University Press, 1954

Evans FJ: The placebo response in pain reduction, in Advances in Neurology, vol 4. New York, Raven Press, 1974

Frank JD: Biofeedback and the placebo effect. Biofeedback Self Regul 7:449-460 1982

Gaarder KR, Montgomery PS: Clinical Biofeedback: A Procedural Manual. Baltimore, Williams & Wilkins Co, 1977

Glucksman M: Physiological changes and clinical events during psychotherapy, in Mind, Body, and the Psychotherapeutic Process (cassette tape). Joint meeting of the American Academy of Psychoanalysis and the American Psychiatric Association, Toronto, Canada, May 15-21, 1982

Glucksman M: Physiological measures and feedback during psychotherapy. Psychother Psychosom 36:185-199, 1981

Graham C, Fotopoulos SS, Cullen HD, et al: The Use of Biofeedback During Acute Opiate Withdrawal: A Double-Blind Evaluation. Proceedings of Biofeedback Research Society, 1976

Green E, Green A, Walters D: Voluntary control of internal states; psychological and physiological. Journal of Transpersonal Psychology 11:1-26, 1970

Green E, Green A: Beyond Biofeedback. New York, Delta Publishing, 1977

Hauri P: Treating psychophysiologic insomnia with biofeedback. Arch Gen Psychiatry 38:752-758, 1981

Hine FR, Werman DS, Simpson DM: Effectiveness of psychotherapy: problems of research on complex phenomena. Am J Psychiatry 139:204-208, 1982

Houde RW, Wallenstein SL, Rogers A: Clinical pharmacology of analgesics: a method of assaying analgesic effect. Clinical Pharmacol Ther 1:163-174, 1960

Jacobson E: Progressive Relaxation. Chicago, University of Chicago Press, 1938

Kamiya J: Operant control of the EEG alpha rhythm and some of its reported effects on consciousness, in Altered States of Consciousness: A Book of Readings. Edited by Tart CT. New York, John Wiley & Sons, 1969

Kiev A: Panic attacks. Medical Tribune, May 11, 1983

Kroger WS: Clinical and Experimental Hypnosis in Medicine, Dentistry, and Psychology. Philadelphia, MJ Lippincott Co, 1977

Landis B: Personal communication, 1983

Lasagna RS, Mosteller F, von Felsinger JM, et al: A study of the placebo response. Am J Med 16:770-779, 1954

LaVallee YJ, Lamontagne Y, Pinard G, et al: Effects of EMG feedback, Diazepam, and their combination on chronic anxiety. J Psychosom Res 21:65-71, 1977

Lazarus RS: A cognitively oriented psychologist looks at biofeedback. Am Psychol 20:553-561, 1975

Levine JD, Gordon NC, Fields HL: The mechanism of placebo anaesthesia. Lancet 654-657, 1977

Lubar J, Shabsin H, Natelson S, et al: EEG operant conditioning in intractable epileptics. Arch Neurol 38:700-704, 1981

Lubar JF, Deering WM: Behavioral Approaches to Neurology. New York, Academic Press, 1981

Luthe W (ed): Autogenic Methods, vols 1-4. New York, Grune & Stratton, 1969

Mathew RJ, Larsen VW, Dobbins K, et al: Biofeedback control of skin temperature and cerebral blood flow in migraine. Headache 20:19-28, 1980

Melzack R, Perry C: Self-regulation of pain: the use of alpha feedback and hypnotic training for the control of chronic pain. Exp Neurol 46:452-469, 1975

Miller NE, Bunuazizi A: Instrumental learning by curarized rats of a specific visceral response, intestinal or cardiac. J Comp Physiol Psychol 65:1-7, 1968

Mittleman B, Wolff HG: Affective states and skin temperature: experimental study of subjects with "cold hands" and Raynaud's syndrome. Psychosom Med 1:271-292, 1939

Pavlov IP: Conditioned Reflexes. London, Oxford University Press, 1927

Pickering TG, Brucker B, Frankel HL, et al: Mechanisms of learned voluntary control of blood pressure in patients with generalized bodily paralysis, in Biofeedback and Behavior. Edited by Beatty J, Legewie H. New York, Plenum, 1977

Rickles WH, Onoda L, Doyle CC: Task force study section report: biofeedback as an adjunct to psychotherapy. Biofeedback Self Regul 7:1-33, 1982

Rickles W: Some Theoretical Aspects of the Psychodynamics of Successful Biofeedback Treatment. Proceeds of the Biofeedback Research Society, 1976

Rossi EL (ed): The Collected Papers of Milton H Erickson, vols 1-4. New York, Irvington Publishers, 1980

Russel H, Carter R: Academic gains in learning disabled children after biofeedback-relaxation training. San Diego, Proceedings of the Biofeedback Society of America, February 1979

Sargent J, Walters D, Green E: Psychosomatic self-regulation of migraine headaches. Seminars in Psychiatry 5:415-428, 1973

Schuster M: Biofeedback control of gastrointestinal motility, in Biofeedback Principles and Practices for Clinicians. Edited by Basmajian JV. Baltimore, Williams & Wilkins Co, 1979

Shapiro D, Tursky B, Schwartz GE: Differentiation of heart rate and systolic blood pressure in man by operant conditioning. Psychosom Med 32:417-423, 1970

Shouse M, Lubar J: Operant conditioning of EEG rhythms and Ritalin in the treatment of hyperkinesis. Biofeedback Self Regul 4:299-312, 1979

Skinner BF: The Behavior of Organisms. New York, Appleton-Century-Crofts, 1938

Steiner S, Dince W: Biofeedback efficacy studies: a critique of critiques. Biofeedback Self Regul 6:275-288, 1981

Sterman MB, MacDonald LR: Effects of central cortical EEG feedback training on incidence of poorly controlled seizures. Epilepsia 19:207-222, 1978

Sterman MB: Neurophysiologic and clinical studies of sensorimotor EEG biofeedback training: some effects on epilepsy. Seminars in Psychiatry 5:507-524, 1973

Stroebel C, Glueck B: Biofeedback treatment in medicine and psychiatry: an ultimate placebo? Seminars in Psychiatry 5:379-393, 1973

Stroebel C: The Quieting Reflex. New York, GP Putnam's Sons, 1982

Stroebel E, Stroebel C, Holland M: Kiddie QR: A Choice for Children (cassette tapes). Wethersfield, Conn, QR Institute, 1980

Szajnberg N, Diamond S: Biofeedback, migraine headache, and new symptom formation. Headache 20:29-31, 1980

Task Force on Biofeedback: Task Force Report 19: Biofeedback, Washington, DC, American Psychiatric Association, 1979

Taub E, Stroebel CF: Biofeedback in the treatment of vasoconstrictive syndromes. Biofeedback Self Regul 3:363,–373, 1978

Toomin MK, Toomin H: GSR biofeedback in psychotherapy: some clinical observations. Psychotherapy: Theory, Research and Practice 12:1-10, 1975

Weiss JM: Somatic effects of predictable and unpredictable shock. Psychosom Med 32:397, 1970

Weiss T, Engel BT: Operant conditioning of heart rate in patients with premature ventricular contractions. Psychosom Med 33:301-321, 1971

Werbach MR: Biofeedback and psychotherapy. Am J Psychother 31:376-582, 1977

Whatmore G, Kohli DR: The Physiopathology and Treatment of Functional Disorders. New York, Grune & Stratton, 1974

Wolpe J: Psychotherapy by Reciprocal Inhibition. Palo Alto, Calif, Stanford University Press, 1958

13
Milieu Therapy

13

Milieu Therapy

INTRODUCTION

Milieu therapy addresses the context within which the management and care of a sick person take place and seeks to change that context so that it will help restore the person to health. Its defining characteristic is the presence of a designed environment, one uniquely intended to provide the conditions necessary for treatment to occur or, more precisely, one that is in itself part of the treatment. Originally, the theory of milieu demanded nothing less than that it be total and comprehensive; subsequently, many partial models have emerged such as day hospital, weekend care, or partial care (as in a therapeutic nursery setting).

Milieu design embraces a large array of variables. Such elements as site, architecture, the allocation of space, the structuring of human interaction, the establishment of channels of communication within the staff-patient matrix, the organization of the power structure, the creation—and maintenance—of an ethos, the sequencing of time allotments, and the assigning of rhythms to the pace of living are all part of the treatment.

In implementing milieu treatment, the therapist is eventually concerned with fine details. Thus, if we consider merely the physical environment, then the impact of the setting, the character of the wall surfacing, the color schemes, the fixtures, the ornaments, the furniture, not to mention the maintenance and replacement policies, the freedom of patients to decorate or otherwise use wall space, in short, everything about the physical ordering of the setting would be recognized to play a role. On that level alone, the wealth of detail that demands attention is of startling magnitude. But that serves merely to restate the elementary truth of milieu therapy: The total environment is part of the treatment.

The roster of significant milieu elements is a long one; indeed, if one were merely to tally the human factors involved, the list would be endless. All of the possible interpersonal interactions within the setting have been pondered by the practitioners of one milieu theory or another; and a host of different devices, e.g., life space interviews, role modeling, limit setting, behavioral rewards, interpretation of behavior, reality orientation, corrective emotional experience, and so on have been shown to be functional and important. In general, it seems fair to say that almost every exchange between staff and patients, as well as those arising among the patients themselves, has been recognized as carrying significant weight.

Therapy can be thought of as the application of a theory of healing within a patterned human interaction. This model clearly applies to milieu therapy with the qualification that in this modality, the number of elements in the pattern is unusually large. Far beyond what is true for any other therapeutic tactic, this treatment approach implies complexity. Its primary mission is the creation of a pattern of interwoven treatment techniques set within an environment designed for repair which will collectively effect the desired change.

Recently, the nature of milieu practices has undergone radical transformation. Historically, in their landmark study, Stanton and Schwartz (1954) spoke of the relatively low prestige accorded to the other 23 hours as compared to the awe in which the psychotherapy hour was held. We have come far since that day. Significant developments in the last few decades have fostered tremendous movement in the nature of hospital psychiatry; and such innovative efforts as partial hospital, day hospital, and other flexible adaptations of theory and method have flourished. These changes have occurred in the context of widespread social transformations that have led us away from the nearly exclusive focus on the intrapsychic dynamics of the mentally ill and on toward an appreciation of the force of biological, interpersonal, and environmental influences. Maxwell Jones (1968a) suggested that " . . . the psychoanalytical model, with its preoccupation with conflicts as it were within the individual and its stress upon a two-person treatment relationship, must be complemented by a much greater understanding of group dynamics, social therapy, and of social organization generally. . . . " Social psychiatry has been defined by the World Health Organization (1959) as "the preventive and curative measures which are directed toward the fitting of the individual for a satisfactory and useful life in terms of his own social environment." The development of community psychiatry has taken place within this broad concept, with an emphasis on such principles as continuity of care, community aftercare services, outreach, crisis intervention, and preventive psychiatry. Milieu therapy has represented the intramural counterpart to these community based efforts (Arthur, 1973; Bettelheim and Sylvester, 1948; Edelson, 1970; Jones, 1976).

Numerous attempts have been made to differentiate among the terms "milieu therapy," "therapeutic milieu," and "therapeutic community," but they continue to be used interchangeably. Rapoport (1960) defines the therapeutic community as follows:

> According to this approach, the hospital is seen not as a place where patients are classified, and stored, nor a place where one group of individuals (the medical staff) gives treatment to another group of individuals (the patients) according to the model of general medical hospitals; but as a place which is organized as a community in which everyone is expected to make some contribution towards the shared goals of creating a social organization that will have healing properties.

As commonly used, however, milieu therapy is based on a more general set of assumptions. These assert that there are social processes in any environment which can be brought to bear therapeutically on the patient; the problem then becomes how best to do so.

The acceptance of this concept is not universal. Thus, Abroms (1969) regards milieu therapy as "clearly a treatment context rather than a specific technique." Van Putten and May (1976), however, state the case as it is more generally accepted:

> Milieu therapy is now commonly prescribed for virtually all mental disorders as a form of . . . treatment on the supposition that the proper environment can exert a therapeutic effect on all who are exposed to it. To this end the patient is expected . . . to participate in a treatment program that includes varying degrees of occupational therapy, group activity, vocational rehabilitation, educational therapy, industrial therapy, resocialization, remotivation, total push . . . patient government, recreational activities, formal individual and/or group psychotherapy, and so forth.

In attempting to give an account of the present status of milieu therapy, this chapter will take a developmental approach. The environmental factors appropriate for work with preschoolers and the techniques of therapy designed to help them differ from the methods and configurations calculated to benefit older children or adults. Each developmental level has its own schools and its own strategies. The role of milieu therapy within the culture is, in many ways, in a state of flux, with terms such as deinstitutionalization, warehousing, and custodial care bearing large admixtures of political, economic—and emotional—significance. In fact, none of these pertains to milieu therapy as treatment; rather they each speak of its abandonment or absence. In any case it is a factor in the treatment of the neediest and the sickest patients; it is expensive and demands much in the present. It also promises much for the future.

HISTORICAL BACKGROUND

In keeping with the developmental approach, we will consider in turn the history of efforts to serve the disturbed preschooler, the child and adolescent, the adult, and the aged. The account cannot be exhaustive, but some of the high points will be mentioned.

The emergence of the therapeutic nursery carried forward at once the traditions of both education and therapy. Each of these fields represents a major cultural current; each is in accord with and in conflict with the other at many points. Presently special education has emerged as a means of integrating expertise in a multi-modal fashion.

One aspect of eighteenth-century enlightenment was an increasing interest in children and a growing belief that early rearing had significant effects on the life pattern. By the mid-nineteenth century the notion of a kindergarten or nursery school had already taken form. The concept included concern for early socialization with peers in a congenial environment. Such nurseries and kindergartens usually consisted of small groups of fewer than 15 children. The youngsters learned some skills and received training in early motor activities via perceptually-oriented games. Together these served to prepare them for the acquisition of later intellectual skills.

The richest advances of the nursery school idea grew out of the severe impact that the two world wars had on children and families. Again and again society had to cope with displaced children who were separated from their families and who had to be cared for in groups. Zigfried Bernfeld (1929) created what he called the "Baumgarten," a type of play setting that used educational methods (based on psychoanalytic techniques) with war orphans. Anna Freud and Dorothy Burlingham (1973) used similar techniques during World War II for children who were displaced and evacuated. In time, the crisis intervention approaches of that earlier day were extended and applied to children with emotional problems. Later, similar measures were introduced for children with retardation and severe mental illness.

Between the two world wars, psychiatric therapy began to be applied to young children. Initially it focused on the preschooler with a symptomatic disorder. The interventions required by such children could often be adapted to nursery school settings—indeed, they could typically be delivered best within that context. One of the great bridging concepts that had recently come into being was the idea that children's play was more than fun or the mere discharge of excess energy; it was communicative and could, in fact, be considered the equivalent of free association. Hence play was a vehicle for therapy and a subject whose content was amenable to study and intervention. With this realization, the field of nursery school behavior became a site for understanding and interpretation. At first this concept was confined to work with individual children; only later were these efforts directed toward groups.

In this way the broad current of educational practice, which for many years had been addressing itself to children in kindergartens, was now intermingled with the powerful stimulus of these newer therapeutic concepts; ultimately each was profoundly affected by the other. Today, normal children in preschool nurseries are managed in part by means of practices derived from therapeutic principles and knowledge. The basic model for such settings has been shaped largely by new developmental and rehabilitative information. Modern nursery school practice shows the influences of Piaget and Montessori as well as the permeating presence of the thinking of Dewey and the insights of Sigmund Freud. For their part, the therapeutic settings also embody these principles; but, of necessity, they lean far more heavily toward the side of the clinical: The therapist has a voice in management as well as the teacher. Within such treatment contexts it seems fair to say that the emphasis now falls far more directly on the search for ways to restore developmental process to its intact state than on any quest for "cure" as such.

Parallel with these trends but quite independent of them there was coming into being a separate universe that concerned itself with the management of the handicapped child. For decades, a whole group of educators and special therapists had been seeking ways to help blind and deaf children. These dedicated practitioners had already established the necessity of special schooling for three- and four-year-olds. They had also underlined how important it was to provide special training to teachers who were to work with such handicapping conditions. The many years of such efforts were finally crowned by national recognition: In 1979, Congress passed a law that gave all handicapped children the right to receive free public education. This federal legislation has created an ever more pressing demand that special educators, social workers, psychologists, and child psychiatrists join forces and work together. The therapeutic nursery has become a major site for such cooperation.

Side by side with these developments, the creation of special environments for older children and adolescents had gone on apace—albeit less rapidly and in a more uneven fashion. Before 1900, most such efforts were in the penal realm where the presence of antisocial behavior thrust the youngsters forcibly onto the consciousness—and the conscience—of the professional world. At the time the theory of managing these troubled teenagers required repentance and reform, which led, respectively, to the creation of the penitentiary and the reform school. From time to time there were isolated independent efforts to seek alternative ways to deal with such troubled youth; thus, the George Junior Republics that were established around the turn of the century sought to use the principles of democracy and self government as the basis for reparative efforts. These created a minor impact but were little more than harbingers of things to come.

In Europe, in 1925, August Aichhorn had written a book that was perhaps the first modern description of milieu therapy (Aichhorn, 1935). It was an account of a project that Aichhorn and his associates had carried on at the institution for delinquents which he directed. In brief, it described the effects of a program of determined nonintervention in the management of these youngsters as they struggled to adapt to this *laissez faire* environment. Although not emulated by later practitioners, it was a model for the creation of a planned environment based on psychoanalytic principles which was to have profound implications for future efforts in this field.

It is of interest that Aichhorn's work was more or less contemporary with the innovations introduced by Makarenko (1940) in the USSR. There, too, the elaboration of a new conceptual structure, the Communist view of man and society, led to the establishment of an institution for vagrant delinquent youth. In the Gorki colony, which he founded, the problem was approached in a new way. Hard work, fair treatment, and the regular inculcation of idealistic principles were the basis of the experiment. Makarenko was an educator who fiercely believed that genetic theories and developmental concepts were fallacious. For him, education was all, and he sought environmental means for creating the new "Marxist man."

In the United States, the first medical settings for children with severe psychological problems came into being in response to organic illness. The epidemic of von Economo's encephalitis which ravaged America in the early 1920's led to the founding of a number of centers for brain injured children. Thus, the Emma Pendleton Bradley Hospital, established in 1931, is said to have been the first psychiatric hospital for children in the country. Withal, however, no general style of treatment had yet emerged.

During the 1920's, the child guidance clinic became part of the American landscape. This was a powerful new movement that caught the imagination of many professionals and had a considerable impact on the public at large. In its wake, a number of orphanages, settings for neglected and dependent children, and agencies for delinquents began to incorporate a mental health professional into their staff structure. Initially this might be an isolated social worker or psychologist, but presently a whole child guidance clinic would be added as part of the staffing pattern. In time the influence of the clinic came to permeate the everyday life of the children, and a new kind of environment began to appear.

The key factor in these centers' functioning was the conscious attempt to apply psychological principles in a consistent way to the children's difficulties. This process involved a particularly intense concern with the details of milieu structuring, and a unique treatment flavor emerged. It was built on the principle of establishing a home-like atmosphere around the disturbed youngsters so that the therapeutic management would be directed as much to their healthy growth as it was to the amelioration of their symptoms. The group of agencies that adopted this course began to call themselves residential treatment centers, and soon a goodly handful of such centers were in practice around the country.

Meanwhile a number of child analysts, many of them influenced by Aichhorn, had begun to direct their attention toward the institutionalized child. In particular, Bettelheim and Sylvester (1948), working at a school for severely sick children, introduced the term "milieu therapy." With this they set the framework for all future efforts in the field. Among other things, they stated the principle that a central dynamic concept should be formulated for each child. This could then be shared and communicated among all staff members so that everyone's approach to the child would be guided by the same basic understanding. More than that, they asserted the need for a consistent caretaker as central to treatment. Shortly after this development, the work of Redl and Wineman (1951) extended the idea to developing specific means for coping with each element in the ego of the delinquent child. A rich growth in theory and method followed. Many authors began to contribute to the field, and residential treatment centers were opened all over the country. By and large they approached their clients within a framework of understanding derived from psychoanalytic thinking. All the children were at least in individual therapy, many were in both group and individual treatment, and most families were in casework.

Toward the end of the 1950's, a new school of psychological intervention made its initial appearance. Behavioral techniques had begun to be described in the literature; and as the 1960's advanced, there was a tremendous flowering of behavioral theory and method. More and more tactics for the management of children based on this approach were introduced and incorporated into even the most conservative, dynamically-oriented settings. The use of behavioral contracts, some sort of level system, a token economy, "time out," and a variety of other devices of that type became commonplace.

Unfortunately, the 1960's saw not only new methods but new problems. Thus, substance abuse became an ever more widespread phenomenon among children and teenagers. This realization brought in its wake a group of settings designed to deal specifically with this problem. These environments used some of the recently developed community approaches, but they turned as well to a set of unusual group strategies and confrontational dynamics in order to achieve their ends. Synanon offered a first model, but other such settings soon appeared. In general these blended elements of the religious-mystical, group survival, and community therapy approaches. Generally speaking, they all used group confrontation—often a form of group denunciation—as a cardinal principle.

During the 1970's, a much wider range of institutional forms emerged along with a decided shift of care toward hospital-type settings. In particular this transition was fostered by economic considerations since it became easier to obtain reimbursement from third-party payors if services were offered within a hospital. Many short-term diagnostic and brief therapy units appeared, psychopharmacological methods became widespread, and novel diagnostic entities such as narcissistic syndromes, childhood depression, and attention deficit disorder became the new foci of interest. Meanwhile, the earlier predominance of the long-term residential treatment center gave way to a far more heterogeneous array of agencies and methods.

As the decade advanced, some of the children who were being treated for these problems—along with the many who needed treatment and failed to get it—were growing up and becoming adults who, in their turn, needed psychiatric help for the later versions or the residual aspects of these difficulties. Let us now turn to an account of the milieu methods in that adult realm.

The moral treatment of psychiatric patients may be considered the first psychiatric revolution. The movement was begun abroad by Pinel, Tuke, and others and was extended to the United States by the early influence of the Quakers and by such reformers as Dorothea Dix (Maxmen et al., 1974; Wolf, 1977). In the early part of the twentieth century, the second psychiatric revolution came about as a result of the impact of the newly emerging psychoanalytic movement on psychiatric thinking. Although it is safe to say that these effects were far reaching, they could not penetrate beyond the walls of the large state hospitals in which the vast majority of the sickest psychiatric patients were "warehoused" under the most overcrowded, understaffed, deplorable conditions. For many years little was done to change this state of affairs. Part of the problem lay in the deep vein of antipathy toward the mentally ill which permeated the culture; another part arose from the lack of effective treatment methods to cope with these chronic conditions (Goffman, 1961). Even in acute-care hospitals, the relatively short-term patients were more often contained and sedated than given any sort of definitive treatment.

A few sites, however, introduced innovative methods and new approaches to management. Ingenious practitioners at a number of small private hospitals began to find ways of applying psychoanalytic ideas to even the sickest patients. The Menninger Clinic, Chestnut Lodge, and Austen Riggs Center were among the leaders in the development of these new strategies. Sullivan (1931) reported on the intensive treatment of a small group of schizophrenic patients at the Sheppard and Enoch Pratt Hospital. He emphasized an interpersonal approach that involved the use of a variety of hospital personnel. Menninger (1936) devised a method of teaching staff how to employ a series of prescribed attitudes to respond specifically to each patient's particular symptom profile. In 1946, Main (1946), at the Menninger Foundation, suggested that the traditional doctor-patient relationship was not a good approach to psychiatric patients because such patients became the *objects* of treatment efforts instead of responsible participants in the work of seeking recovery. He coined the phrase "therapeutic community" to describe a treatment milieu within which all staff and patients joined together to share in the therapeutic task.

In England, Maxwell Jones seized on these conceptualizations and began to apply them in a novel and exciting way. With the powerful example of his efforts to give these ideas substance and method, a therapeutic community movement came into being which some have considered to be a third psychiatric revolution (Dreikurs, 1955). At the same time, a parallel development was emerging which was to be of fundamental importance to all ensuing psychiatric practice—the appearance of a whole universe of psychopharmacologic theory and practice. Thorazine (chlorpromazine) and Serpasil (reserpine) were introduced almost simultaneously; and suddenly, back ward patients who had been silent for years or who were otherwise uncontrollable or unapproachable began to speak rationally and to take an interest in their surroundings. This development, too, has been spoken of as a third psychiatric revolution, although the two developments took place simultaneously.

The therapeutic community movement evolved within the context of the advancing civil rights movement in the United States and took fire from it. Once again the reformers were breaking the chains of the oppressed, in this case the mentally ill. As is typical of such movements, it was a two-edged sword: Ultimately, its benefits will have to be weighed against the problems that came in its train.

With these innovations, state hospitals became quieter but they remained understaffed and gave little heed to the newly developing milieu therapy techniques. Stanton and Schwartz (1954) published a searching study of the mental hospital in which they showed the impact of the environment and the staff on the manifest pathology of the hospitalized patients. Cumming and Cumming (1962) built on these studies and sought to translate ego psychology into a set of milieu principles that could be applied on a hospital ward. Jones (Jones et al., 1953; Jones, 1956, 1957, 1968b) worked initially with military stress syndromes and then with chronic character disorders to develop the principles and methods of community psychiatry which remain indelibly linked with his name. Rapoport (1960) studied the outcome of Jones' work at Belmont Hospital in England and added significantly to the understanding of what went into this approach. At the same time Jones had come to the United States and had worked to further the spread of these ideas to this shore. His approach emphasized such ideals as democratization, the relative elimination of bureaucratic hierarchies, and a blurring of roles among staff members and between staff and patients so that authority could be more equably distributed. Inevitably, these methods flourished in the climate of the 1960's.

In the midst of this ferment, there appeared the report of the Joint Commission on Mental Illness and Health (1961). With the support of President John F. Kennedy, the report's recommendations gave rise to an intensive reorganization of the mental health delivery system in America. Among the many changes that were initiated was the incorporation of many therapeutic principles into treatment facilities for all ages.

This transformation extended even to the most neglected of all patient groups, the aged. Historically, elderly people with psychiatric disorders have not been considered amenable to most forms of psychiatric intervention—including milieu methods. Indeed, the concept that the environment in which the elderly person lives or in which he receives treatment should be structured in keeping with sound psychological principles (i.e., in a fashion that would enhance improved psychological and cognitive functioning) is a relatively new one. When institutionalization did occur, the goal was usually not to provide treatment for the presenting problem but to maintain the patient at the current level of functioning and to meet his or her daily needs at minimal cost in a custodial setting.

The first attempt to treat elderly patients actively in an institutional setting occurred at the Salpetrière in the early 1800's under the direction of Pinel (Hader and Seltzer, 1967). Although this hospital later became famous for its treatment of younger adult psychiatric patients, it was founded originally for the treatment of elderly indigents. Such patients were managed in a separate unit in which environmental manipulation, exercise, diet, and nursing care were considered essential to the treatment of problems associated with old age.

Over the years, however, psychiatric care for the elderly has traditionally been neglected. The general lack of interest in responding to this population arises from a number of factors. It is only recently that a relatively large proportion of the population has survived into old age and, thus, become a focus of both public and psychiatric attention. Formerly, many mental health professionals were reluctant to treat older adults because of a conviction that the elderly are unresponsive to psychiatric ministrations. During the 1960's and 1970's, however, interest increased in developing innovative and effective approaches and in adapting treatment modalities such as milieu therapy for use with elderly psychiatric patients.

THEORETICAL ISSUES AND MODELS

Nursery Schools

The four most influential models to be found in current practice are the therapeutic group, psychoanalytic, behavioral, and educational models. Although they all follow similar principles, the specific programs diverge from one another on key points. Withal, however, if the laws of learning as described by the behaviorists apply to all aspects of human behavior, it would follow that no matter what the care giver's therapeutic predilection, similar tactics might emerge for approaches that stem from widely differing theories.

The Therapeutic Group Model. As applied to preschoolers, therapeutic group work has used play therapy within a group context with or without accompanying observational interaction by mothers. In general, the milieu is designed so that the child's individual emotional expression as he interacts with peers and with play materials can be readily observed. Appropriate interpretations may then be made.

Such an approach is exemplified by the commonly encountered preventive group (so often part of a liaison program). This strategy might be used with children who share some recent or anticipated trauma such as a divorce in the family, impending surgery, or the loss of a parent. The therapeutic methods borrow from insight-oriented and cathartic play models and may last for many months with transfer to individual work as needed (Lopez and Kliman, 1980). It is expected that group play therapy will effect basic changes in the child's intrapsychic equilibrium; his capacity for relationships; and his reality testing through catharsis, insight, sublimation, and/or social group feedback.

This methodology has influenced a variety of group interventions which have been devised to meet the needs of specific preschool populations. Some seek to alter the child's behavior directly, whereas others emphasize parental reorientation. For example, where such problems as retardation, pervasive developmental disorder, or cerebral palsy are present, such youngsters might all too readily be excluded from important dimensions of interactive experience. Hence, groups have been formed to offer these vulnerable children a range of activities appropriate to their age and abilities, especially those forms of expression which bring them into communicative interaction with their peers. An essential ingredient in these groups is the active involvement of the mothers (and often of the fathers as well) to enhance both physical care and parental communication with the child.

In a comparable approach, Nielson (1970) conducts family group sessions for children who range in age between infancy and three years. Mothers meet in a group with a therapist while watching their children interact with teachers and with one another. These meetings focus on the nature of play plus its role and importance in child development. Since play is a form of masked communication, its interpretation remains the responsibility of the therapists. They must explain the behavior as it occurs and convey its meaning to the parent as a means to increase caring and understanding. They must also be alert to the parent's capacity to tolerate such insights and to respond constructively. To do so appropriately, these therapists must have a firm grasp on the child's cognitive and emotional level. Thus, aggressive behavior toward a peer may be imitative of interactions the child has observed, it may be territorial and protective against intrusion, and it may even be a stereotypic pattern that lacks all conscious intent.

Hansen et al. (1969) use modeling theory with socially isolated children of low socioeconomic background to show that they will respond well to peer models. The immediate goal of this group effort is to alter their interactional patterns.

The disorders that tend to isolate children require maximal exposure to peer groups along with sensitive observation and monitoring. Special educators trained in this work watch for affinities with particular materials. These are then used, first in isolation and later in parallel play next to another child. The youngster is given gentle encouragement to acknowledge the presence of the peer. In time, further expansion and generalization of this behavior comes about by adding verbal designations and other representations. These educators are specially skilled at using adult approval as a force making for success.

Psychoanalytic Models. This approach provides an opportunity for using psychoanalytic insights into development in the service of a long-term study of children in need. These practitioners look to children's displaced verbalizations and behavior as their prime source of significant information about the child's longings, underlying conflicts, responses to loss and separation, and peer interaction.

Psychoanalytic theory holds that biologic dependency requires a buffering parent. When the infant's stimulus barrier is faulty or when mothering is inadequate, the infant may withdraw or develop in a deviant direction. Bettelheim (1967), a child analyst, social scientist, and educator, directed the Sonia Shankman Orthogenic School at the University of Chicago where he worked with a large number of autistic children. In considering the etiology of this condition, he suggested that pathological mothers respond to the child's withdrawal with counterwithdrawal and that they then reject their unresponsive child, leaving him empty, autistic, and impervious to social engagement. The child responds to the maternal hostility with rage, feelings of powerlessness, and complete withdrawal. For Bettelheim (1967), the autistic child (and children with similar states) displayed such behavior as self-mutilation, echolalia, insistence on sameness, etc. in an attempt to maintain homeostasis in his psychic environment. The child's autistic behavior was thus regarded as defensive, and treatment efforts based on these theoretical formulations sought to establish an environment within which the child would no longer need to rely on such maneuvers. Thus, Bettelheim required that children be separated from their parents for long periods of time (as long as a number of years in some cases) while they received care in the therapeutic setting. This separation was considered essential to the establishment of trust and autonomy; only when this development had come about could family ties be reinstituted. Within the setting, a large measure of regressive behavior was tolerated. The child was regarded as striving to relive prior experiences in an attempt to free himself from a burdensome past, and the milieu was designed to help him do this. Active pedagogy was intrinsic to the process, and even the sickest children were maintained in school.

Mahler (1952), a child analyst and child psychiatrist, also studied psychotic children in great depth. She described the state of symbiotic fusion which prevails during early development and suggested that in one type of childhood psychosis, the child withdraws into autism if the symbiotic object is lost at a critical period. Under such circumstances the child cannot use mothering; and the goal of treatment, therefore, becomes the re-establishment of the symbiotic tie to the mother. To this end, Mahler suggested a tripartite therapeutic design that includes mother, the autistic or symbiotic child, and the therapist all working together to achieve a "corrective-symbiotic experience." The child communicates his need in the form of deviant behavior; and the therapeutic task is to sensitize and facilitate maternal responsiveness to the child's cues, accomplished by a pattern of close working together. This paradigm serves as well to provide a nursery model because the nursery group becomes a prime site for observation and understanding and thus complements the work with mother and child.

Alpert (1954) treated severe developmental disturbances of preschoolers in a group setting. The central concept in her formulations was the presence in the child of a pathologically exaggerated dependency on the mother. Therapy was, therefore, structured in the form of a "corrective object relations" approach. In the course of this work, the child's dependent needs were transferred from mother to teacher in order to effect a less traumatic disengagement. As treatment got under way, a pattern of "guided regression," which involved the gratification of infantile needs, was used as a starting point for new experiences and achievements. Work with the mother was directed toward relieving both her separation anxiety and her distorted communication with her child.

Behavior Therapy Models. Behavioral theorists have not overly concerned themselves with etiological issues. Instead they have sought to promote changes in specific behaviors, which were then observed and measured directly for any increase or decrease in their frequency of occurrence. This methodology goes back to the basic assumption of behavioral theory, i.e., that the frequency of occurrence of any behavior depends on what follows it rather than on what preceded it. Be they positive or negative, it is the consequences of the behavior which shape its form.

Where other schools of psychotherapy have concentrated on changing the individual's perceptions, feelings, and thoughts, behavior therapists have emphasized the impact of the patient's activity on his environment and the responses he, in turn, receives from his surroundings. In devising a therapeutic plan, the timing and frequency of the positive reinforcers (or rewards) that follow a desirable act are the important components of the treatment schedule. More than that, such therapists try to define any undesirable behavior in operational terms. They observe and analyze the frequency of its appearance, seek any circumstances that seem to reduce the occurrence of that particular behavior, and specify the factors responsible for its termination. Once an appropriate reward system is established and the undesired behavior is eliminated, alternative rewards serve to maintain and to encourage an internal locus of control. Thus, food as reward may be replaced by external praise, which may in turn give way to the child's own vocal self praise or inner speech and control.

At first glance, these measures do not seem to apply to the nursery setting. However, they have, in fact, been used successfully in groups, especially for retarded and deviant children. This technique requires individual assessment of the specific asocial behavior in the groups. Individual interventions may then be devised for the group routines and, over time, the behavior shaped toward more positive social aims. Less severe disorders, including excessive aggression in nursery groups, have also been interrupted successfully by means of reinforcement techniques and reward systems for prosocial behavior. It seems safe to say that an analysis of results with psychoanalytic or general educational methods suggests that an element of reward is operative in those contexts as well.

Historically, behavioral techniques and interventions based on operant conditioning have been derived primarily from the work of B.F. Skinner (see chapter entitled "Behavior Therapy"). Skinner built his work on Thorndike's principle that the environmental consequences of behavior serve to reinforce its occurrence; this holds true for both desirable activities and undesirable behavior. Functional analyses of such events led to systematic programs designed either to reinforce prosocial behavior or to ignore—and thus to extinguish—isolating or disruptive behavior. C.B. Ferster, one of Skinner's students, along with M. DeMyer, a child psychiatrist, were among the first to show that the limited behavioral repertoire of a previously unreachable autistic child could be extended through the use of systematic reinforcement of desired behavior (where food served as the reinforcing agent) (Ferster and DeMyer, 1961). Thus, through the reinforcement of more appropriate patterns, the behavior of an unresponsive autistic child could be made to assume at least the appearance of greater normality. Similar techniques were soon introduced into and became part of the routine practice of all therapeutic nursery group management.

Within this framework, Lovaas et al. (1974) suggest that therapy be directed toward three specific areas: self-destructive, self-stimulative, and language behavior. Thus, in autistic children with low IQ's, self-destructive behavior has been successfully diminished by means of both positive rewards and aversive methods. Such techniques have also been directed toward the delayed and deviant language of these children. Positive reinforcement has been reported to transform echolalic speech into more appropriate communication. It has been noted, however, that the increase is chiefly in the number of lexical items and phrases and not in linguistic complexity. Moreover, when the reinforcement schedules are not maintained, those gains tend to be lost (Lovaas et al., 1966). The same issue arises with the attempts to teach autistic children sign language. One can increase the child's lexicon, but this does not appear to bring about more complex combinations of signs (Tager-Flusberg, 1981).

Aversive techniques require that an unpleasant stimulus be inflicted upon the patient. To say the least, these methods have been controversial, and many practitioners have regarded them as inhumane or unethical. Nonetheless, positive results have been claimed with cases of psychotic children who were treated for headbanging or for self-stimulating rituals that interfered with social interaction. This area requires the most careful weighing of the potential danger or harmfulness of the child's behavior plus the hoped for gains, on the one hand, against the possibly unethical or inhumane character of the suggested intervention on the other.

Educational Models. The educational approach arose from the belief that severely disturbed and deviant children suffered from some form of central nervous system disorder with accompanying cognitive and language deficits. The remedy implicit in this style of intervention takes the form of special educational techniques. To determine the nature of the problem, the child is given an initial interdisciplinary psychoeducational assessment that seeks to evaluate developmental performance in multiple areas. Some of these tests, such as puzzles and blocks, involve motor and intersensory integration; others require the cognitive abilities necessary to manage numbers, distinguish colors, execute fine and gross motor movements, perform adequately at play, etc. With this approach, the child's developmental levels and a profile of abilities are determined; these in turn define areas of strength and weakness for which the academic program is individually designed. Parallel with this undertaking the clinician has been evaluating the emotional and relationship status of the child with an eye to symptoms, interactions with parents and peers, and suggestive biological factors. The special educator and the clinician then work collaboratively to design the child's program.

Schopler and Reichler's TEACCH (Treatment and Education of Autistic and Related Communications for Handicapped Children) approach (1971) aims to provide the interventions necessary to foster growth in three areas in which the autistic child is thought to be especially deficient: (a) human relatedness, (b) perceptual-motor organization, and (c) cognitive functioning. An important component of this strategy is the inclusion of parents in every aspect of treatment and teaching. It is asserted that the use of parents as co-therapists facilitates the acquisition, maintenance, and generalization of the skills taught to the child. This method also serves to increase the child's educational exposure time at home.

Hefner and Balliett* have combined educational approaches with special attention to all varieties of communication difficulties between parent and

*Hefner EC, Balliett E: Utilization of existing community resources for delivery of mental health services to preschool children (unpublished manuscript)

child. This model has been applied to the broadest range of diagnostic groups. These practitioners depart from the assumption that the behaviorally deviant child produces many cues, both verbal and nonverbal. Their goal is to increase parental competence in understanding these messages. The two central components of their approach are thus an increase in confident parenting and the discovery of the communication value of children's behavior.

In practice, the children and their mothers are seen in groups that meet in adjoining rooms separated by a one-way screen. An open door allows easy access from one to the other. The mothers also meet with a group therapist once a week while the nursery class is in session. Within the framework of a semi-structured children's group, communicative competence is fostered by means of an individually designed educational program. Each plan uses a variety of play and educational materials within the context of small social groups that meet for two to three hours daily. The significance of the children's isolated or aggressive play gradually comes to be understood. Natural affinities for a variety of play materials are noted, encouraged, and, where possible, brought into the peer arena. Positive affects are reinforced and mutuality and cognitive growth rewarded.

The parents' reactions to the way the teachers handle the children are discussed in groups, as are the many personal and interpersonal problems that emerge in the group encounters. The group leaders and the teachers do not intentionally act as models. When they are expressed, the parents' feelings of inadequacy, frustration, guilt, and rage are explored as conscious, shared experiences. Ultimately, this experience facilitates acceptance of the child's limitations and enhances appropriate planning. Despair at the slowness of the process and the lack of apparent progress, competitiveness, and meaningful gestures of mutual support are all noted in the parents. Together, these expressions of feeling help the parents face the realities of their children's diagnoses and prognoses; and in time, this process facilitates making plans for future therapy, further education, and remediation.

In general, it may be said that therapeutic nurseries whose patient/pupil populations are predominantly language disordered place particular emphasis on helping the children in the areas of verbal and nonverbal expressive language. In fact, any of the models referred to above allows for complementary language and speech training in addition to the regular program. In a similar fashion, special training in small and large motor skills has also been added to programs.

Finally, mention must be made of a group of research nurseries which have been organized to study specific syndromes or treatment modalities. Thus, in light of the finding that psychoactive drugs influence such target symptoms as excitement, assaultive behavior, self-mutilation, or apathetic withdrawal, programs have been designed to evaluate the drug treatment of psychotic preschool children.

Children and Adolescents

The Residential Treatment Center Model. Amid the many expressions used in connection with milieu therapy for children, the term *residential treatment center* (RTC) has become the preferred designation. In practice, it represents a synthesis that involves both the realm of method and the application of ethic. It implies first a primary love of children so that a sense of hovering care broods over the enterprise. This is characteristic regardless of the details of the particular method of treatment used.

The second common element is the creation of as homelike, i.e., as developmentally normal, an atmosphere as possible. In many ways, the child is offered a setting for normal growth and advance which seeks, in itself, to repair some of the hurt and supply some of the deficits that are presumed to have played a role in begetting or maintaining his difficulties.

The third common element is a basic therapeutic dimension that is built into the way the setting is organized so that treatment efforts weave through the youngster's life on many levels and in a variety of ways.

In the nature of things, there is much room for a measure of conflict among these disparate elements. As a result, the residential therapist for children faces many dilemmas. An important issue arises from the child's need for freedom to grow as well as for channels and directions along which to do his growing. In particular, structure and limits are essential nutrients of childhood; if they are lacking, healthy development will not take place. Although these limits have many roles to play, ultimately they are essential for the formation of inner controls, the critical prerequisite for social adaptation. Theory, therefore, requires that adequate control experiences be provided to the child at the same time that one is trying to deal with him primarily through understanding, insight, acceptance, and empathy. The therapist must somehow find a way to supply the child's developmental needs for freedom (for learning, adventuresome experience, experiments in relationship, moments of dependency gratification, etc.) and to carry on this process simultaneously with the structure-building dimension of the treatment.

An associated problem derives from the emphasis that such treatment settings tend to place on development. After all, the growth of a child is not a matter of treatment; it is a normal process the child should experience as such. Hence, an aware environment that expects to carry a child through a meaningful part of his growing up seeks to emphasize as much as it can of the health and normalcy of the child's interests and adaptations. But it is inherently difficult to do so with a group of sick children within an atmosphere of intensive treatment; hence, some of the insistence on a home-like setting with a strong emphasis on growth and learning rather than on illness and repair.

Another dilemma arises from the inherent tension between the existence of a group of children who need group-oriented rules and regulations and the fact that each child bears his own unique set of personality traits and problems which require recognition as individual issues for care and response. There is a continuing discord between the need to treat each child as a special person in his own right and to require at the same time that all children meet certain basic standards of social behavior in order to learn how to live in society. This conflict is a source of never ending stress for the residential therapist.

A fourth dilemma is the eternal question among staff as to whose work is primary. Does school give way so that the therapist can see the child? Or does the therapist adapt his hours to the school program? Does the teacher "bounce" the eruptive child from class, or does he call in the child care worker to do that? Who conducts the patient group meeting? A good deal of organizational work is basic to running an effective milieu program. Leadership is critical.

Yet another dilemma is the need to sort out how to be both bridge to and barrier between the child and his family. On the whole, staff members tend to be intensely child-oriented. They seek to protect their charges from the seductions, rejections, unreasonable expectations, and double binds emanating from the often highly conflicted parents. At the same time, staff members strive to maintain a working relationship with the entire kinship unit, with the goal of restoring the integrity of family life. One author who has worked primarily with severely ill adolescents regards the first 18 months or so of residential care as the resistance phase. During this time, both the youth and the family need to be engaged in intensive reparative work in order to alter their mutual pathologic interaction enough so that they can embrace the treatment effort (Rinsley, 1968). For many settings, a major dimension of therapeutic effort which seeks to address this dilemma is the inclusion of family approaches in the treatment plan. (This work may take the form of couples therapy, multiple family therapy, network therapy, etc.). Inevitably, different settings vary in the way they deal with these dilemmas.

On a more general level, it can be fairly said that the milieu itself is usually regarded as a sort of external ego that will surround the child in a developmentally supportive and therapeutic environment. To this end, the physical structure of such centers typically involves a relatively small, homelike open setting, usually with eight to 15 children living together in a social unit under the direct care of a number of trained adults. In particular, the cutting edge of therapeutic effect is achieved at the interface of interaction between the caretaking staff members and the individual children. Daytime coverage of not less than one staff person to every three children is usually considered necessary to be effective—although for economic reasons it is not always achieved.

In many settings, each encounter between a staff member and a child is regarded as a potentially therapeutic experience, and the term "life space interview" was coined (Redl, 1959) to indicate the critical character of these contacts. More than that, the entire community within which the child lives and grows comes together at regular intervals (often each morning) to hear announcements, plan group outings, discuss behavioral issues, reward progress publicly, and to enhance the feeling of belonging and participation on the part of each child.

Beyond these activities, a number of additional factors also intensify the treatment power of the milieu structure. Perhaps chief among them is the therapeutic school. Few children are considered too ill to do without schooling altogether; this instrument plays a unique and powerful role in such settings. The role of the school for the emotionally disturbed child is quite different from its place in the life of his healthier counterpart. For the child in residence, the school is a site of essential ego building where social, emotional, and cognitive functions are called upon to interact in a synergistic, integrated fashion to increase the child's adaptive competence on many fronts at once. So central is this role in the child's organization that many settings prefer to consider themselves as a form of school. Or, they may include the word "school" in their name, even though the formal educational process, with the associated emphasis on cognitive structuring, is only a fraction of what they offer the children.

Within the design of the milieu, a major focus of professional effort is on transitions (Whittaker, 1975). The move into residence, the shifts among components, and the eventual transfer to day care or outpatient treatment are critical sites for growth or for failure. Vigorous staff involvement at these junctures is, therefore, essential. For example, to deal with a move from residence to home, frequent home visits, multiple and multi-level contacts with parents, and direct involvement of the child with his home school and other outside agencies are all part of the effort.

As noted, beyond the directly therapeutic quality of the milieu, as such, most agencies use a host of formally structured therapeutic measures. These include speech and language techniques; play therapy and other interview therapies of all sorts; drama, dance, music, and art therapies; activity and recreation group methods; and a variety of special program designs geared to the sublimation potential of individual children. Many behavioral principles are applied in the form of contracts, levels, token economies, and other more individualized approaches. Thus, any given youngster is likely to be in some combination of intensive individual, group, family, and community therapy; an active behavior modification program is likely to be in place to cope with specific symptoms; and a set of privilege levels is present to encourage the child to rise gradually through the levels as his adjustment improves.

With adolescents, a wide variety of group techniques is often added to the mix of available interventions. Most fall within the framework of standard dynamically-oriented group therapy or activity group methods. Some are unusual: For example, Roth (1977) included transactional analysis as part of his work with a group.

Sanctions on disturbing behavior take many forms, the most common of which are verbal reproof, privilege loss, time out, time spent in a "quiet room," or restriction to one's own room. Some settings have a special locked section (a "social skills unit" or a "security unit") with its own assigned staff for the transient custody of a youngster who is on the verge of a major reaction or who has become upset and uncontrollable in the setting and is deemed in need of a period of respite. In a few settings that deal with very disturbed behavioral problems (Marohn, 1980), restraining cuffs may be resorted to as a temporary measure.

Where the loss of privilege is a major component of management, this sanction often applies to visits or weekends at home, and the granting or loss of these privileges has many family implications. When a youngster's behavior becomes grossly or dangerously out of hand, some units (which lack their own security areas) will have him hospitalized briefly in a closed ward setting. The ultimate sanction for the incorrigible or totally unresponsive child is to be dismissed from the residential treatment center.

A commonly enunciated principle is the emphasis on human as opposed to chemical or mechanical controls. Although psychopharmacological agents are now widely used by child psychiatrists, in general their use as part of milieu treatment lags behind the parallel modes with adults. The basic reason for hesitation in the use of these agents is the fear of disturbing the child's development, interfering with his capacity to learn, and altering his fragile sense of initiative and autonomy. New developments in the field (especially in the management of depression and anxiety) are rapidly changing this state of affairs. However, the achievement of behavioral control devolves on staff members as issues of interpersonal skill, the effective use of relationships, and, ultimately, the optimal management of countertransference feelings.

An even harder lesson that staff must learn is to determine when a look or a word is enough, when a child should be asked to leave a group for a while, and when one must intervene physically to protect and to prevent further decompensation. Staff must also learn when the stress they feel comes from within rather than from without. Physical holding of a child is almost universally accepted as a necessary technique at moments of danger or severe regression. The fact that it is often used by children as an opportunity for sensuous stimulation affects the technique of how to accomplish the holding but makes the act itself no less mandatory.

A common means of management is time-out. This involves getting a child to leave a classroom or an activity group until he can compose himself and come back. With conditions requiring more extended intervention, some version of a quiet room is often used. This might entail sending a child to his own room for a bit or placing him in a special chamber designed for the purpose until the storm blows over. He might be left there alone, he might be accompanied by a staff member, and the door might remain either open or closed depending on the needs of that child and the technique favored by that particular setting.

For the youngster with severe eruptive patterns or with major difficulties in managing impulse, "specialing" or "shadowing" is often used. The youngster is required to stay close to a given staff member all the time. Any attempt to move away is countered immediately by the "special"; more severe disruption invites removal from the immediate environment to one's room or to a quiet room.

Overall, the use of programming is basic to residential care. The day is structured for a given patient group, with suitable individual variations for each child. Activities are selected on the combined basis of developmental level and therapeutic need. Therapies are woven into the day and alternate artfully with recreational and educational activities. Throughout, the child care staff members interact with children in natural, spontaneous, and supportive ways; from time to time, in the event of crises, they conduct life space interviews with the children. In aggregate, these experiences are a major dimension of the treatment enterprise.

By and large, residential treatment centers tend to keep children as inpatients longer than do most settings for adults. Thus, for many youngsters, time in residence is likely to run about 18 months to two years. In part this is due to the length of time it takes to wean a child from the intense pathologic family ties that are usually present and to get him to reach out to the residence staff; in part it is due to the need to enable a significant segment of the child's development to go forward within a supportive and therapeutic environment.

There are numerous variations on this model, extending from the total permissiveness described by Aichhorn (1935) and Neill (1960), to the patterns of close confinement and strict supervision on closed wards in specialized hospital units described by Rinsley (1968) and Marohn (1980). However, the essence of the approach is the same, and the major differences are due to the varieties of patients treated and the resulting management emphasis more than to radical differences in treatment philosophy.

Indeed, the question of which children are being served is of central importance in determining the nature of the therapeutic pattern that comes into being. Harrison et al. (1969) have observed that different administrative arrangements might be better for children with different diagnoses. For example, in one setting the psychotherapist might be the key figure in establishing the child's program. The therapist would assign the child's privileges and restrictions, conduct many of the life space interviews at times of stress, supervise the child care workers, and eventually work with the family as well. In another, the therapist is confined exclusively to his office, someone else sees the family, and a unit administrator or the individual child care worker decides on questions of reward or restriction. In fact, the all-inclusive therapist who takes total charge of the program is probably optimal for a schizophrenic child or the more severe borderline problem, whereas the separation of therapist and administrator probably better serves the child with a conduct disorder.

Confrontational Models. Confrontational settings are largely derived from the Synanon experience (DeLeon et al., 1972; Yablonsky, 1965). They serve adolescents and offer a residential style in which the basic emphasis is on group confrontational encounter. The fundamental element in the approach involves a direct challenge to the youngster's primary adaptive stance, his self deception, his evasiveness, his tricks, his efforts at ingratiation or role playing, his manipulation, and his inclination to "con"—it is this array of maneuvers in particular which becomes the treatment target. By and large, primary emphasis in this model is on direct assault on these mechanisms; and much of the confrontation is, in fact, conducted by the youngster's peers. Moreover, in many of these settings, the responsibility for meting out sanctions and privileges is also left largely in the hands of the group, with the adults retaining a reserve veto power that they use sparingly. Such a residential style is not infrequently accompanied by a heavy work program as part of the milieu.

Another variety of this approach is exemplified by a group of programs based within a wilderness type of setting (Loughmiller, 1965) in which the survival of the patient group depends quite literally on the way the youngsters handle the problems of taking care of their own needs. For the most part, these programs are organized in locations that are far from modern conveniences; they may be on an island, in a wilderness, on a mountainside, or in a desert. Group survival is thus a genuine issue, and the rigors of preparing food and obtaining shelter force the youngsters into patterns of mutual dependence as well as requiring them to turn to and rely on the adults to help see them through. Within this ambience the group confrontations are felt to take on added force and immediacy. Young adolescents with drug abuse problems are said to do best in this type of therapeutic milieu.

The RE-ED Model. In the late 1960's, Nicholas Hobbs introduced a milieu approach based on the French *educateur* system. The *educateur* was a trained child care worker who sought to influence his charges largely by modeling good behavior, by empathy, and by offering himself to them as a warm, realistic, common-sense companion. In the version of this idea carried forward by Hobbs, interpretation was avoided and responses to the child's account of previous traumatic events, should these arise, were confined to lending the youngster a sympathetic ear. For the rest, a good school and recreational program filled out the child's day.

Thus, this approach is characterized by a relative absence of the multiple therapeutic modalities that are so typical of the RTC's, and the children are helped primarily through the milieu atmosphere created by the *educateurs*. The time in residence is usually briefer than with the conventional RTC's, and the goals of treatment are achieved chiefly through a form of social learning.

Psychiatric Hospital Units. While some hospital inpatient settings are residential treatment centers, in recent years, the economics of mental health care have led more and more to relatively brief stays of troubled youngsters in hospital units, usually not more than 90 days. Within these settings the primary effort is directed toward diagnosis and short-term therapy. The milieu organization they develop has been strongly influenced by the typical patterns of the RTC's; i.e., there is a therapeutic school, staff nurses and aides often wear street clothes rather than uniforms (even though the unit is frequently part of a larger general hospital setting and white is worn everywhere else), a variety of treatment modalities is the rule, and there are at least some attempts to make the unit as natural and home-like as possible.

Several distinguishing characteristics typify this approach. For one, because of the more active diagnostic emphasis, the children are frequently the focus of numerous testing and examination procedures. For another, in order to obtain rapid reduction of symptoms, an active psychopharmacological program is usually in place along with a rather special devotion to behavioral methods. A major task undertaken by this group of settings is the sometimes complex effort to unravel multiproblem cases.

By and large these are high intensity environments with active programs, a wide variety of diagnostic categories rubbing shoulders with one another, a rich mix of disciplines and programs sharing both quarters and expertise, and rapid turnover. Where a training dimension is present, a diversity of trainees might also be trying to interact with the children in order to have the experience. The use of several rating scales is typical; both trainees and nursing staff make many scaled observations. Not infrequently, the very sick youngsters who pass through these units need continuing treatment thereafter and are referred to a residential treatment center.

Adults

In recent years, the therapeutic community concept has come to permeate the thinking of all who have sought to treat adult psychiatric patients in inpatient settings. Thus, again and again, the various methods that have been described are either versions of this approach or are depicted in terms of the fashion in which they differ from it. Quite simply, the concept has come to dominate this field of endeavor. Nonetheless, in its application it is a method with serious hazards which is prone to many misinterpretations, and it is important to keep in mind these limitations as well as its contribution.

It has been observed (Gunderson, 1980) that in practice no single theory accounts for the way a therapeutic community operates. Rapoport (1959) described the "four themes" of a therapeutic community as democratization, permissiveness, communalism, and reality confrontation. Democratization refers to the principle that traditional hierarchies are replaced with a system of joint patient-staff decision making. Permissiveness refers to the expectation that extremes of what might ordinarily be distressing or deviant behavior will be tolerated and dealt with by group discussions rather than by disciplinary measures. Communalism refers to the importance placed on open communication. Patients and staff are often on a first-name basis, and the expectation is that all feelings and thoughts should be shared openly with others. Staff members as well as patients are expected to be open about their feelings And finally, reality confrontation refers to the belief that patients should be confronted in the "here-and-now" with the effects they produce on others and that interpersonal conflicts should not be smoothed over or denied but openly discussed.

In this connection it might be well to recall the admonition of Sacks and Carpenter (1974) who speak of the dangers of the pseudotherapeutic community. This they define as " . . . a psychiatric unit that subscribes to a particular treatment philosophy, but covertly functions in ways contradictory to the expressed belief. . . . " They suggest five situations that increase such risk: (a) absence of a therapeutic standard, (b) assignment of irresponsibility, (c) the antitherapy leader, (d) absence of therapeutic leadership, and (e) a pathogenic environment. In the light of subsequent research on milieu therapy, it is clear that some of those pitfalls have contributed to the confusion regarding the therapeutic efficacy of the milieu. Ideas derived from one setting have been indiscriminately applied to drastically different settings. Characteristics of the patient population and of the staff have differed widely among hospital settings, all of which have called themselves "a therapeutic milieu." Pathogenic environments—environments "created and maintained by patients attempting to meet the staff's simultaneous expectations of responsibility and irresponsibility" (Sacks and Carpenter, 1974)—may all too often have been the result. Little by little these areas of confusion are being sorted out, clarifying not only research but clinical goals as well. Gunderson (1980) has observed that within the category of milieu therapy there is now a broad diversity of programs. Moreover, these programs have a strong influence on patients, an influence that may be either positive or negative but one that arises from at least three factors: (a) the type of patient being treated, (b) the kind of milieu program being offered, and (c) the length of time the patient stays in the program.

It is in the realm of current acute general hospital psychiatry that considerable variation, if not confusion, has resulted from the therapeutic community movement. In these units patients stay for 30 days or fewer, usually for two to three weeks. As is true of all hospital treatment, milieu therapy is considered to be an important ingredient of the inpatient work in these settings. Indeed, virtually no short-term unit can be found which does not have some form of community meeting, usually at a frequency of several times a week. Yet the theoretical basis for the community meetings stems from the principles of the pure therapeutic community, which, among other things, usually requires a stay of several months with carefully selected patients.

Thus, in addition to the time dimension, the matter of patient selection is critical. Indeed, boundary control is frequently deemed essential for the success of a therapeutic community. As one of the minimal conditions for the operation of a successful milieu unit, White (1972) lists the need for " . . . control over . . . the composition of its therapeutic community. . . . " Rapoport and Rapoport (1959) and Zeitlyn (1967) echo this theme. Hence many issues arise in the actual practice of milieu therapy which remain to be resolved.

The Therapeutic Community Model. Central to the organization of any therapeutic community is the patient government, with standard procedures for the election of officers who will chair the group and community meetings. The community meeting is the hallmark of the therapeutic milieu, and most units begin each day with such a patient led meeting. The agenda of the meeting may change from day to day; eventually it will include a discussion of the patients' problems of everyday living with one another. This is also the site for group decisions (usually by vote) about individual patients' requests for passes, privileges, and often even for medication. Discharge plans may be discussed (or may be referred to small group meetings); decisions about when a patient may be discharged are usually arrived at by consensus vote as well. In cases in which there are separate staff "rounds," they are usually held in an open meeting in which patients may listen and participate. Doors are unlocked, and patients rely on the honor system to abide by unit procedures.

Numerous reports in the literature describe characteristics of typical therapeutic communities (Caudill, 1958; Clark, 1964, 1977; Davis, 1977; Greenblatt et al., 1955; Jones, 1956, 1957; Jones et al., 1953; Karasu 1977; Kennard, 1979; Main, 1946; Wilmer, 1958, 1981; Margolis, 1973; Maxmen et al., 1974; Oldham and Russakoff, 1982; Rapoport, 1960; Schwartz, 1957). "Pure" therapeutic communities usually result in several inevitable additional features although they are not always emphasized in the descriptions of these units (Oldham and Russakoff, 1982). The unit usually retains admission boundary control, and it is often highly selective about who will be admitted for treatment. As a rule, acutely or severely psychotic patients, disabled patients or those who are seriously medically ill, and patients with significant organic brain syndromes are not deemed appropriate. As a natural consequence of these decisions, as well as the unit philosophy, somatic treatments such as medications and ECT and the use of a seclusion room or restraints are also de-emphasized. Little weight is given to the need to establish a medical diagnosis, and the use of individual psychotherapy is rare. Within these settings the average length of a patient's stay tends to be 60 days or more. Many substance abuse treatment centers have tended to maintain the form of these original therapeutic communities.

Milieu Therapy with Schizophrenia. Many methods for the hospital treatment of schizophrenics have been studied. At one time or another, chronic institutionalization, neuroleptic medication, and deinstitutionalization have been in the ascendent position, with milieu approaches playing a role at each stage. Today only a minority of residential centers for schizophrenics are fashioned along traditional therapeutic community lines. Notable among these programs is the Soteria House project (Mosher and Menn, 1978; Wendt et al., 1983) which emphasizes a psychosocial rather than a somatic treatment approach. The patients selected for these programs, however, are generally acutely ill young adults who may be more receptive to such techniques than are the more chronic schizophrenics. Mosher and Keith (1979) and Gunderson (1983) point out the need to differentiate programs for the acute as opposed to the more chronic patients with this condition. Most references to milieu therapy with schizophrenics refer to those aspects of the hospital milieu which can be individually shaped for each patient. Psychiatric nursing intervention, occupational therapy, recreational therapy, vocational rehabilitation, and selected types of group and family therapy are among these specific elements (in addition to the somatic therapies and individual psychotherapy where these are used). There is considerable agreement among clinicians that given the benefit of comprehensive treatment, i.e., a combination of inpatient treatment modalities within a coherent milieu context, these patients achieve a better level of functioning with greater likelihood of being able to advance beyond chronic institutionalization.

The results of deinstitutionalization without adequate planning for continuity of care and the creation of community aftercare resources have been devastating* (Talbott, 1978). This experience has taught psychiatrists that many of the elements of therapy provided by the hospital milieu must not stop when the patient leaves inpatient status. For this group of patients, either extreme, be it chronic institutionalization or radical deinstitutionalization, has its pitfalls. Strauss and Carpenter (1981) point out that our concern with the ill effects of "warehousing" patients should not eclipse the manifold benefits of providing them with good inpatient care.

Mosher and Keith (1979) have summarized the types of milieu characteristics found to be the most effective with schizophrenics. They suggest that acute patients " . . . recover best in highly staffed, accepting, supportive, stimulus-decreasing (at least early in treatment), relatively long stay

---

*Talbott JA: Chronic patients: who, where, and how well are they? Presented at the 135th annual meeting of the American Psychiatric Association. Toronto, May 15-21, 1982

(three to five months) environments in which psychosocial interventions are viewed positively. . . . " In contrast, they find that chronic patients respond optimally when what is to be achieved and how it is to be done are defined for them in specific terms. Some chronic patients may be maintained in stable control over the long run by carefully planned community-based treatment combined with ready access to repeated brief hospitalizations as needed.* Rehospitalization of chronic schizophrenic patients may be more effective if consistent, predictable, and familiar aspects of milieu therapy are provided in a carefully structured way (Oldham, 1982).

Milieu Settings for the Treatment of Substance Abuse. Two apparently independent lines of development have led to the application of therapeutic community principles to treat alcoholism and drug abuse. One source has its origins in Alcoholics Anonymous, and the other arises from within the therapeutic community movement itself. Originally, a major founder of the therapeutic community movement, Maxwell Jones, worked with a heterogeneous group of patients which included chronic neurotics, drug addicts, and character disordered patients who were considered difficult to classify (Jones et al., 1953). Perhaps due to his visibility within general hospital psychiatry, however, Jones later became less clearly associated with the problems of patients with substance abuse. Although occasional reports have linked Jones' ideas with other therapeutic community work with sociopaths (Kiger, 1973) and criminals (Jones, 1968b; Lamb and Goertzel, 1974), little material in the literature reflects direct influence by the therapeutic community movement on the notion of residential treatment for substance abuse (Liebman and Hedlund, 1981). Yet such centers for the treatment of drug abuse are regularly referred to as therapeutic communities. However, it is also true that many of the principles used in such centers have much in common with those described earlier by Jones and his colleagues.

As therapeutic community principles gained widespread acceptance in general hospital work, the usefulness of community meetings, patient government, and patients as active therapeutic agents for themselves became ever more apparent. This success made a profound impression on many who were familiar with active self-help groups, especially Alcoholics Anonymous. As a result, active rehabilitation treatment programs for alcoholics, many of them residential or inpatient, began to incorporate these techniques.

As a direct outgrowth of Alcoholics Anonymous, the first residential treatment facility for drug addiction was established by Charles Dederich; he named it Synanon (Batiste and Yablonsky, 1971; Yablonsky, 1965). Fashioned after AA, this organization had built into it many self-help

*Glick ID, Braff D, Klar H: Which chronic patients most need readmission? Presented at the 135th annual meeting of the American Psychiatric Association, Toronto, May 15-21, 1982

principles along with such familiar features as group techniques. In time, the original Synanon program spread, and a group of similar settings appeared throughout the country. Other drug treatment organizations were created as well, such as Phoenix House (DeLeon et al., 1971, 1972). Many critics have assailed these programs as ineffective and have raised questions about the methodology of the outcome studies that report good results. Nevertheless, residential therapeutic communities for drug problems continue to be used actively to treat these conditions.

Perhaps the most thorough attempt to describe the principles of therapeutic communities as applied to residential programs for substance abuse is presented in the summary of the Proceedings of Therapeutic Communities of America Planning Conference of 1976 (DeLeon and Beschner, 1976). The authors recognize the diversity of the agencies subsumed under this rubric, but they observe that a fundamental tenet of the concept is the presence of a round-the-clock, total influence as basic to rendering stable changes in life-long and socially destructive patterns of behavior. A complete change in life-style can thus be sought, one that includes drug abstinence, elimination of criminal behavior, training or retraining for employable skills, and a transformation of attitudes which would allow the acquisition of new values and behavior. Ultimately the programs seek to make possible an advance toward honesty, responsibility, nonviolence, and self-reliance.

The staff is composed largely of ex-drug addicts and former offenders who have themselves been socially rehabilitated in similar programs. The daily regimen is a busy one and includes encounter group sessions, tutorial learning sessions, remedial as well as standard educational efforts, and in-house work functions. By design, these activities will, in time, prepare the client for conventional occupations in a living out arrangement. The original program required at least 15 months' stay in residence before discharge could be realistically anticipated. After 1975, several programs began to attempt shorter stays varying from six to 15 months.

The Elderly

A number of model programs have tried to adapt the principles of milieu therapy to the treatment of elderly psychiatric patients in psychiatric hospitals (Klein et al., 1980; Roskos et al., 1979) and in nursing homes (Colthart, 1974; Kramer and Kramer, 1976). However, the mental health system in general has been slow to adopt these innovative, expensive, and time consuming approaches. Financial considerations abound and join forces with the well engrained traditions of the biomedical model to maintain long-standing prejudices against providing psychiatric treatment for the elderly. Together these factors hinder the widespread implementation of a milieu therapy approach throughout institutions and communities that care for elderly psychiatric patients.

This problem is all the more unfortunate because, theoretically, there are good reasons to expect milieu therapy to benefit elderly patients. Many of their symptoms reflect social-adaptational failure, i.e., passivity, apathy, and inability to adapt to environmental stresses. As one ages, there is an increasing tendency to use mechanisms of denial and selective inattention to protect oneself from threatening stimuli.

As a result, the elderly may be hesitant to seek psychiatric treatment. They usually engage the mental health system only after difficulties arise in the family or when their problems are recognized by the police, social agencies, senior citizen housing staff, etc. These characteristics indicate the need for a concentrated and all-encompassing means of therapeutic intervention that will impinge on the elderly patient's life in many ways at once—an approach intrinsic to milieu therapy.

In particular, milieu therapy seeks to help the elderly patient (a) develop a more active and assertive stance, (b) maximize remaining intellectual functioning, (c) improve the capacity to interact effectively with others, (d) replace social withdrawal and apathy with increased activity and social participation, (e) build self-esteem, and (f) re-establish ego strength and controls. Such patients' psychiatric problems are frequently reflected in or exacerbated by their interaction with an environment that is perceived as cold and unempathic. Hence, a protective and supportive environment can effectively diminish current stress and prevent future difficulties. Kohut has noted (Lazarus, 1976) that it is more useful to approach the elderly patient by "focusing on the old and his environment as a unit rather than focusing only on the failures of the aged and on the defects of the self." Empirical evidence supports the same view. Reports from the early 1950's indicated that institutionalized geriatric patients responded well to intensive therapy programs aimed at rehabilitation and resocialization (Silver, 1950; Linden, 1953; Donahue, 1950).

In brief, for the elderly, a milieu approach is important. In practice, it involves an integration of multiple treatment modalities, along with individual and family psychotherapy and psychopharmacology, into a cohesive plan designed to meet specific treatment objectives. Such an approach seeks to establish an environment that promotes treatment goals generally appropriate for all elderly patients. At the same time, sufficient flexibility must be built in to address the particular needs of each patient.

It is essential that such a treatment program take place in an environment that facilitates improved psychological functioning. Gottesman and Brody (1975) found that the general atmosphere of the treatment environment should emphasize patient responsibility for his or her behavior and encourage patient freedom. Involvement in the group decision-making processes is also important (Bakos et al., 1980). A milieu therapy program requires careful coordination and teamwork so that staff members work in unison toward agreed upon treatment goals.

Nature of the Milieu for the Elderly. A number of issues are common to all milieu therapy programs for the elderly. To begin with, in order to determine the appropriateness of milieu treatment as well as to establish realistic and individualized treatment goals, the elderly patient requires a comprehensive medical, psychiatric, psychological, and social assessment. The OARS Multidimensional Functional Assessment Methodology developed at Duke University (Pfeiffer, 1975) offers such a comprehensive approach to evaluation. It involves a systematic, quantitative study of five major areas of function: mental health, physical health, social resources, economic resources, and capacity for the activities of daily living.

Physical Structure. A major aspect of milieu therapy for the elderly involves the physical and architectural components of the environment. Modifying the physical environment has been found to be effective in increasing patients' adaptive skills, social participation, and patient-staff interactions. Several investigators have emphasized the importance of using architectural design to create a warm and supportive therapeutic milieu (Proshansky et al., 1970; Schwartz, 1968). The physical features of a ward can be designed to provide privacy, to encourage interaction in social areas, and to combat an atmosphere of sterility and hollowness. In addition, as Whanger and Lewis (1975) suggest, too few facilities caring for the elderly incorporate the appropriate physical, architectural, and environmental features to promote the older adult's pleasure, convenience, and ability to care for himself. Structural features such as handrails, wheelchair ramps, nonslip flooring, and convenient bathroom facilities do much to promote independent self-care. Large type calendars, bulletin board announcements of daily activities, and name plates on room doors serve to increase orientation. Bright wall colors, proper lighting, lack of excessive noise, and comfortable air temperatures all combine to heighten the patient's level of comfort. (Bakos et al., 1980; Melin and Gotestam, 1981; Carp, 1976).

Age Segregation. In evaluating the pros and cons of age-segregated milieu therapy for the elderly, a number of issues need to be considered. The establishment of an age-segregated unit allows for the development of a milieu staff that is educated to the developmental issues of aging and is sensitive to the needs and concerns specific to older patients. Staff biases against the elderly can be dealt with directly and countered through education and training. The elderly's increased needs for thorough medical evaluation and treatment can also be taken into account when developing an age-specific treatment unit.

There are potential problems, however, in structuring such units. One assumption underlying the organization of an age-specific (or for that matter, any single problem type unit) is that the target population has common issues and needs on which to focus treatment. The general therapeutic aims of a unit specialized for the treatment of drug and alcohol abuse patients can be specified fairly easily. Sherwood and Mor (1980), however, believe that it is much more difficult to conceptualize general treatment goals for a group of elderly patients who are placed together primarily because of age. For example, treatment needs of patients with severe cognitive impairment and those with major depression differ markedly, and it is a challenge to establish a milieu therapy program that adequately addresses the needs of both. There are, however, treatment considerations that are important for many, if not all, older adults. These include the need for extensive discharge planning, environmental manipulation, enhancement of cognitive functioning, complete physical evaluation, and strengthening of family and social support systems.

In the course of deciding whether or not to treat a given patient on an age-integrated or an age-segregated unit, the treatment requirements of that particular individual must be among the prime considerations. There is probably more variability among people over age 65 than within any other age group. In respect to health; socio-economic status; and cognitive, personality, and developmental issues, many individuals in the 65- to 75-year-old age group have more in common with 55- to 65-year-olds than they do with those over 75 (Busse, 1980; Neugarten, 1974). As a result, depending on program structure and characteristics of the other patients who are present, particular patients may benefit from treatment on either one type of unit or the other.

Therapeutic Styles. During the past 30 years, a number of innovative and effective treatment approaches have been developed to address the needs of the hospitalized elderly psychiatric patient. These include reality orientation (Folsom, 1966, 1968), attitude therapy (Folsom, 1966), group therapy (Lazarus, 1976), and activity therapy (Herman, 1968). In a more comprehensive sense, therapeutic community patterns have also been used with the aged. All of these modalities are dependent on using and, to some degree, restructuring the total treatment environment.

In attitude therapy one of five basic staff attitudes is prescribed for each patient, depending on the nature of the presenting problems; thereafter, all staff-patient interactions support this attitudinal approach. For example, an attitude of kind firmness may be prescribed for depressed patients and one of active friendliness for those who are withdrawn and apathetic.

The goal of reality orientation is to delay or arrest cognitive deterioration. It works through the use of repetitive stimulation and is specifically designed for use with elderly patients who suffer from organic mental disorders. It is based on techniques that were developed for the treatment of younger patients with traumatic brain damage. Reality orientation involves two components. The first is the use of constant orientation reminders in the milieu and in staff-patient interactions. Staff members frequently address patients by name and discuss current information. Environmental reminders such as date boards are used. The second component is a daily reality orientation class in which the same information is repeated. The effectiveness of this approach in decreasing patient confusion and regression has been substantiated by numerous investigations (Harris and Ivory, 1976; Greene et al., 1979). Modifications of the basic technique of reality orientation have been suggested. These adaptations teach elderly patients to compensate for memory loss rather than seek to arrest the process of loss itself,* or they combine reality orientation with other techniques such as sensory stimulation (Byron, 1978).

Many other modalities have been integrated into milieu treatment approaches. For example, since Linden's (1953) initial work, numerous reports of group therapy have supported its effectiveness for geropsychiatric patients in re-establishing feelings of self-worth and self-esteem, in increasing socialization and assertiveness, in decreasing apparent cognitive confusion, in reducing psychological regression, and in improving problem-solving skills (Lazarus, 1976; Burnside, 1970). In order to address the specific needs of this population, a number of group modalities have been developed. These include remotivation (Bechenstein, 1966), reminiscence (Lesser et al., 1981), predischarge socialization, and coping groups (Whanger, 1980). All of these approaches share in common the fact that they offer the patients an opportunity to discuss problems and past experiences and to interact with a variety of role models.

A range of other treatment modalities has also been adapted for use with the elderly; all of these techniques seek to increase the patients' level of activity, physical exercise, and social interactions as well as to provide additional avenues for their expressions of feeling. Activity therapy (Herman, 1968); art therapy (Finkelstein, 1971); recreational therapy (Hill, 1961); and music, dance, and movement therapy (Boxberger and Cotter, 1968; Palmer, 1977) all appear to have a role in the treatment of the elderly and can be integrated into a milieu therapy approach.

Gottesman and his colleagues at Ypsilanti State Hospital (1973, 1975) restructured the treatment programs for chronic elderly patients according to the principles of the therapeutic community model. Patients in this program averaged 74 years of age and had been hospitalized an average of 16 years. The assumption underlying this investigation was that the patients' impaired behavior reflected the lack of environmental stimulation and the low level of staff expectation as well as the presence of psychopathology. When staff expectations were modified and patients were given the incentive and opportunity to take care of personal hygiene, manage money, and work in a workshop, these elderly people showed an ability to carry out these activities.

Gatz et al. (1979-80) set up a therapeutic community for 55 geriatric patients who had a high potential for self-care and rehabilitation. They found that it was difficult to create program structures that incorporated

*Carroll K, Gray K: Memory development: an approach for responding to the mentally impaired elderly in the long-term care setting. Presented at the 30th annual meeting of the Gerontological Society, 1977

both the ideology of a therapeutic community and a realistic appraisal of both patient needs and treatment goals. For example, modifying the traditional staff hierarchy resulted in contradictory role expectations and confusion about decision making. Efforts to increase the patients' level of competence led to the establishment of unrealistic goals. At the same time, it was difficult to alter many deeply ingrained staff attitudes of wanting to do too much for patients. Other investigators (Goldstein, 1971; Grauer, 1971) have also found that the pervasive passivity and dependency of elderly psychiatric patients discourage those staff members who try to mobilize them. The problem of introducing a milieu therapy approach is further exacerbated by the staff's own investment in the role of "benevolent caretaker" for these patients.

The Problem of Transition. One of the primary goals of inpatient treatment of geropsychiatric patients is their eventual discharge back into the community. Ideally, they would be placed in as supportive and nonrestrictive a setting as possible. For most elderly patients, this means a return to independent living, either alone or with their families. Effective discharge planning involves structuring the home and community environments in order both to maintain the therapeutic gains made during hospitalization and to prevent further psychiatric deterioration. To accomplish these goals, a therapeutic milieu within the community should involve the following five components: (a) linkage between the inpatient facility and the community, (b) coordination of the community services and resources, (c) facilitation of the efforts of family and friends as an effective support element, (d) provision of follow-up outpatient treatment, and (e) access to rehospitalization in the event of relapse.

In order to maintain elderly patients in the community, specific treatment approaches are required. These include counseling, casework and groupwork, protective services, crisis intervention, rehabilitation, and day-care services. During the deinstitutionalization movement in the United States, a nationwide network of comprehensive community mental health centers was established. The mandate of these centers was to provide and coordinate such services to recently discharged patients, including the elderly. As Gurian and Scherl (1972) suggest, "The most promising approach to better mental treatment for older people seems to be flexible, community-oriented preventive services offered through local community mental health centers." Unfortunately community mental health centers have found it difficult to provide comprehensive aftercare services to chronic and long-term psychiatric patients. The provision of psychiatric care for the elderly has been particularly inadequate (Kramer et al., 1978).

Another important resource for discharged geropsychiatric patients is the day treatment center. This facility provides social and rehabilitative activities for frail, moderately handicapped, or slightly confused patients who need supervision during the day. Care-taking family members can thereby be partially relieved of the burden of continuous management and thus be better enabled to retain their elderly family member at home. Some programs focus on meeting their patients' psychosocial and socialization needs, whereas others place more emphasis on caring for physical, emotional, and cognitive impairments (Lowy, 1980). During the transition from the institution to home, patients treated in day treatment centers may require either long-term care or time-limited intense treatment. European countries have had these centers for the elderly for many years; in the United States, however, they are relatively new and still in the process of development.

Another way of using the community as a therapeutic milieu is by working with the patient's family to maximize its effectiveness as a support system. Education of family members regarding psychiatric problems serves to increase their understanding and patience. In cases in which family conflicts have been exacerbated by the elderly patient's psychiatric problems, family therapy can offer a possible channel toward effective relief. Appropriate, well-organized self-help groups can be an additional source of support for families.

An innovative approach has been suggested* for increasing the therapeutic effectiveness of family members and for assuring the transfer of treatment techniques from institution to home. The goal of this program is the elimination or modification of problem behavior. The underlying assumption is that the amelioration of specific behavior problems, e.g., incontinence, can enable families to care for their elderly family member at home. Before the patient is discharged, the relatives are instructed in behavior modification techniques. Beginning soon after discharge, consistent and frequent follow-up is provided in the patient's home to ensure carry-over of the treatment gains.

Following discharge, another important strategy for assuring continuity of care is to assign each patient a designated coordinator or patient-advocate. This individual is responsible for (a) coordinating the available community services, (b) assisting the patient to negotiate the complex health and social service bureaucracy, (c) encouraging the reluctant patient to make use of psychiatric follow-up care, and (d) strengthening and maintaining the patient's family and social support system. Unfortunately, the role of the patient-advocate has frequently been neglected, although some attempts have been made to fulfill this function within the community mental health system and in other inpatient settings (Cotton et al., 1978). Another strategy for coordinating psychiatric treatment in the community is to establish specific clinics that serve the elderly and their families. Reifler and Eisdorfer (1980) describe a clinic that provides psychiatric, medical,

---

*Linsk NL, Green GR, Marlow C: An analysis of community linkage and behavioral treatment strategies with families of the impaired elderly. Presented at the annual meeting of the Gerontological Society, San Diego, 1980

social, nursing, and architectural evaluation and treatment for impaired older adults. In addition, it offers support and practical advice to their families.

Nursing Homes and Foster Care. Because psychiatric inpatient facilities continue to emphasize short-term intervention (even in the case of severely impaired patients), elderly patients in need of long-term care are more and more likely to be treated in alternative settings, particularly nursing homes. Attempts have been made to provide intermediate degrees of care in facilities such as half-way houses and boarding homes, but these agencies are able to give service to only a small number of those in need and usually with little or no direct input from psychiatrists. Community reluctance and antagonism have been implicated in the continuing delay in the growth and development of such facilities (Reifler and Eisdorfer, 1980; Donahue, 1978; Zusman and Lamb, 1977). Efforts have also been made to establish a system of foster care for elderly psychiatric patients, but this too is in the early stages of its development (Lowy, 1980). Ultimately, the vast majority of elderly people with chronic debilitating psychiatric illnesses continue to be placed in nursing homes.

Psychiatric patients discharged to nursing homes experience a number of problems. One of the major sources of stress is the travail of relocation. Investigators disagree as to whether or not relocation is associated with increased mortality (Borup et al., 1979; Goplerud, 1979; Zweig and Csank, 1976). There is, however, no question that transfer is stressful and can have adverse effects (Raasoch et al., 1977; Rodstein et al., 1976). This is particularly true for the most vulnerable elderly patients with severe psychological, cognitive, and physical disabilities. In their study of the effects of transfer on the elderly, Zweig and Csank (1976) identified distinct phases in patient adjustment before and after the move. The most stressful times were, first, the period just before the move when anticipation anxiety was greatest and, then, the four- to six-month period following relocation.

Two factors can lessen the potentially devastating effects of such a move. First, sufficient preparation prior to the actual transfer can alleviate anticipation anxiety and help to reduce the mortality rate while increasing patient adjustment (Whanger, 1980; Zweig and Csank, 1976). The second factor is the nature of the environment into which the patients enter. Slover* and Marlowe† used comprehensive ratings to assess the physical, social, and service-related characteristics of a variety of community and long-term care facilities to which elderly psychiatric inpatients were transferred. They found that following relocation, emotional and physical deterioration was least in environments that promoted individual autonomy and were charac-

---

*Slover D: Relocation for therapeutic purposes of aged mental patients. Presented at the annual meeting of Gerontological Society, San Juan, Puerto Rico, 1972

†Marlowe RA: Effects of environment on elderly state hospital relocatees. Presented at the annual meeting of the Pacific Sociological Association, Scottsdale, Ariz, May 1973

terized by an atmosphere of warmth and caring. Marlowe found that characteristics of the environment predict well-being at follow-up better than any personality characteristics of the transferred patients.

Once the geriatric patient has adjusted to the new nursing home environment, another major problem arises: The advent and expansion of the therapeutic milieu approach in psychiatric hospitals has not extended to most nursing homes. There, treatment continues to be oriented toward the provision of custodial care. Elderly patients are generally seen as disabled and incapable of self-care. Such expectations result in the provision of too much care, which in turn fosters dependency and psychological and cognitive regression, the very characteristics that milieu therapy was designed to combat. Zarit (1980) suggests several reasons as to why the provision of excessive care is ingrained in the nursing home setting. Nursing home staff perceive their role as caretakers and, therefore, assume that the more help given, the better the care. Moreover, if staff, families, and state regulatory agencies perceive patients' independent or self-assertive behavior as potentially risky and, therefore, requiring control, providing too much care can also be self-protective for the nursing home.

To be sure, many nursing homes do provide activity, group, and physical therapy; and some have successfully incorporated principles of the therapeutic community into their management approach. Interventions such as behavior modification (MacDonald, 1978), social skills training (Berger, 1979), activity and group therapy (Kartman, 1979), occupational therapy (Wolk et al., 1965), reality orientation and sensory stimulation (Ernst, 1978), movement and dance therapy (Sandel, 1978), and art therapy (Zlatin, 1979) are used in the better quality nursing homes. These programs can be effective in increasing social skills, alertness, interest, contact with the environment, and cognitive functioning.

The paucity of therapeutic milieus, as well as other aggressive treatment programs, in nursing homes arises from a number of factors. Limited financial resources severely restrict a nursing home's capacity to support innovative programs. High staff turnover, the emotional drain placed on staff by elderly patients with severe physical and emotional problems, little knowledge of psychosocial treatment modalities, and limited opportunities for continuing education undermine staff incentive to participate in program development. In addition, mental health professionals have generally shown little interest in assisting nursing homes to provide treatment for psychiatric patients. The need for psychiatric consultation and the various roles that psychiatrists can and should play in providing assistance to nursing homes deserve more professional attention.

Finally, the goals and techniques of milieu therapy require adaptation in order to be appropriate for use in nursing home settings. The assumption underlying milieu therapy in the hospital setting is that by fostering independence and improved psychological functioning, the patient will be able to be discharged to a less restrictive living environment. However, for many nursing home residents this goal is unrealistic. Either because of the degree of impairment or because of the lack of a sufficient community support system, these patients are likely to remain in a nursing home despite whatever psychiatric treatment is provided. Thus, it may be difficult for nursing home staff to become invested in instituting a demanding therapy program when realistically only limited patient goals can be set.

A few programs that adapt the principles of milieu therapy to nursing home settings have been developed (Colthart, 1974; Kramer and Kramer, 1976). In addition, a few demonstration projects have linked nursing homes to medical centers where the stimulus for training and research is translated into better patient care. In these pilot projects, continuing education programs for nursing home staff and the consultative services of psychiatrists and psychologists have led to the initiation of effective environmental approaches.

INDICATIONS AND LIMITATIONS

Children and Adolescents. In general, to take a child out of his home and remove him to a strange environment to which his family cannot readily follow is a form of major social surgery. There are times when it is desirable, and times when it is essential, even life saving; but it is never a minor form of intervention. To be sure there are children who leave home voluntarily for shorter or longer periods, e.g., to attend summer camp or boarding school. Even such elective experiences as these, however, have been known to provoke untoward reactions in vulnerable children.

In any case, this is the background reality against which indications for residential treatment must be weighed. A number of conditions invite consideration for placement and a few demand it. But in the large majority of instances the final decision is less a matter of a particular diagnosis than it is of a balancing and summing of many social and clinical factors before the outcome falls on the side of residential treatment. To address such issues, some therapeutic settings provide day care or five-day-week rather than full-time care.

Various authors (Rinsley, 1968; Whittaker, 1975) have attempted to list the indications for placement. What it comes down to in many instances is a matter of degree. When the child's pain, the family's pain, or the community sense of intolerable stress rises above a certain level, then the pressure for relief is so great that placement becomes a longed-for solution. There are, to be sure, a number of absolute indications such as dangerousness, be it to self, to others, or to property; such a manifestation is among the paramount imperatives for a protective environment.

In most cases the indications are less absolute. For example, a child may be chronically depressed or show strong tendencies to withdraw from school, friends, and family. Or he may display a level of symptomatic disturbance which is difficult to contain, e.g., a state of chronic anorexia or repeated hospitalizations for unregulated diabetes. In all such instances in which the danger is not too great, a serious attempt should be made at some form of outpatient care before referral for placement is initiated. One important element that determines the appropriateness of the milieu approach is a failure of outpatient treatment.

Adults. Therapeutic communities set great store by such factors as a patient's motivation and ability to live and work on his problems in a group context. It is this rather than any predetermined diagnosis which makes for acceptability into such a treatment setting. Patients who are not voluntarily willing to be admitted are screened out by definition. Motivation for shared work in such a setting must be high, usually including willingness to insist that appropriate family members join in some facets of the treatment.

Critics of these units contend that they are not cost-effective since many of the patients selected for such inpatient treatment could, in the views of some, be treated just as effectively either with shorter periods of hospitalization or with alternative modes such as day hospitalization or crisis intervention, followed by intensive outpatient utilization (Herz et al., 1977). Criticism has also been expressed about the indiscriminate application of therapeutic community principles to inpatient psychiatric units that are fundamentally different from those in which the therapeutic community principles were originally developed.

Thus a pure therapeutic community, emphasizing the usual ingredients such as open information sharing, joint decision making, and permissiveness might be highly inappropriate for certain schizophrenic patients (Bursten, 1973; Rapoport and Rapoport, 1959; Oldham and Russakoff, 1982; Wilmer, 1981). The lack of emphasis on use of medication, ECT, and seclusion and restraint accounts for the frequent—and justified—exclusion of many schizophrenic patients from these settings.

Two general features of acute hospital psychiatry, i.e., the brevity of the average patient's stay and the wide spectrum of diagnoses (including both acutely psychotic and organic conditions), differentiate such work immediately from the type of setting in which the principles of therapeutic community practice originated. It is, therefore, not surprising that numerous reports have criticized the application of such techniques to work with acutely psychotic and schizophrenic patients (Abroms, 1968, 1969; Herz, 1972; Raskin, 1971, 1976; Sacks and Carpenter, 1974; Oldham and Russakoff, 1982; Bursten, 1973; Van Putten, 1973; Van Putten and May, 1976). The usual environment of a therapeutic community, with its expectation of self-revelatory openness, may be overstimulating to some of these patients (Van Putten, 1973). Acutely psychotic and organic patients may not be able to participate effectively in shared decision making or patient government (Bursten, 1973; Wilmer, 1981). The use of neuroleptic medications and the need for security precautions make it vital that clear lines of authority and security containment be firmly established.

Gunderson (1983) has described five variables that must be considered in the structuring of any milieu. These are: containment, structure, support, involvement, and validation. Of the five, there may be a need for special emphasis on containment and aspects of structure for the optimal management of acute inpatient units. This need stands in decided contrast to what is considered best for therapeutic communities.

Rapoport and Rapoport (1959), Quitkin and Klein (1967), Friedman (1969), Brodsky and Fischer (1964), Lehman and Ritzler (1976), and others have cited the perils of permissiveness and the need for limit setting with borderline and character disordered patients. Finally, Herz et al. (1977) have pointed out the usefulness of a traditional medical model when evaluating and diagnosing acutely disturbed patients in a short-term hospital setting. Moreover, Herz (1979) has advocated the abolition of group therapy and community meetings in acute psychiatric hospital work. Recent reports, however, suggest that a "centered" (Wilmer, 1981) or "modified" (Oldham and Russakoff, 1982) model is more appropriate for such work, borrowing those principles of the therapeutic community which are applicable and combining them with more familiar aspects of the medical model. Oldham and Russakoff (1982) have suggested the phrase "medical-therapeutic community" to describe such an acute inpatient service. An emphasis on diagnosis, the use of individual therapy, the prescribing of medications, the use of ECT, the presence of locked doors, and the use of seclusion and restraint would be part of such a model. They suggest that to make such an approach work, the principles of the therapeutic community might well be modified in specific ways, namely:

A. Modified and selective information sharing, individually tailored to each patient's needs;

B. Modified patient government, serving a liaison and advisory function between staff and patients;

C. Modified group therapy requiring all staff to attend and observe (Oldham, 1982);

D. Modified community meetings chaired by staff in a highly structured manner with a carefully planned agenda;

E. Clear hospital identification nameplates (indicating professional discipline) to be worn by staff at all times. At the same time, the staff members would wear street clothes rather than medical uniforms.

Such an approach represents one example of an attempt to retain, yet to clarify and adapt, principles of the therapeutic community for effective use in an acute inpatient setting.

The Elderly. For the elderly patient, a primary issue is whether any treatment program embedded in an institutional framework can overcome the negative impact of hospitalization itself on this population. Institutional-ization has an inherent potential for increasing dependency, producing psychological regression, interrupting the patient's community support system, and undermining self-confidence and coping abilities. Added to this is the disruptive and stressful effect of moving the older person from a known environment into a new and frequently frightening situation. More-over, negative stereotypes about the aged remain, even among mental health professionals. Hence, despite good intentions, their interventions may serve to undermine the patient's sense of self-worth and confidence. In addition, elderly people are frequently referred to psychiatric institutions because of such factors as lack of available alternatives, the tenuousness of their support framework, or someone else's convenience, rather than because their presenting problems could best be treated by inpatient milieu therapy.

There are also problems in instituting a milieu therapy program for elderly patients, particularly when it is to incorporate the principles of the therapeutic community. Initiating a therapeutic milieu within which the attempt is made to break down traditional authority structures would be a difficult accomplishment with any patient group. But changing the psychi-atric care of an elderly population from a traditional, hierarchical biomedical model to a therapeutic community is particularly problematic. Given the increased prevalence of medical problems requiring physical treatment, the greater tendency toward passivity, dependency, and withdrawal in older patients and the long history of experience with the biomedical model, its replacement with a more egalitarian therapeutic community approach is at best a challenging task.

ETHICAL ISSUES IN MILIEU THERAPY

A major ethical problem confronts the therapists who work with nursery school children, arising from the need to maintain therapeutic neutrality in the face of the frequently destructive behavior of the child's primary caretakers. Different workers have taken various stances with these difficult situations, positions that have varied from total focus on the child who is completely separated from the parents for extended periods (as was for-merly the practice in the Orthogenic School program) to some of the family-centered patterns of care that direct attention to the parents as the major targets of therapeutic interest, with the children receiving secondary atten-tion.

Currently, it seems safe to say that the prevailing ethic dictates that, wherever possible, a primary effort be made to preserve the family struc-ture. This position seems to possess both clinical virtue and profound ethical appeal. However, the need for harrowing decisions cannot be glossed over by such comfortable generalizations; there are homes in which children are in grave danger and the situation is beyond remediation by any available means. To some extent, the legal system has made the burden less onerous by mandating the reporting of child abuse. But the number of marginal situations is large, there are many shades of gray, and the area of emotional abuse is far less clearly defined than is the nature of physical battering. In any case, those who deal with preschoolers must sometimes face grave decisions as to when the attempt to resolve problems of parenting can no longer be justified in the face of continuing maltreatment or gross misman-agement of small and helpless children. The ethical burden is not a light one.

Numerous ethical problems attend the placement of children. These difficulties arise at the earliest consideration of adopting such a course and continue through to post-discharge responsibilities. The fact of ethical involvement lies in the potential for harm which is present at each stage of the process.

In effect, by accepting a child for admission, an agency is asserting that it can do more for him than his home has been able to do. This is an exposed position, ripe for challenge, and is inevitably tested by both parents and child to see if they can meet such a challenge. In the nature of things, the en-suing events will probe the moral fiber of the entire staff.

An associated dilemma is when not to take a child. The ethic here is all too clear; a staff should take only those whom it feels reasonably sure it can help. But that means turning away cases in desperate need, which brings the practitioner face to face with a paradox, for the more general value set asserts that all children in need should be helped. Nonetheless, the higher goal in this situation is to admit only those whom that staff can help at that time in that setting.

Generally speaking, people apply for placement of a child when someone in the situation can endure it no longer. Often it is the school that cries "Enough!" Often it is the parents who are pushed beyond their limits of tolerance. Curiously, it is seldom the child who requests the admission; more often than not it is thrust upon him. In any case, the separation of a child from family and familiar surroundings always involves the balancing of the pain it will cost him and his family versus the advantage they all stand to gain by this decision. If the parents do not want the placement but the law requires it, or if the child objects but the parents insist, then the burden on the receiving/treatment agency is all the more onerous—and, where feasible, dictates a lengthy and gradual intake process to try to work through some of the reluctance and distress.

Once admitted, the agency is *in loco parentis* as far as child rearing is concerned and faces all the ethical (as well as the professional) demands of meeting the child's developmental needs. Fun, play, hygiene, exercise, health care, education, privacy, companionship, behavioral guidance, sympathy, tenderness, support, understanding, acceptance, limits, discipline—the full spectrum of what a growing child needs—all must be forthcoming. More than that, however, the complex array of the child's treatment needs must also be met in an equally complete fashion. Given the difficulties posed by these children, it is a heavy burden.

The nature of residential treatment raises certain internal ethical issues as well as a number of external dilemmas. The question of confidentiality of psychotherapeutic material, for example, is clear enough in an outpatient setting; the therapist automatically promises and strives to maintain total privacy. But in inpatient care a good case can be made for sharing such data with the treatment team (with the patient's full knowledge); the therapist is, after all, a member of this team, everyone participates in a united effort, and such mutuality can be basic to good treatment.

The provocative aggressiveness and sexual seductiveness of children are material presences that test the ethical strength of all staff. The temptation to engage in retaliatory or excessively stimulating interactions with a child or adolescent is a continuing source of stress in this work. Active address to the problems raised by these facts of childhood response and rapid, effective action in the face of any violation of this ethic are mandatory.

Externally, the relationships with the families of troubled children tend to generate all kinds of issues concerning control of the children; communication among staff, child, and family; responsibility for disturbing incidents; and the like. The fact is that, despite their preference or their assigned roles, all staff members must often function in a therapeutic way with various family members; this necessity complicates the process considerably. The precise delineation of roles and responsibilities in this realm remains to be described; the ethical problems that arise are not easily resolved. The basic position of staff must be to strive toward as therapeutic a stance as possible with the involved families. Occasionally, the need to defend the child inpatient from the frustrations, unfulfilled promises, manipulations, outright deceit, and overstimulating practices of the family pose substantial challenges to this position—and bring the involved staff members face to face with agonizing ethical choices.

Finally, the matter of discharging patients and setting them on their future course can be a source of considerable stress for the involved professionals. One may have a feeling that the program is not really "reaching" this girl; it is a holding operation, not a course of treatment. However (goes the thinking), if we discharge her (presumably to take in someone more amenable to our efforts), she will go right back into the incestuous home or out onto the street again as a prostitute. The ethical issue is real and not easily settled. Ideally, no child should leave unless there is a good aftercare plan with a maximum of continued support.

But what if the child is ready, but no such plan is possible? Many settings face the danger of becoming custodial care agencies unless they can discharge youngsters who are ready to leave or whom they can no longer help. This chilling quandary of the child with nowhere to go has yet to find a wholesome solution.

Numerous ethical problems are woven throughout the many elements of milieu care for adults and the elderly as well: The initial issues arise when a patient is accepted for hospitalization. For better or for worse in our culture, the fact of a psychiatric hospital stay of any duration will be regarded as good media fare if the individual enters—or is already in—public life. Hence, there is always a danger of potential stigma, and this fact must be balanced against the need for optimal treatment. The question facing the doctor is never merely: What am I doing for this person's illness? It always includes the matter of: What am I doing with this person's life?

If the hospital experience involves any deprivation of freedom (in the sense of involuntary admission or closed ward care), a variety of legal structures are called automatically into play. It is essential that all legal standards be met, both in letter and in spirit. The attendant ethical issues, however, extend beyond the requirements of law. They involve a necessary weighing of all the pros and cons of safety, protectiveness, and responsibility against deprivation of freedom, painful status confrontations, and traumatic wounds to self-esteem; the psychiatrist must act as the pilot who seeks to navigate between the Scylla of protection and the Charybdis of containment.

Within the therapeutic community as such, the ethical issues of group versus private experience are always in the forefront. The primary emphasis on emotional openness and expressivity, aside from its clinical problems, raises ethical issues as well. To what extent may a patient be pressed to reveal himself before a group of others who are not necessarily the audience of his choice? Beyond that, the ambiguities noted above in the authority structuring of such an enterprise can place the staff in a position that is as dubious ethically as it is questionable therapeutically.

Finally, in considering termination of inpatient care, ethical issues attend the question of what to do when the patient's money runs out (whether it be insurance money or funds from any other source). The decision maker is harassed on the one hand by the traditional medical imperative that the relief of suffering and the healing of disease always come first. Within this framework, the physician's recompense, while by no means unimportant, is nonetheless a secondary consideration, something to be attended to after the treatment and not a condition of its offering. On the other hand stand the real financial demands of milieu treatment; the relatively large number of highly trained specialists involved; the complex physical environment to be maintained; and the associated intake, outreach, follow-up, and administrative personnel who are attached—if the agency is to survive at all, all of these people require the most scrupulous protection of the income they earn. In point of fact, in whole or in part, that income usually depends on

patients' fees. Hence the ethic of survival is pitted against the ethic of care—
and in recent years the result has had a revolutionary force in the management of these issues. Due to the relatively large sums necessary to establish
adequate milieu care, the tendency to form corporate structures that are
then required to produce a return on investment has acted to complicate
these already difficult circumstances.

Some elderly patients in their advanced years, especially those in nursing
homes, may be physically frail, have psychological deficits, and be close to
death. Such patients are relatively helpless, totally dependent on others for
elementary self care, and lacking in promise for productive years ahead.
One must respect and value them for their history and their humanity, and
it takes a rather special cast of mind to do this without ambivalence. But it is
only if the dignity and the emotional wellness of such patients are the
primary values of the practitioner that they can be ministered to in adequate
fashion.

There is a long and unhappy cultural tradition of abandonment, neglect,
and exploitation of these elderly, who may be feeble and confused or who
may be mentally alert albeit physically weak. To deal with them and to
manage their treatment in a fully ethical fashion can be an immense
challenge to a treatment environment. To allow a troubled person relief
from distress along with a wholesome and respected place in his small
world for the remaining years has a moral weight that becomes its own
reward for those able to undertake this work.

REFERENCES

Abroms GM: Defining milieu therapy. Arch Gen Psychiatry 21:553-560, 1969

Abroms GM: Setting limits. Arch Gen Psychiatry 19:113-119, 1968

Aichhorn A: Wayward Youth. New York, Viking Press, 1935

Alpert A: Observations on the treatment of an emotionally disturbed child in a
therapeutic center. Psychoanal Study Child 9:334-343, 1954

Ankus M, Quarrington B: Operant behavior in the memory-disordered. J Gerontol
27:500-510, 1972

Arthur RJ: Social psychiatry: an overview. Am J Psychiatry 130:841-849, 1973

Bakos M, Bozic R, Chapin D, et al: Effects of environmental changes in elderly
residents' behavior. Hosp Community Psychiatry 31:677-682, 1980

Batiste CG, Yablonsky L: Synanon: a therapeutic life style. California Medicine
114:90-94, 1971

Bechenstein NI: Enhancing the gains: remotivation, a first step to restoration. Hops
Community Psychiatry 7:115-116, 1966

Bernfeld: Psychology of the Infant. London, Routledge and Sons, 1929

Bettelheim B, Sylvester E: A therapeutic milieu. Am J Orthopsychiatry 18:191-206, 1948

Bettelheim B: The Empty Fortress. New York, Free Press, 1967

Birjandi PF, Sclafani MJ: An interdisciplinary team approach to geriatric care. Hosp Community Psychiatry 24:777-778, 1973

Borup JH, Gallego DT, Heffernan PG: Relocation and its effect on mortality. Gerontologist 19:135-140, 1979

Boxberger R, Cotter VW: Music therapy for geriatric patients, in Music in Therapy. Edited by Gaston ET. New York, Macmillan, 1968

Brodsky CM, Fischer A: Therapeutic programming for the non-psychotic patient. Am J Psychiatry 120:793-797, 1964

Burnside IM: Group work with the aged: selected literature. Gerontologist 10:241-246, 1970

Bursten B: Decision making in the hospital community. Arch Gen Psychiatry 29:732-735, 1973

Busse EW: Old age, in The Course of Life: Psychoanalytic Contributions Toward Understanding Personality Development, vol 3: Adulthood and the Aging Process. Edited by Greenspan SI, Pollock GH. Washington, DC, NIMH, 1980

Byron EM: Reversing senile behavior patterns through RO-Sensory Stimulation group therapy. Journal of the National Association of Private Psychiatric Hospitals 10:68-72, 1978

Carp FM: Housing and living environments of older people, in Handbook of Aging and the Social Sciences. Edited by Binstock RH, Shanas C. New York, Van Nostrand Reinhold, 1976

Caudill W: The Psychiatric Hospital as a Small Society. Cambridge, Mass, Harvard University Press, 1958

Clark DH: The therapeutic community. Br J Psychiatry 131:553-564, 1977

Clark DH: Administrative Therapy: The Role of the Doctor in the Therapeutic Community. Philadelphia, Tavistock, 1964

Colthart SM: A mental health unit in a skilled nursing facility. J Am Geriat Soc 22:453-456, 1974

Cotton PG, Bene-Kociemba A, Kelly CC: A community program for elderly state hospital patients. J Geriatr Psychiatry 11:217-230, 1978

Cumming J, Cumming E: Ego and Milieu, Theory and Practice of Environmental Therapy. New York, Atherton Press, 1962

Davis D: An implementation of therapeutic community in a private mental health center. Dis Nerv Syst 38:189-191, 1977

DeLeon G, Holland S, Rosenthal MS: Phoenix House: criminal activity of dropouts. JAMA 222:686-689, 1972

DeLeon G, Rosenthal MS, Brodney K: Therapeutic community for drug addicts: long-term measurement of emotional changes. Psychol Rep 29:595-600, 1971

DeLeon G, Beschner GM (eds): The Therapeutic Community. Washington, DC, US Dept of HEW, 1976

Donahue W: What about our responsibility toward the abandoned elderly? Gerontologist 18:102-111, 1978

Donahue W: An experiment in the restoration and preservation of personality in the aged, in Planning the Older Years. Edited by Donahue W, Tibbetts C. Ann Arbor, University of Michigan Press, 1950

Dreikurs R: Group psychotherapy and the third revolution in psychiatry. Int J Soc Psychiatry 1:23-32, 1955

Edelson M: Sociotherapy and Psychotherapy. Chicago, University of Chicago Press, 1970

Ernst P: Sensory stimulation of elderly patients: preliminary report on the treatment of patients with chronic brain syndrome in an old age home. Israel Annals of Psychiatry and Related Disciplines 16:315-326, 1978

Ferster C, DeMyer M: The development of performances in autistic children in an automatically controlled environment. J Chronic Dis 13:312-345, 1961

Finkelstein M: Therapeutic value of arts and crafts in a geriatric hospital. J Am Geriatr Soc 19:341-350, 1971

Folsom JC: Reality orientation of the elderly mental patient. J Geriatr Psychiatry 1:291-307, 1968

Folsom JC: Attitude Therapy and the Team Approach. Tuscaloosa, Ala, Veterans Administration Hospital, 1966

Freud A: The Writings of Anna Freud, 1939-1945, vol 3: Infants without Families. Written in collaboration with Burlingham D. New York, International Universities Press, 1973

Friedman HJ: Some problems of inpatient management with borderline patients. Am J Psychiatry 126:299-304, 1969

Gatz M, Siegler IC, Dibner SS: Individual and community: normative conflicts in the development of a new therapeutic community for older persons. Int J Aging Hum Dev 10:249-263, 1979-80

Goffman E: Asylums: Essays on the Social Situation of Mental Patients and Other Inmates. New York, Anchor Books/Doubleday, 1961

Goldstein S: A critical appraisal of milieu therapy in a geriatric day hospital. J Am Geriatr Soc 19:693-699, 1971

Goplerud EN: Unexpected consequences of deinstitutionalization of the mentally disabled elderly. Am J Community Psychol 7:315-328, 1979

Gottesman LE, Quarterman CE, Cohn GM: Psychosocial treatment of the aged, in The Psychology of Adult Development & Aging. Edited by Eisdorfer C, Lawton MP. Washington DC, American Psychological Association, 1973

Gottesman LE, Brody EM: Psycho-social intervention programs within the institutional setting, in Long-Term Care: A Handbook for Researchers, Planners and Providers. Edited by Sherwood S. New York, Spectrum Publishers, 1975

Gottesman LE: Milieu treatment of the aged in institutions. Gerontologist 13:23-26, 1973

Grauer H: Institutions for the aged-therapeutic communities. J Am Geriatr Soc 19:687-692, 1971

Greenblatt M, York RH, Brown EL: From Custodial to Therapeutic Patient Care in Mental Hospitals, Explorations in Social Treatment. New York, Russell Sage Foundation, 1955

Greene JG, Nicol R, Jamieson H: Reality orientation with psychogeriatric patients. Behav Res Ther 17:615-618, 1979

Gunderson JG: A re-evaluation of milieu therapy for non-chronic schizophrenic patients. Schizophr Bull 6:64-69, 1980

Gunderson JG: An overview of modern milieu therapy, in Principles and Practice of Milieu Therapy. Edited by Gunderson JG, Will OA Jr, Mosher LR. New York, Jason Aronson, 1983

Gurian BS, Scherl DJ: A community-focused model of mental health services for the elderly. J Geriat Psychiatry 5:77-86, 1972

Hader M, Seltzer HA: La Salpetrière: an early home for elderly psychiatric patients. Gerontologist 7:133-135, 1967

Hansen JC, Neland TM, Zani LP: Model reinforcement in group counseling with elementary school children. Personnel Guidance Journal 47:741-744, 1969

Harris CS, Ivory PBCB: An outcome evaluation of reality orientation therapy with geriatric patients in a state mental hospital. Gerontologist 16:496-503, 1976

Harrison S, McDermott J, Chethik M: Residential treatment of children: the psychotherapist administrator. J Am Acad Child Psychiatry 8:385-410, 1969

Herman M: Activity programs in personal care homes. Canadian Journal of Occupational Therapy 35:98-100, 1968

Herz MI: Endicott J, Spitzer RL: Brief hospitalization: a two-year follow-up. Am J Psychiatry 134:502-507, 1977

Herz MI: Short-term hospitalization and the medical model. Hosp Community Psychiatry 30:117-121, 1979

Herz MI: The therapeutic community: a critique. Hosp Community Psychiatry 23:69-72, 1972

Hill BH: Here's what recreation can do for geriatric patients. Geriatrics 16:623-625, 1961

Joint Commission on Mental Illness and Health: Action for Mental Health. New York, Basic Books, 1961

Jones M, Baker A, Freeman T, et al: The Therapeutic Community: A New Treatment Method in Psychiatry. New York, Basic Books, 1953

Jones M: Maturation of the Therapeutic Community: An Organic Approach to Health and Mental Health. New York, Human Sciences Press, 1976

Jones M: Beyond the Therapeutic Community, Social Learning and Social Psychiatry. New Haven, Yale University Press, 1968a

Jones M: Social Psychiatry in Practice. Baltimore, Penguin Books, 1968b

Jones M: The treatment of personality disorders in a therapeutic community. Psychiatry 20:211-220, 1957

Jones M: The concept of a therapeutic community. Am J Psychiatry 112:647-650, 1956

Karasu TB, Plutchik R, Conte HR, et al: The therapeutic community in theory and practice. Hosp Community Psychiatry 28:436-440, 1977

Kartman LL: Therapeutic group activities in nursing homes. Health Soc Work 4:135-144, 1979

Kennard D: Limiting factors: the setting, the staff, the patients, in Therapeutic Communities: Reflections and Progress. Edited by Hinshelwood RD, Manning N. London, Routledge and Kegan Paul, 1979

Kiger RS: Treating the psychopathic patients in a therapeutic community, in The Therapeutic Community: A Sourcebook of Readings. Edited by Rossi JJ, Filstead WJ. New York, Behavioral Publications, 1973

Klein S, Frank P, Jacobs J: Token economy program for developing independent living skills in geriatric inpatients. Psychosocial Rehabilitation Journal 4:1-11, 1980

Kramer CH, Kramer JR: Basic Principles of Long-Term Patient Care: Developing a Therapeutic Community. Springfield, Ill, Charles C Thomas, 1976

Kramer M, Taube CA, Redick RW: Patterns of use of psychiatric facilities by the aged: past, present and future, in The Psychology of Adult Development and Aging. Edited by Eisdorfer C, Lawton MP. Washington, DC, American Psychological Association, 1978

Lamb HR, Goertzel V: Ellsworth House: a community alternative to jail. Am J Psychiatry 131:64-68, 1974

Lazarus LW: A program for the elderly at a private psychiatric hospital Gerontologist 16:125-131, 1976

Lehman A, Ritzler B: The therapeutic community inpatient ward: does it really work? Compr Psychiatry 17:755-761, 1976

Lesser J, Lazarus LW, Frankel R, et al: Reminiscence group therapy with psychotic geriatric inpatients. Gerontologist 21:291-296, 1981

Liebman MC, Hedlund DA: Therapeutic community and milieu therapy of personality disorders. in Personality Disorders, Diagnosis and Management (revised for DSM-III). Edited by Lion JR. Baltimore, Williams & Wilkins Co, 1981

Linden M: Group psychotherapy with institutionalized senile women: studies in gerontologic human relations. Int J Group Psychother 3:150-170, 1953

Lopez T, Kliman GW: The Cornerstone Treatment of a preschool boy from an extremely impoverished environment. Psychoanal Stud Child 35:341-676, 1980

Loughmiller C: Wilderness Road. Austin, Texas, Hogg Foundation for Mental Health, 1965

Lovaas OI, Berberish JP, Perloff BF, et al: Acquisition of imitative speech in schizophrenic children. Science 151:705-707, 1966

Lovaas OI, Schreibman L, Koegel RL: A behavior modification approach to the treatment of autistic children. J Autism Child Schizophr 4:111-129, 1974

Lowy L: Mental health services in the community, in Handbook of Mental Health and Aging. Edited by Birren JE, Sloane RB. Englewood Cliffs, NJ, Prentice-Hall, 1980

MacDonald ML: Environmental programming for the socially isolated aging. Gerontologist 18:350-354, 1978

Mahler MS: On child psychosis and schizophrenia: autistic and symbiotic infantile psychoses. Psychoanal Study Child, 7:286-305, 1952

Main TF: The hospital as a therapeutic institution. Bull Menninger Clin 10:66-70, 1946

Makarenko AS: The Road to Life (An Epic of Education). Moscow, Foreign Languages Publishing House, 1940

Margolis PM: Patient Power, the Development of a Therapeutic Community in a Psychiatric Unit of a General Hospital. Springfield, Ill, Charles C Thomas, 1973

Marohn RC: Juvenile Delinquents: Psychodynamic Assessment in Hospital Treatment. New York, Brunner/Mazel, 1980

Maxmen JS, Tucker GJ, LeBow M: Rational Hospital Psychiatry: The Reactive Environment. New York, Brunner/Mazel, 1974

Melin L, Gotestan KG: The effects of rearranging word routines on communications and eating behaviors of psychogeriatric patients. J Applied Behav Anal 14:47-51, 1981

Menninger WC: Psychiatric hospital therapy designed to meet unconscious needs. Am J Psychiatry 93:347-360, 1936

Mosher LR, Keith SJ: Research on the psychosocial treatment of schizophrenia: a summary report. Am J Psychiatry 136:623-631, 1979

Mosher LR, Menn AZ: Community residential treatment for schizophrenia: two-year follow-up. Hosp Community Psychiatry 29:715-723, 1978

Mueller DJ, Atlas L: Resocialization of regressed elderly residents: a behavioral management approach. J Gerontol 27:390-392, 1972

Neill AS: Summerhill. New York, Hart, 1960

Neugarten BL: Age groups in American society and the rise of the young-old. Annals of the American Academy 187-189, September 1974

Nielson GH: A project in parent education. Can J Public Health 61:210-214, 1970

Oldham JM, Russakoff LM: The medical-therapeutic community. Journal of Psychiatric Treatment and Evaluation 4:347-353, 1982

Oldham JM: The use of silent observers as an adjunct to short-term inpatient group psychotherapy. Int J Group Psychother 32:469-480, 1982

Palmer MD: Music therapy in a comprehensive program of treatment and rehabilitation for the geriatric resident. Journal of Music Therapy 14:190-197, 1977

Pfeiffer E (ed): Multidimensional Functional Assessment: The OARS Methodology. Durham, N C, Center for Study of Aging & Human Development, 1975

Proshansky HM, Ittelson WH, Rivlin LG: Environmental Psychology: Man and His Physical Setting. New York, Holt, Rinehart & Winston, 1970

Quitkin FM, Klein DF: Follow-up of treatment failure: psychosis and character disorders. Am J Psychiatry 124:499-505, 1967

Raasoch J, Willmuth R, Thomson L, et al: Intrahospital transfer: effects of chronically ill psychogeriatric patients. J Am Geriatr Soc 25:281-284, 1977

Rapoport R, Rapoport R: Permissiveness and treatment in a therapeutic community. Psychiatry 22:57-64, 1959

Rapoport R: Community as Doctor. London, Tavistock, 1960

Raskin DE: Milieu therapy re-examined. Compr Psychiatry 17:695-701, 1976

Raskin DE: Problems in the therapeutic community. Am J Psychiatry 128:492-493, 1971

Redl F: Strategy and techniques of the life space interview. Am J Orthopsychiatry 29:1-18, 1959

Reifler BV, Eisdorfer C: A clinic for the impaired elderly and their families. Am J Psychiatry 137:1399-1403, 1980

Rinsley DB: Theory and practice of intensive residential treatment of adolescents. Psychiatr Q 92:611-638, 1968

Rodstein M, Savitsky E, Starkman R: Initial adjustment to a long-term care institution: medical and behavioral aspects. J Am Geriatr Soc 24:65-71, 1976

Roskos SR, Lerner S, Kline BE: The elderly patient in a therapeutic community. Compr Psychiatry 20:359-368, 1979

Roth, R: A transactional analysis group in residential treatment of adolescents. Child Welfare 56:776-786, 1977

Sacks MH, Carpenter WT Jr: The pseudotherapeutic community. Hosp Community Psychiatry 25:315-318, 1974

Sandel SL: Movement therapy with geriatric patients in a convalescent home. Hosp Community Psychiatry 29:738-741, 1978

Schopler E, Reichler RJ: Parents as co-therapists in the treatment of psychotic children. J Autism Child Schizophr 1:87-102, 1971

Schwartz B: The social psychology of privacy. American Journal of Sociology 73:741-752, 1968

Schwartz CG: Problems for psychiatric nurses in playing a new role on a mental hospital ward, in The Patient and the Mental Hospital: Contributions of Research in the Science of Social Behavior. Edited by Greenblatt M, Levinson DJ, Williams RH. Glencoe, Ill, Free Press, 1957

Sherwood S, Mor V: Mental health institutions and the elderly, in Handbook of Mental Health and Aging. Edited by Birren JE, Sloane RB. Englewood Cliffs, NJ, Prentice-Hall, 1980

Silver A: Group psychotherapy with senile psychotic patients. Geriatrics 5:147-150, 1950

Stanton AH, Schwartz MS: The Mental Hospital: A Study of Institutional Participation in Psychiatric Illness and Treatment. New York, Basic Books, 1954

Strauss JS, Carpenter WT Jr: Schizophrenia. New York, Plenum Medical Book Co, 1981

Sullivan HS: Socio-psychiatric research: its implications for the schizophrenia problem and for mental hygiene. Am J Psychiatry 10:979-991, 1931

Tager-Flusberg H: On the nature of linguistic functioning in early infantile autism. J Autism Devel Disord 11:45-88, 1981

Talbott JA (ed): The Chronic Mental Patient in the Community. Washington, DC, American Psychiatric Association, 1978

Van Putten T, May PRA: Milieu therapy of the schizophrenias, in Treatment of Schizophrenia: Progress and Prospects. Edited by West LJ, Flinn DE. New York, Grune & Stratton, 1976

Van Putten T: Milieu therapy: contraindications? Arch Gen Psychiatry 29:640-643, 1973

Wendt RJ, Mosher LR, Matthews SM, et al: Comparison of two treatment environments for schizophrenia, in Principles and Practice of Milieu Therapy. Edited by Gunderson JG, Will OA Jr, Mosher LR. New York, Jason Aronson, 1983

Whanger AD: Treatment within the institution, in Handbook of Geriatric Psychiatry. Edited by Busse EW, Blazer DG. New York, Van Nostrand Reinhold, 1980

White NF: Reappraising the inpatient unit: obit milieu. Canadian Psychiatric Assn Journal 17:51-58, 1972

Whittaker JK: The ecology of child treatment. J Autism Child Schizophr 5:223-237, 1975

Wilmer HA: Defining and understanding the therapeutic community. Hosp Community Psychiatry 32:95-99, 1981

Wilmer HA: Toward a definition of the therapeutic community. Am J Psychiatry 114:824-834, 1958

Wolff MS: A review of literature on milieu therapy. J Psychiatric Nurs 15:26-33, 1977

Wolk RL, Seiden RB, Wolverton B: Unique influences and goals of an occupational therapy program in a home for the aged. J Am Geriatr Soc 13:989-997, 1965

World Health Organization Report Series No 177: Social Psychiatry and Community Attitudes. Geneva, World Health Organization, 1959

Yablonsky L: The Tunnel Back: Synanon. New York, MacMillan, 1965

Zarit SH: Aging and Mental Disorders: Psychological Approaches to Assessment and Treatment. New York, Free Press, 1980

Zeitlyn BB: The therapeutic community—fact or fantasy? Br J Psychiatry 113:1083-1086, 1967

Zlatin HP: I never had a chance: art therapy at a geriatric center. Art Psychotherapy 6:19-123, 1979

Zusman J, Lamb HR: In defense of community mental health. Am J Psychiatry 134:887-890, 1977

Zweig JP, Csank JZ: Mortality fluctuations among chronically ill medical geriatric patients as an indicator of stress before and after relocation. J Am Geriatr Soc 24:264-277, 1976

14

Therapies for Psychosexual Dysfunction

14

Therapies for Psychosexual Dysfunction

INTRODUCTION

Recent developments in the theoretical understanding and clinical assessment and treatment of sexual disorders have improved our ability to help sexually dysfunctional patients. One fundamental implication of recent work is that treatment outcome improves as a direct consequence of more accurate diagnosis of sexual pathology. Therefore the evaluation or diagnostic phase of clinical work has increased in significance. It is no longer acceptable simply to label a patient as "impotent" or "frigid"; it is now possible to describe much more accurately whether a patient has a problem with the desire, excitement, or orgasm phase of the sexual response.

It is also increasingly possible to assess the relative influence of psychogenic and organic etiologies. Patients with relatively minor sexual anxieties can be distinguished from those with identical symptoms of sexual dysfunction whose underlying relationship and intrapsychic conflicts are profound and complex. Subgroups of patients who respond only to a *combination* of sex therapy and medication have been identified. Thus, as our diagnostic ability gains precision, we can develop more effective treatment strategies to reduce the pathologic influence of each etiologic factor.

HISTORICAL PERSPECTIVE

Progress in the understanding and treatment of sexual disorders has been erratic but ongoing throughout this century, impeded principally by a socially restrictive moral climate that equated sexual functioning with immorality. Despite this inhibiting social background, which made innovative thought and research difficult, major contributions have been made by Freud, Kinsey, Masters and Johnson, and others. They provided the groundwork for current concepts of the physiology of the sexual response, sexual pathology, and methods of treating sexual disorders.

Freud described the powerful primitive natural urges within human beings. While these urges become convoluted in their manifestations within the context of repressive social attitudes, they nonetheless constitute a compelling force that consciously and unconsciously influences many aspects of our lives. Freud discovered childhood sexuality and called our attention to infantile desires and taboos that shape our adult sexual destinies (Freud, 1905).

Freud's theories—in their classic and modified forms—have dominated our thinking for half a century. Some of his ideas have proved immensely useful and form a cornerstone of modern psychiatric theory. Others have been discarded. But perhaps the critical importance of Freud's contribution to sexual medicine does not hinge on the correctness or error of his propositions but on the fact that he viewed sexuality, an area that had previously been held sacrosanct, from a scientific perspective. He advanced scientific theories about sexuality which could be proved or disproved, argued for or against, dismissed, refined, modified, or extended. These ideas were provocative and controversial, however, and further evidence was needed before the medical community and the public at large would look seriously into sexual health and disorders in a rational and constructive manner.

After World War II progress in sexual medicine accelerated. In the 1940's, Kinsey used structured interviews and statistical methods to survey the intimate sexual habits of ordinary men and women. His poll dispelled many sexual myths and showed, among other surprising findings, that normal American men and women regularly and periodically feel the stirrings of sexual desire and, when these are not satisfied by marital coitus, will express them through masturbation, with diverse partners, and in a variety of other ways, without apparent harm (Kinsey et al., 1948, 1953).

The 1950's saw the development of oral contraceptives for women, and in the 1960's Masters and Johnson took the crucial step that established sexuality as a psychobiological function similar to other human behaviors. They studied the sexual response of human males and females *in vivo*—in the laboratory. For a decade they carefully observed a wide range of human sexual behaviors: men and women having intercourse, masturbating, stimulating each other in various ways, becoming aroused, having orgasms, engaging in heterosexual acts, etc. (Masters and Johnson, 1970). They gave the first accurate description of externally observable physiologic aspects of human sexual response.

Masters and Johnson's contributions to sexual medicine are impressive. Among them are the greater appreciation of female sexual potential and clitoral eroticism and the understanding that some disabling sexual symptoms, such as premature ejaculation, impotence, and anorgasmia, may result from simple anxieties and stresses amenable to rapid, behaviorally-oriented sex therapy methods. They also highlighted the importance of dyadic interactions in the genesis and treatment of sexual disorders.

Some of Masters and Johnson's theories and some elements of their therapeutic method have proved to constitute true and significant advances. Other aspects of their work have been modified, extended, discarded, and criticized. Thus, for example, the basic element of sex therapy, i.e. the combination of structured sexual interactions between the couple combined with psychotherapy, has proved invaluable and has been retained in all subsequent modifications of sex therapy. However, newer forms of sex therapy have, for the most part, discarded some specific concepts and techniques originally advocated by Masters and Johnson. Thus, for example, the new generation of clinicians often does not use the dual sex therapy team but employs a single therapist (Kaplan, 1974), some conduct treatment in a group setting (Barbach, 1974), many now favor a far more flexible treatment program than the standard Masters and Johnson regimen (Kaplan, 1974, 1979; Lief, 1981), and others are more dynamically-oriented (Levay and Kagle, 1977a, 1977b; Levay and Weissberg, 1979). There is also a trend to treat different categories of sexual disorders in a more individualistic and specific manner than was originally used by Masters and Johnson.

By the 1970's the old restrictions had diminished. Sexuality became a legitimate topic for scientific study, and sexual problems were valid medical disorders deserving of treatment. New effective treatments for sexual problems were publicized, and suddenly there was a great international demand for sexual health services. As a result of this ferment, a vast clinical experience has been accumulated in the last decade by clinicians of diverse backgrounds in many cultural settings (Renshaw, 1975; Meyer, 1976; Zussman and Zussman, 1976; Levay and Kagle, 1977a, 1977b; Derogatis et al., 1978; Persky et al., 1978; Lief, 1981; Schiavi, 1981; Wagner and Green, 1982), leading to the construction of new rational concepts of sexual disorders and the development of effective treatment methods. Recent advances in medicine, surgery, and psychiatry have contributed to the maturation of sexual medicine. At long last, the genitals are catching up with the rest of the body.

THEORETICAL ISSUES

The new concepts and clinical developments may be summarized as follows:

Physiology: The Triphasic Concept. The sexual response of men and women is not a single reaction as had been believed in the past but can be understood to be made up of three physiologically distinct subphases: sexual desire, sexual excitement, and orgasm. The orgasm phase in both men and women consists of contractions of genital, perineal, and pelvic smooth and striated muscles, while the excitement phase is characterized by vasodilitation of the genital organs. Sexual desire is a drive state that depends on the activation of neural systems in the brain; however, the brain mechanisms regulating sex drive have not yet been clarified. While it is known that testosterone is essential to the activation of the "sex circuits" and the experience of libido in men as well as women, full understanding of the biological substrate of erotic desire awaits further advances in brain physiology, a field that remains in many respects a mystery despite active research that is beyond the scope of this chapter.

When all goes well, the sexual system operates as a smoothly functioning entity—desire blends with excitement which culminates in the climax of orgasm. But the orgasm and excitement phases and the sex drive (or desire) involve different anatomic structures governed by separate neural systems with their own centers, pathways, and neurotransmitters. This "related but separate" arrangement of neural control makes each subphase of the sexual response vulnerable to a different set of pathogenic influences.

With sufficiently severe trauma, the human sexual response can be totally impaired, with the result that the individual becomes entirely asexual. But this situation is not common. The physiologic organization of the three phases allows each to become impaired discretely and separately from the others, and partial impairment of the sexual response is the more prevalent clinical condition.

Although the triphasic model is a powerful construct, other models are also clinically useful. For example, Lief has subdivided the excitement phase into a mental "arousal" phase and a physical "vasocongestive" phase and has added the separate concept of "satisfaction," which, he points out, can be lacking despite the presence of the other phases. Hence, he finds "DAVOS," or desire, arousal, vasocongestion, orgasm, and satisfaction, as useful subdivisions (Lief, 1981).

Classification of Sexual Disorders. The modern classification of sexual disorders is based on the triphasic physiologic concept (APA, 1980). For the first time the psychosexual dysfunctions have been separated into distinct clinical syndromes or illnesses: the desire phase, excitement phase, and orgasm phase disorders. In the past all sexual disorders, such as premature ejaculation, anorgasmia in women, inhibited libido, impotence, and sexual phobias, were considered as a single clinical entity, which was labeled "impotence" in men and "frigidity" in women. It is more rational to conceptualize the different sexual syndromes as separate disorders because the differences in clinical features are the product of substantially different biologic and psychologic causes. Therefore, the syndromes are amenable to different and specific medical and psychiatric therapeutic interventions, and they carry very different prognoses.

Although *DSM-III* makes no specific provision for doing so, an argument can be made for including sexual phobias and avoidance with the psychosexual dysfunctions because these problems are highly prevalent among patients with sexual complaints and they respond to similar treatment approaches.

Current Concepts of Etiology. It is now clear that sexual disorders are the result of multiple determinants. A wide spectrum of organic and psychological factors can produce identical symptoms of impaired sexual pleasure and disturbances of the genital responses. Sexual disorders are in this respect like other psychophysiologic multidetermined syndromes such as headache, for example, which can also result from organic and psychological factors of diverse kinds and severity.

Psychogenicity. According to traditional views, psychosexual symptoms are always the product of serious psychopathology that originates in early childhood. But the extensive clinical experience of the past decades has shown that psychosexual dysfunctions can often be traced to "minor" psychological determinants, which may be consciously perceived by the patient and frequently have their origins in adolescence, the middle years, or senescence. The recognition that, in many cases, disabling sexual symptoms may occur in basically healthy persons with good marriages—being the product of relatively simple and currently operating psychological causes—is of enormous practical importance because sexual symptoms that are rooted in "minor" causes are highly responsive to the brief new sex therapy methods. Fortunately, a significant portion of sexual disorders falls into this category. Of course, many sexual symptoms are in fact associated with serious or "major" intrapsychic or interpersonal psychopathology. These more serious cases do not have as favorable a prognosis, and they require the more extensive forms of psychotherapeutic intervention which are capable of resolving "deep" and more complex neurotic processes and relationship problems.

DSM-III-defined Psychosexual Dysfunctions (in contrast to the broader category of Psychosexual Disorders) may be considered as psychophysiologic or psychosomatic disorders because they are usually ultimately caused by sexual anxiety. In other words, anxiety that is evoked at some time during love making disrupts the delicate reflexes and brain activity that constitute sexual response.

In general, but with notable exceptions, orgasm phase problems, such as premature ejaculation in men and anorgasmia in women, tend to be associated with relatively mild and comparatively easily modifiable anxiety or conflict, while inhibition of sexual desire (ISD) tends to occur in the most seriously conflicted individuals. Psychogenic impotence (excitement phase disorders) seems to be in the middle of this hypothetical distribution. Many patients who suffer from secondary impotence are the victims of minor performance anxieties, but serious neurotic processes or interpersonal conflicts may be involved in other cases.

As a rough metaphor, the psychological causes of the sexual dysfunctions may be conceptualized as occurring at different mental "levels" (Kaplan, 1979). On the most "superficial level" are the aforementioned "minor" sexual anxieties that occasionally disrupt sexual functioning. These are often consciously recognized and include "performance anxiety" or the fear of sexual failure, obsessive self-scrutiny and harsh judgment of one's sexual performance or attractiveness, the tendency to focus on negative aspects of the sexual situation, overconcern with pleasing the partner, and culturally determined inhibitions that make it difficult for the couple to communicate their erotic preferences and concerns clearly.

Unconscious conflicts about romantic success and intimacy may be considered as "mid-level" conflicts. While usually outside of awareness, they are not deeply repressed, and there is typically little resistance to insight when this material is confronted during brief therapy. These complexes have a "life of their own." They constitute powerful hidden forces that cause many people to sabotage their sexual pleasure and functioning. But success phobias do not arise *de novo*. They likely have their genesis in early repressed sexual and emotional trauma and negative family "messages" and roles. Also included in this class of "mid-level" conflicts may be moderate power struggles and parental transferences which can cause problems in the couple's system.

The most serious or "deepest" conflicts that can give rise to psychosexual dysfunctions include severe early prohibitions against sexual pleasure, which may have cultural or religious roots, and early sexual conflicts that originate during the critical developmental period when the child first tries to integrate his sexual impulses into his psyche—the oedipal period. Or the conflicts may arise even earlier. Disturbances that occur during the "pre-oedipal" period when the child learns the basics of intimacy may result in narcissistic and borderline personality disorders that make it difficult to form pleasurable, unambivalent romantic attachments in adult life (Kernberg, 1976).

The content of the conflicts and fears that lie at the "mid" and the "deepest" mental levels are not specifically associated with a particular dysfunctional syndrome but are, for the most part, nonspecific. In other words, the patient who cannot have an orgasm and the patient whose desire becomes blocked in intimate relationships could both be suffering from an underlying fear of romantic success which has its genesis in unresolved conflicts originating in early childhood. Again it is probable that the severity of this conflict is greater or more crippling for the patient with inhibited sexual desire than for the patient whose only impairment is her inhibited orgasm. But in contrast to the nonspecific nature of the remote psychic causes, the immediate currently operating psychological causes or antecedents are specifically associated with the different kinds of sexual dysfunction (Kaplan, 1974, 1979).

Organicity. Until recently it was believed that 95 percent of sexual dysfunctions were psychogenic. This view has changed in two respects. For one, new evidence indicates that the incidence of organicity may be considerably higher than was believed. Disease states and drugs must, therefore, be given serious consideration during evaluation. Also, the various clinical syndromes are essentially separate disorders that differ with respect to the prevalence of organic etiology. Recent advances in sexual medicine have confirmed the traditional view that orgasm dysfunctions are usually psychogenic (with notable exceptions, such as with certain drugs and autonomic neuropathy), but new insights into the physiologic basis of the excitement phase problems of men and women (impotence and impaired vaginal lubrication) and new discoveries related to libido suggest that these disorders are often due to subtle organic factors. A national cooperative study of 800 middle-aged impotent men indicated that 64 percent had organic impairment of erections (Coleman et al., 1982). Persons over the age of 40 are at especially high risk of developing sexual disorders that have an organic component.

The consideration of the effects of illness and drugs on sexual functioning is relatively new and accounts for the traditional underestimation of organicity in sexual disorders. Until recently only the most obvious organic causes of sexual problems were recognized and diagnosed as such. Sexual symptoms tended to be mislabeled as psychogenic unless they were associated with gross pathology of the sexual organs caused by trauma, surgery or congenital abnormalities, severe deficiencies of testosterone, advanced diabetes, or circulatory deficiencies of the pelvis and the lower extremities as seen in Leriche's syndrome. But there is growing recognition that sexual disorders are often the product of more subtle medical conditions the signs and symptoms of which may be limited to a disturbance of the sexual response or one of its components. Many unsuccessful psychological treatments can be attributed to the clinician's failure to detect the organic roots of the patient's sexual problems.

The recent progress in the understanding of sexual physiology has led to the identification of an increasing number of previously unrecognized medical conditions and drugs that can cause sexual problems. These include alcohol, narcotics, the antihypertensive medications, and beta adrenergic blocking agents, which frequently cause impotence; prolactin secreting micro adenomas of the pituitary, which in early stages may have no other sign except reduced libido and impotence; and arteriosclerosis of the small penile vessels, which spares orgasm and libido and is only manifest by a gradually increasing erectile difficulty. Karacan and colleagues (1978) have compiled a list of more than 100 such contributors to organic impotence.

These new findings, and the fact that identical sexual symptoms can be caused by psychogenic and organic determinants, underscore the need for a comprehensive evaluation of sexual disorders which takes cognizance of both biologic and psychologic causes. As a corollary of the progress in understanding the medical aspects of sexual disorders, improved diagnostic methods are extremely helpful in assessing some of these more subtle organic sexual problems. The most useful of these is the nocturnal penile tumescence monitor, which measures the erections that normally occur during REM sleep when the patient is presumably free of sexual anxieties (Karacan et al., 1978; Wasserman et al., 1980; Schiavi, 1981). This method is extremely helpful in differentiating organic from psychogenic erectile difficulties in those cases in which the clinical pattern is not clear. Nocturnal penile tumescence studies in combination with other tests routinely performed by specialized evaluation centers (Karacan and Moore, in press) can usually detect the etiology of organic impotence. Doppler studies of penile pulse volume and measurements of nocturnal penile segmental blood flow (Karacan, 1983) and penile post-ischemic hyperemia provide extremely useful noninvasive measures of penile circulatory functions. A variety of tests are also available for revealing neurophysiologic impairment and endocrinopathies associated with impotence, such as testosterone and luteinizing hormone deficiencies and hyperprolactinemia (Cunningham et al., 1982). Microscopic studies of the vaginal epithelium have been supplemented by more reliable assays of blood estrogen levels which are of value in differentiating lubrication difficulties caused by estrogen deficiencies from psychogenic inhibition of the excitement phases (Kaplan, 1983).

With these physiologic concepts and an awareness of both psychogenic and organic etiologies in mind, we are prepared for the diagnostic evaluation process.

EVALUATION, INDICATIONS, AND LIMITATIONS

A diagnostic evaluation of a sexual complaint must answer these questions:

A. *Does the patient have a true sexual disorder?* Instead, the complaint may be the presenting symptom of a troubled marriage or another psychiatric disorder. Or the patient may be a normally functioning person who is merely misinformed as to what he or she should expect.

B. *What type of sexual problem is it?* Can it be described as an impairment of desire, excitement, or orgasm? Is it a problem of painful genital muscle spasm or decreased genital sensations? Does it involve sexual phobia, dyspareunia, or unconsummated marriage?

C. *What are the likely causes?* Is it a global problem occurring in all sexual settings and thereby necessitating that organic factors be ruled out? Or is it situational, occurring only with partners or a particular partner, but not under all circumstances, which suggests psychogenicity (with notable exceptions [Karacan and Moore, in press]).

D. *Are there medical factors such as antihypertensive drugs, diabetes, hormone abnormalities, arteriosclerosis, gynecological pathology, or injury which may be contributing organic causes of dysfunction?* Are further examinations or tests indicated?

E. *Are there relevant psychological factors on a superficial, mid, or deep level which may be contributing?* Is there performance anxiety, spectatoring, negative cognitions, fear of intimacy or success, or oedipal anxiety? Is there a lack of knowledge, communication skills, or assertiveness?

F. *What is the quality of the patient's sexual/romantic relationship?* Is there love, trust, power struggle, intimidation, or boredom? What is the nature of mutual transference?

G. *What were the patient's psychosexual background and family messages regarding sexuality?*

H. *Can the immediate cause be identified?* Is it psychological, organic, relational, or technical (including insufficient stimulation); or, as is most often the case, do multiple factors have to be sorted through?

The answers to these questions help to diagnose the problem precisely and to develop a rational treatment plan that will exclude patients who are not likely to be amenable to sex therapy. Some conditions should be excluded from sex therapy because they either do not warrant or will not respond to this approach. Other conditions may be partially helped by sex therapy but are more appropriate for other forms of treatment. More specifically, the evaluation should identify patients whose sexual complaints are not true dysfunctions, those whose problem has an exclusively or predominantly organic basis, and those cases of sexual difficulties which are secondary to major psychopathologic states or severe marital discord.

Conditions to be excluded include:

A. *Normal*—Individuals occasionally will seek therapy due to confusion from lack of information or understanding about sexual functions. These individuals generally need only reassurance and possibly sources of further information.

B. *Obsessions*—Many patients become obsessed with their sexual functioning or the sexual response of their partner and erroneously believe they or the partner has a sexual disorder. These patients defend against other forms of anxiety by dwelling on their obsessions. They need to be reassured about their sexuality and treated for specific obsessive disorders.

C. *Gender identity disorders* (including transsexualism). In general, these do not respond to sex therapy. Such patients should be evaluated in depth and given a trial of psychotherapy prior to any consideration of the irreversible approaches such as hormonal or surgical sex reassignment.

D. Paraphilias—The paraphilias may be considered as special instances of inhibition of desire (Schwartz and Masters, 1983). Traditionally it has been held that such patients, if indeed they desired a change, suffered from deep and profound conflict that required lengthy insight therapy. Recent evidence suggests that some of these patients have developed their variant sexual response pattern on the basis of relatively minor anxieties that are amenable to brief, specific treatment procedures.

Conditions warranting specialized evaluations and treatment prior to or concurrent with consideration of sex therapy include the following:

A. Sexual dysfunctions associated with organic factors, e.g., organically impaired erections or vaginal vasocongestion/lubrication, low sex desire from testosterone deficiencies, hepatic or renal disease, post-coronary syndromes, prolactin secreting pituitary adenomas, and other endocrine dysfunctions. The patients with organic factors may benefit from the educational and communications aspects of sex therapy in terms of sexual rehabilitation, but their underlying physical problem must be addressed directly.

B. Conditions secondary to major psychopathology, e.g., severe depression, severe anxiety, phobic states, and psychosis, which may be the primary cause of sexual disorders and require individual treatment and/or medication.

C. Sexual problems related to substance abuse such as alcoholism or opiate dependence, which will not respond unless these primary conditions are resolved.

D. Sexual problems consequent to severe marital problems requiring conjoint therapy prior to sex therapy.

E. Sexual problems secondary to severe stress of nonsexual nature, e.g., job loss, recent object loss, etc. Stress must be resolved prior to sex therapy.

F. Sexual problems reflecting severe neurotic processes requiring long-term therapeutic interaction.

Once the evaluation is complete and the condition is deemed amenable and appropriate for sex therapy, the clinician can proceed to the treatment itself.

TREATMENT GOALS AND TECHNIQUES

The goals of treatment for sexual disorders are typically quite specific, e.g., the relief of the manifest symptoms such as low sexual desire, absence of or inadequate erection or vaginal lubrication, failure to achieve orgasm, lack of control over ejaculation, unconsummated marriage, the phobic avoidance of sex, or pain in either partner on intercourse. In order to reach these goals, the immediate causes or antecedents of the symptom must be modified. These modifications typically include reduction of sexual anxiety, reduction of anger and ambivalence toward the partner, acquisition of sexual information and techniques, improvement in partner communication about sex, and improvement in sensitivity and loving feelings. Also included are reduction in nonerotic obsessive thoughts; openness to erotic fantasy; and, for premature ejaculation, focusing on the level of arousal. In general, more extensive goals such as personality change, resolution of deep conflict, and fundamental restructuring of the couple's relationship are not pursued unless they are essential to progress toward the specific goal. Sometimes the simple goals described above are attained without major personality change, intrapsychic exploration, or major changes in the marital system. At other times the couple's dyadic difficulties and either partner's intrapsychic conflicts about sex, intimacy, and pleasure must be confronted during therapy before sexual adequacy is possible.

The establishment of symptom relief as a goal became possible as clinical evidence showed that when cases were selected with care many couples were able to obtain symptomatic relief and to go on to enjoy sexual functioning without any adverse reactions. In those cases in which symptomatic relief is not easily obtained and/or in which a great deal of resistance is mobilized by the treatment process, then additional or lengthier and more insight-oriented individual or marital therapy is frequently warranted. Lief (1981) has estimated that in 30 to 40 percent of cases, symptomatic improvement will occur without major psychodynamic changes. He divides the remaining 60 percent as follows: Ten percent need individual therapy; 20 percent need marital therapy, setting aside sex therapy until much later; and 30 percent need a combination of sex and marital therapy. Kaplan's experience (1983) is similar, with the addition that approximately 25 percent of patients receive psychoactive medication for depression or panic disorders concomitantly with sex therapy.

Modern sex therapy uses a combination of behavioral tasks together with psychotherapeutic interventions. The behavior tasks consist of a series of structured erotic interactions conducted by the patient or couple in the privacy of their home. These are integrated with psychotherapeutic sessions conducted in the therapist's office with the individual patient or conjointly with the couple.

In order to cure a sexual symptom it is necessary to alter its immediate cause or antecedent (Kaplan, 1979). If the immediate cause or antecedent is not modified, the symptom will persist, even if the patient gains some insight into the remote or deeper sexual anxieties and conflicts that are ultimately responsible for the genesis of the disorder.

The basic treatment strategy of the new sex therapies is to attempt to identify and modify the immediate inhibitors of sexual functioning—the performance anxieties, lack of confidence and skill, the minor anxieties and relationship difficulties, the tendency to "turn oneself off" by focusing on negative thoughts—but at the same time to be prepared to deal with unconscious conflicts and deeper intrapsychic and dyadic problems that are frequently operative.

The behavioral erotic and intimate tasks and other behavioral techniques such as communication skills and assertiveness training are designed to modify the specific and immediate causes of the symptoms of sexual dysfunction. Since these immediate causes tend to differ for the different dysfunctions, highly specific and different behavioral techniques have been developed for each disorder. Thus the "homework" assigned to the anorgasmic woman is different from the sequence of erotic tasks prescribed for the couple who suffer from sexual avoidance, while the impotent patient and his partner receive yet another set of behavioral instructions. But this emphasis on the behavioral aspects of treatment should not be taken to mean that insight and resolution of unconscious conflict have no place in the modern treatment of psychosexual dysfunctions.

Some sexual symptoms are the product of minor sexual anxieties and are amenable to simple behaviorally-oriented treatment approaches. But more often the symptoms arise from complex intrapsychic conflicts about sex and also from more serious problems in the couple's interaction. These "deeper" or more remote etiologic factors tend to give rise to resistances during the treatment process. The active confrontations of sex therapy, as well as the extremely rapid gains in sexual pleasure and competency, are threatening to the patient with sexual conflicts and to the partner as well. The equilibrium of a previously stable dyadic system may be disturbed in the process. Such complex problems cannot be expected to yield to brief behavioral methods alone. The emotional reactions and psychological conflicts that are evoked by the erotic tasks are dealt with in a psychodynamic framework in the office sessions with the therapist. Here the members of the couple are confronted with their resistances to sexual pleasure and their ambivalence about committing themselves to therapy and to each other. They are supported in their quest for sexual adequacy, their vulnerabilities are gently extracted from their defensive shells, and their unconscious sexual conflicts are explored with the aim of fostering insight and resolution. The integration of behavioral and psychodynamic methods is the key to the success of the new sex therapies and also to their advantage over both insight and behavioral methods alone.

The Sessions

The content of the therapeutic sessions varies from simple education and support to active confrontation and exploration of unconscious material. The psychotherapeutic aspect of treatment is not specifically different for the various syndromes. In each sex therapy session the therapist uses a technique somewhat analogous to crisis intervention strategy, viewing the couple's interaction around the problem or assigned task as a "crisis"

(Kaplan, 1974). The therapist then attempts to balance support and confrontation to facilitate progress. Each session typically includes:

A. A review of the results of the last assigned task;

B. A review of each partner's emotional state, his dreams, and the status of the couple's relationship;

C. Support and encouragement for progress in pleasure, insight, and relating to each other;

D. Careful confrontation of each partner's resistances to progress;

E. Interpretation of possible unconscious intrapsychic or interpersonal conflicts causing resistance; and

F. A new or modified assignment.

The tasks used by Masters and Johnson are similar for all dysfunctions. Recent modifications of sex therapy have retained some of these highly effective maneuvers but have introduced additional interactions that are specifically tailored to each couple and to the particular syndrome. The goal is to select a task that will not create so much anxiety that it is avoided but that will advance progressively toward relief of the sexual symptom. The focus of the tasks is to modify the immediate antecedents of anxiety or conflict which have inhibited normal sexual response in the past. In each individual these immediate antecedents are highly specific and must be identified by the therapist. The behavioral sequences used for the various dysfunctions have been described by Kaplan (1974, 1979) and are summarized below.

Premature Ejaculation. The aim of treatment for premature ejaculation is to facilitate learning voluntary control over ejaculation by fostering the patient's awareness of, and increasing his tolerance for, the pleasurable genital sensations that accompany the intense sexual excitement that precedes orgasm. Any method that encourages the man's concentration on preorgastic erotic sensations, including the "squeeze" (Masters and Johnson, 1970) and the "stop-start" methods (Semans, 1956), can be used to implement this goal.

The following variation of the stop-start method may be used. The patient is advised to concentrate on his erotic sensations only and not to attempt to "hold back."

A. The partner stimulates the patient's penis manually until he feels that he is near climax. He then asks her to stop. A few seconds later when he feels the acute sensations diminish, he asks her to start again. He reaches climax on the fourth period of stimulation.

B. The stop-start stimulation of the penis manually by the partner is repeated, this time using a lubricant (petroleum jelly). This procedure simulates the sensations produced by the vaginal environment.

C. Stop-start stimulation is conducted intravaginally in the female superior position. The woman straddles her partner with his erect penis inside her vagina. His hands are on her hips to guide her motions. She moves up and down until he feels that he is near climax and motions her to stop. Then he signals her to start again. He attains climax on the third period of stimulation. At first he does not thrust during this exercise. After he achieves control he proceeds to thrust.

D. Stop-start intravaginally is conducted in the side-to-side position.

E. Stop-start intravaginally is conducted in the male superior position.

F. Stop-slow intravaginally is conducted. After the patient has learned control by stopping at a high plateau of excitement, if necessary he can improve his control by slowing rather than coming to a complete stop at high excitement levels. This "stop-slow" assignment may be used when the man is having difficulty integrating his new ejaculatory control into his behavior.

Inhibited Orgasm—Men and Women. The objective of the treatment of orgasm inhibition is to modify the patient's tendency to observe his/her pre-orgastic sensations obsessively and to foster abandonment to erotic feelings, which is a necessary condition of orgastic release. These aims can be implemented by structuring the situation so that the patient receives effective penile or clitoral stimulation under the most tranquil conditions that can be arranged. At the same time, he/she is distracted from the obsessive self-observations. The usual means of distraction is fantasy, but external distractions such as reading or observing erotic pictures or films may also be used to circumvent the difficulties some patients experience with fantasy.

The following method may be used, unless the evaluation reveals reasons to modify the treatment plan.

Total Anorgasmia—Men and Women. If the patient is totally anorgasmic, the initial aim of treatment is to have the patient experience an orgasm while he or she is alone, as follows:

A. Self-stimulation of the penis or clitoris. This is first done manually. If the manual stimulation is not sufficient to overcome the resistance to orgasm, the intensity of the stimulus is increased. Toward this end men use a lubricant and women a vibrator.

B. Concomitant distraction by imagery. This may entail concentration on the person's favorite erotic fantasy, reading erotic literature, viewing erotic pictures, or focusing on a nonerotic neutral image. The mental imagery occurs while the patient is stimulating him/herself.

Anorgasmia with a Partner—Men and Women. After the patient is comfortable with his/her own sexual feelings and orgasm, or if orgasm can only be reached when alone, the next step entails learning to have an orgasm in the presence of the partner. Since shared sex is usually far more anxiety-provoking than sex when one is alone, orgasm alone usually precedes shared orgasm unless there is profound resistance to masturbation.

The steps to shared orgasm are:

A. Self-stimulation to orgasm in the partner's presence. This should occur with a gradual increase in intimacy. First the partner turns his/her back while the patient masturbates. Then the partner can hold the patient during the self-stimulation. One partner can masturbate to orgasm after the other has climaxed, but the patient should not attempt to reach orgasm during intercourse at this stage of treatment.

B. Manual genital stimulation to orgasm by the partner, while the patient uses his/her customary fantasy for distraction. (This is preceded by sensate focus I and II as needed. See p. 690.)

Coital Anorgasmia. Treatment for this complaint essentially consists of progressive *in vivo* desensitization to orgasmic release during vaginal containment. The treatment procedures for men and women are slightly different at this point.

Retarded Ejaculation.

A. Orgasm is reached by manual self-stimulation of the genitals in the presence of the partner. This is done progressively nearer to the partner's vagina, until orgasm can comfortably be achieved near the mouth of the vagina.

B. Orgasm is achieved by manual stimulation by the partner.

C. The partner stimulates the man's penis manually to a point close to orgasm. Then the penis is inserted into the vagina at the moment of orgasm.

D. The procedure is repeated but the penis is inserted into the vagina progressively earlier until the need for manual stimulation diminishes.

E. Concomitant manual and vaginal stimulation of the penis. The female stimulates the base of her partner's penis manually as he thrusts in and out of the vagina. This maneuver supplies additional stimulation. It is sometimes used to supplement the progressive desensitization, described in steps A through D.

Partial Ejaculatory Retardation. The immediate antecedents of this syndrome are similar, if not identical, to the immediate causes of general retardation of the entire male ejaculatory reflex, and treatment follows the same tactics: relaxation and stimulation concomitant with distraction by fantasy.

Female Coital Anorgasmia. The aim of the treatment of female coital anorgasmia is to diminish any anxieties, if they exist, that are provoked by penetration in order to lower the woman's orgasmic threshold. In addition, the patient is trained to maximize the relatively low level of clitoral stimulation provided by penetration and to accustom herself to have orgasms in this manner. Most women can learn to have orgasm on coitus with concomitant clitoral stimulation with these techniques. But only a relatively few are successful in achieving coital orgasm without "clitoral assistance."

One suggested method for the treatment of coital anorgasmia uses the following sequence:

A. Self-stimulation with pelvic thrusting. Under usual circumstances women reach orgasm during coitus by actively thrusting the pelvis against the partner's pubic bone and not, as during masturbatory, manual, or oral stimulation, by passive reception of stimulation. Therefore, coitally anorgastic women are first taught to stimulate themselves to orgasm by thrusting their pelvis down against their stationary hand. This pattern of orgasmic release improves the probability of learning orgasm during coitus.

B. The bridge maneuver. This consists of concomitant clitoral stimulation and vaginal intromission. While the penis is inserted, the woman or her partner stimulates her clitoris until she reaches orgasm. This is most comfortable in the side-to-side or rear entry positions. Intromission is delayed until the woman is highly aroused by foreplay.

C. Progressively earlier cessation of clitoral stimulation while the penis is inserted in order to climax without "clitoral assistance."

It is important to communicate to the couple that clitorally induced orgasm is considered to be a normal response pattern. Such couples are counseled to adapt their love making to the woman's pattern of climax, without considering this "settling for second best" or taking it as evidence that the woman is inhibited or that the man is a poor lover.

Inhibited Sexual Excitement—Male (Impotence or Erectile Dysfunction). The performance anxiety that is so frequently associated with impotence can be diminished in many cases by structuring the sexual interactions so that they are nondemanding and reassuring. The patient is encouraged to substitute the nonpressuring goal of pleasure for the stress-producing goal of performance, and the sexual situation is arranged so that it is highly stimulating but has a low level of demand for performance or pressure. The basic Masters and Johnson method accomplishes these goals in a substantial number of patients.

A. Sensate focus I—This step consists of taking turns caressing or "pleasuring" each other's bodies without genital stimulation.

B. Sensate focus II—This step involves taking turns "body pleasuring" and also includes gentle, nondemanding genital stimulation which may proceed to erection but not to orgasm.

C. Brief intromission without orgasm in the female superior position. The woman inserts her partner's penis into her vagina, thrusts a few times, and gets off before there is anxiety or erection loss. The man reaches orgasm by manual stimulation, which is provided by himself or by his partner, depending on which is more comfortable for him.

D. Intromission to orgasm in the female superior position.

E. Intromission to orgasm in the male superior position.

This method is highly effective in those cases in which the etiology is a simple fear of failure. However, many impotent men are basically afraid of sexual success and require a more flexible treatment approach that is designed to accommodate their specific needs. The following tasks may be used to circumvent or "bypass" sexual anxiety that is not related primarily to performance fears. They are designed to reduce the pressure on the man still further and also to provide him with the tools to deal with his anxiety should it arise.

A. The use of fantasy concomitant with genital stimulation, especially during anxious moments.

B. Having the wife learn to accept clitoral stimulation as an alternative to coitus, thus relieving the pressure on the man.

C. Teaching the couple the use of self-stimulation at times of tension.

When partner demands are an etiologic element, treatment focuses on the partner's resistances and on the couple's interactions.

Partial Impotence. It may be speculated that men who cannot ejaculate with a full erection on a psychogenic basis have reinforced the incomplete erections by ejaculating in that state. This reinforcement sequence may be regarded as the immediate cause of the syndrome of partial impotence. Treatment is based on the rationale of extinguishing that response and reinforcing full erection instead.

The man or his partner stimulates his penis. He is advised not to allow himself to reach climax unless he is fully erect. If he feels that he is near orgasm he stops until he is fully erect. Finally, when he has a full erection, he attains climax. This is a frustrating but effective treatment procedure.

Inhibited Sexual Excitement—Female. The aim of treatment of this rather uncommon disorder is to reduce the anxiety that is evoked during the excitement phase and that inhibits its expression. The original Masters and Johnson method is effective, although there are advantages to using some flexibility to accommodate the patient's individual dynamic needs.

A. Sensate focus I—See p. 690.

B. Sensate focus II—See p. 690.

C. Slow, teasing genital stimulation by partner. The vulva, clitoris, vaginal entrance, and the nipples are caressed. This stimulation is interrupted if the woman feels that she is near orgasm; it is continued a little later when arousal has diminished somewhat.

D. Withholding of coitus until the woman is well-lubricated. To avoid frustration and to reduce pressure on the woman, the partner is advised to have extracoital orgasms during this phase of treatment.

E. Slow, teasing, nondemanding intromission in the female superior position under her control, for the purpose of focusing on her vaginal sensations.

When the patient's anxiety does not diminish sufficiently with these desensitizing exercises, it may be helpful to suggest bypass via distracting erotic imagery during stimulation to give her a "tool" for managing her anxiety.

Inhibited Sexual Desire—Men and Women. The sexual exercises used to treat inhibited sexual desire (ISD) are designed to confront the patient with his/her active, though unconscious and involuntary, avoidance of sexual feelings and activities and/or the tendency to focus on negative images and thoughts and to suppress sexual feelings that may emerge despite the patient's defenses against them.

In addition, as has already been mentioned, desire phase disorders seem, with some exceptions, to be associated with more severe and tenacious underlying psychopathology than is typically associated with the genital dysfunctions. Consequently, psychosexual treatment of these disorders often necessitates much more extensive psychotherapeutic intervention than does the treatment of orgasm and excitement phase disorders.

The structured sexual experiences are designed to reduce sexual anxiety and to promote sexual pleasure. At the same time, they play the role of a "probe" to ferret out rapidly and foster the emergence of deeper anxieties and resistances and to make these available for psychotherapeutic exploration in the sessions. The blocks against sexual desire must be clearly identified and resolved or bypassed before sexual desire can return.

In these disorders the sequence of treatment is much more variable than with prematurity, secondary impotence, or inadequate vaginal lubrication. The therapist decides on exercises according to the specific dynamic needs of the couple. However, in order to illuminate these dynamics, it is often useful to begin treatment with the "classical" Masters and Johnson therapeutic sequence that is used in the excitement phase disorders:

A. Sensate focus I—See p. 690.

B. Sensate focus II—See p. 690.

C. Self-stimulation—If the patient is inhibited in desire and is also anorgastic, he/she first learns to have an orgasm alone. If both partners are anorgastic, they masturbate together in each other's presence.

D. Exploring fantasies—In blocked patients the exploration of fantasies is often useful, both to increase desire and to reveal psychological blocks.

E. Sharing erotic fantasies with partner.

F. Sharing erotic material with partner.

G. Slow and nondemanding intromission.

H. Focus on the emotional interaction of the couple before love making.

Functional Vaginismus. The treatment of vaginismus is designed to extinguish the conditioned spasm of the muscles surrounding the vagina by means of systematic *in vivo* desensitization. Any technique that uses gradual dilatation of the spastic introitus is effective. One method uses the following sequence:

A. Inspection of vaginal opening by patient using a mirror.

B. Daily insertion of one of her fingers or a small dilator into her vaginal opening until comfortable. A lubricant may be used in all the dilatation exercises. Also, graduated dilators may be substituted for fingers.

C. Daily insertion of two fingers or larger dilator into vaginal opening until comfortable.

D. Daily insertion of three fingers or largest dilator into vaginal opening until comfortable.

E. Insertion of one or two fingers into vaginal opening by partner.

F. Insertion of penis without thrusting under patient's control. This is usually most comfortable in the female superior position.

G. Insertion with thrusting.

When vaginismus is mild enough to permit penetration but severe enough to make intercourse painful, gradual dilatation of the vagina is also highly effective. The use of a lubricant is helpful.

Ejaculatory Pain Due to Muscle Spasm. The muscle spasm that occurs immediately after ejaculation and that is the immediate cause of this syndrome is treated with a variety of psychological anxiety reduction methods, such as reassurance and explanation. These are used together with procedures that relax muscles by physical means, including diazepam medication and hot sitzbaths.

Sexual Phobias. The immediate cause of sexual phobias and their attendant avoidance behavior is acute anxiety and panic, which is evoked by sexual feelings and/or activities. Sexual phobias respond to the same treatment procedures as other kinds of phobias. When the sexual phobia is part of a panic disorder (phobic anxiety syndrome), treatment with one of several "antipanic" medications is appropriate. Medications that have been found to be helpful include tricyclic antidepressants and MAO inhibitors (Klein, 1980), beta adrenergic blockers and, more recently, alprazolam and trazodone (Sheehan, 1982). Evidence indicates that many sexually phobic patients can be helped by these drugs, which protect them against the panic attacks they experience in the phobic situation. The residual anticipatory anxieties can then be diminished with systematic *in vivo* desensitization by means of gradual sexual exercises and sometimes with systematic sexual assertiveness. It may further be necessary to resolve intrapsychic conflicts about sex and to explore the role that sexual avoidance plays in the couple's relationship. In those cases that require no medication, a combination of very gradual *in vivo* desensitization and psychotherapeutic support and confrontation of resistances is often effective. It is not possible to construct a sequence of tasks which is appropriate for all phobic patients because the anxiety patterns are highly individual (Kaplan et al., 1982).

Unconsummated Marriage. The successful management of unconsummated marriage rests on the accurate diagnosis of the specific immediate causes of the problem. A couple may be unable to have intercourse for a variety of reasons. These include a sexual phobia on the part of either partner, ignorance, dyspareunia, or sexual dysfunction. Treatment will, of course, vary with the specific cause.

Alternative Treatments. The therapeutic goal in the treatment of sexual disorders is to reduce sexual anxiety and conflict to a point at which sexual functioning is adequate and pleasurable. Currently several alternate therapeutic strategies are used to implement these objectives.

Individual Insight Therapy. This may be helpful in resolving some of the basic intrapsychic causes of anxiety, anger, and conflict although even when the patient gains insight into his underlying conflicts, the sexual symptom is likely to persist. It may be speculated that the verbal psychotherapies often fail to modify directly the immediate and specific antecedents of sexual symptoms. When no cooperative partner is available, individual psychotherapy may be a good alternative to sex therapy.

Conjoint Insight Psychotherapy. This is likely to be helpful in enhancing mutual understanding and communication and reducing resentment and the kinds of angers and anxieties that are evoked by marital conflict. However, unless this approach is combined with specific structured sexual tasks that modify the immediate causes of the sexual symptom, it is unlikely to progress quickly or to help resolve many of the immediate causes of sexual dysfunction such as inadequate stimulation, performance anxiety, "spectatoring," or a lack of awareness of each other's tension or arousal. It appears that many mutually cooperative, well meaning partners do not instinctively know how to relax themselves or their partners or how to provide appropriate stimulation. Often much of this behavior must be learned in a gradual structured manner designed to reduce the vulnerabilities and misunderstandings that so frequently are an obstacle to gratifying sexual interactions.

Behavior Therapy. This method is well established in its techniques for analyzing the immediate contingencies of inadequate sexual behavior and in giving patients specific tasks to follow in order gradually to reduce sexual anxiety, acquire new love-making skills, and communicate sexual needs and wishes assertively. Behavior therapists have been highly successful in some cases of sexual phobias, anorgasmia, and sexual avoidance when these syndromes were associated with minor anxieties (Brady, 1976). This approach is less likely to be effective in cases where the roots of anxiety and anger are deeper and not consciously perceived, as in the cases in which issues of fear of competition, fear of success, and fear of intimacy may be involved. In addition, individual behavior therapy is not likely to deal adequately with the more complex "systems" interactional components of many sexual problems.

Medication. Specific and appropriate psychoactive medication is extremely useful in cases of sexual dysfunction in which either phobic anxiety, depression, or psychotic thinking interfere with the ability of patients to progress. While antipanic and antipsychotic medication alone may not produce a remission of sexual avoidance or dysfunction, it may reduce anxiety to a point where treatment can be effective. On the other hand, antidepressant medication, when it effectively treats an underlying depression, may, without specific sexual therapy, produce an increase in libido in the patient who complains of low sex drive. In evaluating a patient for a sexual dysfunction it should always be kept in mind that some cases simply will not progress at all or will be aggravated by sexual tasks attempted in the presence of an underlying psychiatric disorder unless the patient is properly medicated.

Modifications of Sex Therapy. Another strategy practiced somewhat differently by different therapists, this approach generally integrates the use of structured sexual tasks with psychotherapeutic exploration of resistances. This can be done by cotherapists or individual therapists generally working in conjoint sessions with both members of a couple. The frequency of sessions can vary from daily for two weeks, as in Masters and Johnson's approach, to weekly, as many other therapists employ. Brief time-limited treatment is used by some sex therapists, with emphasis on regular progress and efficient use of each therapeutic session either to progress with the structured tasks or to deal directly with resistances. The sex therapy model has been most effective, and clinical experience suggests that unless specific problems exist, it should be tried first in treating psychosexual dysfunctions.

Group approaches, used especially for anorgastic women and men with inadequate ejaculatory control, but also for other psychosexual problems, have also been highly effective (Leiblum et al., 1976; Leiblum and Ersner-Hershfield, 1977; Barbach, 1974; Kaplan et al., 1974). Sex therapy groups also use regular structured tasks that are assigned to each patient, and resistances are worked through via the group process. The choice of a group approach will be influenced by the therapist's experience and comfort with this modality, the patients' preferences, and possibly cost factors, since group treatment may be less expensive. Cases that do not respond fully to group treatment may have individual follow-up.

Additional modifications in sex therapy techniques include bibliotherapy, in which assigned reading may be significantly informative, therapeutic, and in simple cases sometimes curative (Barbach, 1976; Zilbergeld, 1978). Prepared sex therapy films, or the recommendation of selected erotic films and books as a source of information and/or erotic fantasy, may be used to educate and carefully desensitize patients to previously avoided and guilt laden sexual ideas and impulses.

Strengthening of the pubococcygeal muscle in the woman through exercises described by Kegel (1948) has been reported to be helpful to some women with orgasm phase disorders.

The predominant issues of debate surround the theoretical framework that best conceptualizes and treats the various sources of anxiety which contribute to sexual symptoms. Unfortunately, many clinicians who are committed to a particular theory have difficulty acknowledging the value of alternative theoretical approaches. Thus, the strict behaviorists reject the notion of unconscious conflicts, and the orthodox psychoanalysts find great difficulty accepting or using directive desensitization and assertive communication techniques. However, these dichotomies are false. The behavioral and psychodynamic models merely describe human behavior on different levels of abstraction. Sex therapy uses an amalgam of behavioral strategies with intrapsychic exploration. It is hoped that in the future this rigid theoretical bias will fade. But in spite of its theoretical attractiveness, the ultimate acceptance or rejection of an integrated approach will have to wait for the completion of systematic outcome studies comparing it with both "pure" insight and "pure" behavioral methods.

The use of medication is another controversial area. Medication is more likely to be used by clinicians familiar with treating phobic anxiety, depression, and schizophrenic states and rarely used by those not medically trained or biased against medication in psychiatry. Also, there have been some reports that psychoactive medications may cause sexual difficulties. By using reasonable care and flexibility in type of drug and dosage, this potential problem will not arise; in fact, sexual complaints with phobic elements will often remain refractory to sex therapy unless the patient is properly medicated (Kaplan et al., 1982).

TREATMENT CONTROVERSIES AND ETHICAL ISSUES

Although most clinicians have insisted that assigned interactional tasks be done in the privacy of the patient's home, some therapists have described beneficial results from teaching and observing patients conducting mutual hand, foot, and body caressing in the therapist's presence (Hartman and Fithian, 1972). This is a risky therapist involvement and also might be misused by opportunistic "therapists" wishing to engage in sexual activity with patients.

Another controversial technique, not yet studied systematically, is the use of assigned surrogate partners for single patients with sexual dysfunctions. Due to ethical issues, it is unlikely that this approach will be adequately researched.

The treatment of desire disorders is a relatively new concept, is least well understood, and has the least favorable prognosis. No definite statement can yet be made about the treatment of choice. Therefore, inhibited sexual desire is most likely to be overlooked, undiagnosed, or handled quite differently according to the theoretical bias of each treating therapist. As further study of desire problems evolves, it is hoped that treatment techniques will become more effective.

It should be noted that some homosexuals, content with their orientation, suffer from the same kinds of psychosexual dysfunctions in their homosexual activities as do heterosexuals; such patients often benefit as individuals and as homosexual couples from standard sex therapy approaches.

THE RISK/BENEFIT FOR SEX THERAPY

In any individual case a determination must be made as to whether a trial of brief sex therapy can be of advantage and whether any serious negative risks are involved. In general, risks are likely to be minimal except for some of those conditions, mentioned earlier, which should be excluded or which warrant prior treatment. These include conditions secondary to major psychopathology such as severe depression, severe anxiety, phobic states, and psychosis in either partner. In some instances the intimate and erotic tasks of sex therapy are highly threatening to the vulnerable patient and could aggravate anxiety or psychosis by challenging defenses. In a severely depressed patient a "failure" in sex therapy might deepen the patient's depressed mood. Phobic patients might panic as the structured sexual interactions bring them closer to their feared experiences. Thus, all of these psychiatric conditions warrant careful initial management before sex therapy is considered.

When organicity is not evaluated, serious and/or treatable disease states may be neglected. Also, in those patients in whom an underlying organic impairment is a significant factor, unless this is detected and known to the therapist and patient, the stress of slow progress or no improvement in sex therapy might lead a patient to despair or cause a tense relationship to be aggravated. Thus, organicity must be kept in mind to assure that the perspective on the patient's prognosis is a reasonable one.

A final risky situation would be one in which the conflict in a couple's relationship is so intense, and motivation for cooperative effort so slow, that sex therapy is likely to fail. Here the concern might be that the therapy itself could be an additional stressor that would be better deferred until the relationship conflict is further resolved.

On the benefit side of the ledger, sex therapy has the advantages of brevity and symptom focus. A trial of therapy may provide relief in the most efficient manner, and if it does not, the treatment in no way precludes subsequent (or concurrent) individual or couples therapy. In fact the experience of confronting previously avoided sexual issues often elucidates an individual or marital problem that the patients may then wish to explore whether or not sex therapy has been successful.

In cases in which an organic element is only a partial contributing factor, sex therapy may bring surprisingly helpful results by diminishing performance fears that can escalate a partial problem into a total disability. The treatment may enhance communication, sexual discussion, and intimacy between partners and produce an improvement in self-esteem and reduction of the tension that many couples feel over unexplained sexual inadequacy. Often a couple may be relieved just to get "permission" to enjoy new love-making techniques other than the intercourse pattern that has failed them due to organic impairments. Sometimes couples "get in touch with" previously unacknowledged feelings of love for each other and learn to value their relationship more highly.

In general then, except for those severely troubled individuals and couples indicated above, if the problem is clearly psychosexual, a trial of sex therapy seems to be a relatively risk-free approach.

REFERENCES

Barbach LG: For Yourself: The Fulfillment of Female Sexuality. New York, Anchor Press/Doubleday, 1976

Barbach LG: Group treatment of preorgasmic women. J Sex Marital Ther 1:139-145, 1974

Brady JP: Behavior therapy and sex therapy. Am J Psychiatry 133:896-899, 1976

Coleman RM, Roffwarg HP, Kennedy SJ, et al: Sleep-wake disorders based on a polysomnographic diagnosis. A national cooperative study. JAMA 247:997-1003, 1982

Cunningham G, Karacan I, Ware C, et al: The relationship between serum testosterone and prolactin levels and nocturnal penile tumescence (NPT) in impotent men. J Androl 3:241-247, 1982

Derogatis LR, Meyer JK, Vazquez V: A psychological profile of the transsexual, I: the male. J Nerv Ment Dis 1966:234-254, 1978

Diagnostic and Statistical Manual of Mental Disorders, 3rd ed. Washington, DC, American Psychiatric Association, 1980

Freud S: Three Essays on the Theory of Sexuality (1905) vol 7. Complete Psychological Works of Sigmund Freud, standard ed. Edited by Strachey J. London, Hogarth Press, 1953

Hartman WE, Fithian M: The Treatment of the Sexual Dysfunctions. Long Beach, Calif, Center for Marital and Sexual Studies, 1972

Kaplan HS, Fyer AJ, Novick A: The treatment of sexual phobias: the combined use of anti-panic medication and sex therapy. J Sex Marital Ther 8:3-28, 1982

Kaplan HS, Kohl RN, Pomeroy WB, et al: Group treatment of premature ejaculation. Arch Sex Behav 3:443-452, 1974

Kaplan HS: The Evaluation of Sexual Disorders: Psychological and Medical Perspectives. New York, Brunner/Mazel, 1983

Kaplan HS: Disorders of Sexual Desire. New York, Brunner/Mazel, 1979

Kaplan HS: The New Sex Therapy. New York, Brunner/Mazel, 1974

Karacan I, Aslan C, Hirshkowitz M: Erectile mechanisms in man. Science 230:1080-1082, 1983

Karacan I, Salis P, Williams R: The role of the sleep laboratory in the diagnosis and treatment of impotence, in Sleep Disorders: Diagnosis and Treatment. Edited by Williams R, Karacan I. New York, John Wiley & Sons, 1978

Karacan I, Moore C: Objective methods of differentiation between organic and psychogenic impotence, in Male Sexual Dysfunction and Impotence. Edited by Swerdloff RS, Santen RJ. New York, Marcel Dekker, in press

Kegel AH: Progressive resistance in the functional restoration of the perineal muscle. Am J Obstet Gynecol 56:238-248, 1948

Kernberg OF: Boundaries and structure of love relationships. J Am Psychoanal Assoc 25:81-114, 1976

Kinsey AC, Pomeroy WB, Martin CE, et al: Sexual Behavior in the Human Female. Philadelphia, WB Saunders, 1953

Kinsey AC, Pomeroy WB, Martin CE: Sexual Behavior in the Human Male. Philadelphia, WB Saunders, 1948

Klein DF: Anxiety reconceptualized, in Anxiety: New Research and Changing Concepts. Edited by Klein DF, Rabkins JG. New York, Raven Press, 1980

Leiblum SR, Rosen RC, Pearce D: Group treatment format: mixed sexual dysfunctions. Arch Sex Behav 5:313-322, 1976

Leiblum SR, Ersner-Hershfield R: Sexual enhancement groups for dysfunctional women: an evaluation. J Sex Marital Ther 3:139-152, 1977

Levay A, Kagle A: A study of treatment needs following sex therapy. Am J Psychiatry 134:970-973, 1977a

Levay A, Kagle A: Ego deficiencies in the areas of pleasure, intimacy and cooperation: guidelines in the diagnosis and treatment of sexual dysfunctions. J Sex Marital Ther 3:10-18, 1977b

Levay A, Weissberg J: The role of dreams in sex therapy. J Sex Marital Ther 5:334-339, 1979

Lief HI: Sexual Problems in Medical Practice. Monroe, Wisconsin, American Medical Association, 1981

Masters WH, Johnson V: Human Sexual Inadequacy. Boston, Little, Brown, 1970

Meyer JK (ed): Clinical Management of Sexual Disorders. Baltimore, Williams & Wilkins Co, 1976

Persky H, Charney N, Lief HI, et al: The relationship of plasma estradiol level to sexual behavior in young women. Psychosom Med 40:523-535, 1978

Renshaw DC: Impotence in diabetes. Dis Nerv Syst 36:369-371, 1975

Schiavi RC: Male erectile disorders. Annu Rev Med 32:509-520, 1981

Schwartz MF, Masters WH: Conceptual factors in the treatment of paraphilias: a preliminary report. J Sex Marital Ther 9:, 1983

Semans JH: Premature ejaculation: a new approach. South Med J 49:353-359, 1956

Sheehan DV: Panic attacks and phobias. N Engl J Med 307:156-158, 1982

Wagner G, Green R: Impotence. New York, Plenum, 1982

Wasserman MD, Pollak CP, Spiel AJ, et al: The differential diagnosis of impotence: the measurement of nocturnal penile tumescence. JAMA 243:2038-2042, 1980

Zilbergeld B: Male Sexuality. Boston, Little, Brown, 1978

Zussman L, Zussman S: The conjoint physical examination, in Clinical Management of Sexual Disorders. Edited by Meyer JK. Baltimore, Williams & Wilkins Co, 1976

15
Hypnosis

15

Hypnosis

INTRODUCTION

Hypnosis began as part of a pre-Freudian attempt to understand the unconscious; yet, repeated liaisons with legitimate schools of psychotherapy such as psychoanalysis have routinely ended in rejection. Despite this past, hypnosis is finally beginning to achieve recognition as a theoretically interesting and therapeutically useful phenomenon replete with possibilities for scientific investigation. This growth has been coincident with the recognition of hypnosis' limitations: that not all people are capable of experiencing the hypnotic trance and that hypnosis itself is not a treatment. Rather, because it involves enhancement of attention, hypnosis may facilitate a number of psychotherapeutic strategies for some patients with the requisite hypnotic capacity. It can be a useful tool in the treatment of a variety of common symptoms including anxiety, phobias, smoking, obesity, pain, insomnia, psychosomatic conditions, and conversion symptoms. In addition, it has been used in the course of insight-oriented psychotherapy as well as in certain forensic areas.

HISTORICAL BACKGROUND

Hypnosis has been at the root of a variety of movements in psychiatry and psychology. Ellenberger (1970) considers the work of the early hypnotists in the eighteenth and nineteenth centuries to have been the foundation for the first dynamic psychiatry. Their early theories, while encumbered with a mythology involving magnetism, emphasized the understanding of an unconscious mind, a role for the mind in the pathogenesis of a variety of mental and physical diseases, a conception of psychotherapy as a treatment, and an emphasis on the relationship between the therapist and the patient.

The field of hypnosis formally began with Franz Anton Mesmer, an eighteenth-century Viennese physician who developed a substantial reputation by claiming to manipulate the flow of "magnetic fluids" in his patients' bodies. He used a variety of techniques which included the laying on of hands, exposure to large magnets, and suggestion (Ellenberger, 1970). His unusual practices received a favorable response, probably because of growing discontent with the prevailing establishment rationalism characteristic of the Age of Reason (Darnton, 1970). His popularity may have served many patients well, since bloodletting was the major medical treatment of the time, and France was the world's leading exporter of leeches for that purpose. However, Mesmerism was investigated by a French panel of experts at the instigation of the physicians of the day. This panel included Benjamin Franklin, Dr. J.I. Guillotine, and Antoine Lavoisier; it concluded that Mesmerism represented "nothing but heated imagination."

The use of hypnosis was left to practitioners further outside the medical and psychiatric mainstream. Esdaile (1846) in India reported achieving 80 percent surgical anesthesia using hypnosis. Braid (1843) substituted the word *hypnotism*, derived from the Greek root *hypnos*, meaning sleep, for Mesmer's original animal magnetism. Braid and his contemporaries used hypnosis in a rather straightforward and authoritarian way that might best be summarized as "direct suggestion." The idea was that during hypnotic trance the patient's will was subjugated to that of the hypnotist, who instructed the patient to relinquish symptoms.

Early in his career, Freud studied with Charcot and Bernheim, who were engaged in a celebrated debate regarding the nature of hypnosis. Charcot (1890) linked hypnosis with hysteria, calling it *sommeil nerveux*, or nervous sleep, and went on to describe it as an artificial or experimental nervous state, although he recognized that hypnotic phenomena could occur in seemingly normal individuals. He viewed hypnosis as a disorder of the nervous system rather than a functional disturbance. Janet (1920) was greatly interested in hypnosis and supported Charcot's position: "The hypnotic state has never any character which cannot be found in natural hysteric somnambulism." Janet, in fact, believed that recovered hysterics were no longer hypnotizable. Bernheim (1889), on the other hand, performed hypnotic investigations with his staff rather than patients and concluded that hypnosis was a normal phenomenon and was not a disorder of the nerves.

Freud was intrigued by the phenomenon and used it in his early work to explore the unconscious (Breuer and Freud, 1893-95). He used hypnotic regression to help patients relive traumatic events in their past which he felt were connected to their present symptoms. He found that often this reliving and abreaction of the affect connected with a traumatic event were sufficient to dissipate the symptom. However, Freud (1924), too, quickly abandoned the use of hypnosis. As he notes in his autobiography, it was his recognition of transference and his belief that it was the element underlying hypnosis that led him to criticize its use:

> And one day I had an experience which showed me in the crudest light what I have long suspected. One of my most acquiescent patients, with whom hypnotism had enabled me to bring about the most marvelous results and whom I was engaged in relieving of her suffering by tracing back her attacks of pain to their origins, as she woke up on one occasion, threw her arms round my neck. The unexpected entrance of a servant relieved us from the discussion. From that time onwards there was a tacit understanding between us that the hypnotic treatment should be discontinued. I was modest enough not to attribute the event to my own irresistible personal attractions, and I felt that I had now grasped the nature of the mysterious element that was at work behind hypnotism. In order to exclude it, or at all events to isolate it, it was necessary to abandon hypnotism.

Instead, Freud decided to permit the transference to develop in a different fashion by sitting behind the couch that he had been using to induce hypnosis and allowing the patient to free associate. He then shifted his attention to analysis of the transference and made this the focus of the psychotherapy. In work with hypnosis, the transference may be accentuated and is used but not analyzed. In fact, the patient's response to the hypnotic situation can provide a kind of crystallized transference experience that can be usefully explored in later insight-oriented psychotherapy.

In this country, a lively interest in hypnosis was developed by Morton Prince (1975), a neurologist who founded the *Journal of Abnormal Psychology* in 1906 and the American Psychopathological Association in 1910 and who led a Boston group including James Jackson Putnam, Boris Sidis, and William James, among others. Prince took his mother to consult with Charcot and visited with Bernheim in 1893. Both these visits heavily influenced his theories. He accepted Bernheim's (1889) belief that hypnosis was fundamentally a normal phenomenon. He wrote a classical study on a multiple personality patient, Christine Beauchamps, published as *The Dissociation of a Personality* (Prince, 1906). Like Breuer and Freud, he considered hypnosis an important tool in the exploration and understanding of the unconscious. However, he differed from them in emphasizing the diversity of unconscious and instinctual forces, the importance of the will, and the role of education as well as the resolution of transference in the psychotherapeutic process.

Boris Sidis (Sidis and Goodhart, 1905), another member of this group, used hypnosis to produce a theory of hysterical neuroses as recurrent mental states that had as their origin an accidental emotional and mental co-occurrence of events. Later, workers such as Hull (1929, 1933) developed the first measures of hypnotizability. In the 1930's there was a relative lull in interest in hypnosis with a few notable exceptions. One was the clinical work of a physician named Milton Erickson (1967), who developed a variety of ingenious therapeutic strategies using hypnosis which can be summarized as "indirect authority." Rather than seeking to impose his will directly on patients, he developed clever means of outwitting resistance by struggling with the patient's defenses in such a way that the patient came to construe overcoming a symptom as a victory over the therapist rather than submission to him (Erickson, 1960). Erickson did not differentiate between hypnosis as a phenomenon and as a treatment. His thinking and work spawned a large following.

The experience of many psychiatrists in World War II led to a re-examination of the role of symptom-oriented treatment in the spectrum of the psychotherapies. While psychoanalysis had yet to reach its heyday in the United States, a generation of psychotherapists was forced to apply whatever techniques worked quickly in the context of the war. Hypnosis was found to be an effective instrument in treating traumatic neurosis, conversion symptoms, and other psychosomatic problems (Kardiner and Spiegel, 1947). This experience led many to question the psychoanalytic insistence that insight must come before symptom-oriented relief and intrigued others about the workings of hypnotic phenomena.

Several members of the psychoanalytic movement became actively interested in hypnosis and attempted to incorporate what was known about it into psychoanalytic theory. Gill and Brenman (1959) interwove dynamic theory with hypnosis by defining the hypnotic state as regression in the service of the ego, in contrast to Janet's (1920) view of hypnosis as pathological regression. Thus, the phenomena associated with hypnosis could be understood as representations of the unconscious. Wolberg (1948) articulated the use of hypnosis as a tool in medical and psychiatric treatment.

Another development that altered the role of hypnosis was research in the laboratory and the clinic on the measurement of hypnotic responsivity, including that of Hull (1929, 1933) and Friedlander and Sarbin (1938). Methods for simultaneously inducing trance and assessing an individual's ability to experience trance proliferated. Weitzenhoffer and Hilgard (1959) published the first of the widely used Stanford Hypnotic Susceptibility Scales (Forms A and B), and an era of systematic research into the correlates of hypnotic responsivity began in earnest. In the early 1970's, Spiegel and his co-workers (H. Spiegel, 1972; Spiegel and Spiegel, 1978) developed an instrument for assessing hypnotic responsivity in the clinical setting, the Hypnotic Induction Profile (HIP), and attention was directed toward the usefulness of clinical measurements of hypnotic responsivity in selecting treatment and predicting outcome. A scale emphasizing the analogy between hypnosis and the creative use of imagination was developed by Barber and Wilson (1978-79).

Interest in the phenomenon of hypnosis has grown steadily, giving rise to two major national societies* with a combined membership of approximately 6,000, each publishing its own journal, and an international society as well.† Hypnosis is regularly used as a tool in medical, psychiatric, psychological, and dental practice.

THEORETICAL ISSUES

The trance state is a form of aroused, attentive, focused concentration with a sense of parallel awareness and a constriction in peripheral awareness. Associated with this phenomenon are a variety of others that receive varying degress of emphasis, depending on the orientation of the definer. Some emphasize the capacity for imaginative involvement, or believed-in imagination, typical of the trance state (J. Hilgard, 1970); others focus on the importance of trance logic (Orne, 1959), a tendency to suspend critical judgment and accept logical incongruities, and the ability to distort perceptions (Orne, 1959). The reorganization of attention, with the capacity for dividing it (E. Hilgard, 1977), is an important part of the phenomenon; and the role of hypnotic amnesia is often given prominence, enabling a person to seem to forget, but on a certain level of awareness actually remember, instructions given during the hypnotic trance. A hypnotized individual's high level of openness to having his or her experience structured by another is also an important and commonly mentioned attribute. Two important components of the hypnotic experience are dissociation and suggestibility. The former is the subjective sense of increasing the separation between various parts of experience. Suggestibility emphasizes the compulsive compliance aspect of the hypnotic experience, in which an individual is prone to want to please someone and comply without critical judgment. Some individuals are extreme dissociators but not very suggestible, and vice versa.

What these aspects of a definition of hypnosis all have in common is an agreement that the trance state is not a form of sleep but rather an altered form of attention; physiological measures corroborate this view. The trance state is electrophysiologically associated with the production of alpha, an EEG pattern consistent with resting alertness (London et al., 1969). A positive association has been found between the presence of EEG alpha and hypnotizability (Nowlis and Rhead, 1968; Morgan et al., 1974a).

* American Society of Clinical Hypnosis (*American Journal of Clinical Hypnosis*) and Society for Clinical and Experimental Hypnosis (*Journal of Clinical and Experimental Hypnosis*)

† International Society of Hypnosis

Barber and his associates (Barber and Wilson, 1978-79) have carried out an extensive body of research exploring the overlap between hypnosis and what he terms "creative imagination." He emphasizes that groups given formal hypnotic inductions do not perform significantly differently from those given "task-motivating instructions." The critical issue in this research is the spontaneous occurrence of hypnotic phenomena, even without a formal induction ceremony. In recent years, Barber (Barber and Wilson, 1977) has focused greater attention on the minority of individuals who are highly hypnotizable, asserting that they are the only people who demonstrate true hypnotic phenomena.

Sarbin and Slagle (1972) take the more extreme position that hypnosis is nothing more than an example of social compliance. They dismiss the importance of individual differences in hypnotic responsivity by using data showing that individuals can be pressured into carrying out the same social conduct with or without a hypnotic experience. These social-psychological approaches emphasize the analysis of behavior regardless of subjective experience; that is, does the individual comply because of the hypnotic alteration in perception or conviction, or does he comply out of an exaggerated or even a normal desire to please?

The experimental paradigm for these studies is that groups are given either a hypnotic induction and then some instructions or simply are given task-motivating instructions; both sets of performance instructions seem to get comparable results. These theorists argue that there is nothing unique to the hypnotic state. It is, rather, a simple variation in the standard compliance to role pressures. Clearly, social compliance is one aspect of hypnotic phenomena, but what these group studies fail to take into account is the important contribution of individual variance in hypnotizability. Large groups divided randomly will provide an equal spectrum of hypnotizability in both samples, and formal hypnotic induction does not have to occur for reasonably hypnotizable people to respond in hypnotic-like fashion. Indeed, hypnotizability has been found associated with the natural occurrence of hypnotic-like experiences (Shor et al., 1962) and with a tendency for intense absorbing and self-altering experiences (Tellegen and Atkinson, 1974). Likewise, many therapists (Erickson, 1967) believe that all individuals are potentially hypnotizable and that when an individual does not enter a trance in a clinical setting, it is because of a failure of the patient in terms of resistance or of the therapist in terms of technique. Both positions minimize the importance of individual differences in hypnotic responsivity.

A substantial body of evidence has accumulated over the past several decades indicating that hypnotizability is a stable and measurable trait (E. Hilgard, 1965; Spiegel and Spiegel, 1978). Indeed, in one study, hypnotizability was found to be as stable a measure over a ten-year interval as IQ (Morgan et al., 1974b). These data from hypnotizability scales conflict with the previously quoted state theorists and with the position of many clinicians who hold that anyone is potentially hypnotizable. Nonetheless, most people who work with hypnosis concede that there are consistent differences in responsiveness to hypnotic induction. If one takes seriously the concept of hypnotizability as a trait, then the nature of the induction itself is comparatively unimportant as long as it provides the necessary conditions for allowing a demonstration of a patient's ability to shift concentration and to experience some or all of the sensory, motor, temporal, imaginative, and other alterations associated with hypnotic experience. Any of a large variety of brief and competent inductions will enable a hypnotizable person to explore his or her own hypnotic capacity.

On the other hand, the most elaborate inductions, replete with long, "deepening" techniques, will not allow a nonhypnotizable person to experience hypnotic phenomena. Thus, the nature of the induction is less important than the hypnotizability of the subject. One recent study purported to demonstrate that behavioral training significantly increased hypnotizability (Katz, 1979). However, a reanalysis of the data showed that the magnitude of this improvement in scores was dwarfed by the magnitude of the significance in individual differences in hypnotizability (Frischholz et al., 1982) on the Stanford Hypnotic Susceptibility Scale (Weitzenhoffer and Hilgard, 1962).

Clearly, several factors may prevent a given subject from optimally experiencing this hypnotic capacity. If something in the relationship with the person inducing hypnosis makes the subject uneasy or suspicious, he may consciously or unconsciously resist responding to instructions. An atmosphere of respect and trust is an important prerequisite for allowing a person to explore his hypnotic capacity. Likewise, motivation is important. If the subject does not take the occasion seriously and expend a reasonable effort, it is less likely (though by no means impossible) that he or she will respond with full attentional resources.

While there exist a wide variety of induction techniques (Weitzenhoffer, 1957; Spiegel and Spiegel, 1980), the crucial point is that they provide a necessary but not sufficient condition for hypnotic experience. It is only the combination of a reasonable induction technique and a hypnotizable person that allows a hypnotic event to occur.

What is most interesting about the phenomenon from a therapeutic point of view is that this capacity for focused concentration and parallel awareness can be used to help patients focus on a therapeutic strategy. As such, hypnosis is not a treatment but a facilitator—an adjunct to a primary treatment strategy. The hypnotic experience is associated with and is measured by a variety of alterations in usual psychosomatic functioning. These include changes in sensation such as tingling numbness or a sense of lightness, changes in movement with an associated attenuated sense of control, changes in memory with amnesia for events occurring during the trance state, intense experiences of imagination including visual and auditory hallucinations, and experiences of dissociation. For example, a highly hypnotizable subject may write as though the hand that is writing were disconnected from the rest of the body and mind. All of these alterations are theoretically interesting but also have therapeutic potential in that the subject is exploring and expanding the relatedness between mind and body. The capacity to alter somatic reactions using psychological means has obvious therapeutic potential in dealing with anxiety states, conversion symptoms, and psychosomatic problems. Some therapists tend to be more authoritarian, others permissive; some believe that all subjects are equally hypnotizable and emphasize the importance of countering resistance; others emphasize the importance of measuring hypnotic responsivity and recommend approaches other than hypnosis for those found to be nonhypnotizable.

BASIC SCIENCE AND RESEARCH

Hypnotic techniques generally rely on a combination of conviction, compliance, concentration, and comprehension in the service of internalizing change, rearranging resources, and developing a sense of mastery. Subjects are initially induced into a trance by the therapist and then may be given a series of "suggestions" regarding control of the problem. They may also be instructed in self-hypnotic procedures or encouraged to return for further reinforcement. The experience of entering into the trance is often relaxing; in addition, it is frequently a sufficiently surprising experience that it helps give the patient the conviction that he or she will be able to undertake major changes. An induced and experienced sense of lightness, dissociation, and lessened control may convey to the patient an impression that other changes are possible. This element of surprise may help carry on whatever momentum the patient brought to the therapeutic encounter.

Hypnotic treatments clearly contain an element of compliance. Patients often expect to deliver themselves to a therapist who uses hypnosis and to be programmed to do whatever is best, as though the trance experience were analogous to general anesthesia. They are often surprised to discover that they are alert and aware throughout the hypnotic experience. Nonetheless, given the tendency of individuals in a trance to suspend critical judgment, it is clear that hypnotized patients are prone to comply, at least in the short term, with the instructions of the therapist. In this sense, the trance experience optimizes the patient's attention on the therapeutic strategy, whatever it may be.

Concentration is likewise an important aspect in hypnotic therapies. The intensity of focal concentration enables the patient to identify with and absorb the material presented in the hypnotic session. This is a way of mobilizing and optimizing a patient's resources for change and developing a sense of mastery.

Research in clinical and experimental hypnosis has burgeoned. A comparatively recent review of the field selectively cites 215 studies (E. Hilgard, 1975), and much work has occurred in the intervening years. There is an advanced and interesting literature on neurophysiological correlates of hypnosis and other psychological correlates of the phenomenon which can be addressed only superficially here. The trance state has been examined as a laboratory model with analogies to a variety of normal processes including amnesia, memory, concentration, and creativity. Hypnosis has been used as a vehicle for exploring the relationship between emotional state and intensity of memory recall (Bower, 1970), and it has been shown that affect congruence between the mental state at the time of recall and the mental state at the time of being recalled enhances the accurate retrieval of content. These data are consistent with the general theory of state-dependent learning. Recent research on mechanisms of hypnotic amnesia has provided evidence that psychological mechanisms for information retrieval are disrupted, especially those that involve temporal sequencing, that is, the embedding of events into a temporal order (Evans, 1980).

The concentration model of hypnosis has been supported by a study by Van Nuys (1973), who observed that more highly hypnotizable individuals show fewer distractions from a single perceptual focus than less hypnotizable individuals. In addition, the work of Tellegen and Atkinson (1974) shows that hypnotizability is correlated with a characteristic style of concentration: "a full commitment of available perceptual, motoric, imaginative, and ideational resources to a unified representation of the attentional object." J. Hilgard (1970) defines this mode of concentrating as "imaginative involvement" in which, for example, the highly hypnotizable individual suspends the customary temporal and spatial orientation while reading a book and enters the story. The intense involvement characteristic of hypnosis has been explored as a mechanism for creative experiences, characterized as "effortless experiencing" (P. Bowers, 1978). Bowers and van der Meulen (1970) obtained a significant correlation between hypnotizability and scores on tests of creativity.

Considerable interest has emerged in the relationship between hemispheric laterality and hypnotizability, the hypothesis being that hypnotizability involves some selective activation of the nondominant hemisphere. Supportive data have come from a series of studies on laterality of eye movements which show that highly hypnotizable individuals are more likely characteristically to look to the left than to the right in response to a question, indicating a preference for the use of the right hemisphere (Bakan, 1969; Gur and Gur, 1974). Interestingly, Bakan and Svorad (1969) found a negative correlation between resting EEG alpha and the tendency to look to the right in response to questions. They confirmed the association between less hypnotizability and looking to the right.

There is some evidence (Hernandez-Peon and Donoso, 1959; Guerrero-Figueroa and Heath, 1964; Clynes et al., 1964; Wilson, 1968; Galbraith et al., 1972) that sensory evoked responses may be altered in response to instructions in highly hypnotizable individuals. What these studies indicate is that the electrophysiology of the hypnotic trance is more akin to resting alertness than to sleep, that there may be some preferential involvement of the right cerebral hemisphere in hypnotic functions, and that there may be a capacity to alter the electrophysiological responsiveness to sensory input among hypnotizable individuals in a trance.

Several different hypnotizability scales have been used in both laboratory and clinical studies. Each has its proponents and detractors. The Stanford Hypnotic Susceptibility Scales (Weitzenhoffer and Hilgard, 1959, 1962; E. Hilgard, 1965) were developed using college student populations and have been the standard laboratory measure. However, recently the senior author of the scales (Weitzenhoffer, 1980) has pointed to serious limitations in them.

The need for shorter measures for clinical use has been addressed by several condensations of the Stanford Hypnotic Susceptibility Scale (Morgan and Hilgard, 1979; Hilgard et al., 1979) and by a measure developed using a clinical population, the Hypnotic Induction Profile (Spiegel and Spiegel, 1978), which assesses eight aspects of a single hypnotic experience. The relationship of one of these, the eye-roll, to measured hypnotizability has been questioned (E. Hilgard, 1982), as has his critique (Spiegel et al., 1982a). The relationship between the Stanford Hypnotic Susceptibility Scale and the Hypnotic Induction Profile has been found to be moderate, with correlations ranging from .19 to .45 in one study (Orne, 1979) and .6 in another (Frischholz et al., 1980).

There is a large literature on the relationship between measured hypnotic responsivity and responsiveness to treatment using hypnosis or other related techniques. Hypnotic responsivity has not been found to be predictive of treatment outcome in all circumstances (Wadden and Anderton, 1982).

Hypnotic responsivity has been shown significantly to predict responsiveness to treatment for smoking (Spiegel and Spiegel, 1978), asthma (Collison, 1975), flying phobias (Spiegel et al., 1981), pain (Hilgard and Hilgard, 1975), migraine (Andreychuk and Skriver, 1975), and psychogenic impotence (Crasilneck, 1979). Several studies have even indicated that hypnotic responsivity is a significant predictor of response to acupuncture analgesia (Katz et al., 1974; Moore and Berk, 1976). These findings are of both theoretical and practical interest. The fact that hypnotic responsivity can predict outcome for a variety of treatments suggests that hypnotic processes are, indeed, important in the treatment procedure. From a practical point of view, these findings suggest that screening to test hypnotic responsivity can be of practical use in selecting patients for hypnotic treatment. Those who have intact hypnotic capacity are more likely to respond to the intervention, and patients who are not hypnotizable might well be referred for other treatment approaches. For example, a phobic patient who is highly hypnotizable would likely do well with a self-hypnosis technique. On the other hand, since such techniques as systematic desensitization have been shown to be efficacious, this approach can be recommended to those patients who, on formal testing, prove not to be hypnotizable.

These findings provide exciting prospects for the future, since the screening for hypnotic responsivity is brief and well accepted by patients (Mott, 1979; Frankel et al., 1979). It provides one systematic means for assessing those characteristics of the patient which make him or her more likely to respond to a specific treatment strategy. Such an approach has potential for making more efficient use of existing treatment resources by effectively identifying and mobilizing special patient capacities for hypnotic experience when they exist or occur spontaneously. This experience includes an ability to dissociate, concentrate intently, use vivid imagery, enhance access to unconscious material, and become especially receptive to new ideas and feelings. Hypnotic responsiveness is a naturally occurring patient resource with important theoretical and therapeutic potential.

CLINICAL ISSUES

Uses of hypnosis can be summarized as part of three broad categories: (a) symptom control, (b) uses in uncovering psychotherapies, and (c) uses in clarifying differential diagnosis and choosing among treatment strategies.

Symptom-Oriented Approaches

The oldest uses of hypnosis have been to help patients control symptoms. The most straightforward of these approaches is direct suggestion. Patients are instructed to enter a hypnotic trance and are then given a suggestion that the experienced symptom (e.g., pain) or habit (e.g., desire for cigarettes) will disappear. Great emphasis is placed on the rapport and trust established by the therapist, and the success of the intervention is considered largely dependent on a patient's uncritical acceptance of the instructions. More recently, therapists have added a series of supportive and self-enhancing suggestions, emphasizing that the patient will feel better about himself as he complies with these instructions (Crasilneck and Hall, 1975).

Another approach can be classified as indirect suggestion, or symptom prescription. Erickson (1967) felt that he constantly had to outwit a patient's resistance to taking a therapeutic step, including resistance to entering a hypnotic state and to complying with hypnotic instructions. Erickson, therefore, developed a series of ingenious strategies to overcome this resistance to the hypnotic experience, for example, the so-called "confusion technique," in which he attempted to exhaust the patient's efforts at rationally comprehending the instructions; or the "my friend, John, technique," in which he spent a great deal of time giving hypnotic instructions to an imaginary person so that the patient's competitiveness would be stimulated enough to attract him to the instructions he had previously rejected. Erickson then dealt with resistance to therapeutic instructions by instructing the patient to develop or intensify symptoms already present, for example, instructing an overweight patient to gain weight. In this way, he taught the patient to dissociate the psychological experience of overeating from the act of consuming a given quantity of food. The patient could still feel rebellious against Erickson while at the same time actually eating less and losing weight. Implicit in both these strategies is a recognition that the nature of the relationship between the therapist and the patient is important insofar as it may either reinforce or undermine the content of the hypnotic instruction and the therapeutic effect. Indeed, sensitivity to the therapist-patient relationship is one of the hallmarks of practitioners of hypnosis, although the uses of the doctor-patient relationship have varied enormously. Sophisticated uses of hypnosis involve a recognition that the nature of the therapeutic relationship has an important effect on the content and outcome of the hypnotic instructions. If a therapist is telling a patient to take control over his life but, at the same time, is making the patient feel helpless, this double signal can undermine the overall therapeutic impact.

Recent developments in the use of hypnosis for symptom control have emphasized more active patient participation, both in learning to restructure perspectives by practicing a series of self-hypnosis exercises and in formulating the hypnotic instructions in such a way that their implementation involves an affirmation experience rather than fighting a symptom (Spiegel and Spiegel, 1978).

Thus, while most modern practitioners of hypnosis conceptualize it as a collaborative effort in which the patient works out, with the therapist, a strategy that he or she then uses in a combination of instructed and self hypnosis, there is an important educational component: The patient is taught by the therapist how to use the hypnotic state in the service of an agreed upon treatment goal.

Considerable research has also been done on mechanisms of hypnotic efficacy. The Hilgards (1975), for example, found evidence that the mechanism of hypnotic analgesia involves hypnotic amnesia. In essence, the patient forgets to remember the incoming pain signals. They also found that hypnotic responsivity is a good predictor of treatment response in the case of hypnotic analgesia. To look at the problem from another point of view, the phenomenon of hypnotic dissociation is compatible with the ability to use denial and repression as defenses. Analogies have also been drawn between hypnosis and placebo analgesia, although McGlashan et al. (1969) found that while placebo and hypnotic analgesia were comparable among individuals with low hypnotizability levels, highly hypnotizable individuals obtained significantly greater pain relief in the hypnotic state than they did from a placebo condition.

Uses of Hypnosis in Uncovering Psychotherapies

Hypnosis is commonly used to uncover repressed memories. There is a special application of hypnosis in uncovering traumatic amnesias. Interest in this use flourished during World War II when hypnosis was used to help soldiers suffering from the effects of combat to overcome the excessive repression of combat experience and its subsequent debilitating effects such as anxiety, depression, and conversion symptoms (H. Spiegel, 1944; Kardiner and Spiegel, 1947). Often, these individuals are able, in a hypnotic state, to recover large portions of the memory of the combat or other stress experience. Earlier work in these areas emphasized the importance of abreaction, that is, simply expressing the repressed emotions of fear, horror, rage, and anxiety associated with physical assault and a threat to life. In some cases, the mere expression of this affect and the admission of the repressed material into consciousness resulted in relief of debilitating symptoms, including conversion symptoms, reduced ego functioning, nightmares, anxiety states, irritability, insomnia, personality changes, and depression. More recent work has emphasized additional curative factors such as corrective transference experience with an understanding therapist (Brende and Benedict, 1980) in treating combat-related distress, using imagery to facilitate mourning (Fromm and Eisen, 1982), and restructuring the stressful experience by balancing the loss with some aspect of the experience which emphasizes the patient's attempts at mastery (D. Spiegel, 1981).

In general, efforts to retrieve memories in hypnosis involve two broad techniques. One is hypnotic age regression, in which the patient relives the previous experience as though it were happening in the present. This technique is available to a minority of hypnotizable individuals who are extremely hypnotizable. Most people with low and mid-range hypnotic responsivity can relive past events in the trance state but not in the present tense. For many of these individuals a technique involving an imaginary screen on which events are portrayed is more useful. They maintain their temporal orientation but view the event with more vivid perception and affect.

Hypnosis has also been used as a tool to enhance available memories, most often in the course of long-term psychotherapy. In these instances, similar techniques can be used, but the goal is less resolution of specific symptoms than adding to the general body of information that the patient and therapist are uncovering. This is often helpful when the patient and therapist feel stuck and believe that some resistance is being encountered which cannot be overcome in the usual ways. The ceremony of a hypnotic induction may be useful in attesting to the patient's motivation to overcome the resistance and in providing a mode of intense concentration which at the same time helps the patient to control the anxiety stimulated by the repressed event. The use of the screen technique, in particular, gives the patient a means of placing distance between himself and the repressed material, which may likewise alleviate anxiety. The therapist may introduce the hypnotic technique in the course of long-term therapy if both patient and therapist are comfortable with it; otherwise, the therapist may refer the patient to an outside therapist for the hypnotic exploration.

Hypnotic age regression techniques can be especially helpful when patients suffer amnesias regarding traumatic events, for example in fugue states or post-traumatic stress disorders. Hypnosis can be a useful tool in helping the therapist and patient uncover repressed material and link it to present symptoms such as anxiety and depression. Finally, the trance state can also be helpful in enabling the patient to reintegrate the previously repressed material in a new way that is less anxiety provoking and damaging to self-esteem (D. Spiegel, 1981; Fromm and Eisen, 1982).

Since at least as far back as Breuer and Freud's (1893-95) early work, hypnosis has been thought to provide special access to the unconscious, just as dreams are thought to be special representations of it. Hypnosis does not provide any entirely unique access to unconscious process. However, since some patients who seek psychotherapy are ambivalent about their symptoms, the trance state may provide a ceremony that offers a face-saving exit from a conflict. Conscious resistance may, to some extent, be bypassed via the hypnotic experience, and unconscious anxieties may be allayed through the relaxation and anxiety-control aspects of the hypnotic experience. This use of a different technique also makes previous failures less of a burden.

Many hypnotic interventions involve combinations of rational and irrational appeals. For example, Erickson's (1960) previously mentioned apparently irrational instruction to an obese patient in a trance that she would overeat until she lost the required weight allowed the patient to fulfill an emotional hunger while at the same time controlling the physical one. Thus, the trance state may allow the therapist to speak in metaphors that are appealing to the unconscious but would not ordinarily pass conscious scrutiny.

Gill and Brenman (1959) view the trance state as a regression in the service of the ego. It is well known that in the process of remembering, repeating, and working through unconscious conflicts, regression will occur in intensive psychotherapy, with the patient experiencing primitive feelings toward the therapist which are associated with parental and other early introjects. Because of the intensity of the hypnotic experience, it may crystallize the transference relationship. The patient may experience a particular regression as having elements that are dynamically important, for example, a strong desire to let the therapist structure his experience and, at the same time, a great resentment of him for doing so. If such feelings are aroused in a hypnotic induction—and this is more likely to occur when the patient has a long-standing relationship with the therapist—they can be worked on during the ongoing psychotherapy.

Hypnosis has been used, as well, as a facilitator of psychoanalytic psychotherapy, often as an alternative to the free association process; to stimulate dreams, which may then be analyzed; or to provide imagery for the purposes of stimulating associations and analysis of them (Wolberg, 1948). The hypnotic experience may be conceptualized as a crystallized transference (H. Spiegel, 1959) in which a patient's tendency to depend on others for the structure of his beliefs or experience is accentuated and thereby can be examined in the analysis of the transference. Fantasies aroused by the hypnotic experience may likewise be explored. These uses of hypnosis may provide means of working with patient resistance or responding to a specific request from a patient for assistance with difficult material. For example, the physical relaxation often associated with the hypnotic trance coupled with the capacity for dissociation may be useful in enabling the patient to work with emotionally painful material by dissociating somatic from psychological distress. The analyst may be able to help the patient more comfortably face and work through difficult early life experiences and fantasies. In this setting, hypnosis is a tool used to facilitate the analytic process by fostering the examination of fantasies, memories, resistance, and the transference.

Hypnosis in symptom-oriented treatment can likewise be a facilitator of insight-oriented psychotherapy. As Greenson (1965) has noted, it is often important in developing a therapeutic relationship for the therapist to do something that shows the patient that he can be of help. A successful collaboration in overcoming a symptom such as a phobia or anxiety state may make the patient more curious about the reasons for the symptom and also convince him that this therapist can be of help in exploring them. Likewise, if later in the course of therapy a patient develops a symptom or feels immobilized, hypnosis for the purpose of helping the patient overcome a symptom or problem may facilitate further movement.

Uses of Hypnosis in Clarifying Differential Diagnosis

Recently there has been interest in the idea that hypnotic responsivity is the vehicle for the expression of a variety of symptoms. This observation is rooted in very old literature that identified all hysteria with hypnosis but that viewed the hypnosis itself as a sign of illness (*sommeil nerveux*) (Charcot, 1890; Janet, 1920). A syndrome associated with high hypnotizability in psychiatric patients, which has been described (H. Spiegel, 1974), includes a tendency to comply with others compulsively, a nonrational inner sense of inferiority, and a variety of spontaneous dissociative symptoms. A structured and supportive, rather than insight-oriented, psychotherapy has been recommended for such problems. Frankel and Orne (1976) reported that the hypnotizability of a group of phobic patients was higher than that of a group of smokers and speculated that phobic symptoms may be spontaneous trance states in which the patient focuses intently on the irrationally feared object. Later work, however, failed to confirm higher hypnotizability (D. Spiegel et al., 1981) or the absence of low hypnotizability in all phobics (Gerschman et al., 1979).

The literature on multiple personality syndrome likewise proposes that high hypnotizability is a prominent factor in the diagnosis. Such patients, who have a sense of splitting into two or more different selves which they have great difficulty reconciling, may be experiencing spontaneous trance dissociations (Sutcliffe and Jones, 1963). These patients are frequently described as having suffered rather severe stress in their early lives and their current circumstances, often in the form of physical, sexual, or emotional abuse. Psychotherapy has involved the use of hypnosis to provide access to various dissociated aspects of the self, which have been described by some authors as different from one another on psychological and physiological testing (Ludwig et al., 1972). Hypnosis has been further used to explore these different dissociated personalities and to teach the patient a process of reintegrating them (Prince, 1906, 1975).

Likewise, some authors have suggested that high hypnotic responsivity may be consistent with a syndrome of acute psychotic decompensation, characterized by rapid and dramatic onset of symptoms in the face of severe environmental stress and rapid recompensation with psychotherapy and without recourse to antipsychotic medication (Spiegel and Fink, 1979). This syndrome of hysterical psychosis has been described in many settings (Hollender and Hirsch, 1966; Siomopoulos, 1971), but interest in it was increased with the growing recognition that acute schizophrenic symptoms are significantly different from chronic and borderline schizophrenia (Kety et al., 1971). Despite continued disagreement in the field (Pettinati, 1982), evidence is accumulating that the most seriously disturbed psychiatric patients, for example schizophrenics and patients with major affective disorders, are less hypnotizable than patients with milder psychoneurotic symptoms or no symptoms at all (H. Spiegel et al., 1975; Lavoie et al., 1973; Lavoie et al., 1976; Lavoie and Sabourin, 1980; D. Spiegel et al., 1982a). These data are consistent with observations of a concentration deficit in schizophrenia (Shakow, 1974).

Gross (1980) has reported that the capacity to experience hypnosis may be used to differentiate between hysterical and grand mal seizures. Measuring a patient's capacity for hypnotic experience may be a useful device for organizing information about his or her symptoms as well as a means for teaching the patient symptom control (Spiegel and Spiegel, 1978; Frankel et al., 1979; Mott, 1979). Such symptoms as hysterical conversion, multiple personality, fugue states, and hysterical seizures can be understood as spontaneous, undisciplined trance dissociations. Demonstrating to the patient his or her capacity to experience more traditional hypnotic phenomena such as hand levitation may be a way to emphasize the ease with which he or she can provoke somatic and psychological alterations. This understanding can make the symptoms less frightening to the patient since he or she now sees them from a new point of view with greater possibilities for inherent control.

INDICATIONS

Since hypnosis is often effective in facilitating brief treatment, its use is recommended in conjunction with psychotherapy for such problems as circumscribed phobias, performance and other anxiety states, conversion symptoms, pain unresponsive to somatic interventions, and certain habit problems such as smoking (Crasilneck and Hall, 1975). Hypnosis is used in treating these specific somatic and habit symptoms as an adjunctive tool in the implementation of a primary treatment strategy.

Anxiety and Phobias

Anxiety. Hypnosis has a place, along with psychotherapy and psychoactive medication, in the management of anxiety and phobias. Patients with extremes of anxiety may not be hypnotizable. In general, it is the patients with mild to moderate anxiety who are capable of hypnotic experience. For them, the dissociation in the trance experience can be especially helpful. They can be taught to separate the mental experience of anxiety from the somatic concomitants of it: the churning in the stomach, the sweaty palms, the muscular tension, etc. Some approaches emphasize variations on the theme of progressive muscle relaxation; others emphasize teaching patients to develop a physical sense of floating while picturing their problems on an imaginary screen. This technique gives them a sense of facing their preoccupations but in a distant and less immediate way that allows them to dissociate somatic from psychological stress. Just the act of having something to do when anxiety strikes is, in itself, anxiety reducing.

Hypnosis has been used successfully in the treatment of specific kinds of performance anxiety, for example psychogenic impotence. Crasilneck (1979) used hypnosis exercises in conjunction with couples therapy aimed at clarifying and working through unconscious hostility between husband and wife while facilitating relaxation during sexual activity.

Phobias. In treating phobias, hypnotic techniques have the advantage of being brief and learnable by the subject so that most of the treatment is handled by the patient himself. Hypnosis can be used both to induce physical relaxation in the face of the anxiety-provoking stimulus and also to teach patients how to prepare themselves for such an encounter by focusing on aspects of the experience which are less anxiety-provoking. For example, individuals with fear of flying can be shown that rather than focusing on feeling trapped and thus fighting the plane, they can relate to the plane as an extension of their bodies and float with it. Viewing the pilot as the intermediate agent gives them a greater sense of being in control (D. Spiegel et al., 1981).

Pain Control

Perhaps the oldest medical use of hypnosis has been in the treatment of pain. Just before the discovery of inhalation anesthesia, a Scottish surgeon named Esdaile (1846) reported 80 percent surgical anesthesia using hypnosis. Both acute and chronic pain conditions have been successfully treated with the help of hypnosis. Beecher's (1956) classic observations on the relationship of the meaning of an injury to the amount of pain experienced provide strong evidence that all pain consists of two components, somatic and reactive. Anxious or depressed individuals with the same amount of physical discomfort as normals experience more pain, and a kind of vicious cycle can be set up in which the pain and disability produce depression and/or anxiety, which in turn worsens the pain. Many chronic pain patients notice that the pain is worse on evenings and weekends when they are less distracted by their work and other activities. This variability in the pain experience based on mood and attention is a fertile area for hypnotic intervention.

Patients who are hypnotizable can be offered a variety of treatment strategies tailored to their degree of hypnotizability. Highly hypnotizable patients are often able to eliminate pain completely. Some patients tolerate the dentist by simply vividly imagining that they are somewhere pleasant. They feel totally dissociated from the physical experience. Others use the metaphor of dental analgesia as a way of making an affected body part numb. Moderately hypnotizable patients often find it useful to use a metaphor involving an alteration in temperature, developing a sensation of warmth or icy cold tingling numbness in the affected body area. Less hypnotizable individuals often find it helpful to focus on a competing sensation, such as the sense of touch in a nonaffected body area, or to reinforce the hypnotic experience with actual warmth or cold. All of these individuals can be taught to "filter the hurt out of the pain" by focusing on a competing or superseding sensation. This technique helps to shift the attention away from the painful stimulus, and patients can be instructed to use self-hypnotic exercises to reinforce this hypnotic analgesia.

Hypnotic mechanisms may underlie a variety of treatments for pain.

Several studies (Katz et al., 1974; Moore and Berk, 1976) have reported that hypnotizability is a factor in responsiveness to acupuncture analgesia, although this finding has been questioned. In rare cases, major surgical procedures have been performed with hypnosis as the sole anesthetic. This experience underscores the point that an individual's responsiveness to hypnotic analgesia is by no means an indication that the pain is functional. Indeed, many highly motivated patients with real somatic disease are more likely to obtain pain relief using hypnosis or related procedures than patients with a pain of more functional origin or those invested with greater secondary gain.

Conversion Symptoms

Some patients with either pure conversion symptoms or, as is much more common, disability with a physical and psychiatric component, can use hypnosis as a face-saving way to achieve rehabilitation. Patients with problems ranging from skin and seizure disorders to muscle weakness and contractures have been helped. It is rarely productive to confront a patient directly with a doctor's suspicions that he or she is "malingering" or having a "conversion symptom" since, from that point on, the patient is in the position of dishonoring himself by getting better. Because the physician is seldom absolutely certain about the etiology of the dysfunction anyway, it is often best to take a stance of offering rehabilitation. The experience of parallel awareness, which is a central feature of hypnosis, can be a transition point for the patient at which he learns something new that enables him to begin rehabilitation. This process provides him with a way to rationalize why rehabilitation could not have begun earlier and at the same time offers a means of exploring his capacity to alter somatic sensation. The trance experience of developing tingling, numbness, lightness, or a change of motor control in an extremity can provide a model for altering physical function. A patient can be instructed to develop a tremor and restless movement sensation in the affected limb, for example, and to work on increasing these tremors as a way of building up circulation and strength so that he may eventually return it to full function.

Habit Control

Hypnosis has been used as an adjunctive tool in treating a variety of habit problems. In general, the effectiveness of hypnosis in this area is proportional to the effectiveness of other treatments. The most successful area has been smoking control, less so with weight control, and even fewer positive reports emerge with alcohol and drug abuse. In general, the results of hypnosis in the control of smoking have been as good as other areas, ranging from a low of four percent to a high of 88 percent (Holroyd, 1980).

There are several problems with outcome research in this area:

Comparability of Populations. Individual differences in hypnotizability and motivation are generally not taken into account.

Lack of Standardized Outcome Criteria. Some report a decrease in smoking as success rather than the more appropriate goal of abstinence. The use of chemical confirmation is rare. Some researchers do not distinguish between short- and long-term results despite the fact that abstinence is not likely to be stable before six months (Hunt and Bespalec, 1974). Also, treatment drop-outs are sometimes ignored.

Differences in Treatment. More extensive treatment requires greater motivation on the part of the patient, and these differences in patient participation and other characteristics are not taken into account. The less intensive treatments tend to have lower long-term outcome results but are simpler to administer. Outcome six months after a single session of self-hypnosis treatment for smoking has been reported at 17 to 25 percent effective (Spiegel and Spiegel, 1978), and the finding has been replicated (Berkowitz et al., 1979). Responsiveness is associated with hypnotizability. A variety of approaches have been used. In general, aversive techniques have little to recommend them since they are not self-reinforcing. Effective treatments have included encouragement and reinforcement from the doctor, concentration on the health effects of smoking (Crasilneck and Hall, 1975), and a restructuring strategy that encourages the patient to view himself as protecting his body from poison (Spiegel and Spiegel, 1978). Approaches that encourage the patient to focus on what he is in favor of, rather than fighting smoking, seem to be intrinsically more self-reinforcing.

LIMITATIONS

There are no absolute contraindications to the use of hypnosis per se. The trance experience is not dangerous, and it occurs spontaneously anyway. If there is a danger, it is to allow such phenomena to occur unrecognized or mislabeled. The few available reports in the literature of deleterious side effects related to hypnosis address the issue of symptom substitution but fail to distinguish the therapeutic technique used for the induction of hypnosis per se. In one widely cited case (Joseph et al., 1949), the patient, a rather disturbed young woman, was coerced with hypnosis into relinquishing neurodermatitis and had an acute psychotic episode. It was likely the coercive technique and her underlying psychopathology rather than the use of hypnosis per se which led to her decompensation. The data presented did not establish a cause and effect relationship. Given the widespread use of hypnosis, there have been relatively few reports in the literature of problems with it.

There is little evidence that the removal of symptoms by hypnosis results in the emergence of a new symptom unless it is expected by the therapist or patient. Far more commonly, patients simply do not respond to treatment or respond initially and then regress. The risk of symptom substitution can therefore be minimized by de-emphasizing the older authoritarian use of hypnosis. If a patient, for whatever conscious or unconscious reason, is unwilling to relinquish a symptom but feels extreme pressure from the therapist to do so, symptom substitution may be the way out of this transference-countertransference dilemma. On the other hand, if the patient is offered an opportunity to overcome a symptom but feels consciously free to choose not to avail himself of the opportunity, complying by substituting a symptom becomes unnecessary.

In fact, the literature contains some evidence of what has been called a ripple effect (Spiegel and Linn, 1969). That is, when patients use self-hypnosis to master one area of their lives, for example a phobia, they find themselves making other positive changes using similar techniques, for example, losing weight or stopping smoking. Since the trance capacity is inherent in the individual, he or she is then free to use this resource more fully once it has been identified and mobilized.

The primary limitations on the uses of hypnosis for symptom-oriented treatment have more to do with the ability of the patient to experience the trance state than anything else, although this issue is still debated in the field (Barber, 1980; Frischholz et al., 1981).

Hypnosis should never be used in a coercive or deceptive manner. The nature of hypnosis should be explained briefly and the patient's cooperation elicited. If the patient refuses, he or she should not be pressured to undergo a hypnotic experience. An atmosphere of clinical respect and informed consent is critical. Except in acute emergencies, euphemisms for hypnosis should be avoided, since patients often suspect that nonhypnotic techniques involve hypnosis and a relationship of trust can be undermined by misleading a patient. Usually a simple explanation about the modern understanding of hypnosis and an invitation to the patient to explore his or her hypnotic capacity in the service of the treatment goal will elicit full cooperation.

Additional precautions should occasionally be taken. Some paranoid patients, for example, will have difficulty understanding the difference between compliance with hypnotic instructions and mind control and may elaborate a projective framework around the person attempting to induce hypnosis. It is especially important with such patients to be rather diffident about using hypnosis. Most such patients make the problem easy by refusing the procedure. In addition, research shows that schizophrenics are, in general, less hypnotizable than normals (D. Spiegel et al., 1982; Lavoie and Sabourin, 1980). However, numerous researchers have attempted to hypnotize populations of schizophrenics and have reported no untoward effects. It is also important to use hypnosis with caution among depressed and suicidal patients. Since patients often invest considerable irrational hope in hypnosis as a cure-all, a failure to experience relief from the trance state may become an additional disappointment that constitutes a pretext for a suicide attempt. Diffusing excessive expectations is important, along with careful clinical examination.

There is some apprehension on the part of the public and professionals that an individual may panic during a hypnotic induction or be unable to re-emerge from the trance state. Such reactions may take one of two forms: a nonspecific anxiety state during the induction and/or an abreaction of some affectively laden event.

No patient has ever been irretrievably lost in a trance state. At worst, if left in a trance by an inept hypnotist, such a subject will eventually fall asleep and will reawaken in a normal, nontrance condition. However, hypnotizable individuals are especially sensitive to the anxiety of the therapist inducing the trance, and it is possible for a kind of snowball effect to occur in which the subject senses the therapist's anxiety and becomes more anxious, which only makes the therapist even more anxious. Such an effect may be exemplified by the patient who says, "I can't open my eyes. I can't come out of the trance." Calm reassurance and the avoidance of a power struggle are sufficient to handle such situations. The subject can be told, "When you are ready, you will find that you are able to open your eyes. Just take a few deep breaths and you will find a time when you are ready to exit from the trance state."

It is not uncommon for powerful affects to be remobilized when a highly hypnotizable individual relives a traumatic event in a hypnotic age regression. This is more likely to happen when the therapeutic work involves the treatment of a post-traumatic stress disorder. However, sometimes an apparently innocent regression may happen upon an affect-laden moment. It is usually wise to begin a hypnotic regression with a new patient by experiencing with him or her a presumably neutral period in the patient's life, for example, an early birthday, as a way of establishing control over the regression and the patient's response to the procedure. Occasionally, the patient will happen to have been, for example, in the hospital even at a seemingly neutral time. It is important to allow reasonable expression of the affect and to bear in mind that a kind of traumatic transference develops in which the patient identifies the therapist with either the circumstances of the unpleasant event or as one of the characters in it, for example, a doctor inflicting pain or a parent physically assaulting him or her, etc. The therapist may be called upon, in a sense, to role play as part of the regression. Unwittingly, one can slip into the most anxiety-producing position of acting out the role of the person inflicting the trauma, for example by telling the patient, harshly, to be quiet or not to worry. It is important to allow the subject to experience the discomfort and at the same time to reassure him that no additional harm is being inflicted on him. The trance experience can ultimately be helpful in enabling the patient to face aspects of the painful experience intensely for a while and then to put it aside at other times.

The rare untoward panic reaction in a trance state can be handled by a skilled clinician if one bears in mind that the trance state is a means of intensifying concentration on certain aspects of experience, accompanied by an exquisite sensitivity to the person providing the structure. Calm reassurance and acknowledgment of intense affect will help maintain control of the situation and enable the patient to exit from it having learned something.

In general, individuals capable of responding to hypnotic instructions must exhibit some capacity for trusting another individual. Some foundation experience of other-relatedness and trust is usually a prerequisite for the ability to experience trance. J. Hilgard (1970) has noted that a family history of imaginative involvement and firm but fair discipline seems to be a further prerequisite for higher hypnotizability in adult life. In order to enter a trance, a patient must be able to suspend, at least temporarily, a posture of extreme vigilance and allow the person structuring the experience for him to take over in a presumably protective fashion. This trust creates a special responsibility for the therapist using hypnosis, especially when the patient is extremely hypnotizable.

Countertransference Issues

Because of the tendency of individuals in a hypnotic trance to suspend critical judgment and be relatively receptive to input, the trance state can be seen as a magnifier of therapeutic technique. This means that an inept, deceptive, or exploitative therapist can inflict more damage on a patient if the patient is in a trance. It is especially important, therefore, that a practitioner using hypnosis be aware of countertransference problems and use sound evaluation, differential diagnosis, and therapeutic strategies. Countertransference problems can arise in any clinical situation, and, while none is unique to the hypnotic encounter, the relative posture of trust and proneness to uncritical acceptance characteristic of the hypnotized patient may limit the patient's ability to correct for countertransference problems or conscious exploitation on the part of the therapist. Irrational desires to manipulate or control patients, or to obtain gratification from them rather than offer help, have been acted out by therapists using hypnosis with deleterious results to patients. This misuse has included cases of sexual and financial exploitation. Using hypnosis in therapy is in some ways analogous to driving a car at high speed: The same mistake may have greater consequences. It is incumbent upon training programs and therapists in training to scrutinize their own motivations.

In addition, the more recently developed, less authoritarian approaches to hypnosis, which emphasize the teaching of self-hypnosis and an educational model of the use of hypnosis, are less prone to elicit such countertransference control problems since the patient is taught to use an exercise only if he or she chooses.

Some therapists who use hypnosis sometimes come to feel as though they do indeed control the patient. They may develop the illusion of imposing their ideas upon the patient, and they may foster dependency rather than help the patient discover new resources within himself for coping with stress. This can be a particular problem when the state of being in a trance is confounded with psychotherapy. The mere act of helping a patient enter a trance state is erroneously considered therapeutic when, in fact, it is simply a transition into a state of receptive, attentive concentration. The therapist and patient may struggle at two extremes of the hypnotic spectrum. A highly hypnotizable patient may frighten the therapist by appearing ceaselessly plastic and willing to respond to any instruction. This extreme compliance also gives the therapist an exaggerated sense of his own power. On the other hand, a nonhypnotizable patient may be viewed as "resisting." The therapist may take the patient's failure to respond to the hypnotic induction as a narcissistic injury and may become angry with the patient. Thus, it is particularly important to clarify the difference between patient resources for responding to hypnosis and psychotherapeutic strategy in order to minimize the tendency for hypnotic encounters to deteriorate into power struggles.

One of the main dangers of using hypnosis in psychotherapy is that it is such an intriguing phenomenon that it may be used, especially in a highly hypnotizable patient, when it is not really necessary. Simply because an individual is capable, for example, of age regressing to a traumatic incident and reliving it with dramatic and intense affect does not mean that the process of doing so is either necessary or relevant to the problem at hand. There may be times when the therapist will be satisfying his own curiosity rather than helping the patient solve a problem by using hypnosis to delve into periods of past conflict. A tendency to compliance, which typifies the highly hypnotizable individual and which may especially plague those who seek psychotherapy (H. Spiegel, 1975), may make it especially difficult for the highly hypnotizable patient to challenge the therapist's curiosity. Thus, it is especially important that the therapist have a clear conceptual view of the use of the hypnotic exploration and its place in the overall treatment plan.

The overriding issue is that sound clinical history-taking, evaluation, and formulation are the necessary prerequisites for work with hypnosis. With these basic considerations taken into account, there is no reason to fear that the use of hypnosis will harm patients or the therapeutic relationship.

AGE RELATED ISSUES

Sound evidence suggests that hypnotic responsivity is significantly age-related. Morgan and Hilgard (1973) have shown that hypnotic responsivity is highest in late childhood. Children seem to be quite hypnotizable from the time they are old enough to understand and follow instructions, so much so, for example, that Jacobs and Jacobs (1966) suggest that if, on examination, a child is found not to be able to experience hypnosis to some degree, one should begin to suspect neurological dysfunction. Hypnotic responsivity begins a gradual decline through adolescence and the adult life span. Morgan and Hilgard (1973) noted the decline to become more acute in the third and fourth decades. They found that approximately two-thirds of a large adult psychiatric outpatient population was hypnotically responsive to some degree. About one out of ten normal individuals is extremely hypnotizable in his or her adult years.

What these survey findings indicate is that hypnosis may be a particularly useful tool among children old enough to respond to instructions. A number of ingenious therapeutic techniques have been developed for helping children with such problems as pain, conversion symptoms, anxiety, seizure control, and enuresis (Gardner and Olness, 1981; Williams et al., 1978; Hilgard and Hilgard, 1975). The vivid imagination of young children combined with their high hypnotic responsiveness makes the use of imaginative hypnotic techniques an extremely valuable tool, for example, in allaying anxieties regarding painful medical procedures. Many physicians use a technique known as misdirection, in which they have a young patient focus on an imaginary television show which they recount, an imaginary baseball game, or an imaginary animal while suturing or injections are performed.

J. Hilgard (1970) believes that certain kinds of parent-child interactions may facilitate the development of hypnotic responsiveness, for example, experiences of imaginative involvement with a parent in which a child learns to develop intense imaginative experiences. Hilgard also points to the importance of a strong relationship with the opposite sex parent and firm but fair discipline as being associated with high hypnotizability in later years.

At the other end of the life cycle, the prevalence of high hypnotizability is far lower, but a sufficient number of older patients are hypnotizable to some degree to make testing for responsiveness worth the effort unless concentration is overwhelmingly impaired.

PROFESSIONAL AND ETHICAL ISSUES

The use of hypnosis as a therapeutic technique has been officially sanctioned by the American Psychiatric Association and the American Medical Association (1958), and its use by a licensed physician or therapist is legal in every state of the United States. All but a few malpractice insurance policies provide coverage for hypnosis, although some insist that practitioners who use it indicate that they do so as a special procedure. Written informed consent for the use of hypnosis is not required unless special exigencies of the clinical situation would make it advisable. It is necessary to audio or video tape hypnotic sessions only in certain special circumstances such as forensic uses. When hypnosis is used for legal purposes to help a victim or witness uncover information, it is crucial that all interactions between examiner and subject be recorded, preferably on video tape, so that all influence on the subject can be evaluated by the court.

The fundamental training issue is that anyone using hypnosis should have competence, training, and licensure in a primary specialty field. The two official hypnosis societies sanction training only for physicians, doctoral level psychologists or social workers, and dentists. These two societies have recently opposed training nonprofessionals to use hypnosis in the course of interrogation. The professional hypnosis community is virtually unanimous in condemning the licensing and practice of lay hypnotists who are trained only in hypnotic induction techniques since they lack the clinical skills for diagnosis and treatment as well as the knowledge of various treatment strategies.

Specialized training in hypnosis is offered in courses at a number of medical schools to medical students, residents, and practicing physicians; in a number of clinical psychology programs; and in a variety of workshops, some in association with the two hypnosis societies. A fully trained professional can learn to begin using hypnosis in his or her practice after one or two weeks of intensive training, but supervision from someone skilled in the clinical discipline of hypnosis is recommended as a supplement. Basic training in hypnosis should include a discussion of hypnotic induction techniques, methods of evaluating patients' responsiveness, limitations, and treatment strategies.

Co-therapists are not necessary for the use of hypnosis, but there is no reason to exclude other people from the room where hypnosis is performed if their presence is appropriate to the overall therapeutic context. Thus, hypnosis has been used with co-therapists or with appropriate family members in the room with the consent of the patient. It is important in these situations for the therapist to structure the situation carefully, since the patient in the trance state is in a somewhat vulnerable position. One useful key to the appropriateness of the presence of others when hypnosis occurs is the therapist's and patient's sense of comfort or discomfort with the arrangement. If there is any question that the patient may feel frightened of experiencing hypnosis alone with the therapist or that the patient may be prone to charge the therapist with some form of seductive or inappropriate behavior, it is wise to have a third party in the room. This occurs rarely.

The risk-benefit ratio of hypnosis is exceedingly favorable. There are no significant side effects. Since the trance state occurs naturally in individuals capable of experiencing it, the greatest risk is simply that the procedure will not work, in which case little other than some time has been lost. On the other hand, when the procedure does work, the benefits can be considerable, not only in terms of symptom relief, but if the strategy is structured appropriately, in terms of enhanced self-esteem and a sense of greater mastery on the part of the patient.

The uses of hypnosis in the United States are myriad, and clearly some practitioners are inept and even unethical. Several have been prosecuted for using hypnosis to exploit patients. The patient in a trance state is prone to be receptive, uncritically accepting, and vulnerable to manipulation of perception. This does not mean that the patient is unable to disagree with the therapist or reject suggestions. It does mean that to the extent that the patient is hypnotizable and in a trance state, he or she is less prone to disagree, especially over a short period of time.

FINANCIAL, LEGAL, AND SOCIAL-POLITICAL ISSUES

Fees for the use of hypnosis vary widely, but in general they should be based on the appropriate reimbursement for the services provided by someone with a comparable professional background. Especially when self-hypnosis is taught, treatment techniques using hypnosis are usually brief, and therefore the treatment is cost-effective.

There are growing interest and controversy regarding the role of hypnosis in forensic work (Orne, 1979; H. Spiegel, 1980). It is of obvious interest in enhancing the recall of witnesses and victims of crimes and has proven to be dramatically effective in unearthing otherwise repressed information. For example, the bus driver who was kidnapped along with a school bus full of children in Chowchilla, California, was hypnotized. In the hypnotic regression he was able to give police most of the license numbers of the car used by the abductors, information that led to their arrest and conviction. However, some (Diamond, 1980) insist that hypnosis in forensic work is more of a danger than a help because of the possibility of contaminating the memory of witnesses. There is evidence that, used improperly, hypnosis can make an honest liar of a subject (H. Spiegel, 1980), who can be artificially instructed in the trance state to testify to events that did not occur. Another danger is that the ceremony of hypnosis will provide a setting in which an individual can either deliberately deceive the examiner or can become convinced of his own error because the information was given in a trance state. There is no agreement in the field on these issues, but most responsible practitioners concur that if hypnosis is used, care should be taken to record all aspects of hypnotic work and the contact with the professional using hypnosis, preferably on video tape, so that overt or subtle influences can be studied by all parties (Orne, 1979). The Supreme Court of the United States has ruled that to use hypnosis without the consent of a defendant is a violation of First Amendment rights (*Leyra* v. *Denno*, 1954). Courts vary in their willingness to allow hypnosis or admit evidence based on hypnotic testimony (*State* v. *White*, 1979; *People* v. *Shirley*, 1982; *State* v. *Mack*, 1979; *People* v. *Hurd*, 1980; *Kline* v. *Ford Motor Co.*, 1975).

The primary social and political issues associated with hypnosis involve its availability, indications, and costs. While some patients are frightened of its use or object to it, it is in general a growingly popular technique.

REFERENCES

American Medical Association: Report on medical use of hypnosis. JAMA 168:186-189, 1958

Andreychuk T, Skriver C: Hypnosis and biofeedback in the treatment of migraine headache. Int J Clin Exp Hypn 23:172-183, 1975

Bakan P, Svorad D: Resting EEG alpha and asymmetry of reflective lateral eye movement. Nature 223:975-976, 1969

Bakan P: Hypnotizability, laterality of eye movements and functional brain asymmetry. Percept Mot Skills 28:927-932, 1969

Barber J: Hypnosis and the unhypnotizable. Am J Clin Hypn 23:4-9, 1980

Barber TX, Wilson SC: The Barber Suggestibility Scale and the Creative Imagination Scale: experimental and clinical applications. Am J Clin Hypn 21:84-96, 1978-79

Barber TX, Wilson SC: Hypnosis, suggestions, and altered states of consciousness: experimental evaluation of the new cognitive-behavioral theory and the traditional trance-state theory of "hypnosis." Ann NY Acad Sci 296:34-47, 1977

Beecher HK: Relationship of significance of wound to pain experiences. JAMA 161:1609-1613, 1956

Berkowitz B, Ross-Townsend A, Kohberger R: Hypnotic treatment of smoking: the single treatment method revisited. Am J Psychiatry 136:83-85, 1979

Bernheim H: Hypnosis and Suggestion in Psychotherapy: A Treatise on the Nature of Hypnotism (1889). Translated by Herter CA. New Hyde Park, NY, University Books, 1964

Bower GH: Mood and memory. Am Psychol 36:529-533, 1970

Bowers KS, van der Meulen SJ: Effect of hypnotic susceptibility on creativity test performance. J Pers Soc Psychol 14:247-256, 1970

Bowers P: Hypnotizability, creativity and the role of effortless experiencing. Int J Clin Exper Hypn 226:184-202, 1978

Braid J: Neurypnology (1889). New York, Julian Press, 1960

Brende JO, Benedict BD: The Vietnam combat delayed response syndrome: hypnotherapy of "dissociative symptoms." Am J Clin Hypn 23:34-40, 1980

Breuer J, Freud S: Studies on Hysteria, vol 2 (1883-95), in Complete Psychological Works of Sigmund Freud, standard ed. Translated by Strachey J, Freud A. London, Hogarth Press, 1955

Charcot JM: Oeuvres Completes de JM Charcot, tome IX. Paris, Lecrosnier et Babé, 1890

Clynes M, Kohn M, Lifshitz K: Dynamics and spatial behavior of light-evoked potentials, their modification under hypnosis, and on-line correlation in relation to rhythmic components. Ann NY Acad Sci 112:468-509, 1964

Collison DR: Which asthmatic patients should be treated by hypnotherapy? Med J Aust 1:676-681, 1975

Crasilneck HB, Hall JA: Clinical Hypnosis: Principles and Applications. New York, Grune & Stratton, 1975

Crasilneck HB: The use of hypnosis in the treatment of psychogenic impotency. Australia Journal of Clinical and Experimental Hypnosis, commemorative issue, 1979

Darnton R: Mesmerism and the End of the Enlightenment in France. New York, Schocken Books, 1970

Diamond BL: Inherent problems in the use of pretrial hypnosis on a prospective witness. California Law Review 63:313-349, 1980

Ellenberger HF: Discovery of the Unconscious: The History and Evolution of Dynamic Psychiatry. New York, Basic Books, 1970

Erickson MH: Advanced Techniques of Hypnosis and Therapy: Selected Papers of Milton H Erickson, MD. Edited by Haley J. New York, Grune & Stratton, 1967

Erickson MH: The utilization of patient behavior in the hypnotherapy of obesity: three case reports. Am J Clin Hypn 3:115-116, 1960

Esdaile J: Hypnosis in Medicine and Surgery (1846). New York, Julian Press, 1957

Evans FJ: Phenomena of hypnosis: 2: posthypnotic amnesia, in Handbook of Hypnosis and Psychosomatic Medicine. Edited by Burrows GD, Dennerstein L. New York, Elsevier/North Holland Biomedical Press, 1980

Frankel FH, Apfel RJ, Kelly SF, et al: The use of hypnotizability scales in the clinic: a review after six years. Int J Clin Exper Hypn 27:63-73, 1979

Frankel FH, Orne MT: Hypnotizability and phobic behavior. Arch Gen Psychiatry 33:1259-1261, 1976

Freud S: An Autobiographic Study, vol 22 (1924), in Complete Psychological Works of Sigmund Freud, standard ed. Translated by Strachey J, Freud A. London, Hogarth Press, 1959

Friedlander JW, Sarbin RT: The depth of hypnosis. J Abnorm Soc Psychol 33:281-294, 1938

Frischholz EJ, Blumstein R, Spiegel D: Comparative efficacy of hypnotic behavioral training and sleep/trance hypnotic induction: comment on Katz. J Consult Clin Psychol 50:766-769, 1982

Frischholz EJ, Spiegel H, Spiegel D: Hypnosis and the unhypnotizable: a reply to Barber. Am J Clin Hypn 24:55-58, 1981

Frischholz EJ, Tryon WW, Vellos AT, et al: The relationship between the Hypnotic Induction Profile and the Stanford Hypnotic Susceptibility Scale, Form C: a replication. Am J Clin Hypn 22:185-196, 1980

Fromm E, Eisen M: Self-hypnosis as a therapeutic aid in the mourning process. Am J Clin Hypn 25:3-14, 1982

Galbraith GC, Cooper LM, London P: Hypnotic susceptibility and the sensory evoked response. J Comp Physiol Psychol 80:500-514, 1972

Gardner GG, Olness D: Hypnosis and Hypnotherapy with Children. New York, Grune & Stratton, 1981

Gerschman J, Burrows G, Reade P, et al: Hypnotizability and the treatment of dental phobic behavior, in Hypnosis. Edited by Burrows GD, Dennerstein L. New York, Elsevier, 1979

Gill MM, Brenman M: Hypnosis and Related States: Psychoanalytic Studies in Regression. New York, International Universities Press, 1959

Greenson RR: The working alliance and the transference neurosis. Psychoanal Q 34:155-182, 1965

Gross M: Hypnosis as a diagnostic tool. Am J Clin Hypn 23:47-52, 1980

Guerrero-Figueroa R, Heath RG: Evoked responses and changes during attentive factors in man. Arch Neurol 10:74-84, 1964

Gur RC, Gur RE: Handedness, sex, and eyedness as moderating variables in the relation between hypnotic susceptibility and functional brain asymmetry. J Abnorm Psychol 83:635-643, 1974

Hernandez-Peon R, Donoso M: Influence of attention and suggestion upon subcortical evoked electric activity in the human brain, in First International Congress of Neurological Sciences, vol 3. Edited by Van Bogaert L, Radermecker J. London, Pergamon Press, 1959

Hilgard ER, Crawford HJ, Wert A: The Stanford Hypnotic Arm Levitation Induction and Test (SHALIT): a six-minute hypnotic induction and measurement scale. Int J Clin Exper Hypn 27:111-124, 1979

Hilgard ER, Hilgard JR: Hypnosis in the Relief of Pain. Los Altos, Calif, William Kaufmann, 1975

Hilgard ER: Illusion that the eye-roll sign is related to hypnotizability. Arch Gen Psychiatry 39:963-966, 1982

Hilgard ER: Divided Consciousness: Multiple Controls in Human Thought and Action. New York, John Wiley & Sons, 1977

Hilgard ER: Hypnosis. Annual Review of Psychology 26:19-44, 1975

Hilgard ER: Hypnotic Susceptibility. New York, Harcourt, Brace and World, 1965

Hilgard JR: Personality and Hypnosis: A Study of Imaginative Involvement. Chicago, University of Chicago Press, 1970

Hollender MH, Hirsch SJ: Hysterical psychosis: clarification of the concept. Am J Psychiatry 120:1066-1074, 1964

Holroyd J: Hypnosis treatment for smoking: an evaluative review. Int J Clin Exper Hypn 28:341-357, 1980

Hull CL: Hypnosis and Suggestibility: An Experimental Approach. New York, Appleton-Century-Crofts, 1933

Hull CL: Quantitative methods of investigating waking suggestion. J Abnorm Soc Psychol 24:153-169, 1929

Hunt WA, Bespalec DA: An evaluation of current methods of modifying smoking behavior. J Clin Psychol 30:431-438, 1974

Jacobs J, Jacobs J: Hypnotizability of children as related to hemispheric reference and neurological organization. Am J Clin Hypn 8:269-274, 1966

Janet P: The Major Symptoms of Hysteria. New York, Macmillan, 1920

Joseph ED, Peck SM, Kaufman R: A psychological study of neurodermatitis with a case report. Mt Sinai Hospital Journal 15:360-366, 1949

Kardiner A, Spiegel H: War Stress and Neurotic Illness. New York, Paul Hoeber, 1947

Katz NW: Comparative efficacy of behavioral training, training plus relaxation, and a sleep/trance hypnotic induction in increasing hypnotic susceptibility. J Consult Clin Psychol 47:119-127, 1979

Katz RL, Kao CY, Spiegel H, et al: Acupuncture and hypnosis. Adv Neurol 4:819-825, 1974

Kety SS, Rosenthal D, Wender PH, et al: Mental illness in the biological and adoptive families of adopted schizoprenics. Am J Psychiatry 128:82-86, 1971

Kline v Ford Motor Co, 523 Fed 2d 1067, 9th Cir, 1975

Lavoie G, Sabourin M, Ally G, et al: Hypnotizability as a function of adaptive regression among chronic psychotic patients. Int J Clin Exper Hypn 24:238-257, 1976

Lavoie G, Sabourin M, Langlois J: Hypnotic susceptibility, amnesia, and IQ in chronic schizophrenia. Int J Clin Exper Hypn 21:157-167, 1973

Lavoie G, Sabourin M: Hypnosis and schizophrenia: a review of experimental and clinical studies, in Handbook of Hypnosis and Psychosomatic Medicine. Edited by Burrows GD, Dennerstein L. New York, Elsevier/North Holland Biomedical Press, 1980

Leyra v Denno, 347 US 556 (1954)

London P, Hart JT, Leibovitz MP: EEG alpha rhythms and susceptibility to hypnosis. Nature 219:71-72, 1969

Ludwig AM, Brandsma JM, Wilbur CB, et al: The objective study of a multiple personality. Arch Gen Psychiatry 26:298-310, 1972

McGlashan TH, Evans FJ, Orne MT: The nature of hypnotic analgesia and the placebo response to experimental pain. Psychosom Med 31:227-246, 1969

Moore ME, Berk SN: Acupuncture for chronic shoulder pain. Ann Int Med 84:381-384, 1976

Morgan AH, Johnson DL, Hilgard ER: The stability of hypnotic susceptibility: a longitudinal study. Int J Clin Exp Hypn 22:249-257, 1974b

Morgan AH, MacDonald H, Hilgard ER: EEG alpha: lateral asymmetry related to task and hypnotizability. Psychophysiology 11:275-282, 1974a

Morgan AH, Hilgard JR: The Stanford Hypnotic Clinical Scale: adult. Am J Clin Hypn 21:139-147, 1979

Morgan AH, Hilgard ER: Age differences in susceptibility to hypnosis. Int J Clin Exp Hypn 21:78-85, 1973

Mott T: The clinical importance of hypnotizability. Am J Clin Hypn 21:263-269, 1979

Nowlis DP, Rhead JC: Relation of eyes-closed resting EEG alpha activity to hypnotic susceptibility. Percept Mot Skills 27:1047-1050, 1968

Orne MT: The use and misuse of hypnosis in court. Int J Clin Exper Hypn 27:311-341, 1979

Orne MT: The nature of hypnosis: artifact and essence. J Abnorm Soc Psychol 58:277-299, 1959

People v Hurd, Sup Ct NJ, Somerset Co, April 2, 1980

People v Shirley, 31C 3d 18, modified 918a, 1982

Pettinati HM: Measuring hypnotizability in psychotic patients. Int J Clin Exper Hypn 30:404-416, 1982

Prince M: Psychotherapy and Multiple Personality: Selected Essays. Edited by Hale NG Jr. Cambridge, Harvard University Press, 1975

Prince M: The Dissociation of a Personality. New York, Longmans, Green, 1906

Sarbin TR, Slagle RW: Hypnosis and psychophysiological outcomes, in Hypnosis: Research Developments and Perspectives. Edited by Fromm E, Shor RE. Chicago, Aldine-Atherton, 1972

Shakow D: Segmental set: a theory of the formal psychological deficit in schizophrenia. Arch Gen Psychiatry 6:1-7, 1974

Shor RE, Orne MT, O'Connell DB: Validation and cross-validation of a scale of self-reported personal experiences which predicts hypnotizability. J Psychol 53:55-75, 1962

Sidis B, Goodhart SP: Multiple Personality. New York, Appleton-Century-Crofts, 1905

Siomopoulos V: Hysterical psychosis: psycho-pathological aspects. Br J Psychol 44:95-100, 1971

Spiegel D, Detrick E, Frischholz E: Hypnotizability and psychopathology. Am J Psychiatry 139:431-437, 1982a

Spiegel D, Frischholz EJ, Maruffi B, et al: Hypnotic responsivity and the treatment of flying phobia. Am J Clin Hypn 23:239-247, 1981

Spiegel D, Tryon WW, Frischholz EJ, et al: Hilgard's illusion (ltr). Arch Gen Psychiatry 39:972-974, 1982

Spiegel D, Fink R: Hysterical psychosis and hypnotizability. Am J Psychiatry 136:777-781, 1979

Spiegel D: Vietnam grief work using hypnosis. Am J Clin Hypn 24:33-40, 1981

Spiegel H, Fleiss JL, Bridger AA, et al: Hypnotizability and mental health, in New Dimensions in Psychiatry: A World View. Edited by Arieti S. New York, John Wiley & Sons, 1975

Spiegel H, Linn L: The "ripple effect" following abjunct hypnosis in analytic psychotherapy. Am J Psychiatry 126:53-58, 1969

Spiegel H, Spiegel D: Induction techniques, in Handbook of Hypnosis and Psychosomatic Medicine. Edited by Burrows GD, Dennerstein L. Amsterdam, Elsevier North-Holland/Biomedical Press, 1980

Spiegel H, Spiegel D: Trance and Treatment: Clinical Uses of Hypnosis. New York, Basic Books, 1978

Spiegel H: Hypnosis and evidence: help or hindrance? Ann NY Acad Sci 347:73-85, 1980

Spiegel H: The Grade 5 syndrome: the highly hypnotizable person. Int J Clin Exper Hypn 22:303-319, 1974

Spiegel H: Manual for Hypnotic Induction Profile: Eye-Roll Levitation Method, rev ed. New York, Soni Medica, 1973

Spiegel H: An eye-roll test for hypnotizability. Am J Clin Hypn 15:25-28, 1972

Spiegel H: Hypnosis and transference: a theoretical formulation. Arch Gen Psychiatry 1:634-639, 1959

Spiegel H: Preventive psychiatry with combat troops. Am J Psychiatry 101:310-315, 1944

State v Mack, Minn Sup Ct No 50036 (Pretrial probable cause hearing certified as important and doubtful question January 30, 1979, by Dist Ct Co of Hennepin, 4th Judicial Dist, under Minn Rules of Crim Proc No 29.02, subd 4)

State v White, No J-3665 (Cir Ct, Branch 10, Milwaukee Co, March 27, 1979, unrep)

Sutcliffe JP, Jones J: Personal identity, multiple personality, and hypnosis. J Clin Exp Hypn 40:231-269, 1963

Tellegen A, Atkinson G: Openness to absorbing and self-altering experiences ("absorption"), a trait related to hypnotic susceptibility. J Abnorm Psychol 83:268-277, 1974

Van Nuys D: Meditation, attention, and hypnotic susceptibility: a correlational study. Int J Clin Exper Hypn 21:59-69, 1973

Wadden TA, Anderton CH: The clinical use of hypnosis. Psychol Bull 91:215-243, 1982

Weitzenhoffer AM, Hilgard ER: Stanford Hypnotic Susceptibility Scale, Form C. Palo Alto, Calif, Consulting Psychologists Press, 1962

Weitzenhoffer AM, Hilgard ER: Stanford Hypnotic Susceptibility Scale: Forms A and B. Palo Alto, Calif, Consulting Psychologists Press, 1959

Weitzenhoffer AM: Hypnotic susceptibility revisited. Am J Clin Hypn 22:130-146, 1980

Weitzenhoffer AM: General Techniques of Hypnosis. New York, Grune & Stratton, 1957

Williams DT, Spiegel H, Mostofsky DI: Neurogenic and hysterical seizures in children and adolescents: differential diagnosis and therapeutic considerations. Am J Psychiatry 135:82-86, 1978

Wilson NJ: Neurophysiologic alterations with hypnosis. Dis Nerv Syst 29:618-620, 1968

Wolberg LR: Medical Hypnosis, vols 1,2. New York, Grune & Stratton, 1948

16

Narcosynthesis

16
Narcosynthesis

INTRODUCTION

Narcosynthesis is a form of therapeutic intervention in which a pharmacological agent is introduced intravenously to facilitate emotional abreaction and communication. Its effects are achieved through alteration of the state of consciousness, appropriately directed stimulation, or suggestion to induce derepression of affective states associated with psychologically traumatic experiential memory traces. The term narcosynthesis, introduced by Grinker and Spiegel (1945), implies that the material derepressed through the abreactive experience becomes consciously available for integration and synthesis by the personality.

Others have called this procedure narcodiagnosis, narcotherapy, or narcoanalysis, depending on the primary intent of the psychiatrist in prescription of parenteral injection of drugs in treating patients. Many recent publications pertaining to the prescription of intravenous drugs are restricted to the use of a particular drug (e.g., sodium amytal or pentothal, etc.).

HISTORY

The use of pharmacologic agents to facilitate abreaction arose from the earlier application of barbiturates and other agents to effect prolonged narcosis as a method of treating and/or managing excited, agitated, or insomnic patients. Blackwenn (1923) generally is credited with the first publications pertaining to this technique. Lindemann (1932) reported the marked effect of small doses of sodium amytal injected intravenously into both healthy and mentally disordered persons. He showed that such prenarcotic dosages of the drug altered subjects' mental states to produce serenity and a sense of well-being. This state of disinhibition seemed to facilitate friendliness and drive to contact others in which the subjects spoke easily of their intimate thoughts.

During World War I, Simmel and others (see Freud et al., 1921) observed that hypnosis was effective with some traumatized soldiers in inducing abreaction of subjectively traumatic combat experiences and noted that their symptomatology resolved thereafter. It was recognized, however, that hypnotic induction was impossible in many men and that many relapsed after this treatment. With the onset of World War II abreactive treatment using intravenous barbituates was attempted. The earliest reports were those of Sargent and Slater (1940) and Mallinson (1940), who described the rapid resolution of such symptoms as stupor, mutism, confusion, and various conversion paralyses. Many men so treated were returned to the lines. Horsley (1936), applying psychoanalytic insights to this treatment, designated it as "narcoanalysis." This term is now used to describe the recall of repressed material with abreaction during the drug induced states and when one gives dynamic interpretations and provides post-hypnotic suggestions.

Since World War II narcosynthesis has been prescribed mostly for treatment of acute post traumatic stress disorders, particularly when expressed in seriously impairing social symptoms. Many attempts to use abreactive narcoanalysis to assist in the treatment of psychotic and neurotic conditions were made during peacetime when communication was blocked through mutism or other resistances. The technique has been modified in that other psychopharmacologic agents are now sometimes used to alter cerebral functioning and states of consciousness. To effect certainty of later recall and open the possibility of personal confrontation, more recent researchers have begun to video tape the narcosynthetic session so that the subject may later review his recorded behavior.

Alteration of consciousness by intravenous injection of drugs is used less frequently to facilitate diagnosis, elicitation of history, and free association. These applications extend beyond treatment of the post-traumatic states.

THEORETICAL ISSUES

Narcosynthetic treatment appears to have its roots in the long record of catharsis as a means of bringing relief to sufferers with a variety of forms of disturbing behavior. Through their rituals, medicine men and shamans seemed to try to bring about emotional abreaction in those they were called on to help. Hypnotically induced abreaction assumed a recognized place in the armamentarium of medicine during the nineteenth century. Freud's abandonment of the hypnotic technique with the development of free association did not do away with catharsis as one of the principles influencing effective treatment.

In his summary of the use of abreaction as one of the major therapeutic techniques, Bibring (1954) states that the single abreaction experience came to be recognized as indicated only in the simplest of the three forms of hysteria—that is, retention hysteria—in which the abnormal behavior is hypothesized to exist as the outward expression of attempts at massive repression of affect. Freud defined three types of hysteria: retention, hypnoid, and defense. In the latter two, in contrast to retention hysteria, splitting of consciousness was thought to occur. For these complex hysterical constellations, abreaction with discharge of affect in association with reminiscence of the traumatic event was conceived as incomplete. Partial dissociation persisted; the additional therapeutic step needed was the conduct of the ideas associated with the trauma into full consciousness to bring about an ego associative adaptation.

Derepression of acutely induced affectively charged complexes constitutes the psychodynamic indication for the use of drug induced narcosynthetic treatment. But for those with personality organization that disallows full affective discharge through abreaction, as in the hypnoid and defense hysterias, "working through" beyond abreaction is necessary to effect complete symptom resolution. Yet tension relief in emotional catharsis remains a cardinal principle in all therapeutic interventions.

Theorists have given little attention to the interpersonal aspects of cathartic treatments. Beyond the individual's clearer, more objective perspective of his experience, Bibring (1954) refers to the sufferer's sense of being "understood and accepted" as well as his receiving narcissistic gratification through personal exposure of his predicament before the therapist or others.

Kolb (in press) conceives of abreaction as an interpersonal event in which the sufferer is set, even beforehand, to act out his repressed complex. He has come for help to a healer generally recognized as one who attempts both to relieve distress and to accept it realistically for what it is without adverse judgment. The therapist thus may be considered as an alter ego. Abreactive exposure usually releases affects of primitive fear, rage, and helplessness— all associated with shame as well as other affects of anxiety, sadness, guilt, and sometimes triumph and revenge. The therapist's exposure, understanding, and acceptance of these affects relieves superego condemnation associated with intrapsychically repressed shame, guilt, personal condemnation, or humiliation. Tension is usually reduced immediately as the result of the affective discharge and relief from shame and guilt engendered through critical assessment of the actions committed or omitted during the traumatic incidents.

Beyond the psychodynamic and interpersonal explanations for the therapeutic value of narcosynthesis, this psychopharmaceutic intervention releases cerebral cortical functions concerned with the control of conscious inhibiting processes.

PROCEDURE

The patient and/or his surrogates, if available, are advised of the reasons for proposing narcosynthesis, the nature of the procedure, and the potential outcome.

Generally, sodium amytal or sodium pentothal have been the drugs of choice. Other agents that have been used are methohexital, methylphenidate, and amphetamines. The only data available support the earlier impression that abreaction with recall will be achieved more effectively with the barbiturates than with other administered agents.

The drug is administered intravenously using either the bolus or drip technique. Preferably using a butterfly needle, gauge 21, the intravenous insertion may be made into the dorsal veins of the hand or those in the antecubital fossa. A 10% solution of a barbiturate containing 500 mg of sodium pentothal is injected at the rate of approximately 1 cc for the first two minutes. The rate of injection and the amount of drug injection are then varied depending on the patient's state of consciousness.

During initial introduction the psychiatrist casually initiates contact with the patient by advising him of the technique and of the somatic sensations he may notice. The patient may be told that the medicine to be injected will help him to relax and to express himself about his experiences and feelings, that he may feel as though he has been drinking, that he will experience pleasurable relaxation and drowsiness. The patient is asked to report when he begins to notice relaxation and warmth.

To examine the changing level of consciousness the patient is instructed to count backward from 200 and to comment when he first feels subjective bodily change. When he begins to slur his speech and to make errors in counting the therapist will know that cerebral functioning is altered appropriately to receive either the suggestion for abreaction or selected stimuli to induce the response.

Stimulation

The usual stimulus to abreaction is given in a vigorous voice. The therapist, addressing the patient by his familiar name, loudly tells the patient he is at the scene of the traumatic event. If this event is not known and in the case of a post-traumatic event due to war the therapist will loudly depict a combat scene—mortars or artillery shells are coming in; tanks, planes, or helicopters are approaching. Kolb and Mutalapassi (1982) have found that one may obtain immediate time regression to the traumatic scene by playing 30 seconds of audio tape of combat sounds without any use of verbal suggestion.

Abreaction

The amount of verbal stimulation needed to induce abreaction is variable. Some patients respond immediately with the initial stimulus; others appear resistive. The response may vary from highly dramatic attempts to escape, fight, or verbally express intense rage or hopelessness to a longer, more verbal account of feelings, actions, and reactions. There often occur simultaneous crying or yelling, evidence of neuromuscular tension, rapid respiration, perspiration, and pupillary dilation. Injection of the drug is terminated once abreaction is under way.

Exploration

The therapist will attempt further exploration of both action and affect through following the patient's behavioral response. This will be done with questions to clarify the meaning of his behavior and that of others mentioned in the events recounted. Some therapists (DeAguiar, 1982) continue the session both over several hours and through repeated sessions.

Termination

When ready to terminate the session, the therapist will indicate sympathetically and firmly that the experience is over and that it has been a dream. The opportunity now exists to provide supportive, compassionate, and interpretive statements regarding the revealed affective and behavioral acting out. As the patient recovers consciousness he is encouraged to rest in bed and sleep for a period.

Confrontation and Interpretation

Later, on recovery of clear consciousness, the therapist will ascertain what memories the patient has of the experience. The extent of recollection is variable from individual to individual, yet reports of immediate tension reduction are usual. The therapist will review his observations of the abreaction with appropriate interpretations. To effect a more certain potential for recollection Metzger and Grinker* and others† record the narcosynthetic session and later review the recording with the patient, thus presenting him with a confrontation of his total response. The therapist is with the patient at the time of the confrontation. In the case of those with war-induced post-traumatic states, the patient may be asked if he wishes to expose his tape to others significant to him (wives, girlfriends, other family members, or friends). Many patients have done so. Once again the therapist attends the viewing with the patient and friends and offers interpretations as indicated.

CLINICAL ISSUES

Narcosynthesis is used to treat the seriously impairing acute symptoms of post-traumatic stress disorders such as mutism, amnesia, confusional states, and paralysis as well as repetitive dissociative expressions of the delayed and chronic forms of these disorders, now commonly spoken of as "flash-backs."

The aim of narcosynthesis is symptom reduction, particularly for those behavioral expressions mentioned above. It is not curative since the personality conflicts that predisposed to the dissociative states usually remain unmodified. Generally patients treated with narcosynthesis are engaged thereafter in additional individual or group therapy and may receive indicated psychopharmaceutical support to alleviate continuing affective distress.

Repeated narcosynthetic abreactions have been used to treat resistive symptoms of acute psychological trauma. Repeated interviews under sodium amytal have been used to diminish initial resistance to verbalization in psychotherapy, to facilitate history taking, and to discriminate diagnostic features.

LIMITATIONS

The major physiological risk in undertaking narcosynthesis using the barbiturates is respiratory delay or paralysis. It is advisable to have readily available support and advice from trained anesthesiologists as well as appropriate equipment to abort any respiratory embarrassment. The thera-

---

*Metzger JR, Grinker R: Videotape self-confrontations after narcotherapy. Presented at the 130th annual meeting of American Psychiatric Association, Toronto, May 2–6, 1977

†Kolb LC: Uses of videotape for therapeutic confrontation. Presented at 7th World Congress of Psychiatry, Vienna, Austria, 1983

pist should have knowledge of and be capable of assuring restitution of pulmonary ventilation.

Psychological risks center around possible breakdown of the patient's defenses with occurrence of a psychotic regression. Such a risk is possible in those with a pre-psychotic personality make-up. It may be avoided through a careful diagnostic study, including psychological testing, prior to consideration of the procedure.

In those with post-traumatic stress disorders of war, the potential of a post-narcosynthetic depressive affective state should be assessed, particularly when there is likelihood of revelation of commitment of atrocities. Finally, for the same group of patients, occasional prolongation of the abreactive state may occur in which the patient acts and lives out a state of terror. Such rare abreactive conditions simulate a psychotic reaction. Some may be aborted by inducing deep sleep through administration of a further hypnotic dose of a barbiturate or benzodiazepine. To assure care in such eventualities the therapist should have made arrangements for admission to a psychiatric unit, if necessary, to allow protective treatment and working through.

Narcosynthesis should not be undertaken in those with severe cardiac, pulmonary, liver, or kidney disease. Narcosynthesis should be avoided absolutely in those with porphyria.

DEVELOPMENTAL ISSUES

This technique has been and continues to be applied throughout the adolescent-adult age range.

ETHICAL ISSUES

It is advisable to obtain signed consent for the treatment after explaining the reasons for the recommendation and describing the technique and its risks. If the patient's response is to be recorded electronically in any way the uses of the recording should be described and the patient allowed to define the limits or extent of public exposure. It is desirable to review such definitions again after the patient has been confronted with his behavioral response.

LEGAL ISSUES

Amytal interviews have been used to facilitate development of information from suspects of crimes and also potential witnesses of crimes. Seemingly pertinent data may become available as well in the course of a narcosynthetic abreaction. It must be recognized that fantasy as well as fact may erupt in narcosynthesis. The reviews of Adatto (1949), Gerson and Victoroff (1948), and the experimental work of Redlich et al. (1951) indicate the dubiousness of testimony gained by amytal interviewing or narcosynthesis.

REFERENCES

Adatto CP: Observations on criminal patients during narcoanalysis. Arch Neuro Psychiatry 62:82-92, 1949

Bibring E: Psychoanalysis and the dynamic psychotherapies. J Am Psychoanal Assoc 2:745-770, 1954

Blackwenn WJ: Narcosis as therapy in neuropsychiatric conditions. JAMA 95:1168-1171, 1923

DeAguiar AP: Personal communication, 1982

Freud S, Ferenczi S, Abraham K, et al: Psychoanalysis and War Neurosis. Vienna and New York, International Psychoanalytic Press, 1921

Gerson MJ, Victoroff VM: Experimental investigation into the validity of confessions obtained under sodium amytal narcosis. Journal of Clinical Psychopathology 9:359,–375, 1948

Grinker RR, Spiegel J: Men Under Stress. Philadelphia, Blakiston, 1945

Horsley JS: Narco-analysis. J Ment Sci 82:416-422, 1936 Lancet 1:55, 1936

Kolb LC, Mutalapassi LR: The conditioned emotional response: a sub-class of chronic and delayed post-traumatic stress disorder. Psychiatric Annals 12:979-987, 1982

Kolb LC: The place of narcosynthesis in the treatment of chronic and delayed stress reactions of war, in Psychiatric Problems of Vietnam Veterans. Edited by Sonnenberg SM, Blank A, Talbott J. Washington, DC, American Psychiatric Press, in press

Lindemann E: Psychological changes in normal and abnormal individuals under the influence of sodium amytal. Am J Psychiatry 11:1083-1091, 1932

Mallinson WP: Narcoanalysis in neuropsychiatry. J Roy Nav Med Serv 26:281-284, 1940

Redlich RD, Ravitz LF, Dession GH: Narcoanalysis and truth. Am J Psychiatry 107:586-593, 1951

Sargant W, Slater E: Acute war neuroses. Lancet 2:1,–2, 1940

17
Creative Therapies

17

Creative Therapies

INTRODUCTION

The creative arts therapies, which include dance, music, art, movement, and drama therapy, developed after World War II when there was a great expectation that society would address the problems of the mentally ill and would do extraordinary things in bringing such patients back to full production, function, and mental health. A large number of different types of interventions were developed during that period and have flourished throughout the past several decades.

These therapies have several theoretical and therapeutic factors in common. First, they are introduced to both the patients and the system through the nonverbal aspects of their work. Second, they use fine arts media to foster expression and to stimulate communication between the therapist and the patient. Third, they enhance knowledge of and use the symbolic process. Since the creative arts therapies began at the height of the psychoanalytic era, the fundamental concepts of psychoanalysis were part of the underpinnings of these therapies. Fourth, because of their background in the nature and meaning of art, these therapists are highly sensitive to and acutely aware of the therapeutic value of the creative process. In addition, each of these professions has roots in the care of the chronic patient.

The past 25 years have seen all creative arts therapy groups develop

749

professional organizations and journals and establish advanced levels of training. In the art and music fields, there has been an ongoing controversy between the role of education versus that of therapy. Factions have taken various positions on this subject—some therapists feel that their role is to do primary therapy, and others see themselves only as educators in the area of arts, music, dance, and drama. Other controversies over accreditation, certification, licensure, and role continue. Issues of ethics, reimbursement, and private versus institutional practice are far from being resolved. Nevertheless, modern patient care systems recognize the need for and value of these therapists and their techniques. Whether their relationship with the physician is supervisory, collaborative, or consultative, the ability of these therapists to provide useful and often otherwise unavailable input into both diagnosis and treatment has been found to be helpful to other members of the therapeutic team.

These fields began as ancillary and adjunctive paraprofessions and have evolved into autonomous, independent professions. While most creative art therapists work in institutions, some do develop an independent practice and are often primary therapists, both in institutions and in private practice.

The questions of the role of creative arts therapists as members of a team, their relationship with physicians and other mental health specialists, and their ability to practice their fields independently will be discussed in the following sections of this chapter.

ART THERAPY

Art therapy as a discipline has grown rapidly over the last 20 years, and the definition of this new discipline has gone through many evolutions. Kramer (1958a) states, "Since the time of the caveman, men have created configurations which serve as equivalents for life processes." She also describes art as a means of widening the scope of human experience by providing a way to express these experiences through various art media.

The current definition, as described by the American Art Therapy Association, is as follows:

> Art therapy provides the opportunity for nonverbal expression and communication. Within the field there are two major approaches. The use of art as therapy implies that the creative process can be a means both of reconciling emotional conflicts and of fostering self-awareness and personal growth. When using art as a vehicle for psychotherapy, both the product and the associative references may be used in an effort to help the individual find a more compatible relationship between his inner and outer worlds.

> Art therapy, like art education, may teach technique and media skills. When art is used as therapy the instruction provides a vehicle for self-expression, communication, and growth. Less product oriented, the art therapist is more concerned with the individual's inner experience. Process, form, content, and/or associations become important for what each reflects about personality development, personality traits and the unconscious.

As can be noted from the above, definitions have gone from the specific to the more general interpretation of art therapy. While the current one seems to suffice in most areas, the field continues to grow and develop not one, but several, approaches to the process of art therapy. Consequently, there may eventually be a demand for several specific definitions rather than one encompassing one.

Historical Background

Kraepelin and Bleuler suggested that drawings be considered in making a diagnosis (Harms, 1975). Printzhorn's book, published in 1922, spurred psychopathologists to use the art expressions of their patients to diagnose their pathological condition. Hammer states:

> From these casual diagnostic beginnings, a great number of systematic diagnostic methods have been developed which today we call tests; and the method has been designed as a projective technique (in Harms, 1975).

In 1925 Nolan C. Lewis began to use free painting with adult neurotics. Stern, describing free painting in psychoanalysis with adult neurotics, stated that one of the reasons this modality had not generally been adopted may have been in part a lack of understanding of the use of the technique and its results (Fink et al., 1967).

Art therapy as a profession was first defined in America in the writings of Margaret Naumburg (Levick, 1973), who was trained as a psychologist with a psychoanalytic orientation. She dates her awareness of the relationship between children's drawings and psychotherapy to her early years of experience as director and art teacher of the Walden School, which she founded in 1915. She became convinced that the free art expression of children represented a symbolic form of speech which was basic to all education. As the years passed, she concluded that this "form of spontaneous art expression was also basic to psychotherapeutic treatment" (Naumburg, 1947, 1966).

Under the direction of Nolan C. Lewis she initiated an experimental research program in the use of spontaneous art in therapy with children with behavior problems at the New York State Psychiatric Unit. In 1958 graduate courses in the principle and methods of her concept of dynamically-oriented art therapy were instituted at New York University. Her prolific writings, lectures, and seminars throughout the country spearheaded growing interest in the field and stimulated mental health professionals and educators to question and explore the possibilities of a broader conceptual framework in the application of art as a diagnostic and therapeutic tool.

Subsequent art therapists added significant impetus to the development of this modality. Eleanor Ulman originally defined her profession as an art teacher but later took training in psychiatry and attended a series of lectures in art therapy by Naumburg (Ulman, 1966). In 1961 she published the first issue of the *Bulletin of Art Therapy*, which has continued to be a major publication in the field.

Ben Ploger has been both an art teacher and art therapist. He began his career in 1935 and was persuaded to volunteer time to teach art to mentally disturbed nuns cloistered in the religious unit of the DePaul Hospital in New Orleans. He soon began to introduce and implement his own particular expertise throughout the hospital and was made director of art psychotherapy there in 1966.

In 1950, Edith Kramer initiated and for nine years conducted an art therapy program at Wiltwick School for Boys in New York. Her first book, *Art Therapy in a Children's Community*, was written in 1958 (Kramer, 1958b).

Don Jones, a World War II conscientious objector working at a New Jersey State Institution, became interested in the graphic projections of patients covering walls. He shared his ideas with Karl Menninger, M.D.,which resulted in his being employed as an art therapist at the Menninger Foundation and marked the beginning of the art therapy program at that institution.

In 1967 the late Morris Goldman, M.D., and Paul Fink, M.D., at Hahnemann Medical College and Hospital, proposed the first graduate training program in art therapy in the world, leading to a master's degree at that institution. In 1968, the college hosted a lecture series in art therapy and a reception for practicing art therapists throughout the country. At that meeting, an ad hoc committee was elected to develop guidelines for the organization of the National Art Therapy Association. The committee members were Eleanor Ulman, Don Jones, Felice Cohen, Robert Ault, and Myra Levick. In 1969, the American Art Therapy Association was officially launched in Louisville, Kentucky.

Theoretical, Philosophical, and Basic Science Issues

Current training in the field of art therapy embraces many orientations; therefore, it follows that the philosophy of art therapists coming from theoretical frameworks such as behavioral modification, Gestalt, patient-centered, humanistic, etc. would be different from that originally put forth by Naumburg.

The psychoanalytic approach to ego mechanisms of defense is the basis of Naumburg's treatment methods (Naumburg, 1966). She maintains that spontaneous art expression releases unconscious material and that the transference relationship between patient and therapist plays an important role in the therapeutic process. Further, the encouragement of free association in pictures closely allies dynamic art therapy with psychoanalytic therapy (Ulman, 1966). "Most drawings of the emotionally-disordered express problems involving certain polarities, e.g., life-death, male-female, father-mother, love-hate, activity vs. passivity, space rhythm, color, some being specialized and others being generalized in composition," Naumburg (1947) wrote.

More recent proponents of Naumburg's original premise maintain that the patient's artistic productions, like the dream brought to the analyst, cannot be interpreted without the patient's associations. Condensation, displacement, symbolism, and secondary elaboration, components of dreams and graphic productions, plus the patient's associations, provide more information than is often observable in the clinical setting (Fink, 1967).

For dynamically-oriented art therapists, the goal is to develop the transference relationship so that, through the patients' associations to their spontaneous drawings, insights into conflictual areas of the psyche may be uncovered. In the process of making verbal what was nonverbal, conscious what was unconscious, the art psychotherapist makes connections and clarifications in an effort to help the patient interpret his/her own symbolic images.

In 1958, a second and widely respected theory of art therapy was formulated by Edith Kramer. While recognizing the unconscious as a determinant of behavior, she believes that the very act of creating is healing; that the *art* in therapy provides a means of widening the range of human experience by "creating equivalents for such experiences" (Ulman, 1961). Kramer places great emphasis on the process of sublimation and feels that the arts are to be highly valued in the treatment of the mentally ill. She clearly identifies her role with patients as different from that of the art teacher in that process takes precedence over product (Ulman, 1961). In emphasizing the healing aspect of the creative process, the goal of art therapy is to provide a means, according to Kramer, " . . . wherein experiences can be chosen, varied, repeated at will" (Ulman, 1961). It also provides an opportunity to re-experience conflict, resolve, and integrate the resolution.

The art therapists who have adopted the Naumburg ideology are viewed as psychotherapists by the followers of the Kramer ideology; the art therapists who, like Kramer, place emphasis on the healing quality of the creative process are viewed as art teachers by Naumberg's followers (Ulman, 1961). The current literature, which primarily consists of case studies, reflects a wide variety of theoretical concepts somewhere between Naumburg and Kramer. Many of these theoretical formulations and methodologies have evolved as the result of the many different graduate training programs that have been established throughout this country in the past decade. As was briefly suggested above, a number of individuals who were pioneers in the field developed their own unique art therapy theories. No longer are there just two accepted but divergent viewpoints but many valid frames of reference which lead to as many valid goals. In summary, a list of goals that would be acceptable to all art therapists includes: (a) provide a means for strengthening the ego, (b) provide a cathartic experience, (c) provide a means to uncover feelings, (d) offer an avenue to reduce guilt, (e) facilitate a task to develop impulse control, (f) introduce an experience to help develop the ability to integrate and relate, and (g) help patients use art as a new outlet (Levick, 1967). Additional values of art therapy with groups and families may include: (a) to help patients focus their attention through structured art experiences; (b) to help patients increase tolerance for group situations; (c) to facilitate active and creative group problem-solving through the use of inanimate art materials; (d) to facilitate communication by all members through the art media; and (e) to serve as an equalizer with patients who are functioning at different levels due to age, severity of illness, etc.

Clinical Issues

Art therapy sessions may be conducted on a one-to-one basis, in small or large groups, and with families. The location of the work is contingent on the needs and ideology of the institution that employs an art therapist or the orientation and style of the art therapist in private practice.

The art therapist must have a sound knowledge of and considerable experience with all art media in order to carry out treatment goals in the art therapy session. For example, finger paint, oil paints, and clay are tactile media that foster the compulsion to smear. If the treatment goal is to provide structure toward helping the patient gain internal controls, these supplies would be problematic. A more protective choice of media might be felt-tip markers or crayons. Patients who need to be encouraged to communicate with others but cannot do so verbally often benefit from some form of group mural activity. For the child who has become either withdrawn or presents a behavior problem because of a specific learning disability, the therapist's acceptance and valuing of a first drawing by the patient may be the initial step toward self-acceptance.

For all patients, art therapy provides a way to gain distance from disturbing thoughts and feelings. The art product promotes externalization of one's inner psychic life. For the psychotic patient, it often helps to separate fantasy from fact; for the severe neurotic patient, it may help connect feelings and thoughts. For troubled families, art therapy may dispel family myths and uncover denied scapegoating. Unhealthy alliances can be confronted and changed, and healthy separation of generations and consequent individuation can be reinforced. When verbal interaction is not offered by the patient, the team may turn to the art therapist for an understanding of the patient's nonverbal statements.

The length of art therapy varies according to the setting in which it is conducted and the orientation of the therapist. For example, just as any other form of psychotherapy conducted in a short-term hospital unit, art therapy must be consistent with the treatment goals of the milieu. In a one-to-one situation, the length of therapy would reflect both the needs of the patient and the therapist's clinical application of his/her particular orientation.

Art therapy's role has been demonstrated with a variety of populations diagnosed with an equal variety of mental disorders. The most prevalent of these is schizophrenia, probably because the schizophrenic patient suffering an acute episode is usually in a severe state of regression and "seems compelled to express himself compulsively and continually through any art media" (Levick, 1975).

Many mental patients who have been hospitalized for years have learned that "doing something is good for them." Art therapy can provide an activity that may alleviate anxiety but does not necessitate verbalization. Gratification is obtained in the act of participating in the creative process. It also provides a form of resocialization for the chronic patient who feels isolated from society.

The involutional-depressed patient usually resists any request to perform a task that might reflect his/her feelings of helplessness and inadequacy. Therefore, the art therapist must be cognizant of this state and not offer any activity or project that would cause frustration or anxiety. To engage such a patient in any activity, the goals must be tasks that will foster ego enhancement.

Obsessive-compulsive neurotic patients rely heavily on their ability to intellectualize and often resist involvement in an activity, particularly a nonverbal one, such as drawing or painting. Here, too, the art therapist must be skilled in therapeutic techniques in order to establish a therapeutic relationship. It is sometimes helpful to draw with this type of patient, projecting thoughts and ideas onto the same piece of paper in a shared experience.

Numerous articles in the literature describe work with alcoholics, prisoners, and children, both physically and emotionally handicapped. A great deal of work has been done with families, particularly using the art therapy evaluation designed by Kwiatkowska (1967) many years ago. This evaluation is used widely by art therapists working with different kinds of populations, both child and adult. The evaluation consists of six tasks and provides a considerable amount of data about individual ego strengths and weaknesses and family interactions. Often material elicited through the art therapy evaluation will provide direction for future therapeutic interventions for the members of the therapeutic team.

Greater awareness on the part of educators of learning disabilities has reinforced early writings by Kramer (1958b) and Naumburg (1966) regarding the knowledge that can be gained about developmental sequences and intrapsychic conflicts from children's drawings. They and other well known art therapists have shown that the spontaneous drawings of both children and adults reveal normal and pathological evidence of fears, fantasies, thoughts, and affects stimulated by internal and external pressures, ego strengths and weaknesses, id derivatives, and normal and abnormal defense mechanisms (Levick et al., 1979). Through the use of children's drawings, the trained art therapist can "guide the therapeutic team in pinpointing developmental, motoric, perceptual, or emotional problems that may interfere with learning" (Levick, et al., 1979).

Artistic products may be addressed in terms of both form and content, with formal qualities providing important information about cognitive functioning, its level, and quality; content tells much about the areas of greatest concern for the individual. Close observation of the working process provides further developmental information if viewed with an understanding of normal growth in modes of using materials. Without a solid and clear understanding of normal development, many characteristics of product or process may be misinterpreted, leading to diagnostic confusion rather than clarification (e.g., transparencies in drawings are pathogenic for adults but not for children in a "pre-schematic" stage of development). Assessing a patient at any age level requires a high degree of sophistication and knowledge in understanding and organizing the available data; an art therapist can make a major contribution to developmental and psychodynamic assessment, but only with a sound developmental framework.

Developmental issues in art therapy are certainly present, for what one offers a three-year-old is often different from what one offers a 30-year-old. Most basic media (chalk, pencil, marker, clay, plasticine, tempera paint, etc.) are usable by all age levels past two or three. However, some are most appealing to the very young (such as play dough) and others are too difficult to manage until the individual has developed sufficient fine-motor control (such as water color). While a choice of media works well with all age levels, an awareness of which materials are most related to issues germane to specific developmental phases is also useful to the art therapist, who, for example, will want to be sure to have available clay or fingerpaint for children dealing with conflicts around control and aggression. An awareness of the technical demands of media and processes is equally valuable, enabling the art therapist to suggest or offer appropriate materials to meet specific expressive needs, consonant with the skills of the individual. While an armature certainly helps a clay figure to hold its shape, for example, it would not be a helpful adjunct for a very young child whose probable way of modeling would be additive and whose technical skills would make it more frustrating than useful.

Professional and Ethical Issues

The American Art Therapy Association (AATA) has designated professional entry into the field to occur at the master's or graduate level training in institute or clinical programs. Graduate training must include didactic and practicum experience, but the emphasis may vary depending on the facility in which the student is trained.

The association has also developed specific standards for registration, and art therapists who have met these standards receive a certificate of registration by the AATA and may use the initials A.T.R. This registration system, administered by the AATA Professional Standards Committee, is the major mechanism for quality control of art therapists. Currently, the association has approximately 2,000 members. While no states license art therapists, several have civil service job classifications for them. At the present time there are no continuing education requirements for re-registration.

MUSIC THERAPY

The presence of music in all ages and cultures attests to its relevance to all human beings, individually or in groups. Primitive people used music in their shamanistic practice to heal and placate a variety of nonhuman forces. The Hellenic Greeks heard music as a means of expressing the opposing human forces of reason and emotion personified in the incongruous pair of gods, Apollo and Dionysus. The music of ancient Greece represented logic, balance, and harmony. "The music of the cult of Dionysus was, on the other hand, that of pure emotion and was employed in rites marked by exhilaration, ecstasy, and near savagery" (Graham, 1982).*

During the Middle Ages, the clerics recognized *musica humana*, a method by which the human being was attuned to harmonies of the universe. Sinful and religious musical structures were dictated by the church. And, according to Graham,*

> In spite of the efforts of the Medieval Church to proscribe certain music to its congregation, the need for all music did not escape notice of the physicians of the time. While prayers were being chanted to the sick by priests, medical students at Salerno learned to employ lively tunes and to prescribe music along with their initial efforts at dissection. When a great personage of the day was purged, bled, or treated for disease, the appropriate music accompanied the procedure.

> During the Renaissance, musicians and physicians revived the Hellenic Greek concepts which held that opposing forces could be revealed through music (Dionysian vs. Appolonian) when they proceeded to match appropriate musical modes to the four humors of Hippocrates for the purpose of stabilizing the moods of their patients.

*Graham, Richard M., "Music Therapy as a Psychiatric Therapy," unpublished paper, the University of Georgia, Athens, Ga 1982.

Modern music therapy shows elements of all parts of the history of music as a form of aesthetic behavior. Music is used in the therapy session as a means of expressing either raw emotion or self-control. It has been used through the history of humankind to soothe or to excite. It affords the diffident, the anxiety-ridden, and the depressed a means of expression and nonverbal communication.

Music therapy is the specific use of music and its elements—rhythm, pitch, melody, harmony, and dynamics—to accomplish therapeutic goals. The symbolic elements of music in the therapeutic situation must be appreciated. Masserman (1981) points out that these elements arouse specific feelings and emotions, e.g., rhythm (heart beat, melody), harmony (interpersonal accord), and counterpoint (interpersonal supplementation). The application of music in a therapeutic setting and through the therapeutic relationship allows the music therapist to treat an individual or group. The trained music therapist uses an understanding of human development, psychodynamics, and music to structure a relationship for understanding, insight, and/or behavior change. Two of the major reasons for referral to music therapy are (a) the patient's previous appreciation or skill in music and (b) the nonverbal communicative nature of the treatment. The music therapist is a contributing member of a therapeutic team and can function as both primary and/or secondary supportive therapist.

Music therapy as a unique system of psychotherapy provides opportunities for a patient to experience relations with other human beings without the fear of harm or hurt associated with verbal experiences. The structure of the music provides for an individual or group experience within structure and self-organization and a means for relating to others (Sears, 1968). These persons may use the nonthreatening setting of the music group to practice new stratagems for dealing with their respective difficulties. During the course of music therapy one has the opportunity for aesthetic experiences and high points, which the patient himself helps to bring about but with the intimate assistance of other human beings.

An individual in music therapy works with the therapist on designated therapeutic issues through the music. This work might take the form of singing, original songwriting, instrumental improvisation, structured performance, sound role playing (Green, 1978), guided imagery and music (Bonny and Savary, 1973), music for relaxation, music for biofeedback (Wagner, 1975), or acquisition of musical skills for use in leisure time.

Historical Background

During and immediately following World War II, individuals who were using music in varied therapeutic settings, predominantly veterans' hospitals, began to share their work. A music therapy community began which led to the organization of the National Association for Music Therapy (NAMT) in 1950. In its fourth decade, NAMT remains a strong, growing organization that has created standards for training and registration in music therapy. NAMT grants registration (R.M.T.) to individuals who meet the academic and clinical requirements the organization upholds. In 1970, the Urban Federation of Music Therapists began and is now known as the American Association for Music Therapy. This organization also sets standards for training and grants certification (C.M.T.) to those who qualify. Both organizations affiliate with colleges and universities that provide music therapy training and support, and both offer conferences and seminars for continuing education.

Theoretical Issues

Although music therapy has its roots in the chronic adult psychiatric inpatient setting with a traditional psychodynamic theoretical base (Gaston, 1968), the field has expanded to include and embrace a varied range of theoretical positions. The *Journal of Music Therapy* has been published quarterly for nearly two decades and illustrates the interest in research and theory which has always been a part of the profession.

While the practice of music therapy has not grown from a well established theoretical base, education (particularly music education), medicine, psychology, and philosophy have all influenced music therapists. The most important influence comes, however, from the long history of the music performer, for it is the ability of the music therapist to produce music that makes this specialist both unique and valuable in psychiatric settings.

When one considers the disciplines that have influenced the development of music therapy, it is not surprising that current techniques reflect many influences and areas of emphasis. Over the past four decades, one can easily track shifts in attention beginning just after World War II, when emphasis was placed solely on music, with little regard for the role of the therapist in music therapy. A major shift in emphasis within the field saw the music therapist emerge as an important factor in one-to-one relationships with the patient, with music being little more than a means of creating a pleasant background for verbal psychotherapy. In more recent years, a third position has developed between these two extremes, finding the music therapist and the music as roughly equal factors in the music therapy procedure.

The most predominant theoretical framework in the profession is the behavioral theories (Ruud, 1980). The largest body of data within the discipline available in research and clinical work is related to music as a stimulus for behavior change and music as a reinforcer in the behavioral model.

A major component in understanding music therapy is that of music as the art form that shares the same developmental milestones in physical sound as speech. The infant begins life using sound as a signalling device to get his primitive needs met and continues to develop the neurological and physiological structures and systems needed to become a communicator of continually more subtle ideas, needs, and feelings (Oswald, 1963). Through stages such as vocal contagion, sing-song babbling, changing rhythms, and eventually planned musical production, the human organizes sound for affective and cognitive communication. Music's close tie with the most frequent way in which humans communicate, i.e., the written and spoken word, makes the elements and structures of music a language that individuals can use as an alternative sound communication (Nordoff and Robbins, 1977).

Volumes of research have tried to measure and validate the physiological response to music. Using planned music listening, the physiological measure of electroencephalograph, electrocardiogram, galvanic skin response, blood pressure, and pulse have been applied. There are data to support the concept that manipulation of musical elements can effect specified changes (Zimney and Weidenfeller, 1978; Furman, 1962). Broad categories such as stimulative versus sedative music have been researched, but the best predictor of precise physiological responses remains the individual, and responses are determined more on the basis of preference. The issue of preference has been well studied and seems to be a pivotal point of music therapy. Be it environmental, developmental, physiological, memory, taste, or training, the preferences of an individual appear to play an integral part in applying music in therapy (Cotter and Toombs, 1968).

Ruud (1980) has explored the relationship of music therapy to psychoanalytic, behavioral, and humanistic/existential theories. He sees music therapy as a natural extension of the philosophy, psychology, and sociology of music and warns that the human and his or her music cannot be understood through any single theory and certainly not if the model is centered on pathology. Other music therapists and theoreticians disagree and, while borrowing from many theoretical approaches, recognize and use principles of unconscious mental functioning as a major presumption in the application and use of music as a vehicle to the understanding and treatment of the mentally ill.

Many psychiatrists have explored music and its form and role in therapy. Among them are Kohut (1957), Miller (1967), Masserman (1958), and Reik (1953).

Music as Nonverbal Communication: Clinical Application

Music is a form of nonverbal communication which has its roots in the human organism's desire to express that which goes beyond words. There would be no music and no need for it if it were possible to communicate verbally that which is easily communicated musically (Gaston, 1968). The power of music as a major medium for the expression of emotions can be seen in the research of Hannett (1964), who categorized popular music of the past century and showed that the largest percentage of songs were about love and family.

Music provides for a patient-therapist interaction without the threat of words. When people interact in music, the cues between them include harmonic cadences, melodic contour, the dynamics of sound, and volume. These cues can become a language for patients who do not use spoken language effectively.

As noted by Graham*:

> Of course there are many different musical languages (Asian music, African music, European music) and each of these have [sic] their dialects (e.g., classical music, folk music, jazz). The effective therapist must communicate in the language of the patient and—in the case of the music therapist—this requires flexibility and a willingness to attempt the production of as many musics as any situation might demand. The success of music therapy will depend, to a great extent, upon selection and use of the correct music as part of the music therapy procedure.

All adjunctive psychotherapies, including music therapy, use verbal as well as nonverbal techniques. In music therapy, the work with music may stand alone or serve as a vehicle to affective and/or verbal expression.

In using music in assessment, emphasis is placed on the elements of music and how an individual uses or responds to specific musical parameters. The ability to reproduce rhythmic and melodic patterns of increasing difficulty; the capacity to remember lyrics and melodies; previous exposure and training in music; and even instrumental, artistic, or style preferences are all important components of assessment. The patient who demonstrates compulsive drum beating may be indicating anxiety or organicity, and further examinations of related behaviors should be done. The autistic child who sings on pitch and uses song fragments to communicate and the mentally retarded individual who has perfect rhythmic synchrony are both displaying musical skills with functional implications that go far beyond music.

The establishment of a therapeutic relationship between the music therapist and the patient or patients is the initial task in treatment, as in any psychotherapy. Some music therapists begin the therapeutic relations by performing musically for the patient, while other music therapists initiate the therapeutic process by presenting an array of instruments and instructing each member of a group of patients to select an instrument of his/her choice which can be used to express feelings or ideas. This method is more nondirective, and the selection and use of the instrument by the patient

---

*Graham, Richard M., "Music Therapy as a Psychiatric Therapy," unpublished paper, the University of Georgia, Athens, Ga, 1982.

reveal unconscious material that may be useful to the music therapists in formulating a plan for the patient. The development of a relationship between the music therapist and the patient is not precisely the same as in other psychotherapies, for a relationship is based on music as a communicae. As Graham* noted:

> The patient or patients in music therapy may not talk about their pathologies, they perform them (play, sing, compose, or dance). Or if the manifestation is not precisely a musical one, it can be seen in the social behaviors attendant to the performance of music. The performing ensemble or even the music discussion group permits the music therapist and patients to become involved in the patient's inefficient, self-defeating strategies but from a completely different perspective, one not based on words.

Psychiatric patients place the music therapist in the role of an authority based on other experiences in music, allowing the music therapist the transference needed to facilitate the therapeutic process. For some music therapists, the patients' best efforts are encouraged, for individual commitment toward an aesthetic end is an essential of the music therapy procedure. For others, the product is much less important since the essential goal is therapeutic engagement.

The process of music therapy is the most difficult aspect of the treatment, as the music therapist must learn to confront patients with the defenses or destructive behaviors they are using in music therapy. The therapist must learn to indicate to the patient that his behavior in music therapy is a repetition of the behavior patterns used in other areas of his life. The music therapist must offer the patient new behaviors that can then be practiced in the music therapy setting where support can be offered. The emphasis in these sessions is less on perfection of musical performance and acquisition of facts about music than on opportunities for acquiring new and better responses to inner and outer pressures.

Professional Issues

All registered and certified music therapists are required to have extensive formal training in music, including music literature, theory, history, and performance. A music therapist must also have specified coursework in psychology, human development, physiology, and supervised clinical experience with varied patient populations. Requirements are continuously upgraded, and continuing education is encouraged.

Music therapy qualifies for third-party reimbursement in only a few isolated states and situations. Although both the National Association for

---

*Graham, Richard M. "Music Therapy as a Psychiatric Therapy," unpublished Paper, the University of Georgia, Athens, Ga, 1982

Music Therapy and the American Association for Music Therapy monitor training and confer certification, there is presently no procedure for licensure of music therapists. While some music therapists conduct private practices, most are affiliated with institutions and agencies that provide a range of services.

DANCE THERAPY

Historical Background

In her article entitled "Dance Therapy: A New Profession or Rediscovery of an Ancient Role of the Dance," Bartenieff (1972) expresses the viewpoint that perhaps our roots extend back to the shaman who used dance as a means of exorcising evil spirits or evoking good spirits. One does not have to search far in anthropological literature to find many examples of man using primitive dance forms for expressive events within the community.

It is clear that the intuitive and creative aspects of the dance choreographer are the elements that proved useful with early dance therapy pioneers such as Irmgard Bartenieff, Mary Whitehouse, Marian Chace, and Trudi Schoop. These women applied the skills used to train a dancer to work with psychiatric patients: the ability to "see" the essence of a body moving, the intuition of the feeling state attached to the gestalt, and an understanding of the possibilities for modulating the movement to produce communication. It was their success that laid the groundwork for the beginnings of the profession of dance therapy. In the early 1940's, the publishing profession had not heard the words "body language," but it was literally this language that reached hundreds of back ward patients (Chaiklin, 1975).

The evolution of dance therapy has been influenced by psychotherapists as well. Freud's descriptions of his patients' physical manifestations of neurosis, particularly the evolution of those manifestations during the process of analysis, are exquisite movement descriptions; and Freud clearly related the psychic material to the physical. Deutsch (1959), Reich (1949) and, with children, Anna Freud (1946) and Margaret Mahler (1975) have given attention to nonspeech behavior as it relates to the psychological development of humans. Even though psychiatry's interest in nonverbal behavior did not produce an uninterrupted stream of investigation, it nevertheless influenced those who were using this behavior in clinical activities.

Dance therapists also claim social science ancestry. Social scientists whose interest has been centered around investigation of cultural differences in movement behavior share that interest with those members of the profession who have investigated that parameter within the dance form. One outstanding piece of research, a collaborative project by Alan Lomax,

Irmgard Bartenieff, and Forestine Pauley proposed a method of examining movement style so that dance form could be compared cross-culturally (Pauley, 1970). Their study provides an excellent reflection of how differences in dance style reflect differences in social structures.

The roots of our most commonly used method of notating movement observation sprang from the work of Rudolph Laban and those who continued his work, Warren Lamb and Marion North in England and Irmgard Bartenieff in America. Laban (1950) wrote:

> The artist must realize that his own movement make-up is the ground on which he has to build. The control and development of his personal movement habits will provide him with the key to the mystery of the significance of movement.

This quote encapsulates the key element of the Laban system of notation, that of understanding movement in one's own body first. This system provides a consistent and objective framework from which to view movement. In addition, it provides the ability to describe both content and quality. When we begin to understand the observation in terms of use of time, space, and force in the service of basic drives, the cognitive and emotional states are manifested as well as the individual's characteristic means of coping.

An excellent tool for quantifying observable movement behavior has developed through the use of Laban's Labanotation System (1960). The system provides a conceptual framework for the possibilities in human movement and descriptive terms with tested inter-rater reliability which have significantly improved precision in movement description.

Summarizing the evolution, dance therapy has collectively grown and developed from a cross-disciplinary background and is deeply rooted in the clinical realities of patient work. The field's growth and development have not been through the traditional academic evolution. Pioneers in the field were engaged because of their clinical interest. The movement therapist has attempted to reflect and decode the inner state of the patient by observing, experiencing, internalizing, translating into secondary process thinking, and evaluating his movement.

In 1966, when the American Dance Therapy Association was chartered, there were approximately 50 members. Today, there are more than 1,000 members working with patients in clinics all over the world. Dance/movement therapists may be found working with an autistic child, a geriatric patient, a person whose last 20 years were spent rocking in a chair in a back ward, or a child with learning disabilities. The tool that is used in dance therapy—and, in fact, its focal point—is the body itself as the vehicle for communication and expression of feeling. It is also a language that is difficult to distort or conceal. It speaks honestly about the self for those who wish to observe (Chaiklin, 1975).

Dance/movement therapists have specific training that enables them to use movement as a psychotherapeutic agent in the process of furthering emotional, physical, and intellectual integration of the individual. Dance therapists work with individuals who have social, emotional, cognitive, and/or physical problems. They are employed in psychiatric hospitals, clinics, day-care facilities, community mental health centers, developmental centers, correctional facilities, and special schools and agencies. Therapists work with people of all ages individually and in groups.

The stated goal of dance/movement therapists is the growth of the total individual beginning at the level of present functioning and moving toward a greater level of functioning.

Theoretical Issues and Clinical Applications

The most important component of dance movement therapy is the connection between mind and body. The assumption is that working with a person on a bodily level can affect the overall functioning of the person.

The profession developed from an intuitive dancer's view of life from birth to death as an endless stream of movement with other humans and objects. The dancer knows that the manner in which he/she walks onto a stage signals affect, information, and symbolic meaning. The eclectic beginnings of synthesizing new knowledge from a creative art with known information about human behavior has produced a new discipline.

Movement interaction between people in a therapeutic relationship provides the possibility to organize behavior, bring it to conscious awareness, examine behavior's symbolic meaning, and clarify communication signals. It is the vehicle of movement interaction which is unique to dance movement therapy. A good dance instructor knows exactly how to build complex rhythms, combinations, and steps to develop the dancer's highest mobility and potential. The means by which a dance/movement therapist joins in this interaction has become a technique variously called "replication," "interactional synchrony," or "movement empathy." It is the tuning in of one body to another, analogous to the theory of physics which describes the synchronous attunement of pendulum clocks spaced closely on a wall. These skills enable the therapist literally to "tune in" and communicate.

Humans use their bodies to cope with feelings. The angry person may become "rigid" with rage or "wild" with anger—either motor state being a reflection of the person's response to a feeling. An internal phenomenon seems to be expressed in the body. Other motor responses to anger can be taught, such as sublimation or structured aggressive discharge, with the additional benefit of talking about the feeling rather than acting out in a nonproductive manner.

Sometimes another person can evoke the pathway in reverse. One example might be a group of people moved into a trance-like state by a movement such as "the whirling dervish." The dance movement therapist uses this theory in assisting a person to move into structured task-oriented movement or to move toward being in contact with emotions dependent on the therapeutic goal. In this way the therapist can assist in trying more constructive ways of coping and handling emotions and functional behavior.

Words originally possess a concrete meaning. For example, the concept of "mouth" is felt by an infant before it becomes an abstraction. Although we become verbal beings, if we are fortunate we do not lose the concrete connection during our adult years. However, words often become disconnected from their bodily experiences, or they are used in a manner in which the meaning seems to be incongruent at first glance. For instance, if a patient said, "My husband *burst* into the room," the therapist might ask, "How does one burst into a room—knocking the furniture down—his body exploding—how do you feel entering a room in a rage?" The dance therapist explores and converts verbal imagery into bodily movement. Each of us has kinesthetic attachments to words, and those meanings do not always remain conscious. Often, memories are sparked by the movement activity within the session. Using nonverbal means to evaluate, understand, and treat is the essence of all adjunctive therapies using art forms. In dance therapy, the therapeutic component can remain totally nonverbal, allowing alterations in kinesthetic activity to be essentially therapeutic by themselves, or it can capitalize on movement to lead to verbal interaction with clarification of bodily activity, exploration of meaning of movement, and/or discussion of feelings and ideas alone.

Kestenberg's *Children and Parents* (1974) gives a complete description of the stages of development seen from a movement perspective based on 20 years of research. She describes characteristic movement stages corresponding to Freud's stages of psychosexual development. North's *Personality Assessment through Movement* (1974) examines the development of normal English school children in longitudinal studies comparing the movement perspective with standardized psychological and educational tests, establishing connections to movement parameters and personality traits.

Kalish et al.'s contribution of the *Behavioral Rating Instrument for Atypical Children* (1977) provides a movement scale for assessment of age-appropriate behavior of the pre-school child. The movement scale is one of seven scales in functioning correlated in a long-term research project at the Developmental Center for Autistic Children in Philadelphia, Pennsylvania. The work of these researchers provides a tested theoretical basis for evaluating such parameters as functioning in development, locating the emotional age of children, and examining their developing personality traits.

In the clinical setting, the dance/movement therapist must determine whether the symptoms should be directly addressed or treated as a signal of some unconscious conflict whose meaning will be pursued during the course of treatment. The decision to maintain a supportive therapeutic posture is not uncommon. The therapist offers the healthy aspects of himself to the patient who is repressed and unable to cope. On the other hand, the decision may be made to use a more expressive or investigative mode. Often dance movement therapists work in clinics dealing with high-risk children, early intervention programs, and day-care centers supporting age appropriate mastery and a personal growth model. It is critical to treatment outcome that the therapist develop clinical judgment through adequate training and supervision.

Professional Issues

Dance therapy is included as a related service under PL 94-142, the Education for All Handicapped Children Act. The federal Office of Personnel Management has recently established a new professional occupation and separate register for dance therapy for use by federal medical facilities and agencies. Some states identify dance therapists on civil service lists, while others are in the process of creating separate job lines.

The 1978 President's Commission on Mental Health recommended greater use of dance therapists in federally assisted facilities, community mental health centers, and programs reimbursed by third-party payment. Representation of dance therapy on the arts task panel of the President's Commission on Mental Health and at the proposed White House Conference on the Arts, as well as the endorsement of dance therapy in the proposed Mental Health Systems Act, reflect the growing recognition of its importance in the field of mental health (ADTA, 1979).

There are six approved masters' degree programs in dance therapy, a journal, and a considerable body of literature. As must be true for many relatively new professions that have emerged from the innovations of a few creative personalities, dance therapy has not been rigorously assessed as to underlying theories, specific methods, and outcome.

DRAMA THERAPY

Drama therapy can be defined as the intentional use of creative drama toward the psychotherapeutic goals of emotional and physical integration and personal growth. Drama therapy, like other creative art therapies, is the application of a creative medium to psychotherapy. Specifically, drama therapy refers to those activities in which there is an established therapeutic understanding between the patient and therapist and the therapeutic goals are primary, and not incidental, to the ongoing activity. Thus, creative drama in a strictly educational setting, for example, though probably helpful to the participants, should be differentiated from drama therapy. Likewise drama therapy is not the same as the more tightly structured psychodrama, which seeks to alter cognitive patterns through action methods. Drama therapy, broadly defined, includes any therapeutic use of role-playing. However, the term "drama therapy" is best used for those approaches that stress the appreciation of creative theatre as a medium for self-expression and playful group interaction and that base their techniques on improvisation and theatre exercises.

History

In the past decade in the United States, drama therapy has emerged as a profession that spans both creative and mental health disciplines and offers great potential for further research into the nature of theatre and interpersonal processes (Irwin, 1979; Schattner and Courtney, 1981). The current development of drama therapy is the result of many influences. Foremost among these is Jacob Moreno, whose *psychodrama* was the first use of theatre for curative purposes (Cole, 1975; Moreno, 1945) (see full chapter entitled "Psychodrama"). He developed a very specific, structured approach in which the client portrays himself and significant others in reenactments of important life events. In the 1950's, pioneers of child drama such as Peter Slade (1954) and Brian Way (1969) in Great Britain and Winifred Ward (1957) in the United States began applying theatre techniques in children's education. They stressed the *process* of creative drama rather than merely the production of scripted plays. A parallel trend in child psychotherapy was occurring with the development of play therapy approaches that used role-playing and pretend games (Axline, 1947; Moustakas, 1953). In the 1960's, Viola Spolin (1963) and others applied many principles of creative drama and story theatre to the creation of theatre games and improvisational forms of theatre. At the same time, Jerzy Grotowski's (1968) experiments became known in the United States. Together, these advances influenced a generation of American theatre artists such as Chaiklin (1972) and Schechner (1973), who began experimenting with new forms of theatre and increasingly focused on the experience of the *actor* instead of the audience.

The social upheaval in the 1960's in the United States also influenced the emergence of drama therapy. New humanistic techniques that departed from traditional psychoanalytic approaches were being created; many of these used fantasy, physical activity, or role-playing. In addition, the increased sensitivity to socially deprived groups, as well as the increased scarcity of jobs in the theatre, sent many trained theatre artists into hospitals, schools, prisons, and nursing homes, where they began to adapt their techniques to these special populations. The result has been a new recognition in the United States of the therapeutic applications of theatre and other creative arts. The National Association for Drama Therapy was established in 1979.

Drama therapy is currently used in the treatment of both groups and individuals, children and adults, in hospitals, outpatient clinics, prisons, and schools. It has been used with psychiatric patients of all diagnoses, alcohol and drug abusers, the handicapped, and the elderly. Drama therapy seems to be able to reach more severely disturbed or handicapped populations who are less available to insight-oriented verbal psychotherapy. Finally, drama therapy is also increasingly being appreciated for its evaluative applications, both as a projective device and as an indicator of the individual's communication style.

Basic Science and Theoretical Issues

Drama therapists base their work on theories of emotional and cognitive development (Johnson, 1982a; Jennings, 1974), with some therapists adopting a psychoanalytic perspective (Irwin and Rubin, 1976) and others an educational orientation (Wethered, 1973). The developmental paradigm has obvious relevance to the processes encountered in drama therapy.

The developmental perspective sees disorder as a blockage or a halt in development. Treatment first involves an assessment of where in the developmental sequence the person has stopped himself/herself and then starting the journey again with the therapist as a companion and guide. Thus, the drama therapist with a developmental approach works with processes and sequences, always sensitive to the subtle transformations in the *forms* of a patient's behavior, which signal a developmental advance or retreat. Johnson (1982a) has described the importance of four developmental processes in drama therapy:

Structure. To the extent that one lacks internal organization, an external organizing environment is necessary to support one's adaptive functioning. Studies of children have shown that those with greater imaginativeness and more articulated inner lives could sit longer in a chair without being distracted or requiring attention. The basic principle here seems to be that as development proceeds, the need for the external environment to be structured with clear boundaries, rules, and expectations decreases.

The external environment in a drama therapy session is made up of the physical location, the spatial arrangements of the members, the dramatic activities, and the nature of the roles of therapist and group members (Johnson and Sandel, 1977). Initially, these aspects of the external environment need to be more structured, stable, and clear than later in the group's development, when members can tolerate greater reliance on their own abilities to structure the experience.

Media. Developmentalists (e.g., Piaget, 1951; Bruner, 1964; Werner, 1948) describe the development of thought (i.e., representation) in essentially three stages: a *sensorimotor* or enactive stage in which thoughts are represented by bodily movements and expression; a *symbolic* or iconic stage in which symbols (visual, sonic, or postural/gestural as in mime) are the units of representation; and a *reflective* or lexical stage in which representation is accomplished through words, language, or other abstract symbols.

The media of movement, drama, and verbalization, respectively, correspond to these three stages of representation. Thus, at least in this regard, one can place movement and sounds, images and drama, and verbalization on a developmental continuum. In drama therapy, the therapist uses this sequence to order the sessions. He usually begins with pure movements and adds sounds as a bridge to imagery, which is then acted out in a dramatic way and finally discussed verbally (Johnson, 1982a). Since this procedure follows in some measure the progression of thought from preverbal to verbal forms, it may serve to facilitate verbal communication in patients for whom pure verbalization has otherwise been difficult (e.g., children, schizophrenics).

Interpersonal Demand. A person's perception of others also develops over the course of life. Initially, self and others exist inseparably from one another in an undifferentiated state (Blatt et al., 1976). As development proceeds, self and others slowly emerge as separate entities. Others initially are barely different from objects, then may be equated with animals or other simple forms of otherness. The attainment of a full appreciation of others as separate, feeling, reacting beings occurs with difficulty.

In drama therapy, the identities of characters chosen by patients may vary from physical forces to objects, animals, monsters, and people. Likewise, interactions can vary from passive (e.g, guided fantasy) to reactive (e.g., mirror game) to fully active (e.g,. improvisations). The degree of interpersonal demand on the participants will fluctuate throughout a session, though in general one would expect it to rise from simple interactions in warm-ups to the more developed interactions of scenes and improvisations.

Transitional Processes. People tend to be comfortable within very narrow ranges of expression, and they naturally expend energy keeping social interaction within these boundaries. In a drama therapy session in which the modes of expression are varying widely along this developmental continuum, it is not surprising that difficulties arise for many people at points of transition between developmental levels. Shifts between media from simple to complex activities, or from one structure to another, challenge each person to shift his/her relation to the environment and, thus, cause a shift in his/her organization of self.

Basic Techniques

At the heart of many therapists' technique is the use of improvisation and spontaneous role-playing to encourage individual self-expression. The therapist aims to create a supportive, "free play" environment in which the individual's feelings and thoughts become reflected in the improvised roles. The therapist usually participates in the activities and serves as a relatively nondirective facilitator of the "play." His interventions (either verbal or nonverbal) are always focused on the *processes* within the group or individual which are inhibiting free expression and not on the various *products* created (i.e., the quality of the individual's performance in the role-playing). Depending on the type of patient involved and the specific goals of therapy, a variety of techniques are used to encourage the individual's growth and insight.

Role-playing is a process of identification in which the actor assumes the identity of another personality. Usually this "other" personality is defined by a text or script that the actor studies and attempts to understand. The actor will often try to relate certain aspects of his own experience to that of this other personality in order to impersonate it better. Such a role may be called a *scripted role*.

Another type of role, however, is the *improvisational role*. Here, a vague situation or general label (such as "doctor" or "nurse") is all that has been defined, and the actual personality to be played is spontaneously created by the actor. Thus, the actor must use more of his own resources to create and maintain a coherent role identity. He draws on memories, habits, mimicry, and also more intangible aspects of his own personality, both conscious and unconscious. The result is a characterization that truly is a self-expression; the unstructured nature of the role-playing allows many aspects of the self to emerge, some under the control of the individual, some not. In this way, the improvisational role is a powerful one that stimulates self-expression on several levels; yet, because of the structure of the situation ("acting"), it is not usually experienced as a complete revelation of the self.

In drama therapy, the behavior produced by the patient is often attributed in part to the identity of the role or character, not the self. The role, if scripted, may be quite unlike the actual self of the client. Improvisational roles reflect more of the self and, if psychodramatic, are of course very much like the client's self. Nevertheless, since the self is not *directly* identified with the behavior, the need to restrict this behavior defensively decreases. For this reason, drama therapy has been found to be a powerful intervention in that it allows people to express aspects of themselves which they normally restrict.

A major focus of drama therapy is on stimulating the individual's creativity and spontaneity. Here, the therapist's interventions are directed at the disruptions in the patient's spontaneous play. Anxieties with individuals and conflicts among group members inevitably arise and interfere with the ongoing flow of the session and the spontaneity of the members. For example, the play may become blocked and repetitive (known as the "impasse"), may break down entirely, or may actually become confused with reality. These inhibitions in the role-playing are experientially quite vivid to both patient and therapist and can serve as indicators of the individual's specific difficulties.

One way of addressing these difficulties is through *role analysis*. In improvisational role-playing, one's role is intimately connected to one's real self, as there is no script to give it any other content. Over the course of a drama therapy experience, recurring patterns of behavior emerge in the role-playing of each individual which are crystallized versions of his basic interpersonal stances. The person often feels powerless to change them, even though they often dissatisfy him. The therapist can help the individual to become aware of these patterns and then to examine the reasons he continues to choose them. Drama therapy attempts to increase the individual's self control by providing the opportunity and group support to experiment with other, more satisfying roles.

Another set of techniques in drama therapy is oriented toward the goal of developing interpersonal relationships and group values. For most people, and especially for severely disturbed patients, forming a group is an exceptionally difficult and threatening task. The use of creative drama and movement has been found both to engage people who are hesitant to join groups and to encourage group formation in general. The focus of drama therapy is not usually on the relationships that members have had in the past or with people outside of the group but rather on the development of interpersonal relationships within the group itself. The group's activities, by being relatively unstructured, encourage each individual's interpersonal style to emerge and his problems with others or the group to be expressed. The therapist's goal is to help the group develop methods of examining these problems as they arise and to explore them further in the role-playing itself.

Drama therapists may use a variety of props or costumes and may emphasize movement, mime, or art work. Many also use scripts and even produce plays with their patients, though in these cases, too, their goal is to examine the process that develops between the individual and his assigned roles.

Evaluative Applications

Due to its "power to reveal" role-playing has been used for evaluation purposes (Johnson, 1981; McReynolds and DeVoge, 1977). Aspects of the patient's personality traits will reveal themselves as consistent patterns across many situations in his role-playing. Once these patterns are perceived, it is possible to see variations in them as reflective of current fluctuations in the person's thoughts or feelings. It is possible to show how both relatively stable traits and more transient, unconscious thoughts combine to determine the particular content of a person's role-playing.

The following styles are but a few that can be explicated through drama therapy. One group finds participation in pretend activities extremely difficult, and individuals with this *inhibited* style often refuse to join; when they do role-play, it is extremely restricted, with minimal involvement. In the most severe cases, the person simply cannot personify roles, either because he is no longer able to represent other people as having any solidity or reality or because, by becoming another personality, even in play, he would no longer know who he was. The *over-involved* style is characterized by high degrees of physical and emotional involvement in the role-playing. The neurotic individual wishes to be identified with the role although he secretly realizes he is not really the role; the schizophrenic is apt literally to define his identity by aspects of the role and can no longer distinguish between them.

The *compulsive* styles are those in which concern for detail and perfection and efforts to maintain self-control by the repetition of actions are especially evident. This style may be distinguished by the degree to which such attention seems to serve efforts at self-control instead of communication. In its most common manifestation, the development of a compulsive style can be recognized in an over-concern about props or the details of mimed objects, over and above the development of the relationship to other people. The extremely compulsive person is unable to function smoothly at all and is severely hindered by rigidity in his body, actions, and role-playing.

Impulsive styles are characterized by a general lack of control over actions, unpredictability, and hyperactivity. Generally, one finds this style more often in children; but it is observable in many adolescents and even adults, for example, when "pretend" fights or love scenes become all-too-real ones, causing the therapist to intervene lest someone get hurt or mishandled. In its mild forms, the impulsivity is contained within the role-playing: The person plays impulsive characters, while others play the controlling, authoritative roles (e.g, police, teacher, parent). Occasionally the person may play these authoritative roles also but does so in an especially threatening and tyrannical way, usually stimulating rebellious behavior in the others.

The identification of these styles by the drama therapist can be useful in determining which problems to focus on and which methods might be most appropriate.

Interactions Among Actors

While much attention has been placed on the relationship between the actor and his role, researchers in the United States have also been studying the nature of interactions *among* actors in a role-playing scene (Johnson, 1982b; McReynolds and DeVoge, 1977). In a scene between two actors, four relationships exist: (a) between the two actors, (b) between the two characters, (c) between each actor and his own character, and (d) between each actor and the other actor's character. When the characters are from a script in which the setting, plot, and dialogue are predetermined, then the actors must struggle to learn their roles while mutually coordinating their efforts. However, when the scene is an improvisation, that is, when character, plot, dialogue, or setting must be determined by the actors spontaneously, each actor tends to experience some anxiety about how to relate to the other actor. Each actor then seems to create a characterization that in part protects him from this anxiety but at the expense of listening to the other actor. Difficulties inevitably arise since the actors are out of touch with each other. In this way, problems in the actor-actor relationship become expressed more or less directly in the character-character relationship.

One problem that often emerges is that each actor "clings" to his own characterization in order to feel secure in the improvisation. When the scene calls for a mutual decision by the two actors concerning the development or ending of the scene, each actor, fearful of losing his reasonably clear identity, resists any change that would affect his character adversely. The scene inevitably moves to an uncomfortable stalemate, called the "impasse," in which little action occurs and the actors repeat themselves, feel anxious, and often end the scene abruptly.

Spolin (1963) has defined criteria to avoid this crisis by insisting that each actor "keep the ball rolling" and maintain a "point of concentration," that is, an explicit focus or goal in the scene. In contrast, Johnson (1982b) has begun to use this phenomenon therapeutically by allowing impasses to develop and then helping the actors understand how they fall into impasses and how to work through them creatively. This work necessitates a real confrontation of the person's interpersonal difficulties. Thus, the impasses often reflect problems patients have in other real-life relationships.

Legal, Ethical, and Organizational Issues

Drama therapy as a profession is in a period of rapid growth in the United States. The National Association for Drama Therapy (NADT) has developed standards of training and competence for drama therapists who, when qualified as registered drama therapists, may use the initials R.D.T. Drama therapists are required to have an intensive background in the theatre arts, preparation in psychology and psychotherapy, and several years of experience in treatment settings. Training programs at the bachelor's and master's levels are developing rapidly. NADT's goals are to encourage training and research in drama therapy, to define standards of competence and ethical practice, and to represent the interests of drama therapists in the mental health field.

LEGISLATIVE ALLIANCE OF CREATIVE ARTS THERAPIES (LACAT)

In the past four years, the call for action in the legislative arena has provided the forum through which the therapies have worked together toward common goals. The Legislative Alliance of Creative Arts Therapies (LACAT) is a group of representatives from the executive boards of the American Art Therapy Association (AATA), the American Dance Therapy Association (ADTA), the National Association for Music Therapy, and the Federation of Trainers and Training Programs in Psychodrama (FTTPP) who are committed to improving the ability of these professions to be of greater service in meeting the mental health needs of the nation. This umbrella organization, through a legislative advocate, represents these organizations on legislative matters of common concern and coordinates legislative activities. It provides information to legislators and others regarding creative arts therapies and keeps the creative arts therapists abreast of new legislation and political issues related to the profession.

In 1978, the Veterans Administration (VA) and the Office of Personnel Management (OPM) initiated a revision of an existing civil service job classification with serious implications for the creative arts therapies. Working closely with OPM and the VA, LACAT was able to assist in developing a new classification title with specific categories for each of the creative arts therapies (art, dance, music, and psychodrama). This title, GS638: Recreation Therapy/Creative Arts Therapies, is of major significance in making available creative arts therapies services within the federal system. Accordingly, LACAT has been working closely with the VA regarding implementation of creative arts therapies programs in veterans' hospitals.

The creative arts therapies were written into the final report language of the Mental Health Systems Act as follows:

> Many persons who could benefit from the creative arts therapies do not have access to them. It is hoped that greater use of the creative arts therapies will be facilitated through this legislation, especially through the provision of services for the chronically mentally ill and severely disturbed children and adolescents, funding for innovative projects meeting mental health service needs and development of bicultural programs. Furthermore, the Committee expects the Secretary to examine the barriers to the provision of creative arts therapies to prioritize population groups and to recommend steps to alleviate or remove such barriers.

Following enactment of this legislation, the creative arts therapies were included among those services designated as reimbursable in a three-year Medicare Demonstration Project initiated in 1981 through a joint effort between the National Institute of Mental Health (NIMH) and the Alcohol, Drug Abuse, and Mental Health Administration (ADAMHA) in cooperation with Medicare.

CONCLUSION

The application of the creative arts to therapy is a relatively recent event that has had significant value in the treatment of the hospitalized mentally ill. In some instances, these techniques have been expanded to include outpatient therapy and treatment of families in addition to individuals and groups. With some variation, all of these therapies have begun to develop structured graduate level training programs and have organized on a national basis in order to set standards of training, membership, and practice in lieu of the self-ordained talented individuals who gave birth to the fields.

REFERENCES

ADTA Brochure, 1979

Axline V: Play Therapy. Boston, Houghton Mifflin, 1947

Bartenieff I: Dance therapy: a new profession or rediscovery of an ancient role. Dance Scope, 7:6-18, 1972

Blatt S, Brenneis B, Schimek J, et al: Normal development and psychopathological impairment of the concept of the object on the Rorschach. J Abnorm Psychol 85:363-373, 1976

Bonny HL, Savary LM: Music and Your Mind. New York, Harper and Row, 1973

Bruner J: The course of cognitive growth. Am Psychol 19:1-15, 1964

Chaiklin H: Marian Chace: Her Papers. Columbia, Md, American Dance Therapy Association, 1975

Chaiklin H: The Presence of the Actor. New York, Atheneum, 1972

Cole D: The Theatrical Event. Middletown, Conn, Wesleyan, 1975

Cotter VW, Toombs S: A procedure for determining the music preferences of mental retardates, in Music In Therapy. Edited by Gaston ET. New York, Macmillan, 1968

Deutsch F: Correlations of verbal and nonverbal communication in interviews conducted by the associative anamnesis. Psychosom Med 21:123-130, 1959

Fink PJ, Goldman MJ, Levick MF: Art therapy: a new discipline. Pennsylvania Medicine 70:60-66, 1967

Fink PJ: Art as a language. Journal of Albert Einstein Medical Center 15:143-150, 1967

Freud A: The psychoanalytic study of infantile feeding disturbances. Psychoanal Study Child 2:119-132, 1946

Furman CE: The effect of musical stimuli on the brainwave production of children. Child Dev 33:891-896, 1962

Gaston ET (ed): Music in Therapy. New York, Macmillan, 1968

Green AD: Sound-Roleplaying: A Technique Used in Music Therapy Assessed through Sound and Movement Quality Scales (master's thesis). Philadelphia, Hahnemann Medical College, 1978

Grotowski J: Towards a Poor Theatre. New York, Simon and Schuster, 1968

Hannett F: The haunting lyric. The personal and social significance of American popular songs. Psychoanal Q 33:226-269, 1964

Harms E (ed): The development of modern art therapy. Leonardo 8:241-244, 1975

Irwin E, Rubin J: Art and drama interviews: decoding symbolic messages. Journal of Art Psychotherapy 3:169-175, 1976

Irwin E: Drama therapy with the handicapped, in Drama, Theatre and the Handicapped. Edited by Shaw A, Stevens C. Washington, DC, American Theatre Association, 1979

Jennings S: Remedial Drama. New York, Theatre Arts Books, 1974

Johnson D, Sandel S: Structural analysis of movement sessions: preliminary research. American Journal of Dance Therapy 1:32-36, 1977

Johnson D: Developmental approaches in drama therapy. Int J Arts in Psychotherapy 9:183-190, 1982a

Johnson D: Principles and techniques of drama therapy. Int J Arts in Psychotherapy 9:83-90, 1982b

Johnson D: Some diagnostic implications of drama therapy, in Drama in Therapy, vol 2. Edited by Schattner G, Courtney R. New York, Drama Book Specialists, 1981

Kalish B, Ruttenberg BA, Wenor C, et al: Behavioral Rating Instrument for Atypical Children. Philadelphia, Staelting, 1977

Kestenberg J: Children and Parents. New York, Jason Aronson, 1974

Kohut H: Observations on the psychological functions of music. J Am Psychoanal Assoc 5:389-407, 1957

Kramer E: Art Therapy at Wiltwyck School. School Arts 58:5-8, 1958a

Kramer E: Art Therapy in a Children's Community. Springfield, Ill, Charles C Thomas, 1958b

Kwiatkowska H: The use of families' art productions for psychiatric evaluation. Bulletin of Art Therapy 6:52-69, 1967

Laban R: Mastery of Movement. Cedar Falls, Iowa, McDonald Evans, 1950

Levick MF, Dulicai D, Briggs C, et al: The creative arts therapies, in A Handbook for Specific Learning Disabilities. Edited by Adamson W, Adamson K. New York, Gardner Press, 1979

Levick MF: Transference and countertransference as manifested in graphic productions. Int J Art Psychotherapy 2:203-224, 1975

Levick MF: Family art therapy in the community, Philadelphia Medicine 69:257-261, 1973

Levick MF: The goals of the art therapist as compared to those of the art teacher. Journal of Albert Einstein Medical Center 15:157-170, 1967

Mahler M: The Psychological Birth of the Human Infant. New York, Basic Books, 1975

Masserman JH: Personal communication, 1981

Masserman JH: Say id isn't so—with music, in Science and Psychoanalysis. Edited by Masserman J. New York, Grune & Stratton, 1958

McReynolds P, DeVoge S: Use of Improvisational Techniques in Assessment, vol 4. San Francisco, Jossey-Bass, 1977

Miller M: Jazz and aggression. Psychoanal Rev 54:141-156, 1967

Moreno J: Psychodrama, vol 1. Beacon, NY, Beacon House, 1945

Moustakas C: Children in Play Therapy. New York, McGraw-Hill, 1953

Naumburg M: Dynamically Oriented Art Therapy: Its Principles and Practice. New York, Grune & Stratton, 1966

Naumburg M: Studies of Free Art Expression in Behavior of Children as a Means of Diagnosis and Therapy. New York, Coolidge Foundation, 1947

Nordoff P, Robbins C: Creative Music Therapy. New York, John Day Co, 1977

North M: Personality Assessment Through Movement. Great Britain, Rlarp, 1974

Oswald PF: Soundmaking. Springfield, Ill, Charles C Thomas, 1963

Pauley F: Dance and culture. in Proceedings of the Fifth Annual Conference, American Dance Therapy Association, New York, American Dance Therapy Association, 1970

Piaget J: The Construction of Reality in the Child. New York, Basic Books, 1954

Reik T: The Haunting Melody. New York, Grove Press, 1953

Reich W: Character Analysis. New York, Orgone Institute Press, 1949

Ruud E: Music Therapy and Its Relationship to Current Treatment Theories. St Louis, Magnamusic-Baton, 1980

Schattner G, Courtney R: Drama in Therapy, vols 1,2. New York, Drama Book Specialists, 1981

Schechner R: Environmental Theater. New York, Hawthorn, 1973

Sears WW: Processes in music therapy, in Music in Therapy. Edited by Gaston ET. New York, Macmillan, 1968

Slade P: Child Drama. London, University of London Press, 1954

Spolin V: Improvisations for the Theater. Evanston, Ill, Northwestern University Press, 1963

Ulman E: Therapy is not enough: the contribution of art to general hospital psychiatry. Bulletin of Art Therapy 6:13-21, 1961

Wagner MJ: Brainwaves and biofeedback: a brief history—implications for music research. Journal of Music Therapy 12:46-58, 1975

Ward W: Playmaking with Children. New York, Appleton-Century-Crofts, 1957

Way B: Development through Drama. New York, Barnes and Noble, 1969

Werner H: Comparative Psychology of Mental Development. New York, International Universities Press, 1948

Wethered A: Movement in Drama and Therapy. Boston, Plays, Inc, 1973

Zimney GH, Weidenfeller EW: The Effects of Music Upon GSR of Children. Journal of Music Therapy 15:108-117, 1978

18
Psychodrama

18

Psychodrama

INTRODUCTION

Psychodrama is a professional practice based on the therapy, philosophy, and methodology developed by Jacob L. Moreno, M.D. (1889-1974), which uses action methods of enactment, sociometry, group dynamics, role theory, and social systems analysis to facilitate constructive change in individuals and groups through the development of new perceptions or reorganization of old cognitive patterns and concomitant changes in behavior.

HISTORY

The history of psychodrama to a great extent is also the history of its founder, Jacob L. Moreno, M.D. Moreno was born on May 6, 1889, in Bucharest, Romania; moved with his family at school age to Vienna, Austria; and immigrated to the United States in 1925 (Bratescu, 1975). Vienna provided an important foundation for Moreno. It was there that he received a Doctore of Medicine degree from the University of Vienna in 1917. During the years 1908-1925 he formulated his theories of psychodrama, sociometry, and group psychotherapy in Vienna. According to Moreno (1946), the first psychodrama session was held on April 1, 1921.

Sociometry, the measurement of groups, had its beginnings during World War I. Through his connections in Vienna, Moreno secured an appointment as superintendent of a World War I resettlement camp at Mittendorf. The camp was composed primarily of wine growing peasants of Italian extraction. During his tenure as superintendent it became evident that a system to resettle war refugees within the camp was needed. Rather than randomly assigning them to living quarters and work duties, Moreno developed sociometric methods that allowed the refugees to select their living and working partners.

Similarly, his work on spontaneity and role playing was refined and refocused through his work at Das Stegreiftheater in Vienna, 1922-1925, at the Maisedergasse. Prostitutes from the red light district became Moreno's first clients in his pioneering adventure in group psychotherapy. Through his interactions with these women, he discovered the principle of the therapeutic agent: Each member of the group can serve as the therapeutic agent for another, and the therapeutic nature of groups comes from interactions with one another rather than from the group leader.

Moreno's interests were not limited to medicine, psychiatry, or studies in the parks or the theatre. His unbounded energy was also directed to editing a literary magazine, *Daimon*. In 1914, Moreno published "Einladung zu einer Begegnung," which was republished in February 1918, as "Einladung zu einer Begegnung: Die Gottheit als Autor" ("Invitation to an Encounter: The Godhead as Author"). Martin Buber was a contributing editor of *Daimon*; and their articles on encounter, existentialism, and interpersonal relations appeared side by side.

At some point in his practice in Vienna, Moreno became impatient with the slow reception of his ideas within the professional community. He searched for a country in which new ideas would be accepted and could be tested and chose America.

By 1927 Moreno was actively engaged in the practice of psychiatry; and from then until 1938 he worked at the New York State Training School for Girls in Hudson, New York, and conducted a private practice in New York City.

Moreno developed important friendships and relationships with other members of the scientific and professional community. One of his greatest benefactors was William Alanson White, M.D., superintendent of St. Elizabeths Hospital in Washington, D.C. White wrote the foreword for Moreno's first major American work, *Who Shall Survive?*, and was instrumental in obtaining a publisher for the book. White also saw to the establishment of a psychodrama theater at St. Elizabeths in 1939. Members of the St. Elizabeths Hospital staff were visitors at Beacon where Moreno had his sanitorium. Moreno was a frequent lecturer and consultant to the hospital (Buchanan and Enneis, 1981).

Moreno was intricately involved in the research, training, and dissemination of information on psychodrama, sociometry, group psychotherapy, role theory, and social systems analysis throughout his life. He devoted the years 1930-1950 to the development of his theories and techniques through phenomenological and empirical research conducted while director of research under the New York State Social Welfare Department (Moreno, 1953); the New York State Training School for Girls at Hudson, New York (Jennings, 1950); and his sanatorium in Beacon (Moreno, 1951).

Moreno founded *Sociometry, A Journal of Interpersonal Relations* in 1937 (currently titled *Social Psychology Quarterly*) and transferred ownership of the journal on its eighteenth anniversary to the American Sociological Society (Moreno, 1966). He founded the journal *Sociatry* (later renamed *Journal of Group Psychotherapy and Psychodrama*) in 1947. He also established the first professional association for group psychotherapy in 1942—the American Society of Group Psychotherapy and Psychodrama.

Moreno was instrumental in founding the First International Committee of Group Psychotherapy in Paris in 1951. This committee planned the First International Congress of Group Psychotherapy, which was held in Toronto in August of 1954 (Moreno, 1962). He also founded the International Psychodrama Congress, whose first meeting in Paris in 1964 attracted 1,500 psychodramatists from around the world. Ironically, today psychodrama is probably more respected and used in several other countries (West Germany, Japan, Australia, Argentina, Brazil, and France) than it is in the United States (Buchanan, 1979).

Toward the end of his life, Moreno began to receive respect and admiration from the mental health community (Z.T. Moreno, 1969). His pioneering efforts and seminal contributions were recognized and credited by such leaders in the field as Benne and Muntyan (1951) and Schutz (1971). In fact, Berne (1970) states that all who attempt to use action methods or action techniques are confronted with the "Moreno Problem." Simply put, he stated that any time therapists try to work with action techniques they will find that it has already been done and written about by Moreno. Biddle and Thomas (1966) call Moreno one of the three major founders of role theory, and certainly he is acknowledged as the founder of psychodrama and sociometry.

Moreno died on May 14, 1974, in Beacon, New York. At his request, his only epitath was "the man who brought laughter to psychiatry." While Moreno deserves credit for the germination of the ideas, other colleagues such as William Alanson White, Gardner Murphy, Stagg Whitin, Alfred Adler, Fanny French Morse, Helen Hall Jennings, Zerka Toeman Moreno, Warner Wellman, Ron and Rosemary Lippitt, James Enneis, and Mary Northway all contributed to the overall growth and development of the field. However, if anyone deserves a place as a major force in the development of psychodrama, it is Moreno's wife, Zerka Toeman Moreno. For more than 40 years Zerka Moreno has been researching, writing, directing, and training in the fields her husband created. The Moreno Academy in Beacon, New York, closed in 1983 after 47 years. The Psychodrama Section at St. Elizabeths Hospital, founded in 1939, is now the oldest continually operating center for clinical practice, training, and research in psychodrama, sociometry, and group psychotherapy.

PHILOSOPHY AND THEORETICAL ISSUES

Psychodramatic treatment is based on Moreno's view of a man as a cosmic, social, and singular individual. This triadic conceptualization leads to the three philosophical cornerstones of psychodrama therapy: the idea of the Godhead, sociometry, and psychodrama. The concept of the Godhead, of God as ultimate creator, refers to the spontaneity/creativity potential of each person. Sociometry addresses the basic social structure of all human interaction and provides a method of observation and intervention in group process. Psychodrama develops the concept of man, the "co-creator" and the "actor," and provides action methods and role constructs that reflect this concept. While each base can be addressed individually, psychodramatic treatment cannot be accomplished without the integration that forms the potent synergetic basis for psychodramatic treatment.

Godhead

The most controversial concept espoused by Moreno still remains his idea of the Godhead. Through his search for an understanding of life he developed his belief in the spontaneous/creative God, the interpersonal God. In this area there was a shared influence between Moreno and Martin Buber, the Jewish theologian. Buber's theological statement identified God as the source of "universal relation," and Moreno refers to the God of "emotional expansiveness." Both men refer to the co-creative powers we share with the Godhead.

Psychodramatists have interpreted the image of man as God within the theoretical perspective that each of us is the center of our own world. The people with whom we choose to live and to love, the people whom we ignore, and the people who become our enemies are all chosen by us. We inhabit a world of co-creators. Each of us influences and is influenced by others. We have free will. We have the power to create. We are potentially limitless.

Psychodramatists do not mean that, as creators, we have the power to create at will regardless of the will of others. Each person is encouraged to experience his own creativity and to realize that he is responsible for his own life. The responsibility involved in assuming the role of creator is much too frightening for some; consequently, they retreat to passive ascriptive roles wherein they vest their creative powers to some authoritarian figure. It is the work of a psychoanalyst (Fromm, 1941) which largely explains this "escape from freedom."

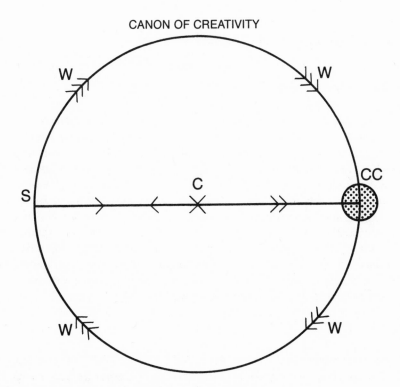

Figure 1. Spontaneity—Creativity—Cultural Conserve

Field of Rotating Operations Between Spontaneity-Creativity-Cultural Conserve (S-C-CC)
S—Spontaneity, C—Creativity, CC—Cultural (or any) Conserve (for instance, a biological conserve, *i.e.*, an animal organism, or a cultural conserve, *i.e.*, a book, a motion picture, or a robot, *i.e.*, a calculating machine); W—Warming up is the "operational" expression of spontaneity. The circle represents the field of operations between S, C and CC.

Operation I: Spontaneity arouses Creativity, C. S ——— >C.
Operation II: Creativity is receptive to Spontaneity. S< ——— C.
Operation III: From their interaction Cultural Conserves, CC, result.
                  S ——— >C ——— >>CC.
Operation IV: Conserves (CC) would accumulate indefinitely and remain "in cold storage." They need to be reborn, the catalyzer Spontaneity revitalizes them. CC ——— >>>S ——— >>>CC.

S does not operate in a vacuum, it moves either towards Creativity or towards Conserves.

Total Operation

Spontaneity-creativity-warming up act$<^{\text{actor}}_{\text{conserve}}$

Source: Moreno JL, 1953. Reprinted with permission.

The "Spontaneity-Creativity-Cultural Conserve" (Figure 1) shows the interrelationship and interaction of spontaneity and creativity with the status quo. According to Moreno (1956), spontaneity-creativity is the most important problem of psychology. He further postulates that spontaneity and the creativity factor are available to everyone, and the success of our adventures in the world is directly related to our ability to be spontaneous. Spontaneity is the human ability that enables us to develop adequate responses to life situations. Adequacy encompasses the concepts of appropriateness, competency, and skill in interacting within the given situation. A person can be creative without being spontaneous, and responses may be dramatic and original without necessarily being spontaneous. Likewise, if a person always responds with the same rote patterns, there is likely to be little spontaneity operating.

Spontaneity can be thought of as the readiness for an action, and creativity as the response (act). The twin concepts of spontaneity and creativity are responsible for the formation of our cultural conserves. Cultural conserves are the given patterns, relationships, or products of our society. They define the norms, mores, and folkways of our culture and help transmit these normative patterns to future generations.

Sociometry

Sociometry is the second philosophical base of psychodramatic treatment. Sociometry is derived from the Latin "socius" meaning social and the Latin "metrium" or the Greek "metron" meaning measure; it literally means the measurement of social groups.

Moreno viewed man as a social being who develops his identity through interactions with the individuals around him. Therefore, he postulated that the larger society is composed of units made up of each individual and the essential persons in his or her life. Moreno named this smallest unit of society the *social atom*. Blatner (1973) defines the term as the "complex of all the significant figures, real or fantasied, past or present, who relate to a person's psychological experience."

From birth every individual has a set of relationships around him— mother, father, brothers and sisters, lovers and antagonists, students and mentors. The volume of the social atom expands during the course of human development as the child moves from the nuclear family to society, and with old age the social atom generally begins to shrink as the persons in it move or die and are not replaced by others. The social atom is a dynamic construct.

Each of us has certain feelings toward members of our social atom. Some individuals attract us, some repel us, and with some we are neutral in our feelings. Moreno refers to this range of feelings between persons as *tele* (from the Greek meaning "at a distance"). He conceptualizes that each social atom is composed of numerous tele structures, defined as the smallest units of social feelings that enter our awareness. These intangible communication channels between individuals are the basis for the formation of larger social groups.

Sociometry applied as a quantitative measure of social interactions is basically value free. Sociometrists measure social choice patterns without reference to moral interpretation (Hale, 1981). Rejection and acceptance patterns are neither right nor wrong but merely reflect the value systems of a specific culture. It is the task of the sociometrist to set up criteria that allow all group members to explore and clarify the sociometric connections within a given group. Once this information is made available, an examination of implications for individuals in the group is possible. Through psychodramatic and sociodramatic enactment, mixed messages and distortions in transference and countertransference are clarified. Through application and analysis of sociometric data the sociometrist facilitates the group process so that each individual can focus his own spontaneity and creativity within the structure.

Psychodrama

The philosophy and methods associated with psychodrama comprise the third cornerstone of psychodramatic theory. Moreno (1946, 1953) has called psychodrama the science that explores the truth by dramatic methods. Adaline Starr (1977) refers to psychodrama as a rehearsal for life. Psychodrama is an action therapy because Moreno believed that life itself evolves from action and interaction. Psychodramatic treatment was designed to approximate life closely. Consequently a psychodramatist helps the patient to recreate his world in the course of a psychodrama session. Certain terms assume a unique meaning when applied to the psychodramatic method and need to be understood within this specific context. The subject or patient in a particular psychodrama is referred to as the protagonist, and the therapist is called the director. The actors who participate in the role-playing as significant others in the drama are referred to as auxiliary egos.

Role theory, as developed by Moreno, enables the director to involve the patient in a situation that elicits a collection of behaviors and affective states. According to Moreno (1946), "Every individual just as he has at all times a set of friends and foes, has a range of roles in which he sees himself and faces a range of counter roles in which he sees others around him."

Catharsis is another essential psychodramatic concept that has a different definition than may be associated with it by others. The genesis of the term *catharsis* can be traced to Aristotle, who, in his *De Poetica*, discussed the purging, emptying, or cleansing of the emotions which occurs in a spectator when watching a drama. Breuer and Freud revived the term for use in psychoanalytic treatment. Their definition of catharsis, which is still the most common use of the term, was as "a treatment of psychoneurosis to bring about abreaction, by encouraging the patient to tell everything that happens to be associated with a given train of thought, thus purging the mind of the repressed material that is the cause of the symptoms" (Dorland, 1974).

Moreno (1946) identified three major forms of catharsis: (a) the aesthetic, that is, the experiencing of beauty; (b) spectator, as described by Aristotle; and (c) actorial catharsis or catharsis of integration through action. It is the last that is of primary importance to psychodramatists and to psychodramatic treatment. Instead of the person's recounting the story, the protagonist is encouraged to experience his participation in the event. The psychodramatist creates an existential situation in which the events dramatized all occur in the here and now. Thus, in the enactment the protagonist is holding the hand of a "dying parent," experiencing once again the break-up of a "marriage" or the loss of a "child." The other group members serving as auxiliary egos are also experiencing actorial catharsis; instead of passively observing a play through role reversal with the protagonist, they are experiencing life from the role of the dying parent, the abandoning spouse, or the departing child. The goal is not a catharsis of abreaction but one of integration. As Z.T. Moreno (1971) states, "We know from psychodrama that the greatest depth of catharsis comes not merely from re-enactment of the past, however traumatic or instructive, but from embodying those dimensions, roles, and interactions which life has not, cannot and probably never, will permit." In her summation of her classical article on catharsis, she states that the final lesson from the catharsis of integration is to teach the protagonist to discard his old role construct to redo his life here and now.

One final important psychodramatic construct is the concept of *surplus reality*. Moreno refers here to aspects of our life, our everyday reality, which are not fully experienced or expressed. In the psychodrama experience, reality is magnified and amplified to provide a different and fresh perspective. Role reversal is the principal surplus reality technique used in psychodrama.

While each of the branches of Moreno's philosophical system may stand on its own, they are intended to be applied concurrently in order to provide an integrated treatment program.

PSYCHODRAMATIC COMPONENTS

Five elements are vital to psychodrama: the stage, the group members, the auxiliary egos, the protagonist, and the director (Yablonsky and Enneis, 1966). The psychodrama theatre, designed so that every phase and structure of the human organism can be enacted, prepares the individual to interact with significant others. By entering the psychodrama theatre, the participants are "warmed up" for the therapy process, just as the architecture of a church warms up the participants for a religious experience (Z.T. Moreno, 1965).

In earlier experiences with psychodrama, members of a person's social atom were physically present in the therapy. The first use of auxiliary egos to portray roles in a psychodrama session occurred because a dead person was an important part of the drama. Consequently, Moreno assigned a therapeutic actor to play the role of the deceased person within the family treatment session. Later in other group sessions, it became apparent that not all individuals could be physically present in all treatment sessions, thus Moreno began to use auxiliary egos to portray the roles of absent or missing social atom figures (Z.T. Moreno, 1982). He considers these roles tangible and observable units of an individual's personality. In this way the psychodramatist works with the patient to explore the pathological and the healthy aspects of the personality structure. Role is a dynamic concept, and therapeutic change occurs through improvement in the individual's role structure.

PSYCHODRAMATIC RULES AND PROCEDURES

Z.T. Moreno (1965) has compiled a list of basic psychodramatic rules and techniques for a typical psychodrama session, which include:

Psychodrama can be a method of restraint as well as expression. It is not always therapeutic or appropriate for every psychodrama to help the client express his unexpressed feelings or behaviors. Psychodramatists should structure the production so that it facilitates a change from typical behavior patterns. If the client screams hysterically as a regular and routine behavior, it would be important to help the client develop new ways of expressing his emotions.

All psychodramas occur in the here and now. For Moreno (1966) time in psychodrama is a function of the past, present, and future. We interact in situations based upon our past experiences, present observations, and future expectations. Consequently, time is a here and now experience. Whether a person is enacting a role from childhood, present life, or some anticipated future role, he acts "as if" it is occurring in the here and now.

Reality is a subjective experience. Neither the psychodrama director nor the client has a complete knowledge of reality. Each of us views the world from our own perspective. Through facilitation and role reversal, we are more able to view the world from other perspectives. When we are able to view a given situation from a number of different perspectives, we will be closer to reality than when viewing it from only one.

In addition to these rules and techniques, several key definitions are essential to the understanding of the concepts of psychodrama. They are:

Protagonist. The central character in the psychodrama. The subject. The client.

Auxiliary Egos. Individuals who assume a role in a psychodrama to help facilitate production of the session. Auxiliary egos may be fathers, mothers, dogs, tombstones, doubles, or devils (Zinger, 1975).

Therapeutic Agents. The other group members. Moreno (1946) states that the therapy comes from the group members through their interactions with each other and not from some mystical omnipotent leader.

Director. The psychodrama group leader, the therapist. Moreno (1946) chose this term because of his belief that the leader of the group facilitates expression among group members and guides and directs those experiences rather than "curing" patients. In this context, Z.T. Moreno (McCrie, 1975) coined the metaphor of the psychodrama director as the midwife. The director is responsible for assisting in the birth of a production but not for the genesis of the production.

Scripts. Psychodramatists work from the scripts of the mind. Directors are not interested in the individual's creating the words of a playwright but are concerned with helping the individual rewrite his own life scripts. Almost all psychodramas are spontaneous, that is, they arise from the emergent interactions of the group members without assigned roles and scripts from a pre-planned written document.

Surplus Reality. Surplus reality is an expansion of a person's perceptions of reality. As a technique it is the dramatization of an individual's internal reality. For example, if the protagonist states that his parents are tearing him apart, the director would literally instruct the auxiliary egos portraying the parents to begin tearing at the protagonist. If a suicidal patient states that he is at the end of his rope, the director would enact a scene where the protagonist is literally at the end of his rope and explore the scenes leading up to his reaching the end of his rope. Dramatization and concretization of metaphors are used to help increase the psychological reality of the situation. Because many of life's major scenes are condensed into a relatively few short minutes on a psychodrama stage, it becomes necessary for the director to "magnify" the scenes through the use of surplus reality techniques. Surplus reality also is an integral part of any role reversal when the protagonist steps out of his own role to view the world from the role of the other.

Role Reversal. The most commonly used technique, role reversal, occurs when two individuals switch roles. "A" becomes "B" and "B" becomes "A." Role reversal is indicated for a variety of reasons including (a) helping the person understand the role of the other, (b) learning how one's interactions affect the roles of others, (c) providing information about the individual's social system, and (d) making the subject cognizant of discrepancies in nonverbal and verbal communications. Role reversal encourages a shift in perception and reorients the personal experience through a process of "ego-borrowing."

Double. The assignment of one group member to "double" another group member, to physically and verbally become a psychological twin. The double's job is to express feelings that the subject cannot or will not express. Sometimes a double is used as an amplifier, at times a double is used to help a subject express his feelings, and at other times doubles may be used to help more impulsive clients integrate cognitive functions (Toeman, 1948).

Soliloquy. This technique is used to help an individual express thoughts and concerns during a particular scene and to break through resistance. It is similar to the concept of free association except that the client expresses his feelings while engaged in the situation from which the feelings derive (e.g., a client may be asked to soliloquize about his feelings and expectations as he is walking into his home or office).

Future Projection. The technique wherein the protagonist acts "as if" he is in the future. This technique is valuable in helping a client rehearse or prepare for future situations (e.g., job interviewing, community placement, retirement, etc.).

Structured Warm-Ups. A structured warm-up is a preplanned exercise that helps the group focus on a particular theme or concern. A large variety of structured warm-ups have been developed to aid the psychodrama director in exploring the concerns of a group. This exercise differs from a "spontaneous" warm-up where the structure emerges spontaneously from the group. Weiner and Sacks (1969) have developed a lengthy list of structured warm-ups ranging from courtroom scenes to fantasy explorations.

PSYCHODRAMA SESSIONS

There is no such thing as a typical psychodrama treatment session because the individual resources of each director and the specific needs of each group and client vary. However, there is a general model for the direction of a psychodrama group. Most sessions are composed of three main phases: warm-up, action, and sharing.

Warm-Up

The warm-up is the initial phase of the group therapy session. For a spontaneous warm-up, the director and group members join together (usually in a semi-circle or circle) and discuss their common concerns or participate in a structured warm-up exercise. Channels of communication are established among group members, and a theme and area of concern are uncovered. The basic goals and objectives for the treatment session are mutually negotiated between the protagonist, group members, and director.

A person (the protagonist) is selected who can best represent the concerns of the group.

There are two basic forms of psychodramatic treatment: the protagonist centered model (Moreno, 1946) and the central concern model (Buchanan, 1980). In the protagonist-centered model one individual volunteers or is requested to volunteer to be the protagonist in the drama. This model works well with neurotic populations and with persons who are highly motivated for therapy and have established some of their own ideas concerning treatment.

The central concern model was developed at St. Elizabeths Hospital, Washington, D.C., and is used mostly in the treatment of hospitalized populations. The central concern model devotes more attention to establishing interaction patterns between individuals and facilitating communication channels among the group members. A common concern and theme are selected which best represent the here and now concerns of the group. Then a protagonist is selected to represent the central concern of the group.

Action

After a protagonist has been chosen, he acts out the issue by interacting with the various persons, roles, and themes. Psychodramatic techniques are used to clarify and concretize the concern. The action is structured in a way that facilitates catharsis, action insight, clarification, and behavioral change. New roles are explored and alternate affective and behavioral styles are encouraged.

Sharing

The final phase of a typical psychodrama session is called sharing or closure. This is the process during which other group members share their own reactions to the scenes that were enacted during the action phase of the psychodrama session. Members of the group have the opportunity to express their feelings and concerns about similar situations they have or might have to confront. Clients are drawn out of their patterns of isolation and self-centeredness and again resume interacting with one another.

The Hollander psychodrama diagram (Figure 2) (1978) offers a pictorial representation of the psychodramatic processes that occur during psychodrama enactment.

CLINICAL INDICATIONS AND LIMITATIONS

Psychodrama has been used with the full range of psychiatric populations (Buchanan and Dubbs-Siroka, 1980). It has also been used for the specific

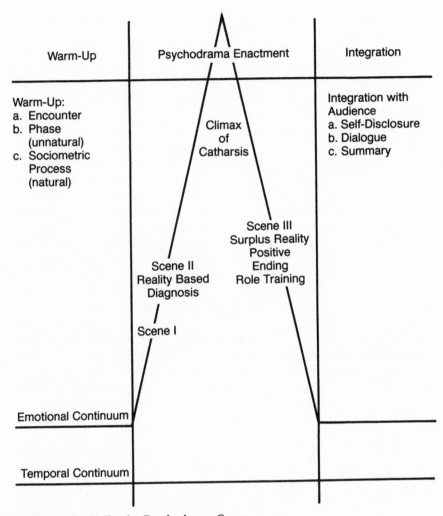

Figure 2. The Hollander Psychodrama Curve

Source: Hollander C, 1978. Reprinted with permission.

treatment of alcoholic (Starr, 1977; Weiner, 1966; Zimberg et al., 1978), blind (Routh, 1957; Altman, 1981), deaf (Robinson and Clayton, 1971; Swink, 1980), drug addicted (Eliasoph, 1955; Olson, 1972), elderly (Buchanan, 1982), and dying (Weiner, 1975) patients and with children and adolescents (Jennings, 1950; Rowan, 1973; Altschuler and Picon, 1980). For a complete description of the psychodramatic literature relating to different clinical populations, the reader is encouraged to consult Gendron (1980).

Psychodramatists are usually flexible in their orientation to treatment; sessions can focus on abstract goals (e.g., increase in spontaneity and creativity) or highly measurable objectives (e.g., the client will sit erect and maintain eye contact in role enactment of a prospective job interview). In most cases the psychodramatist facilitates the development of both affective and behavioral roles. Psychodramatic methods can be used as part of a preventive program, i.e., helping clients cope with stressful situations and helping them plan alternative roles to cope with those stressful environments or to treat specific symptoms (e.g., psychodramatic desensitization techniques to enable clients who are claustrophobic to travel by bus, etc.).

Psychodrama is not recommended when an individual client is not ready to participate in a group experience. Traditional precautions used to place patients in group therapy are applied to the placement of patients in psychodrama groups. Psychodrama has been used with the full range of psychiatric patients, but adjustments in the methodology are needed so that goals for the group match the needs of the patients. For example, chronic schizophrenics have benefited greatly from psychodramatic social skills training. Patients with fragile ego boundaries are often assigned to psychodrama groups that focus on behavioral skills and the development of social-emotional relationships. Individual psychodrama therapy may be indicated for a client in preparation for or in conjunction with psychodrama group therapy.

It should be emphasized that in the hands of an appropriately trained and experienced psychodramatist, psychodrama has the flexibility and creativity to respond to most clients' needs. The techniques available to the psychodramatist are carefully selected to meet the needs of specific individuals in the group. Psychodrama enactment can take many forms, from a sociometric investigation of choice patterns to an interpersonal exploration of cultural issues (e.g., racism, sexism) or a highly structured intrapersonal exploration of childhood development.

PROFESSIONAL AND ETHICAL ISSUES

Psychodrama is a potent therapeutic modality that offers benefits for the treatment of psychiatric populations. Its greatest disadvantage occurs when persons who are inappropriately trained or experienced attempt to use the psychodrama action methods with their clients. It is imperative that practitioners of psychodrama be trained and experienced in the use of psychodrama, sociometry, and group psychotherapy.

The American Board of Examiners in Psychodrama, Sociometry, and Group Psychotherapy has established criteria for certification as a practitioner (1982). To be eligible for the certification examination (written and on-site), the applicants must have (a) completed 780 hours of training from an accredited psychodrama training institute, (b) had one year of supervised experience, and (c) have a master's degree or acceptable equivalent in the field of mental health. The board has also established requirements for persons seeking certification as trainers and educators of psychodrama. Naturally the requirements for this certification level are based on higher educational, experiential, and training requirements.

The American Society of Group Psychotherapy and Psychodrama (ASGPP), established in 1942, is the general membership organization for psychodramatists. It has a code of ethics and standards of practice that members are expected to follow. However, membership in the ASGPP is not an endorsement of professional competence. The ASGPP encourages broad membership from clients to students. There are no educational or training requirements necessary for membership.

The Federation of Trainers and Training Programs in Psychodrama was established in 1975 for persons who are trainers in psychodrama. Only individuals certified by the American Board of Examiners in Psychodrama, Sociometry, and Group Psychotherapy are eligible for membership. It is a consortium of trainers and training institutes which meets yearly to discuss innovations and issues in training. The federation also has a code of ethics and standards of practice for trainers in psychodrama, sociometry, and group psychotherapy. Continuing education and quality control are important issues for the professional associations, and emphasis is placed on a continual interface between present and emerging knowledge.

REFERENCES

Altman KP: Psychodrama with blind psychiatric patients. Journal of Visual Impairment and Blindness 75:153-156, 1981

Altschuler CM, Picon WJ: The social living class: a model for the use of sociodrama in the classroom. Group Psychotherapy, Psychodrama and Sociometry 33:162-169, 1980

American Board of Examiners in Psychodrama, Sociometry and Group Psychotherapy: Examination Information Pamphlet, 1982. (Available from PO Box 844, Cooper Station, New York, NY 10276.)

Benne KD, Muntyan B: Human Relations in Curriculum Change. New York, Dryden Press, 1951

Berne E: Gestalt therapy verbatim: a review. Am J Psychiatry 126:1519-1520, 1970

Biddle BJ, Thomas EJ (eds): Role Theory: Concepts and Research. New York, John Wiley & Sons, 1966

Blatner HA: Acting-In. New York, Springer Publishing, 1973

Bratescu G: The date and birthplace of JL Moreno. Group Psychotherapy and Psychodrama 28:2-4, 1975

Buchanan DR, Dubbs-Siroka J: Psychodramatic treatment for psychiatric patients. Journal of National Association of Private Psychiatric Hospitals 11:27-31, 1980

Buchanan DR, Enneis JM: Forty-one (41) years of psychodrama at Saint Elizabeths Hospital. Journal of Group Psychotherapy, Psychodrama & Sociometry 34:134-147, 1981

Buchanan DR: Psychodrama: a humanistic approach to psychiatric treatment for the elderly. Hosp Community Psychiatry 33:220-223, 1982

Buchanan DR: The central concern model, a framework for structuring psychodramatic production. Group Psychotherapy 33:47-62, 1980

Buchanan DR: Psychodrama: an overview of the first fifty-eight years, in Conference on Creative Arts Therapies: The Use of the Creative Arts in Therapy. Washington, DC, American Psychiatric Association, 1979

Dorland's Illustrated Medical Dictionary, 25th Ed. Philadelphia, WB Saunders, 1974

Eliasoph E: A group therapy and psychodrama approach with adolescent drug addicts. Group Psychotherapy 8:161-167, 1955

Fromm E: Escape from Freedom. New York, Holt, Rinehart & Winston, 1941

Gendron JM: The Roots and the Branches and Bibliography of Psychodrama, 1972-1980; and Sociometry, 1970-1980. Beacon, NY, Beacon House, 1980

Hale AE: Conducting Clinical Sociometric Explorations: A Manual for Psychodramatists and Sociometrists. Roanoke, Va, Author, 1981

Hollander C: A Process for Psychodrama Training: The Hollander Psychodrama Curve. Denver, Snow Lion Press, 1978

Jennings HH: Leadership and Isolation: A Study of Personality in Interpersonal Relations. New York, Longmens, Green, 1950

McCrie E: Psychodrama: an interview with Zerka T Moreno. Practical Psychology for Physicians, December 1975, pp 45-48, 68-79

Moreno JL: Psychiatry of the 20th century: function of the universalia, time, space, reality, and cosmos. Group Psychotherapy 29:146-158, 1966

Moreno JL: The roots of psychodrama. Group Psychotherapy 19:140-145, 1965

Moreno JL: The group psychotherapy movement, past, present and future. Group Psychotherapy 15:21-23, 1962

Moreno JL (ed): Sociometry and the Science of Man. Beacon, NY, Beacon House, 1956

Moreno JL: Who Shall Survive? 2nd ed. Beacon NY, Beacon House, 1953

Moreno JL: Sociometry, Experimental Method and the Science of Society. Beacon, NY, Beacon House, 1951

Moreno JL: Psychodrama, vol 1. Beacon, NY, Beacon House, 1946

Moreno ZT: Personal communication, Sept 8, 1982

Moreno ZT: Beyond Aristotle, Breuer and Freud: Moreno's contribution to the concept of catharsis. Group Psychotherapy and Psychodrama 24:34-43, 1971

Moreno ZT: The seminal mind of JL Moreno and his influence upon the present generation, in Psychodrama, vol 3. Edited by Moreno JL, Moreno ZT. Beacon, NY, Beacon House, 1969

Moreno ZT: Psychodramatic rules, techniques and adjunctive methods. Group Psychotherapy 18:73-86, 1965

Olson PA: Psychodrama and group therapy with young heroin addicts returning from duty in Vietnam. Group Psychotherapy and Psychodrama 25:141-147, 1972

Robinson LD, Clayton L: Psychodrama with deaf people. Am Ann Deaf 116:414-419, 1971

Routh TA: A study of the use of group psychotherapy in rehabilitation centers for the blind. Group Psychotherapy 10:38-50, 1957

Rowan PJ: Psychodramatic treatment of death fantasies in adolescent girls. Handbook of International Sociometry 8:94-98, 1973

Schutz WC: Here Comes Everybody. New York, Harper and Row, 1971

Starr A: Psychodrama: Rehearsal for Living. Chicago, Nelson Hall, 1977

Swink DF: Psychodrama: an action psychotherapy for deaf people. Mental Health in Deafness 4:14-19, 1980

Toeman Z: The double situation in psychodrama. Sociatry 1:436-448, 1948

Weiner H: Living experiences with death. Omega 6:251-274, 1975

Weiner HB, Sacks JM: Warm-Up and Sun-Up. Group Psychotherapy 22:85-102, 1969

Weiner HB: An overview on the use of psychodrama and group psychotherapy in the treatment of alcoholism in the United States and abroad. Group Psychotherapy and Psychodrama 19:159-165, 1966

Yablonsky L, Enneis JM: Psychodrama theory and practice, in Progress in Psychotherapy. Edited by Fromm-Reichman F, Moreno JL. Beacon, NY, Beacon House, 1966

Zimberg S, Wallace J, Blume SB: Practical Approaches to Alcoholism Psychotherapy. New York, Plenum, 1978

Zinger NG: A working paper for group auxiliary egos. Group Psychotherapy and Psychodrama 28:152-156, 1975

19
Occupational Therapy

19

Occupational Therapy

INTRODUCTION

Occupational therapy is the application of goal-oriented, purposeful activity in the assessment and treatment of individuals with psychological, physical, or developmental disabilities. These services address the development and maintenance of adaptive skills and performance capacities that enable the patient to achieve optimal levels of function in such activities of daily living as work, self-care, socialization, and leisure time pursuits. The occupational therapist's functional assessment and treatment/rehabilitation methods are concerned with specific performance components that include, but are not limited to, motor, sensory-integrative, perceptual-cognitive, psychological, and social-interpersonal functions, as well as those environmental factors that inhibit performance.

Reference to occupation in the title is in the context of goal-directed use of time, energy, interest, and attention to foster adaptation and productivity, to minimize pathology, and to promote the maintenance of health (*American Journal of Occupational Therapy*, 1972). Assessment and treatment services may include, but are not limited to:

- Independent living skills: self-care/self-maintenance;
- Task-oriented treatment using creative-expressive modalities, crafts, education, leisure-time, play, socialization and other role related activities;
- Pre-vocational and work adjustment programs (employment and academic preparation, homemaking, child care/parenting);

- Sensorimotor, including neuromuscular and sensori-integrative assessment and treatment;
- Design, fabrication, and application of orthotic devices;
- Adaptation to physical environment, guidance in the use of adaptive equipment;
- Therapeutic exercise to enhance functional performance;
- Discharge planning and community re-entry;
- Patient/family education and counseling (NY State Occupational Therapy Association, 1970).

Occupational therapists work in a broad range of practice areas and settings. Within the scope of general psychiatry, services are provided to children, adolescents, adults, and the elderly of all functional levels and diagnostic categories in institutional, community-based, partial hospitalization, residential treatment, and forensic programs. These programs are offered in general and psychiatric hospitals, nursing homes, psychosocial and physical rehabilitation centers, sheltered workshops, clinics, public and private schools, group homes, correctional institutions, home health agencies, community mental health centers, day-care centers, private practice physician's offices, and in industry and business.

HISTORICAL BACKGROUND

Belief in the meaning and value of purposeful activity, or "occupation," in the care and treatment of the mentally ill has a lengthy history. Today's practice of occupational therapy has evolved over a 65-year period of professional service to both the physically and mentally disabled. The formal birth of the profession in the early 1900's found its historical roots in an interest in the healing potential of activities documented in Biblical stories, Greek legends, and the early medical teachings of Hippocrates. The enlightened efforts of Pinel and the Tukes further demonstrated the conviction that activities linked to the needs, interests, and skills of individuals had beneficial effects. The "moral treatment" of the eighteenth and nineteenth centuries brought a disciplined and humanistic philosophy to the care of the mentally ill. During this era, work, exercise, games, arts, and crafts were prescribed as regular therapeutics to develop a consciousness of society and for:

> . . . diverting the attention from the unpleasant subjects of thought . . . in tranquilizing the mind, breaking up many associations of ideas and inducing correct habits of thinking as well as acting. (Jones, 1983)

The twentieth century neuropathologist Adolph Meyer identified a more substantive rationale for the use of socially acceptable work and leisure involvements. His holistic view of the patient, in which adaptation was derived from a balance of work, rest, play, and sleep within the context of the individual's broader social environment exerted an important influence on pioneering occupational therapists. Early practitioners, infused with Meyer's conviction that "performance is its own judge and regulator and therefore the most dependable and influential part of life" (Meyer, 1922) used graded, planned, and purposeful activities emphasizing attention and habit formation to promote self-care, social behavior, and work skills. These objectives were realized through the use of a highly organized regimen of normal activities of daily living, selected arts and crafts, and the intervention of a "masterful teacher" who was "alert to determine the means by which each patient learned best: visually, orally, and kinesthetically" (Gillette, 1971).

The principles embodied in these early methods represent significant but rudimentary precursors of a contemporary model for occupational therapy in which the patient's individual style, needs, and assets, and the objects, actions, and interpersonal relationships within purposeful tasks serve as interlocking components of treatment philosophy and process. Important distinctions, however, must be made between this earlier period's emphasis on habit formation and today's greater concern for the complexities of sensorimotor and cognitive skills, personal motivation, self-determination, and adaptation.

Theoretical shifts and the technical and educational developments within occupational therapy over the years have been influenced by many factors. World War II and the return of disabled veterans stimulated support for the rehabilitation movement. The belief that the disabled could achieve independence, and that such achievements were economically advantageous, had a salutary effect upon the role of occupational therapy with the physically disabled. Equally strong advocacy did not emerge on behalf of the mentally ill, even though federal legislation in 1943 and 1954 authorized the extension of vocational rehabilitation for psychiatric patients. These events did, however, influence the development of pre-vocational units in psychiatric facilities where occupational therapists assumed a major role in generating principles and techniques of pre-vocational exploration and treatment (Granofsky, 1959).

The rich content of psychodynamic thinking did not find significant application within occupational therapy until the 1950's and 1960's. These psychodynamic concepts emphasized a view of activities as catalytic agents giving impetus to the development of relationships and intrapsychic experiences, which are used by the therapist and patient collaboratively to eliminate or alter pathology (Fidler and Fidler, 1963). While based on Freudian and Sullivanian theories originally applied to the "talking cure," the commitment to nonverbal communication with its self-expressive and interpersonal potential remained extremely important to the integrity of occupational therapy. The literature of that period underscores that commitment through its emphasis on the meaning of nonhuman object relationships and a more thorough use of the properties of activity and activity analysis. These approaches enhanced the therapeutic fit between activity selection and patient needs and balanced that period's preoccupation with the "therapeutic use of self."

As psychoanalytically-oriented therapists pursued these themes, an "occupational behavior" model perpetuated Meyer's earlier allegiance to performance, adaptation, and health by concentrated examination of work and play behaviors. Assessment of strengths as well as areas of dysfunction constituted a "functional diagnosis"; treatment was directed at improving innate and previously learned skills in the service of concepts of role and socialization (Gillette, 1971). The assumption that "man, through the use of his hands, as they are energized by mind and will, can influence the state of his own health" became key to this rehabilitation orientation (Reilly, 1962).

The historical commitments to psychodynamic and rehabilitation concepts continue to influence occupational therapists. Contemporary neurobehavioral approaches that emphasize sensorimotor components of task performance and the many other theoretical, technical, and cultural changes of the past 20 years have, of course, influenced and enriched practice. None has altered the original essential premise that "performance is its own judge and regulator and therefore the most dependable and influential part of life" (Meyer, 1922).

CONTEMPORARY THEORETICAL AND PHILOSOPHICAL ISSUES

As history indicates, the basic philosophy and practice of occupational therapy are derived from concepts relating to the neurobiological, psychological, and sociocultural nature of man. Concern for the totality of human behavior continues to influence the view of human performance and adaptation as determined by dynamic and complex interrelationships among physical, psychological, interpersonal, and sociocultural processes (King, 1978). Practice is therefore conceptualized both from the internal components of mind, motion, and maturation and from external structures in which man occupies a physical, temporal, social, and symbolic world (Kielhofner and Burke, 1977).

The innate drive to master the environment and the capacity to engage in purposeful activity are viewed as the products of the brain's ability to formulate and symbolize concepts and the ability of human hands to translate concepts into action (Clark, 1979). The ability to adapt, to cope with the demands of everyday living, and to fulfill age specific life roles requires a rich reservoir of experiences gathered from direct engagement with both the human and nonhuman objects in one's environment. "Doing," or purposeful activity, is a critical normative part of a life-long process of stimulation, investigation, and response to the world around us; it also provides the evidence of our capacities to deal with the challenges and demands of that world. The feedback generated from purposeful activity allows the individual to know the potential and limitations of self and the environment and to develop a sense of competence and worth (Fidler and Fidler, 1978).

Occupational therapy places primary emphasis on the use of such purposeful activity to produce a range of desired behavioral changes in clinical situations. The selection and adaptation of activities are based on the needs of the individual patient and on identifiable frames of reference and theoretical assumptions. Contemporary frames of reference developed by occupational therapy include, but are not limited to, neurobehavioral, biomechanical, developmental, psychodynamic, adaptive performance, and occupational behavior models. Those that currently generate the most interest among mental health specialists merit some elaboration.

Adaptive Performance Model. This frame of reference reflects the complex integration of psychodynamic and rehabilitation concepts. Fidler and colleagues used the accepted psychoanalytic belief in the unconscious as a motivating mechanism of behavior but developed treatment strategies that addressed the manifestations of internal conflicts. Assessment and treatment techniques focus on the development or reactivation of ego adaptive skills. These bio-psycho-social skills, more recently referred to as performance components, are inherent and learned elements of behavior which permit the individual to satisfy human needs and meet environmental demands (Mosey, 1968). They are the focus of a therapeutic process in which purposeful, goal-directed activities are "selected from play, work and self-care categories and used for organized, controlled stimulation of adaptive behavior" (Clark, 1979). Changes in skill competency are facilitated by the therapist in one-to-one or group settings and through active involvement in learning by doing "which provides a microcosm of lifework situations which can be seen and explored as they occur rather than in retrospect" (Fidler, 1969).

Occupational Behavior Model. As indicated, the occupational behavior approach found its earliest influence in Meyer's interest in the performance of "those categories of human activities that occupy time, energy, interest and attention" (Clark, 1979). Currently grounded in social role theory and psychological theories of achievement motivation, problem-solving, and personality development (Matsutsuyu, 1971), its primary concerns are with the skills and behaviors necessary for adequate role performance in a given social/environmental context. Such roles include those of worker, student, parent, spouse, and retiree. Therapists provide opportunities for patients to try out tasks representative of specific roles. These are structured to enhance the adaptive capacity of the individual and the adaptable nature of the task

(Heard, 1977). Concerns with intrinsic gratification as a determinant of task performance and the ability to use time in the planning and performance of tasks are notable characteristics of this frame of reference.

Neurobehavioral Model. The neurobehavioral frame of reference focuses on the effects of basic biological functions on task performance. Its theoretical premise is that normalization of sensory and motor patterns, and their integration for interaction with the environment, will promote adaptive development of body integration, cognitive orientation and conceptualization, and manipulative and social skills (Clark, 1979). Its theory emanates from the neurosciences, the cognitive psychology of Piaget, physiological psychology, and other experimental branches of the behavioral sciences (Ayres, 1972). The methods used in this approach involve developmentally sequenced sensorimotor activities and special techniques and equipment that inhibit or excite the neural mechanisms, in keeping with the assumption that the state of dysfunction in a variety of conditions (i.e., schizophrenia and minimal brain dysfunction) reflects the inability of the body to process or correctly respond in an efficient, appropriate way to information received from the environment (Clark, 1979).

While these dominant models of theory and practice reflect some diversity in emphasis, there is an underlying constancy and overlap in actual practice and several common themes emerge:

A. The first, *the importance of purposeful activity*, is evident in practice and well documented in the literature. The overriding focus on actual engagement in a task or activity distinguishes occupational therapy from the verbal psychiatric therapies.

B. The second constant theme is the overall goal of *maximizing independent function in keeping with individual potential.*

C. The third is the belief that *the patient is more than his illness* and that activities are used to discover and develop assets even in the presence of profound and continued illness (Fine, 1980).

CLINICAL ISSUES

Occupational therapists work in a variety of psychiatric settings in collaboration with other health care professionals. Upon referral, or as members of an ongoing multidisciplinary team, occupational therapists participate in identifying problems, establishing overall treatment objectives, and developing treatment and discharge plans. In all instances, specific activities and techniques are selected, based on knowledge of the patient (functional evaluation) and the resources of the discipline (purposeful activity) (NY State Occupational Therapy Association, 1980).

Functional evaluation determines the patient's abilities and deficits related to performance of basic life tasks and fulfillment of roles within work, family, home, and community settings. It pursues several basic questions: What are the activities of daily living which are required of this individual in his or her environment? What skills are intact and what areas of dysfunction exist? What internal and external factors are impeding the ability to function and adapt? (Fidler et al., 1981) The answers to these questions are pursued through a systematic, individualized evaluation of past and current performance levels. Data are gathered through actual task performance and standardized tests, as well as through interview and activity histories that review educational, occupational, leisure time, self-care, and time management capacities. Assessment tasks usually involve a combination of formal structured activities and open-ended, or projective, problems, all chosen to elicit a range of bio-psycho-social skills essential for performing activities of daily living. Assessment is not limited to a simple, factual identification of achievements, interests, and failures. Because the simplest of life tasks (preparing a meal, using a telephone, or filing a letter) represents the complex integration of multiple factors, a systematic consideration of these components facilitates a fuller understanding of patterns of past, current, and potential function. A full-scale evaluation is not indicated for all patients, but a systematic screening of functional capacities and needs is important.

When the collection, review, and interpretation of data are completed, problems are identified within the context of short-term and long-range goals in collaboration with the treatment team. The therapist and patient select activities for the purpose of controlled stimulation of appropriate adaptive behaviors. Tasks are analyzed and chosen on the basis of their inherent characteristics; the required antecedent skills; and their relevance to patient needs, interests, role expectations, and the likelihood of addressing specific treatment goals (Clark, 1979). They are used both for remediation of specific performance components and for the development and integration of those components within work, self-care, leisure time, and social settings. For example, a given activity may be chosen to provide appropriate sensory alerting stimuli to improve the ability to organize responses, to clarify cause and effect, to alter disorders in thinking and problem-solving, to provide structure and external control, to encourage self-expression and exploration, or to reinforce work skills and encourage independent functioning in activities of daily living (Fidler et al., 1981). With regard to the latter, special services such as pre-vocational programs are offered to evaluate vocational interests, aptitudes, and attitudes and to provide remedial work adjustment experiences dealing with work habits and related interpersonal behaviors. In all instances, desired changes in behavior are facilitated by the therapist in one-to-one or group settings through the structure, cues, "intervening objects," and interpersonal contacts inherent in activity-oriented experiences (Fine, 1980).

In addition to these remedial or treatment programs that address specific pathology, symptoms, and the residuals of illness by aiming at behavioral change, occupational therapy provides services directed toward sustaining and protecting intact functions and abilities and preventing further disability. In such instances, the primary concern is to provide activities that make it possible for the individual to use existing skills and interests; experience intrinsic gratification; and meet basic needs for acceptance, achievement, creativity, autonomy, and social interaction. In keeping with such goals, the occupational therapist's understanding of tasks, group process, and the importance of involvement provides many opportunities to organize and stimulate an active therapeutic milieu.

These categories of practice are not mutually exclusive but most often occur simultaneously. Their availability and use is, of course, modified by such factors as patient need (including developmental and age related issues), length of stay, and institutional priorities. For example, while short-term acute care settings cannot provide lengthy remedial experiences promoting ambitious rehabilitation outcomes, occupational therapists serve a particularly important and versatile role with regard to functional assessment, mobilization for rapid return to community living, and discharge planning. In many settings, they also are involved in providing transitional and long-term care in outpatient clinics and partial hospitalization programs so as to help newly discharged patients consolidate gains made during hospitalization and to work on longer-term issues revolving around vocational performance, independent living, and social-interpersonal skills.

PROFESSIONAL ISSUES

Founded in 1917, the American Occupational Therapy Association (AOTA) now represents more than 35,000 registered therapists, certified assistants, and students. The profession and its association have shown evidence of concern for quality of patient care by extensive involvement in developing professional ethics and formal standards of practice in mental health, developmental and physical disabilities, home health, and schools. The association has also placed a high priority on quality assurance as a means of monitoring practice. Standards of practice emphasize outcome studies and quality assurance. Sample quality review criteria for specific diagnoses have been prepared by AOTA and numerous state associations. In addition, active support for quality review, required by professional standards review organizations and the Joint Commission on Accreditation of Hospitals, occurs at both national and local levels.

Reimbursement for occupational therapy varies according to the setting in which it is provided. Public policy, as set forth in federal programs, generally emphasizes institutional care, although alternative care settings are now being explored. A medical referral for occupational therapy is usually a prerequisite to reimbursement from federal, state, and private reimbursement sources. Occupational therapy as a mental health specialty usually falls under the same limitations as other mental heath services outlined in federal, state, and private plans. Medicare, Medicaid, and private insurance companies generally reimburse for occupational therapy when the patient is in the hospital or is participating in an organized outpatient setting. Federal programs do not cover occupational therapy provided in private practice settings. However, private insurance companies will sometimes cover physician-referred treatment of this nature.

Occupational therapy practitioners are graduates of more than 60 professional educational programs offered at colleges and universities throughout the country. These programs meet standards approved by the American Occupational Therapy Association and the Committee on Allied Health Education and Accreditation of the American Medical Association. A combination of academic and field work characterizes basic professional training at both baccalaureate and master's degree levels. All preparation acknowledges the bio-psycho-social components of performance and adaptation. The basic sciences (anatomy, kinesiology, physiology, neurophysiology, neuroanatomy), the behavioral sciences (psychology, sociology, and human growth and development), occupational therapy theory, the study of medical and psychiatric conditions, and health care systems comprise the foundation of all academic programs. Occupational therapy theory and application involve studies of human performance and its sensory, biomechanical, cognitive, psychological, and social components; the meaning and impact of activity on normal states as well as illness; its application to neonatal, pediatric, adolescent, adult, and geriatric populations; and the therapeutic use of activities of daily living, leisure, social, prevocational and vocational activities, tests and measurements, and a range of creative-expressive and craft modalities. Didactic and supervised field work experiences integrate basic knowledge with clinical practice skills (i.e., functional assessment, treatment planning and implementation, therapeutic use of self, activity analysis, discharge planning, task-oriented group process, and documentation skills). A minimum of six months of full-time field work is required for basic professional education. Certification as a registered occupational therapist requires graduation from one of the aforementioned programs and successful completion of the National Certification Examination. Licensure is required in many states.

There are also more than 50 technical education programs for occupational therapy assistants. A certified occupational therapy assistant completes either a certificate course or an associate degree program approved by the American Occupational Therapy Association. Didactic course work provides an orientation to basic and behavioral sciences and emphasizes techniques and procedures for using the media and modalities of occupational therapy. Certification involves graduation from an approved program, completion of two months of required field work, and successful completion of the assistant level certification exam.

Master's and doctoral degree programs for registered occupational therapists are available. These prepare the therapist for specialized practice, for administrative/managerial roles, as educators, and for research.

REFERENCES

Ayres AJ: Sensory Integration and Learning Disorders. Los Angeles, Calif, Western Psychological Services, 1972

Clark PN: Human development through occupation: a philosophy and conceptual model for practice. Am J Occup Ther 33:505-514, 1979

Fidler GS, Fidler JW: Doing and becoming: purposeful action and self-actualization. Am J Occup Ther 32:304-310, 1978

Fidler GS, Fidler JW: Occupational Therapy: A Communication Process in Psychiatry. New York, Macmillan, 1963

Fidler GS: An overview of Occupational Therapy. White Paper. American Occupational Therapy Association, 1981

Fidler GS: The task-oriented group as a context for treatment. Am J Occup Ther 23:43-48, 1969

Fine SB: Psychiatric treatment and rehabilitation: what's in a name? J NAPPH 11:5,8-11, 1980

Gillette NP: Occupational therapy and mental health, in Occupational Therapy, 4th ed. Edited by Willard H, Spackman C. Philadelphia, Lippincott, 1971

Granofsky J: A Manual for Occupational Therapy in Pre-Vocational Exploration. Dubuque, Iowa, William Brown Book Co, 1959

Heard C: Occupational role acquisition: a perspective on the chronically disabled. Am J Occup Ther 31:243-247, 1977

Jones RE: Moral treatment: the basis of private mental hospital care. The Psychiatric Hospital 14:5-9, 1983

Kielhofner G, Burke JP: Occupational therapy after 60 years: an account of changing identity and knowledge. Am J Occup Ther 31:675-689, 1977

King LJ: 1978 Eleanor Clarke Slagle lecture: toward a science of adaptive responses. Am J Occup Ther 32:429-437, 1978

Matsutsuyu J: Occupational behavior: a perspective on work and play. Am J Occup Ther 25:291-294, 1971

Meyer A: The philosophy of occupational therapy. Archives of Occup Ther 1:1-10, 1922

Mosey AC: Occupational Therapy: Theory and Practice. Medford, Mass, Pothier Brothers, 1968

Occupational Therapy: Scope of Practice. New York, Metropolitan District-New York State Occupational Therapy Association, 1980

Occupational therapy: its definition and functions. Am J Occup Ther, 26:204-205, 1972

Reilly M: 1961 Eleanor Clarke Slagle lecture: occupational therapy can be one of the great ideas of 20th century medicine. Am J Occup Ther 16:1-9, 1962

20

Self-Help Groups

20

Self-Help Groups

INTRODUCTION

"Law, say the gardeners, is the sun" (Auden, 1953). Law, biologists might say, is change. We humans, like all other living organisms, conceal constant change within an envelope of apparent stability. And when people do show overt changes no one really knows *why* they occurred *then* and whether they will be maintained over time.

Each of the psychosocial therapies surveyed in this volume is based on theories about how people can and do change planfully. The "Reprise" provides a synthesis of the common elements of psychosocial interventions and reviews some prior formulations by many thoughtful colleagues. Minimum planning for such psychosocial interventions entails (a) positive expectations or hope on the part of both the helper and the helped, (b) exposure to one or more persons who are models for alternate behaviors or who otherwise expand the potential repertoire of the person being helped, and (c) cognitive and affective learning anchored by positive feedback after improved interpersonal experience(s). It should not surprise the reader that similar resources are often provided in self-help groups.

Somehow the phrase "self-help" seems strange when our psychiatric focus customarily is already on the "self." We know that induced change is better maintained over time when the changed persons feel that they, themselves, are responsible for whatever shifts have occurred. Yet "self-help" is at least a partial misnomer: The context provided by others always is a crucial factor for personal reorganization, for overcoming demoralization, and for embarking on new life paths. "Self-help" mostly refers to the fact that the helping others are not trained professionals. A widely used description/definition is:

> Self-help groups are voluntary, small group structures for mutual aid in the accomplishment of a special purpose. They are usually formed by peers who come together for mutual assistance in satisfying a common need, overcoming a common handicap or life-disrupting problem, and bringing about desired social and/or personal change. The initiators and members of such groups perceive that their needs are not, or cannot be, met by or through existing social institutions. Self-help groups emphasize face to face social interactions and the assumption of personal responsibility by members. They often provide material assistance as well as emotional support; they are frequently "cause"-oriented, and promulgate an ideology or values through which members may attain an enhanced sense of personal identity. (Katz and Bender, 1976)

Moreover, their defining attributes—which usually include starting from a condition of powerlessness, mandating personal participation (often associated with an underlying antibureaucratic tenor), and providing a reference group for affiliation and self-identification—differentiate such groups from service and philanthropic organizations, from various economic and political "mutual aid" groupings (unions, boards, cliques, etc.), and from natural associations of neighbors working together in an emergency or disaster or in transient encounter groups, etc.

HISTORICAL BACKGROUND

Sociologist Alfred Katz (Katz and Bender, 1976) writes: "Self-help through natural or created 'lay' groups and networks is both the oldest and the most pervasive system of care for human ills." He even cites anthropological studies suggesting that common interest groups, not based on kinship or propinquity, were widespread in ancient societies. Clearly, people have helped (and hurt) each other since the beginnings of humankind. The helping part did not receive much special notice. Various religious groups, orders of samaritans, and community organizations offered aid and asylum to those in need, but these activities clearly do not lie within our focus for this chapter. As Katz points out, even after Peter Kropotkin (1901) wrote *Mutual Aid: A Factor In Evolution* in 1901, little more about self-help and mutual aid appeared in the academic literature for the next 60 years.

Early studies include Bales' (1944) inquiries into the therapeutic role of Alcoholic's Anonymous (AA) groups, Wechsler's (1960) review of Recovery, Inc., Katz's (1961) discussion of Parents of the Handicapped, and Volkman and Cressey's (1963) examination of Synanon. Yet it was not until the 1970's that self-help groups and the "self-help movement" commanded more attention from both academic literature and public media. Self-improvement became widespread in paperback form, and the "movement" was noted in a variety of media affirmations and satires. At the same time professional resistance to self-help groups began to subside, as professional limitations for curing alcoholics, addicts, and chronic schizophrenics became more apparent. In the recent past years, we have seen the self-help movement flourish with varying degrees of success.

AA, which was organized in 1934, served as a template for a number of "anonymous" groups which have since been organized into self-help groups for gamblers (Gamblers Anonymous and Gam-Anon, 1957 and 1962) and neurotics (Neurotics Anonymous, 1965), to name just a few. AA probably remains the most frequently studied self-help group. Since its inception 50 years ago the format of this organization has endured essentially unchanged. AA is now estimated to have more than 500,000 members and 25,000 chapters around the world.

The Recovery method (Low, 1950; Wechsler, 1960; Lee, 1971) was originally initiated by psychiatrist Abraham Low, M.D., as a research project in 1937 at the University of Illinois Medical School. It subsequently was formed into the Association of Nervous and Former Mental Patients and became Recovery, Incorporated in 1941. It is the largest of all of the ex-patient self-help organizations in the mental health field, with a membership that includes approximately 15,000 persons in about 1,000 Recovery groups. The primary objectives of Recovery are to help prevent relapses or chronicity. After organizing and developing major precepts for Recovery, Low intentionally stepped aside from the group so that it would function as it does now, almost totally as a lay organization.

Another well noted self-help group, Synanon, functions as an alternative community in the drug abuse field. Synanon was founded in 1958 by an ex-alcoholic and AA member who had rejected the spiritual implications of AA. Synanon views itself as a "secular religion" with an obligation to influence its members beyond the drug abuse sphere by maintaining continued participation in Synanon's "community life." Their community approach to drug abuse has influenced the formation of such programs as Day-Top in New York City, Delancy Street in San Francisco, and others. Synanon attempts to facilitate and strengthen in-group bonds through the use of the "Synanon Game," a powerful exercise of intensive group confrontation with the individual whereby the group demands that the former drug user shed the web of deceit (of himself and others) which usually characterizes users' lives and relationships. It is unfortunate that in recent years, and perhaps because of such controversial confrontation techniques, Synanon has experienced leadership problems and lawsuits because of accusations of violent actions and fiscal abuses.

Katz and Bender (1976) estimated that nearly one-half million self-help groups exist in North America alone, embracing many millions of participating members. Even when lobbying groups such as United Cerebral Palsy or National Cystic Fibrosis or weight watching groups such as Weight

Watchers or Take Pounds Off Sensibly (TOPS) are discounted, there remain a multitude in number and diversity of bona fide self-help groups.

Self-help groups now exist for people labeled in a variety of categories: ex-addicts, alcoholics, gamblers, prostitutes, and prisoners; people who are designated by various mental and psychological categories such as neurotics and anorectics; people who are medically stigmatized, who have special surgeries, various -ostomies, or suffer from malignancies; people who are concerned about their offspring, such as parents of gifted children and parents of handicapped children; and parents without partners. In addition to the 500 or so national organizations and derivative chapters, there also exist many ad hoc local groups. Reports from countries such as West Germany, Holland, Australia, Poland, Yugoslavia, the United Kingdom, and South America indicate the ubiquitous nature of self-help groups formed in the last three or four decades. Although differing in clinical focus, these self-help groups have common elements such as facilitating access to treatment and preventing disability, fostering ideologies, forming social institutions, and helping to develop empowerment strategies.

THEORETICAL ISSUES AND PHILOSOPHY

It is difficult to know exactly what has led to the proliferation of self-help groups. Many theorists carry their own distorting lenses with which they speculate. One condition that seems to promote the development of such groups is a dissatisfaction with professional care givers or a feeling that the latter have failed to meet the needs of these particular patient groups. Most self-help groups appear to have been founded by people who were unsuccessfully treated in traditional professional programs (e.g., alcoholics, addicts, abusing parents, etc.). On the other hand, some groups were formed because of the very success of the professional discipline (e.g., burn patients, persons who have had "heroic" surgeries, etc.) although these groups are far fewer.

The initiation of lay groups into the health care field may represent popular reactions against the dysfunctional aspects of the present health care system, particularly its dehumanizing, fragmenting features. Moreover, nonprofessional groups that offer the possibility of having more control over one's life attract many. More recently we have seen the emergence of "holistic health" progams, which embrace a variety of alternative therapies including diet, exercise, meditation, and biofeedback, among others. It has also been suggested that such groups develop in response to the increased sense of isolation of the individual in our expanded urban society. Groups facilitate the socialization and support derived from cohesive structure.

From an economic perspective, some theorists hypothesize that an exploitative system fosters the creation of self-help groups. When cases are either too "tough" for professional care or not economically rewarding, the patient then is "blamed" and is ostracized. Thus, alcoholics, addicts, and chronic mental patients become suitable candidates for self-help groups after seeking and failing at traditional health treatments. A curious paradox becomes evident when we examine the plight of the individual who seeks help. If the situation is bad enough, professionals are sought who are presumed to have refined the healers' art. Yet, if professional treatment is unsuccessful and the situation worsens, some individuals then turn to fellow sufferers in a final attempt to obtain help.

Our expanding population, mobility, increased urbanization, and technology have markedly altered old kinship patterns and rituals. Self-help groups add significant identifications for those who feel alienated. Clearly, these groups function as needed support systems and social networks. They can provide an enduring pattern of ties that improve adaptive competence by offering guidance, promoting emotional mastery, and offering peer support and validating feedback. Self-help organizations represent intentionally created social units rather than the family, work, or friendship-generated spontaneous social networks.

The organizational structure of the self-help group shows how group members may function alternatively as givers and recipients of "care." This is true of many forms of peer counseling whereby the counselor and counseled are involved in a mutually beneficial relationship. Perhaps the process of labeled deviants' forming social groups has a normalizing effect on the group itself. Levy (1976) maintains that cognitive restructuring is an integral part of how self-help groups work. Such restructuring includes demystification, information exchange, expansion of alternative perceptions, consensual validation, and elaboration of a substitute culture. Caplan and Killilea (1976) suggest that organizing into a group also helps to extend an individual's ego strength by sharing with the *group* his/her miseries and discomforts and by providing a community in which friendships take on a new meaning. Inherent in the structure and process of self-help groups such as Recovery and many others is the opportunity to practice resocialization.

What one thinks determines the possibilities for action. Cognitive and affective sets (readiness to respond in a particular direction) are mental constructions developed over time which function in the same way as any other ideological facilitators or constrainers of action. Although ideological and cognitive approaches as used by self-help groups are important, changes are promoted particularly through "peer psychotherapy."

In many self-help groups, the apparent incongruities are similar to those observed in conventional therapy. The member first acknowledges that he is helpless to overcome the problem by himself, yet he is obliged to take responsibility for his actions; he is reminded that he is free, yet a particular set of behaviors and treatment regimen are obligatory; and finally, while responsibility is focused on the individual, it is the helping peer group or the therapist-patient unit (in therapy) that provides the working intervention. Gartner (1979) suggests that it may be this very combination of an individual seeing himself as helpless while concurrently seeing a powerful group (or other) as having *the* way which may enhance therapeutic effectiveness.

Our first intimates, i.e., family members, clearly serve as the most powerful matrix for nurturance, growth, and potential healing; self-help groups may be understood as "quasi-families" (Foote and Cottrell, 1965). The other members of the group appear as surrogates for and perhaps more adequate extensions of those kinds of supportive relationship patterns. A context emerges in which there is a reciprocal equality in the self-help group quite different from the hierarchical authority that typifies professional-patient relationships. In the latter, boundary demarcations between helper and helped are evident, even if parenthetical: "I am okay (you are not), and I will help you find out how to be okay." The nonprofessional or self-help group diminishes those boundaries: "I personally know about your experience of feeling under water because *I* have been right there next to you." With some exceptions, self-help groups empower the direct knowledge of the membership and facilitate egalitarian rather than hierarchically structured leadership. Moreover, the lack of strong hierarchical organization itself may elicit membership activity and competencies.

COMMON ELEMENTS

A common element in many self-help group activities is to raise the member's sense of control and mastery over the environment, thus increasing self-confidence. Active participation is almost always a basic program element. The inevitable consequence of certain relationships (parent-child, professional-patient, etc.), no matter how benignly intended, is that the professional is always in a superordinate position, perpetuating a hierarchical relationship that sometimes serves to diminish the competence of the helped person: One becomes a passive recipient of the help, which inadvertently prolongs dependent relationships. "Participation in a self-help group more nearly simulates the stuff of adult life" (Katz, 1981), i.e., collateral rather than hierarchical relationships. There is nothing so competence-engendering as the bona fide experience of deserved success.

Perhaps the single most significant common denominator in self-help groups is the fact that one or more significant others, who have themselves lived through many of the same disheartening experiences, now are side-by-side with the supplicant. The other knows what the old experience is like *and* is demonstrating how he also has learned to play the required new role, e.g., as *ex*-addict, *ex*-mental patient, *ex*-off-the-wagon alcoholic, etc. And that person also has achieved valued status in the self-help organization. Synanon and a number of other self-help groups demand that the participant play a new role without necessarily understanding it: The person is required to act as if he understands, as if he is responsible, mature, and caring about others. The notion of a person being forced to adopt and necessarily then experience a new role may serve as a central explanation for how self-help groups (or even other therapies) are effective. Rather than knowledge, action precedes change. If one can be "socialized into the patient role" then perhaps self-help groups also can be used to socialize ex-patients into a "well role" (Parsons, 1951; Lee, 1971).

Mowrer's (1971) Intensity Groups' motto, "We alone can do it, but we cannot do it alone," is a pithy expansion of the self-help concept to emphasize human mutuality and communality. Within the various groups there generally is a united "we" that binds the group's members together. AA members proudly accept the stigma of "I am an alcoholic." Conversely, Recovery, Incs.' members are taught to normalize their experience, perceiving themselves as average and life as consisting mainly of trivialities. A common difficulty among fellow group members is in permitting themselves to be average and to envision life as trivial. Members are instead encouraged to become just human, rather than uniquely special, which may result in both disappointment and at the same time relief for many—for in the Recovery philosophy, problems can be approached in scale because all human beings are capable of both making and correcting mistakes.

It appears that a continuum of psychodynamic processes can be traced from individual therapy to family or group therapy to self-help. One difference, of course, resides in the presence or absence of a "trained" therapist. Yet in some self-help groups, lay persons, acting out of intuition, experience, and identification, achieve "therapeutic" results.

SOME SPECIFIC TECHNIQUES

The common elements of self-help groups were considered in the previous section. Although many commonalities exist among self-help groups, these groups maintain a variety of different intervention techniques. The overview for this section will begin with a detailed look at the Recovery, Inc., format and will then examine intervention techniques in a more generic sense.

Recovery is largely based on Low's (1950) book *Mental Health Through Will Training*. It attempts to teach participants to gain confidence in themselves and to come to the realization that since external situations cannot be controlled they must work on something over which they do have control (e.g., how they feel and react to situations). The size of Recovery groups varies; about 60 percent of all groups have six to 15 members. Mutual aid goes beyond the actual meeting so that if a member is experiencing problems for which he/she needs help, the member can call another member; calls are limited to five minutes but there is no restriction on the number of calls.

Groups meet weekly. After reading a chapter from Low's book or other materials or hearing Low on tape, each person is encouraged to recount examples of recent life situations and how using Recovery's principles has helped resolve attendant stresses. Sharing "trivial experience" is emphasized, and intimate personal details need not be disclosed. A special terminology is used as well as clear emphasis on taking responsibility for one's self. The structure of the meeting, the leadership, and the language prevent members from slipping into judgmental and/or treatment models in the meeting. Any discussion of doctors or medical problems is forbidden during the meetings. When members are under a doctor's care, Recovery, Inc., encourages them to follow their doctor's orders. Recovery, Inc., is overt in its disclaimers: It does not try to replace the member's therapist, physician, or counselor; it does not offer diagnosis, treatment, or professional advice or make professional referrals (although these obviously occur informally). Recovery, Inc., seems to have a good relationship with medical and other professionals.

The group's use of special language is informative about its philosophic and pragmatic orientation. For example, *averageness* refers to what one would strive for in handling the trivialities of everyday life, insofar as average people have both successes and failures. The *trivialities of everyday life* are those average daily experiences that cause people to get worked up rather than large occurrences. *Sabotage* is to undermine one's mental health; and *exceptionality* is a form of sabotage in which a person thinks of what is happening as being exaggerated and different from what happens to others. When high or unrealistic goals are set and are not accomplished, a feeling of exceptional failure develops. Good mental health demands that one have the *courage to make mistakes*. The two forms of temper are *angry temper* when one blames someone else and *fearful temper* when one blames oneself when something goes wrong. It is important to give oneself compliments or pats on the back, but such *self-endorsements* are directed at the effort rather than at the accomplishment itself. Members are taught to *use their muscles*, relax them or control them. Muscles are seen as being able to teach the brain (e.g., "If you think you cannot get up out of bed, you can move your muscles to get up even if the brain has been unwilling!").

Reading Low's works, regular meeting attendance, and practicing the techniques are a necessary part of the protocol. Members listen to each other's recountings of current life events with the guidance of the group leader. Leaders are veteran members who have received six months of training in demonstrating the method. Mental health professionals are welcome to attend meetings but may not participate as leaders. Recovery, Inc., emphasizes the similarity of the distressed person with all other people. Explicitly and implicitly, it suggests that normalcy, averageness, and destigmatization are important routes to reasonable functioning. The in-house jargon helps prevent the use of professional therapy language. Although there are many long-term members, one can get better and not need to continue in the group. About one-half of Recovery's members have not been hospitalized, and a quarter have had no psychiatric treatment. The underlying notion is that will-power can be strengthened usefully. Group members' attention is maintained on those things they can do to exercise and strengthen their competencies in will and action.

Most self-help groups have in common the anonymity of members, rotating lay leadership, and ritualized confessional formats of varying length and intensity. Often, the particular group's literature achieves a kind of sacrosanct quality. Low's taped voice, Dederich's Wisdom, and AA's Twelve Steps become canons of faith. The groups demand overt acknowl-edgment of the need for help, the desirability of taking only one event or one day at a time, and the primacy of taking responsibility for one's own be-havior.

AA's views of the alcoholic (i.e., one is an alcoholic for life) and the idea that it may be important for the person to hit rock bottom before he can change successfully stand in contrast to Recovery, Inc. The former promotes the assumption of a chronic defect model (the alcoholic is always only one drink from drunk) versus the normative citizen model of Recovery. The core question is whether problems are "cured" or merely "controlled." AA and Synanon members apparently are not encouraged to outgrow the self-help group, and such groups may assume a messianic form: Their active proselytizing of others reflects the organizations' view that they provide an alternative way of life, significantly different from the normal track. The activities of the program become central in members' lives, and the group's "way" must be acknowledged as the only solution for the member.

According to Gartner and Reissman (1977), AA's major features are common to a number of self-help groups: a high degree of authoritarianism, a form of blaming the symptomatic person, acceptance of societal stigmati-zation, and a need for behavioral reform by the individual who accepts the prevailing cultural and social values. Members are enjoined to abstain from the prohibited behavior and publicly shamed for backsliding; yet the organization balances those punitive sanctions with status rewards for meritorious action. Each anonymous member is held responsible for his conduct (three-quarters of AA members are men) and is to accept the proposition that while the individual is powerless over alcohol, his problem can be overcome through careful and searching self-appraisal, public disclosure, and specific responsible behaviors.

Relatives of identified, stigmatized, or deviant people also participate in many self-help groups. Al-Anon, Gam-Anon, Alateen, Mended Hearts, Prison Families Anonymous and other groups are designed to inform the relative of the nature of the problem and to help the relative cope by providing understanding and support to the symptomatic person. The groups provide lectures, literature, and open discussion. Some organizations, involving both relatives and identified patients, have considerable political potency (National Association for Retarded Citizens, United Cerebral Palsy, etc.). Relatives emphasize the value of realizing that they are not alone and that there is a place where they can address their negative feelings about the identified patient without necessarily feeling guilty. Other groups such as Parents Without Partners and various widows' associations also are helpful in combatting the social isolation the person otherwise experiences when placed in a (temporarily) deviant role in society. Parents Without Partners implicitly recognizes the practical hardship of the single parent role position and addresses the inferred belief that the prevailing social norm, parents *with* partners, is morally better, rather than only practically advantageous.

Gamblers Anonymous, established in 1957 by AA members, similarly follows a simple, unvarying format. The credo is read aloud; and each member gives a "weather report," a recounting of past sins and an endorsement of current progress via Gamblers Anonymous activities. Many other "anonymous" groups have adopted AA's Twelve Steps or other ritualized credos, processes, or language. One extreme example of ritualization might be the "Synanon Game," which forces powerful personal confrontation of "total honesty," going several steps beyond the self-confessionals of most anonymous groups.

A relatively recent source of additional impetus to the self-help trend has been the feminist movement. In the past, women's traditional role in the social hierachy has served as a constraint on the development of autonomy and self-reliance. Data suggest that such factors play a significant role in the higher incidence of depression in women (twice that of men) and their greater use of tranquilizers, barbiturates, and physician visits. The "Women's Movement" maintains that the persistence of those stereotypes perpetuates dysfunctional conditions for women today. Increased dissatisfaction has led to the development of supportive or "rap" groups which include various women's health coalitions. Emphasis is on learning about one's own body and taking responsibility for and making informed decisions about one's health. Consciousness-raising groups (usually consisting of about six to ten women who meet on a regular basis) are the mainstay of these groups. A facilitator may be present to help the group in its formation, but often the groups proceed without advice, interpretation, or expertise. The consciousness-raising format is also used to address specific problems (e.g., abortion, rape, battering, etc.). During consciousness-raising meetings members share personal experiences that are often painful and guilt-ridden. The groups provide support by enhancing members' reality testing, self-esteem, individuation, and plans for assertive action. One of the strongest advantages of such groups is that women's need for bonding becomes a source of strength rather than a vulnerability. Professional help is looked upon with suspicion by many consiousness-raising groups. Some groups support and value members' continuing or initiating psychotherapy, while others tend to frown upon it. Co-counseling in which two individuals exchange the roles of client and counselor is particularly helpful to women who have felt patronized by patriarchal professionals.

CLINICAL ISSUES—INDICATIONS AND LIMITATIONS

According to Katz and Bender (1976), self-help groups also are especially useful for persons whose social networks have been disrupted, those in significant life transitions or crisis, or for the parents and relatives of chronically ill or handicapped persons. They further suggest that self-help groups can be effective in helping to reduce a large variety of normative stresses (changes of social status, moving, etc.).

AA's growth and use by professional referrers may either reflect its effectiveness or the relative ineffectiveness of other interventions. There are some data that suggest that those who do well in the "will power" model of Recovery are often poor candidates for the AA treatment paradigm in which the individual concedes powerlessness (Trice, 1957).

Do self-help groups treat "merely" symptoms? Can they be helpful in avoiding disability or preventing new problems. These questions reflect a more general uncertainty in defining "illness" versus symptoms and in trying to formulate whether a whole host of psychosocial treatments, including self-help, are synergistic, adjunctive, alternative, or substitutive.

Although anecdotal examples of self-help successes abound, there is little in the way of hard research on which to base our evaluations. Hanus Grosz, M.D., professor of psychiatry at Indiana University, reported in *Psychiatric News* (Grosz, 1972) on a random sample of 100 recovery groups. Forty percent of participants had been attending for more than two years, and over 25 percent fewer than six months. Approximately half the respondents in his survey had been hospitalized for a psychiatric illness before they joined Recovery, Inc., and 25 percent of the group had more than two hospitalizations. Grosz' view is that it is in the area of chronicity that Recovery, Inc., is most helpful and especially in the development of psychological skills to cope with symptoms and to promote attitude change.

Although data are not available, common sense dictates that patients not be placed in positions of unnecessary conflict and divided "loyalties." If a patient is seeing a therapist who is uncomfortable with adjunctive "self-help," or if the group is covertly anti-professional and views itself as a frankly preferred substitutive treatment, one would speculate that the resulting situation would be unfavorable for the patient. Presumably, therapists prefer to see, cure, and discharge patients. Certain self-help groups (e.g., AA, Synanon, etc.) view membership as a lifetime proposition. Stable membership in the other self-help groups may reflect dissatisfaction with professional processes or point out deficits in what the organized service system offers.

DEVELOPMENTAL AND AGE RELATED ISSUES

Four-fifths of the members of Recovery, Inc., are between ages 30 and 65. Young persons are not usually represented in self-help groups (exception: Alateen and other specially designed groups), probably because such groups often draw membership from people who have already "made the rounds," i.e., been involved with a number of therapies and therapists. Young people are just not "chronic" enough. This situation may change in view of the recent apparently expanded number of street-loose psychotic young people who cannot be held in institutions for treatment.

PROFESSIONAL AND ETHICAL ISSUES

There is no apparent consensus among self-help groups as to the extent of their collaborative efforts with professionals. Some groups are strictly nonprofessionally oriented while others work in a synergistic fashion with professionals. Perhaps a third of the members of self-help organizations use professional services. Recovery, Inc., for example, stresses that it provides services that are quite different from those of professionals. Interestingly, approximately one-third of Recovery's members are referred to the group by professionals.

Ethical issues that must be addressed by both professional and non-professional groups include quality control, treatment efficacy, possible harm to group members, breach of the group's rules about confidentiality, and undue prolongation of dependent relationships.

Self-help group leaders typically are group members who have worked successfully within the group and have then had some additional training, usually quite limited. Obviously, harm can result when well-meaning nonprofessionals (or insensitive professionals) go too far or too fast with group members. Another potential harm is self-help group attrition. When people drop out of self-help therapy they may tend to devalue themselves and intensify negative self-concepts, self-blame, and feelings of inadequacy and alienation.

The groups usually function on a first-name basis and require that what is reported/confessed/revealed in a group meeting be held in confidence.

Despite the ready possibilities of breaches (or even blackmail), no reports of such have been found.

Therapeutic efficacy is a complicated issue. Widespread belief and some data suggest that results achieved in self-help groups for some forms of addiction, alcoholism, and perhaps delinquency are better than those obtained in more conventional psychosocial therapies. Clearly, the self-selecting nature of self-help groups tends to ensure that those who remain feel most comfortable and positive about the group and may be those who are most likely to be helped. Similar arguments can be posed about all self-selected therapies.

SOCIAL/POLITICAL ISSUES

In times of economic hardship, legislative and administrative bodies diminish funding for public mental health services, causing already short-staffed clinics to increase group work and reduce one-to-one sessions. Paraprofessional training and services are then justified by several rationales. Undoubtedly similar changes occur in the private sector as well. But it is clear that economic factors as well as treatment efficacy determine what types of treatment are used.

The spread of nontraditional health maintenance models, self-care, and self-help groups has added to the need for serious review in the planning of cogent social policy. Most self-help groups are both instrumental and expressive in that they provide services in addition to social support and can be viewed as alternative service systems, sometimes competing with currently institutionalized systems.

SUMMARY

Self-help groups are a useful addition to contemporary psychotherapy. Their common theme is that it is helpful to work in a group context with peers who have had similar life-stressing experiences. Confessional and inspirational motifs are frequent in such groups, while successful peer models are available for identification. The focus on present relationships, problems, and activities takes priority. Cognitive learning, experiential shifts (sometimes through enforced behavioral change), and effective group interactions all contribute to the self-help group's impact. The significant commonalities for such groups appear to be acceptance, emotional support, and availability. Indeed, self-help groups serve also to remind us all that an effective preventive measure against emotional dysfunction is the establishment and maintenance of social ties.

REFERENCES

Auden WH: Law, say the gardeners, is the sun, in Concise Treasury of Great Poems. Edited by Untermeyer L. New York, Doubleday, Permabooks, 1953

Bales R: The therapeutic role of alcoholics as seen by a sociologist. Q J Stud Alcohol 5:267-278, 1944

Caplan G, Killilea M (eds): Support Systems and Mutual Help: Multidisciplinary Exploration. New York, Grune & Stratton, 1976

Foote N, Cottrell L: Identity and Interpersonal Competence. Chicago, University of Chicago Press, 1965

Gartner A, Riessman F: Self-Help in the Human Services. San Francisco, Jossey-Bass, 1977

Gartner A: Self-help and mental health. Reflections 14:25-49, 1979

Grosz H: As cited in "Study Indicates 'Recovery' Doing Well as Self-Help Program," Psychiatric News 7(14):10, 1972

Katz AH, Bender EI (eds): The Strength in Us: Self-Help in the Modern World. New York, Franklin-Watts, 1976

Katz AH: Self-help and mutual aid: an emerging social movement? Annual Review of Sociology 7:129-155, 1981

Lee DT: Recovery Inc: a well role model. Mental Hygiene 55:194-198, 1971

Levy LH: Self-help groups: types and psychological processes. Journal of Applied Behavioral Science 12:310-313, 1976

Low AA: Mental Health Through Will Training. Boston, Christopher, 1950

Mowrer OH: Peer groups and medication: the best "therapy" for professionals and laymen alike. Psychotherapy: Theory, Research, and Practice 8:44-54, 1971

Parsons T: The Social System. Glencoe, Ill, Free Press, 1951

Trice HM: A study of the processes of affliction with Alcoholics Anonymous. Quart J Study Alcohol 18:39-54, 1957

Volkman R, Cressey D: Differential association and the rehabilitation of drug addicts. Am J Sociol 69:129-142, 1963

Wechsler H: The self-help organization in the mental health field: Recovery Inc: a case study. J Nerv Ment Dis 130:297-314, 1960

21

Psychotherapy Outcome Research

21

Psychotherapy
Outcome Research

INTRODUCTION

Reviews of the psychotherapy outcome literature which have been published during the past three decades reveal a steady growth in the number of research studies dedicated to measuring the outcome of psychotherapy. In addition, they show an increasing preoccupation with the details of methodology and a growing concern with meeting rigorous research standards.

Over the years we can detect an increase in the degree to which various aspects of the research have been made explicit. For example, research diagnostic criteria are more and more frequently used to diagnose patients; and psychometric tests are often added to provide precise figures on the degree of a patient's symptomatology. There has also been an increase in the number of manuals prepared by advocates of particular modalities of psychotherapy to enable clinicians to conduct therapy in a comparable manner. In addition, audio or video tape recordings are made so that independent assessors can determine whether the therapists are, in fact, following the guidelines provided by the manuals. Attention has also been given to the more precise specification of outcomes and to defining the personality of the therapist. Finally, increased attention has been paid to the problem of control or comparison groups.

Thus, we have an apparent picture of robust growth of research, healthy skepticism, increased precision, and more sophisticated methodology.

EFFICACY ISSUES

Historical Trends

Many people identify the beginning of the critical evaluation of psychotherapy outcome research with the review by Eysenck (1952), which was based on 24 reports that he collected from various sources, most of which did not describe any controlled investigations of psychotherapy. The arguments were indirect and inferential, and statistics were uncritically pooled. Instead of being ignored, the review, which threw doubt on the efficacy of psychotherapy, stimulated despair, anger, criticism, and rebuttals. Despite the belief of some (e.g., Bergin and Lambert, 1978; Meltzoff and Kornreich, 1970; Vandenbos and Pino, 1980) that Eysenck's arguments have been undermined and defeated, it is interesting to note that a paper published in 1980 in a prestigious psychological journal has essentially resurrected Eysenck's critique and argued that his claims have never been adequately dealt with (Erwin, 1980).

To illustrate some of the diversity of opinion resulting from the various reviews of the literature, a number of authors may be quoted or cited. In 1964, Cross stated that the "efficacy [of psychotherapy] has not been scientifically demonstrated beyond a reasonable doubt." In 1966, after reviewing 14 controlled studies of psychotherapy, Dittman stated that his own "conclusions are modest, and are, moreover, diluted by confusion." On a more optimistic note, Meltzoff and Kornreich (1970) concluded that "controlled research has been notably successful in demonstrating more behavioral change in treated patients than in untreated controls." More cautiously, Bergin (1971a) stated that "psychotherapy, as practiced over the last 40 years, has had an average effect that is modestly positive." Malen (1973) arrived at a mixed conclusion after his review of the literature. He stated that "there is considerable evidence that dynamic psychotherapy is effective in psychosomatic conditions; but, that the evidence in favor of dynamic psychotherapy . . . [for] neurosis and character disorders . . . is weak. . . . "

The review by Luborsky et al. (1975) concludes that "everyone has won and all must have prizes," meaning that no one psychotherapy is more effective than any other. Frank (1979) concludes from his review of the literature that "psychotherapy . . . [is] more effective than informal, unplanned help."

That these conclusions do not apply only to individual therapy may be illustrated by citing several reviews of other modalities. In a survey covering 42 years (1921-1963) of group psychotherapy with psychotic patients, Stotsky and Zolik (1965) concluded: "The results of controlled experimental studies do not give clear endorsement for the use of group therapy as an independent modality." In 1971, a review by Bednar and Lawlis came to the same conclusion. More recently, Parloff and Dies (1977) reviewed the group psychotherapy outcome literature for the period 1966 to 1975. Because they were particularly concerned with "real" patients rather than volunteer college students or growth potential groups, their analysis covered group therapy as used with schizophrenics, psychoneurotics, offenders, and addicts. They concluded that the research evidence indicated that group therapy had little or no effect on schizophrenics or addicts and that the evidence was too limited or irrelevant to make any decisions about its effects on delinquents or psychoneurotics. They wrote: "Very little can be concluded regarding the efficacy of group psychotherapy." Essentially similar conclusions of little or no *proven* efficacy have been reached in reviews of the literature on family and marital therapy (Gurman and Kniskern, 1978) and social and milieu treatments (Mosher and Keith, 1980). The only recent reviewers of the literature who present their conclusions in positive and stronger terms are Smith et al. (1980).

Controlled Studies

Over the years, the general trend has been for the recent and more comprehensive reviews to conclude that psychotherapy is effective for a variety of symptomatic and behavioral problems, i.e., chronic moderate anxiety states, simple phobias, depressive symptoms, sexual dysfunctions, adjustment disorders, family conflicts, and communication difficulties.

A large number of studies have been concerned with combined treatment for various diagnostic conditions. Research on schizophrenia has not shown that traditional psychotherapies significantly enhance the benefit of pharmacotherapy, but the effects of the psychotherapy are much more difficult to quantify than are the drug effects. However, token economy therapies and psychosocial rehabilitation are valuable as an adjunct treatment for schizophrenics. Studies of drug/psychotherapy interactions for major affective disorders reveal that psychotherapy for some depressed patients produced better results and that the effects of psychotherapy plus drugs are basically additive in treating depression. Studies of psychotherapy for medically ill patients suggest that psychotherapy plus a medical regimen is more effective in influencing some of the target symptoms for certain medical illnesses than is medical treatment alone. Psychotherapy is especially useful for post-illness psychosocial rehabilitation. A general conclusion about interaction effects is that drugs affect symptoms relatively early whereas psychotherapy has an influence on interpersonal relations and social adjustment, especially at a later stage of treatment.

Relatively little research has been directed toward the question of the effectiveness of psychotherapy with patients of different ages. The limited findings suggest that children show both higher "spontaneous remission" rates and higher rates of improvement due to psychotherapy. Variables such as parent levels of motivation, the children's symptoms and diagnoses, and types of therapy are probably important but have not been systematically studied. Only about 15 investigations have been reported for adolescents which compare a treated group with a control group. Results indicate that about two out of three adolescents benefit from psychotherapy, while about one out of three improve in the control conditions. The available data strongly support the role of psychotherapy for adolescents. Unfortunately, the literature on psychotherapy for the aged is largely anecdotal and greatly in need of expansion.

Although a number of papers have proposed the possibility of deterioration effects due to psychotherapy and anecdotes on this topic have been reported by clinicians, research data on the subject are limited. In addition, the idea of negative effects is fraught with conceptual as well as research problems. The most extensive review of this literature comes to the conclusion that about five percent of patients in psychotherapy get worse (Sloane et al., 1975).

A few investigations have dealt with the aspects of the cost-effectiveness or cost-benefits of psychotherapy which are, at best, difficult to measure and perhaps are immeasurable. These studies have examined variables related to the delivery of care, have compared alternative treatment programs, and have determined the effects of psychotherapy on medical utilization. The results support the conclusion that community-based programs are more cost-effective than institutional treatment. Several studies have shown that the provision of minimal amounts of psychotherapeutic contact tends to decrease the use of medical services over a short time period. Overall, it appears that the economics of delivering psychotherapy, including salary and rent costs, determine measurable cost-effectiveness more than the techniques used.

Controversy still reigns over the question of whether certain types of therapy are more effective than other types for certain kinds of problems. Another issue that also has not been adequately studied is what aspects or elements of the complex therapeutic interaction are relatively the most effective. Then there is the question of spontaneous remission, which may be high in certain conditions.

In addition, the comparability of therapies bearing the same generic labels has been challenged, and many investigators have noted that relatively little is known about the actual process of psychotherapy and about the degree of variation that exists in the way it is carried out. Attempts are now being made to create manuals designed to provide guidelines for the therapist on the conduct of different modes of therapy. Such guidelines may be useful in controlled research settings but are believed by many clinicians to be largely unsuitable to the operation of their day-to-day practice. It is unclear at the present time whether this apparent conflict between the research demands of reproducibility and standardization will ever be reconciled with the clinicians' need for flexibility, creativity, and sensitivity to the uniqueness of individual patients.

Among the important conclusions of the various reviews of psychotherapy outcome is that better controlled studies do not show that therapy is more (or less) effective than do the less well controlled studies. The demonstrable effectiveness of psychotherapy appears to depend, at least in part, on the type of outcome measure used.

The Relation Between Research and Practice

Do research data have any substantial impact on the practice of psychotherapy? Parloff and Dies (1977) have given their answer: There is "indisputable evidence that clinicians have long been able to resist the offerings of the researcher. . . . " Garfield (1981) points out that "in spite of repeated and often harsh criticisms of psychotherapy's effectiveness, psychotherapeutic activities have continued to grow and develop in various ways." This growth is evidenced in several areas. The first is the large increase in the number of people providing psychotherapeutic services. They include not only psychiatrists and psychologists but social workers, nurses, pastoral counselors, and lay people with various types of training. A second sign of growth is the large increase in the types of psychotherapies which have become available, including such therapies as transactional analysis, transcendental meditation, primal scream therapy, and dozens of variants on these themes.

PROBLEMS IN PSYCHOTHERAPY RESEARCH

There are many reasons for the ambiguous picture of the field of psychotherapy in relation to research. Some are sociological, some economic, some psychological, and some methodological. The reviews of the literature have continued to reveal many methodological problems in much of the published research, so that the conclusions reached, whether positive or negative, have an air of ambiguity. The following sections will describe some important methodological issues in order to shed light on this source of uncertainty in judging and using the findings of psychotherapy research.

Description of Patients

A critical issue encountered in research on psychotherapy concerns an adequate description of the population selected for investigation. Patients coming to psychotherapy, far from being relatively homogeneous, are quite heterogeneous on almost every measure that one could devise (Kiesler, 1966). They differ on a host of dimensions, including intelligence; age; the nature, duration, and severity of their problems; as well as degree of motivation for therapy. These differences make them differently receptive to different forms of therapy (Strupp and Bergin, 1969).

It has been argued by some (Kazdin and Wilson, 1978; Marks, 1969) that in carrying out research, homogeneity of patient samples is desirable for a number of reasons. First, there is little to be gained by subjecting to a given treatment a group of patients representing a mixture of diverse syndromes, only some of whom may be expected to respond to that treatment. The nonresponding patients might very well mask an effect on the one syndrome that is improving.

Once the characteristics of a given form of treatment and the type or types of patient populations who are likely to respond to it are relatively well established, the results of outcome studies are less ambiguous and more clearly interpretable if samples of patients are selected who are relatively homogeneous in their personal characteristics, the nature of their difficulties (Fiske et al., 1970), or their situational contexts (Horowitz, 1976). This strategy is most likely to lead to studies showing differentiated successful treatment (Bordin, 1974a, 1974b). A second reason for choosing a relatively homogeneous sample that is explicitly defined is that meaningful comparisons may be made across studies (Paul, 1967). Also generalizations to other samples can be relatively unambiguous (Klein et al., 1980).

One important difficulty may arise in the attempt to assemble a homogeneous sample of patients, particularly if the disorder under consideration is an uncommon one. That is, in any one setting only a small number of patients may be suitable for inclusion in the sample one wishes to study. In practice, this means that the process of selecting patients could take a very long time or that collaboration with other investigators would be the best strategy.

There is, however, another side to the issue of the desirability of homogeneous patient samples which is seldom mentioned. When, for example, a treatment, be it psychosocial or psychopharmacological, is relatively new and untried, it would be more advantageous to give it to a random sample of patients with a wide range of symptoms in order to determine those for whom it is most efficacious. Conceivably, patients with more than one type of disorder could be responsive, and that fact would be obscured and generalizations reduced by strict adherence to homogeneity of sample selection. It is evident, therefore, that the desirability of a homogeneous or a heterogeneous sample of patients depends to a great extent on the level of development and usage of the particular therapeutic modality under consideration.

Standardizing Diagnoses

In 1972, Feighner, Robins, Guze, Woodruff, Winokur, and Munoz provided diagnostic criteria for 14 psychiatric illnesses. The aim of this approach was to provide a framework for comparison of data gathered in different centers and to promote communication among investigators. These criteria, modified and expanded expressly for research purposes by Spitzer et al. (1978), became the Research Diagnostic Criteria (RDC). They were designed to enable researchers to apply a consistent and standardized set of criteria for the description or selection of relatively homogeneous samples of subjects with functional psychiatric illnesses. Many of the terms and criteria found in RDC have been incorporated into the *Diagnostic and Statistical Manual of Mental Disorders, Third Edition (DSM-III)*, the revised nomenclature of the American Psychiatric Association (Karasu and Skodol, 1980).

Even with standardized diagnostic schemas, it is clearly desirable to have diagnoses made by two or more clinicians, at least until such time as it has been determined that there is a high degree of agreement among them. Also, although researchers are fundamentally in agreement that the criteria provided by *DSM-III* represent an improvement over previous idiosyncratic schemas, it is desirable to use multiple measures relating to diagnostic issues, particularly in studies in which diagnosis is a significant variable. Diagnosis could, for example, be supplemented by additional criteria based on scores obtained on standardized rating scales, i.e., those measuring symptoms or personality traits (Garfield, 1978).

There is still a clear need for better methods of assessing the totality of a patient's functioning in terms of both strengths and weaknesses (Strupp, 1978). One recent attempt to develop measures of strengths as well as of dynamic factors is given in the report on Sequential Diagnostic Evaluation by Plutchik et al.,* which includes scales for measuring ego strength, ego function, ego defenses, and coping styles.

Description of Therapists

Another research concern is the appropriate definition or description of the therapist. Like patients, therapists differ on a multitude of dimensions including age, sex, cultural experience, psychological sophistication, and social values (Strupp, 1978). They also differ among themselves on such factors as professional discipline, training, professional experience, belief in the efficacy of treatment, personal therapy, interests, and personality (Fiske et al., 1970; Meltzoff and Kornreich, 1970; Sundland, 1977).

It is difficult to understand, at least since Kiesler (1966) presumably laid to rest the "therapist uniformity assumption," how therapists can be considered interchangeable units. Yet it is the rare study that even provides information on the competence of the therapists (Luborsky et al., 1975) or that defines the therapist sample in any greater detail than "experienced,"

---

*Plutchik R, Karasu TB, Conte HR, et al: Sequential psychodiagnostic evaluation. Presented at the 11th annual meeting of the Society for Psychotherapy Research, Pacific Grove Calif, June 17-20, 1980.

"senior clinicians," or "inexperienced" therapists. As May has pointed out, even the definition of experience may be a good deal more complex than it first appears. "Counting patients previously treated or hours of patient contact will not satisfy those who insist on a judgment of skill. But how reliable and valid are judgments of skill? . . . Skill in doing what?" (May, 1974). At the present time there seems to be no consensus on how to describe adequately the "therapist qua therapist" or on how to assess the impact of therapist characteristics on the efficacy of treatment.

Nevertheless, it is obvious that such personal characteristics of therapists as adequacy of adjustment, liking of and regard for the patient, genuineness, empathy, and nonpossessive warmth (Bergin, 1971b; Lambert et al. 1978; Truax and Mitchell, 1971) are all relevant to the extent to which a therapist can form a helping relationship with the patient. It is, therefore, unfortunate that to date, serious research problems vitiate the findings of studies that attempt to relate patient change to selected therapist characteristics or qualities (Parloff et al., 1978; Schaffer, 1982). Efforts to characterize the therapist and his or her role in influencing the outcome of psychotherapy are important. Perhaps the therapist contributes equally with the patient to the outcome of the interactions that occur between them. However, "the exact contribution of relationship variables, their interaction with client characteristics, and their relative importance in contrast to specific techniques remains an area of continuing debate" (Lambert and Utic, 1982).

Description of Therapy

There can be little doubt that psychotherapy as currently practiced does not refer to a uniform, homogeneous process (Kiesler, 1966; Strupp, 1978). Further, although it might seem to be belaboring the issue, general categories of therapy such as behavior therapy and dynamic psychotherapy obviously include different techniques. Yet these global entities have been compared empirically (Sloane et al., 1975) and in reviews of outcome (Luborsky et al., 1975) as if one could make a general conclusion about "behavior therapy" or "psychotherapy" per se.

One of the major difficulties in psychotherapy research is that of adequately specifying and describing what actually goes on during treatment. However, relying on the therapist's description of his treatment without further documentation does not provide sufficient definition of the treatment factor. When established treatment procedures are under consideration, this problem becomes even more complex because most experienced psychotherapists have developed their techniques in more or less idiosyncratic ways (Paul, 1976). In addition, therapists who are part of a strong theoretical tradition develop ways of discussing their therapeutic efforts which may or may not be direct translations of what they actually do in their therapeutic encounters (Bordin, 1974a, 1974b).

The therapist's description of therapy is insufficient by itself. It must be supplemented by other specifications in order to evaluate whether or not a technique has been properly conducted. For example, supervisors' reports may be included to correct for biases in the therapists' observations, but supervisors themselves may be subject to theory-dictated observational biases. Independent observers may provide descriptions based on audio or video tapes of selected therapy sessions or portions of sessions. However, the problem of definition of treatment still is not completely solved inasmuch as even with video taping, only a relatively limited aspect of the therapist's behavior is selected for observation (Bordin, 1974a, 1974b). In addition, the process of analyzing tapes is time-consuming and costly. Nevertheless, these independent observations are indispensable to an adequate definition of the actual therapeutic process. However, few, if any, psychotherapists are prepared to welcome independent observers into their offices.

Nature of Control Groups

Once the population under investigation has been defined, it is then necessary to specify the appropriate control or comparison groups and to determine how to draw the total sample. During the time period represented by a psychotherapeutic intervention, patients are experiencing many other influences, and any change noted may be due to any or all of these influences. Studies purporting to show that a particular treatment has produced changes must permit the inference that had the treatment not been introduced, the observed changes would not have taken place. This means that controls must be introduced to rule out plausible alternative hypotheses.

The most straightforward strategy for controlling extraneous factors that could account for experimental findings is to use an untreated control group. Methodologically, a group receiving no treatment serves to control for such factors likely to jeopardize internal validity as history, maturation, the effects of repeated testing, and statistical regression (Campbell and Stanley, 1963).

In actual fact, however, the term "untreated controls" is probably a misnomer, particularly in psychotherapy research (Frank, 1966; Imber et al., 1966) because of the serious ethical and practical obstacles that would be encountered were an attempt made to use a genuine "untreated" control group. For example, if patients selected for the untreated group were truly comparable to those in the experimental group in terms of symptomatology and diagnosis, could a conscientious investigator refuse them treatment? Also, on the practical side, it is difficult to conceive of many patients in enough discomfort to seek treatment who would not look elsewhere if they were refused therapy in one setting. It thus seems evident that a true no-treatment group is virtually impossible to set up and maintain.

One way of circumventing the problems posed by attempts to use no-treatment controls which has been proposed by a number of investigators is the somewhat modified procedure of using "drop-out" patients or "waiting list" patients. Actually, however, these are not particularly adequate controls.

Drop-outs, sometimes called "terminator controls," are defined as those individuals who requested treatment but who, for one reason or another, did not keep any appointment or terminated very early during treatment, usually without the approval of the therapist (Imber et al., 1966). While they may be considered an essentially untreated group, a group composed of "drop-outs" has serious disadvantages. Not only do they drop out of treatment for different reasons and at different times, but they are also different kinds of people with potentially different eventual outcomes (Baekeland and Lundwall, 1975). The flaw involved in using these patients as controls lies in the fact that some unknown selection factor is operative in their termination and that, therefore, they represent a self-selected sample whose motivation for help is obviously different from patients accepting and receiving treatment (Gottman and Markman, 1978; Imber et al., 1966; Meltzoff and Kornreich, 1970).

Waiting list controls have advantages over those previously discussed. First, because most treatment centers are unable to offer therapy immediately, except possibly to acute cases, a waiting list is a natural aspect of their operation. Therefore, the investigator has the advantage of a naturally formed control group of patients, presumably no different from those currently in treatment. Second, because they have been guaranteed therapy, they are less likely to seek help elsewhere, particularly if therapy has been scheduled for a specific time in the future (Gottman and Markman, 1978). Third, while a waiting list control group does not control for expectancy effects (i.e. patients' expectations that the treatment will help them), it does provide crucial information regarding the natural history of the disorder. It is, therefore, particularly useful in the early stages of research with most clinical problems (O'Leary and Borkovec, 1978). For all its advantages, one problem with this type of control is that it permits a comparison of treatment with no treatment for only the period during which treatment is not provided (Sloane et al., 1975). No long-term comparisons between treatment and no treatment groups are possible because the waiting list group eventually receives treatment.

Another type of control group that has been used in both drug studies and studies in psychotherapy has been called an attention or placebo group. The term "attention" is usually used when the intervention is nonpharmacological, whereas the term "placebo" is generally reserved for drug studies. Whichever it is called, this type of group serves to control for such factors as the frequency of contacts and other nonspecific factors such as the patients expectation of improvement and faith in the value of the treatment they are receiving (Hampton, 1973; Kazdin and Wilson, 1978). Patients see a "therapist" with the same frequency as the group receiving treatment, but the content of their sessions is not designed to be therapeutic. At the very least, it should be neutral. The disadvantage in the use of attention/placebo controls lies in our supposed knowledge of what is therapeutic. These patients believe they are being treated, and there is a good deal of evidence that the physical and emotional status of patients in placebo groups can change significantly (Bergin, 1971a; Imber et al., 1966; Rosenthal and Frank, 1956). It is questionable, therefore, whether these patients are actually receiving "no treatment."

As another approach to the control problem, alternative treatment groups, with or without a "treatment-as-usual" condition, can be used. If, for example, the question is whether a new therapeutic approach is better than an old one, then the old one is the appropriate control (Meltzoff and Kornreich, 1970).

One additional and innovative type of alternative treatment control is the "PRN contact" group used by the Boston-New Haven collaborative depression study and briefly described by Weissman (1979). Treatment for patients in this group is provided only at the patients' request and not at a regularly scheduled time. This type of control group probably falls somewhere between a "waiting list" group and a regularly scheduled "low contact" group in terms of therapeutic interaction.

Another type of control group is implicit in the use of a crossover design. With this method, for a given period of time one group serves as the control while the other serves as the active treatment group. At the end of this period, the roles of the two groups are reversed. At the end of the course of treatment for the group that previously served as the control group, a comparison is made between the treatment and control conditions. There are basically two drawbacks to this method of obtaining a control group. First, it is possible that the group that first receives treatment improves sufficiently to be unable to provide an adequate control once treatment is discontinued. Second, while it is not likely, it is possible that patients in the initial control group could improve spontaneously to the point that when they are finally given treatment, there is no room for further improvement.

One way to circumvent the problem of obtaining an equivalent sample of patients for a control group is to use the experimental patients as their own controls. With "own-controls" designs, changes in a patient's behavior during a waiting period are compared with changes in that same patient after treatment. However, while having the advantage of requiring a smaller total sample, this approach has at least two serious drawbacks. One is that the pretreatment waiting period is almost invariably shorter than the treatment period itself, and this lack of temporal equivalence reduces the validity of comparisons (Imber et al., 1966; Paul, 1976). A second drawback to this type of control group is that for the design to be valid, one of two conditions must be met. Either one must have comparative data on the natural history of the disorder, obtained for a large number of patients; or a long period of baseline data must be obtained. Only if it can be shown that behavior remains relatively stable over time and then rather abruptly changes when treatment is introduced can one be fairly certain that the intervention is responsible.

Selection and Assignment of Patients to Groups

Let us assume that the population to be investigated has been decided upon and the type of control group or groups to be used has been established. One important issue that still remains is *how* to assign patients to the groups.

One of the most frequently used methods is random assignment. Basically, this means that patients are assigned to treatment and control groups on the basis of a method that prevents bias, such as through the use of a table of random numbers. This method of assignment assumes that in the long run, all significant variables will be equally distributed among the groups so that any differences found at the end of the study can be attributed, within statistically definable probability limits, to treatment effects rather than to extraneous patient variables. This is a good method so long as a sufficiently large pool of patients is available.

A second way to select individuals for groups is matching in pairs, particularly if one member of each pair is randomized to each treatment. This method involves matching control and treatment populations, patient by patient, on certain variables believed to be relevant such as age, sex, race, education, and family income. However, "since each additional matching variable greatly increases the size of the population that must be screened, this approach is hopelessly impractical in outpatient studies" (Frank, 1966). Furthermore, because a large number of potential subjects will not meet the matching criteria, such matching requires discarding a sizable percent of the total population, thereby endangering the representativeness of the samples.

A variation on this procedure of matched pairs is to assign individuals to groups in such a way as to ensure that group means for the variables in question will not be significantly different. This version of the matching procedure still presents formidable real-life difficulties. May (1974) emphasizes just how frustrating an experience matching can be as he describes the difficulties Rogers and his colleagues (1967) experienced in trying to match on six variables. Another drawback of this method is that when patients are matched on a number of supposedly relevant variables, they may, in fact, be mismatched on variables of equal or even greater importance.

RESEARCH DESIGNS FOR PSYCHOTHERAPY EVALUATION

Conceptual Problems

Research designs for investigating the effectiveness of a particular mode of psychotherapy or for studying the comparative efficacy of two or more therapeutic modalities cannot be classified into simple types since they may be characterized along a great many dimensions. For example, Campbell and Stanley (1963) discuss the pretest post-test control group design, factorial designs, and the equivalent time-samples design, among others. Meltzoff and Kornreich (1970) describe empirical, inductive, and hypothetico-deductive studies, univariate and multivariate designs, as well as prospective and ex post facto studies. Fiske et al. (1970) state that there are basically two types of approaches: experimental and correlational. Horowitz* describes three types of research paradigms: the contrast group design, the relational paradigm (correlational), and the descriptive approach. Plutchik (1968) describes random and matched groups designs; counterbalanced designs; and bivalent, multivalent, and parametric experiments. Kazdin and Wilson (1978) present a large number of treatment evaluation strategies, among which are constructive and dismantling strategies, comparative, and process strategies. It is evident that a number of different descriptive terms have been used to categorize the various approaches to the evaluation enterprise.

These different terms reflect the fact that research designs may be described in terms of levels of inference permitted, time period under consideration, type of sampling procedures used, number of variables considered, number of levels of each variable, and type of strategy employed. Therefore, the research design itself could be considered a variable that determines the level of inference of the results and their generality. As the design permits increasing control over possibly irrelevant or confounding variables, the number of alternative explanations to account for observed changes is reduced. While the researcher can never prove unequivocally that a particular therapeutic effort caused a particular outcome (Cronbach, 1978; Gottman and Markman, 1978), the reduction of alternative explanations increases his confidence that results are due to a specified intervention. Unequivocal conclusions about causal connections are never possible in psychotherapy research because psychotherapy is not a simple stimulus that produces a simple response. Psychotherapy is a highly complex set of interactions between two or more individuals extending over a period of time. Therefore, the selection of any one piece of this complex in-

---

*Horowitz MJ: Strategic dilemmas and the socialization of psychotherapy researchers. Presidential address delivered at the meeting of the Society for Psychotherapy in Aspen, Colorado, June 1981.

teraction as a causal agent is extremely questionable. However, as pointed out by Fiske et al. (1970), the objective should not be the impossible one of providing controls for every possible relevant variable but providing a framework that is replicable and that can provide at least a partial answer to an important question.

Research designs may be conceptualized as existing on five different and increasingly complex levels. At each succeeding design level, the possible confounding of variables is reduced and the resulting level of knowledge obtained is increased.

Design Level I (the one-shot case study). Level I is one in which a single group of patients is studied only once after some intervention and can be considered the lowest design level, inasmuch as studies using such a design have a total absence of control (Campbell and Stanley, 1963). It is, however, the only one possible if a course of treatment or program is already ongoing.

Design Level II (the one-group pretest post-test design). Level II involves measurement before, during, and after treatment. It is thus possible to determine with some precision the changes that occur during the period of treatment; however, there is still no control or comparison group, which prevents making adequate inferences about important variables that might influence outcome. No follow-up is planned to determine how lasting any observed changes may be.

Design Level III (extended baseline A-B design). Level III uses patients as their own controls. Repeated measurements of a behavior or symptom to be modified are made until a stable baseline is obtained. Treatment designed to be therapeutic is then introduced and continued for a period of time. If a fairly abrupt change is noted, and behavior had been relatively constant before therapy, in all likelihood the change is due to the treatment variable. There is, however, at least one drawback to this design: It will only show the effectiveness of therapies that produce rapid changes. Slow changes will not be evident. This type of design is also referred to as a single-case design.

Design Level IV (pretest post-test control group design). Level IV is what most people tend to think of as an adequately controlled study. Studies at this level involve one or more pre- and post-tests and one or more assessments during the follow-up period. The use of this level of design provides considerably more precise information than is provided by lower level designs. However, its biggest advantage is that it provides a control group whose purpose is to rule out alternative explanations for research findings, such as maturation and other changes produced by the passage of time. Furthermore, the inclusion of follow-up assessment permits determination of the duration of the effects noted at the end of treatment.

Design Level V (multivariate design). Level V involves the use of multiple pre-test measures, standardized intervention procedures, one or more control groups, process measures, and post-treatment and follow-up evaluations. The central advance at Level V is the opportunity to examine interactions, either within treatment, patient, or outcome factors, or across more than one domain of factors.

Each type of design has advantages and limitations, and not all good research need be conducted at Level V. Because of the tremendous investment in terms of personnel, time, money, and number of patients required by Level V designs, investigations at a lower level may be conducted prior to the initiation of these more complex designs. Their use is more properly reserved for investigations of the differential effects of treatments whose parameters are well specified and which are known to be effective for specific types of patients.

PRAGMATIC AND ETHICAL ISSUES

Research in psychotherapy poses a number of practical and ethical problems for which there are at present no truly satisfactory solutions. One concerns the issue of privacy and confidentiality. A second issue relates to the need for no-treatment or placebo/attention control groups; a third issue involves the use and implications of informed consent.

Privacy and Confidentiality

With regard to this first issue, the relationship between patient and therapist has traditionally been a confidential and privileged one (Karasu, 1980; Meltzoff and Kornreich, 1970). Yet increasingly in recent years, there has been external intrusion on this traditionally confidential relationship. The need for unbiased, objective data for the purposes of evaluation and research has led to the use of such devices as one-way screens, tape recorders, and motion picture cameras.

Some therapists hold that these intrusions constitute a violation of the intimate, private atmosphere of the therapeutic relationship. Furthermore, it is argued that the use of observational or recorded data for research purposes so alters the behavior of the participants that generalizations to sessions in which strict privacy is maintained are weakened. This position obviously tends to discourage research and hinders the acceptance of research findings.

No-Treatment and Attention/Placebo Controls

The second issue that has both pragmatic and ethical implications concerns the use of no-treatment or placebo/attention control groups. While the advantages of such experimental methods are well known and widely accepted, they raise a number of problems.

As previously discussed, one problem concerns the ethics of withholding treatment from those patients in the control group who are actively seeking help, even if the purpose is to advance our knowledge, with the ultimate goal of benefiting an even greater number of individuals. This problem is compounded when one considers the possibility that treatment prohibition for control patients could continue over several months or even years. There is, in addition, the practical difficulty of retaining patients assigned to a no-treatment group. Attrition over time is likely to be high, leaving the investigator with a sample certain to be biased in significant ways.

One solution to this problem is to use the "waiting list" approach. By randomly assigning a number of individuals to what amounts to a delayed treatment group, the ethical issue is surmounted. There are, however, problems with this solution, too, as already noted. First, this option is possible only when therapy is of relatively short duration. Second, it would only be viable for those patients who do not seek help elsewhere; and third, what does one do with an acutely psychotic or suicidal patient? He could be treated out of turn, but this would compromise the research design. He could be treated immediately and simply be dropped from the study. This approach, however, is likely to destroy the representativeness of the sample by restricting its range of severity of illness.

A second solution is to use an attention/placebo condition. This has the advantage of permitting randomization of patients and of controlling for patients' expectations. However, even if it were possible to develop a theoretically inert placebo condition, it is unlikely that therapists would be willing to implement it over any length of time; and even if they were willing, their expectations about the success of this treatment condition relative to other credible conditions would differ. Such differences would serve to confound results.

Informed Consent

A third issue having both pragmatic and ethical implications which arises in the conduct of research in psychotherapy, although not unique to this type of research, is the requirement for informed consent. To ensure that a patient's rights are not violated, participation in any study or experiment must be voluntary and based on the patient's or the patient's legal surrogate's informed consent. A number of government agencies and professional societies have provided explicit guidelines for the procedures to be followed in obtaining this consent. A practical drawback to the informed consent approach is that it may inhibit participation in some research.

One last problem with the use of informed consent is a conceptual one. How is "voluntary participation" of a committed patient in a state mental hospital or a prisoner in a penal institution to be interpreted? The patient may believe he has no choice, or he may not be fully capable of understanding the situation. In the case of the prisoner, it is not unknown for trade-offs to occur.

It is obvious that the use of informed consent is not a panacea for all the methodological and ethical problems that plague psychotherapy research. It is, however, still the best way of reconciling the conflict between our ethical responsibility to society to evaluate the efficacy of treatment and our ethical responsibility to protect the rights of human subjects.

In summary, there are three areas in which ethical issues lead to pragmatic difficulties and pragmatic issues lead to ethical problems. The invasion of privacy for the purpose of collecting the objective data necessary to evaluate psychotherapy systematically is one area. A second concerns the ethical issues involved in assigning patients with distressing problems to no-treatment or placebo conditions in order to provide baselines for evaluation of experimental treatments. The third area relates to the possible refusal to participate in a study or differential attrition which results from our ethical responsibility to obtain informed consent.

ASSESSMENT ISSUES

The problems relating to such issues as research design, patient selection, and the like can almost be considered as secondary to basic decisions regarding what needs to be assessed. Disagreement exists both on the question of what conditions need treatment (e.g., intrapsychic conflicts, interpersonal problems, and family conflicts, or such social problems as crime and delinquency) and on the question of what outcome criteria should be used to assess the consequences of treatment.

Controversies over outcome criteria have traditionally centered around such issues as how therapeutic change is to be assessed (e.g., subjective ratings, ratings of overt behavior, psychological test results), the source of information on which to base evaluation (e.g., the patient, the therapist, an independent observer, etc.), the generality or specificity of assessment (e.g., global personality ratings, ratings of such specific symptomatology as depression or anxiety, ratings of overt behavior), and whether the patient's status is to be assessed at only one point in time or whether the assessment includes the concept of changes or improvement. However, regardless of the criteria that have been chosen, the lack of concordance among outcome criteria used by different researchers has been a recurrent methodological difficulty.

This state of affairs is partly due to the fact that some investigators have selected criteria for making overall judgments of success or improvement from a specific theoretical frame of reference, and these criteria are likely to be only partially related to those selected from another point of view. For example, investigators with a psychoanalytic orientation, whose main concern is with intrapsychic functioning, are prone to select psychodynamic, cognitive criteria for the assessment of change in their patients. Behaviorists, in contrast, seek as criteria of change alteration in overt symptomatology and observable behavior. Others, perhaps those with a more idealistic value system, might consider as criteria for the success of treatment the enhancement of a patient's quality of life or the fulfillment of his positive capacities. The result is that evidence derived from different criteria is difficult to generalize. The use of different criteria also makes comparisons from one study to another ambiguous.

A recent attempt to deal with this problem has been the development of multiple measurement procedures that are applicable across different types of therapeutic techniques. Consensus exists that divergent processes occur in therapeutic change and that divergent methods of criterion measurement, both objective and subjective, are needed.

In general, research on the effectiveness of psychotherapy would benefit from an expanded set of outcome criteria. Techniques are likely to be differentially valuable across the available criteria so that one specific treatment may be superior to another only on one or a few criteria. Thus, "the treatment of choice for a given patient may vary depending upon the particular outcome criterion relevant to the individual patient's problem" (Kazdin and Wilson, 1978).

Strupp and Hadley's (1977) "tripartite model" suggests that psychotherapeutic outcome be viewed from multiple vantage points: the individual himself, society, and the mental health professional. The term "mental health" has somewhat different meanings when viewed from these different perspectives inasmuch as different value systems are involved. From the standpoint of society, whose concern is primarily with the prevailing standards of sanctioned conduct, mental health tends to be defined in terms of behavioral stability and conformity. The individual himself, however, wishes to be content or happy; consequently, for him mental health is equated with a sense of well-being. For the mental health professional, mental health tends to be defined with reference to some theoretical model of a "healthy" personality structure, the most comprehensive and ambitious of which is psychoanalytic theory.

Whether or not one accepts this model, there is general agreement in the following areas. Change is diverse; therefore, any single study of psychotherapy should incorporate a number of measures in order to enhance the sensitivity of the research and its comparability across studies. In addition, information about changes that have occurred or are occurring should be obtained from as many sources as possible. Among these are the patient, the therapist, independent observers, and significant others (relatives, friends, associates, etc.).

Measurement of Therapeutic Outcome

While an investigator may want to focus on a specific area of interest, e.g., interpersonal relationships, there are advantages to having instruments with a broad coverage which have been shown to be both reliable and valid. Most investigators, for example, would agree on the importance of evaluating subjective distress, overt symptomatology, and impairment in functioning. An advantage to this approach is that because the behaviors of interest can be described in such a way as to avoid theoretical assumptions, a comparison of therapeutic approaches based on different theoretical principles is possible (Spitzer and Endicott, 1975).

There has been a trend toward the development of measurement procedures that can be used across different types of psychotherapy. Notwithstanding the unique goals of particular therapies, there appears to be some support for the notion that changes produced by psychotherapy may be assessed by "batteries" of instruments which, through the use of several types of measurement procedures, attempt to assess the core changes that result from any psychotherapeutic endeavor (Waskow and Parloff, 1975).

While acknowledging that a routine battery such as that recommended by Waskow (1975) could be instrumental in coordinating and accelerating the advancement of knowledge about psychotherapeutic change, Bergin and Lambert (1978) express doubts that a single core battery could be effectively applied because of the differing theoretical and conceptual preferences of investigators as well as differences concerning valued directions of change. Nevertheless, they do not rule out the development of several core batteries that could be applied to treatment situations when appropriate. Gottman and Markman (1978) also express reservations about the "core battery" concept. They consider it a "step backward in psychotherapy research" inasmuch as it persists in viewing therapy and change as uniform concepts. As they see it, change measures should be geared to what the therapy intends to accomplish.

Nevertheless, there appears to be consensus that, when possible, information pertinent to outcome be obtained from multiple vantage points— the patient himself, the therapist, an independent observer, and relevant others.

Issues Related to Follow-Up

Two basic approaches have characterized follow-up research in psychotherapy. The first is what Liberman (1978) calls the "global-archival" one. With this method, a researcher makes an effort to locate patients who were treated and assessed at discharge two, five, or ten years previously in order to make a global assessment of their current condition relative to their status at the termination of treatment. Each patient is given a rating, e.g., "improved," "same," or "worse"; and the percentage of patients in each category is then determined.

Although a large number of studies using this approach have been conducted, primarily in European settings, it is no longer used as frequently as it was in the 1950's and 1960's. While the global-archival approach may provide some valuable information, it suffers from many methodological weaknesses. For example, its lack of a control group precludes making inferences from the data, and only descriptive statements of current status relative to previous status are possible. Further, "even these statements may be of questionable merit as the original assessment procedures used to determine the patient's pathology are frequently no longer in existence or no longer available" (Liberman, 1978).

With the second major approach to follow-up, a study is conducted in which two groups of patients each receive a different form of therapy. The patients are then assessed at the end of treatment and comparisons are made of the relative efficacy of the treatments. These patients are then contacted and evaluated at some future point in time in order to assess the longer-term comparative effectiveness of the treatments. Since comparison groups exist, inferential statements are possible; however, this approach faces many of the same methodological problems inherent in the global-archival one.

For example, the longer the period of time between the end of the study and the follow-up, the greater the likelihood that assessment devices and evaluative procedures will differ. Investigators such as Strupp and Bergin (1969), who stress the importance of having follow-up procedures as thorough, precise, and complete as those that were used during the therapy period, see this as a major drawback. A second problem with long-term follow-up is the likelihood that the personnel making the evaluations will change (Liberman, 1978). Either of these factors alone or in combination can render the data obtained questionable.

Possibly for these reasons, follow-up, when it is conducted at all, has seldom tended to take place more than six months after the termination of therapy (Liberman, 1978). For example, in their examination of four major behavior therapy journals for the year 1973, Cochrane and Sobol (1976) found that only 35 percent of the studies included follow-up assessments. Further, only a third of these occurred as long as six months after the termination of therapy.

There is consensus that the judicious use of follow-up is necessary for an adequate evaluation of the effects of psychotherapy. Even though it may not be possible to arrive at definitive conclusions concerning efficacy, such research may provide useful information regarding the process of therapeutic change. A number of methodological difficulties in the conduct of follow-up research exist. These include: inconsistencies in the use of measuring instruments, differential patient and personnel attrition, and the occurrence of intercurrent events. How long the follow-up period should be remains problematical, but six months appears to be the most frequently used time period. Whatever the period chosen, there should be a careful assessment of events in the lives of patients, both environmental and interpersonal, which have occurred since the end of therapy. An important theoretical and empirical endeavor would be the development of a series of appropriate categories for defining the important events in the lives of patients which are likely to have therapeutic or antitherapeutic impact.

STATISTICAL ISSUES

The interpretation of psychotherapy outcome results is difficult and complex for many reasons, some of which have already been described. In addition, many complicating factors relate to the statistical analysis of data, a few of which will be mentioned here. The measurement of change is not a simple matter. "Indeed, this is a methodological area fraught with booby traps, where intuitive 'doing what comes naturally' is almost certain to lead one astray" (Cohen and Cohen, 1975). Even the methodologists appear to be unable to settle the complex issues centering around what, how, or even whether to measure change.

This section will present a discussion of a number of measures that have been used to assess outcome, their advantages, and their drawbacks. These measures will include direct ratings of benefit or improvement, two types of change scores, and the use of final adjustment status as a criterion.

The most frequently used measure of outcome in the 1950's was therapist ratings of improvement. Their use has survived to the present day. Two advantages of these direct ratings of benefits or change in the form of an overall rating on a simple scale are their flexibility in terms of unique evaluation of each patient and the ease with which they can be obtained. However, the meanings of such ratings are often vague, and it is almost never clear exactly what standards were used for making the ratings. An extreme example of the possible ambiguity to be found in global ratings of improvement would be the case in which the therapist making the initial rating of a patient's condition is not the same person who makes the final rating. In addition, change is multidimensional, and a single global rating of improvement provides no insight into the nature of the change.

The second most frequent method of assessing outcome in psychotherapy research is pretreatment post-treatment difference scores. This "raw-gain" score is the simple difference between final and initial scores. Although intuitively appealing since it takes into account level of patient functioning at two distinct points in time, this method is subject to serious statistical problems.

Raw change scores may be satisfactory when both initial and final scores are perfectly reliable, but measurements of changes associated with psychotherapy possess limited reliability (Fiske, 1977). Therefore, because raw change scores reflect the measurement error of both initial and final scores, their reliability is likely to be substantially lower than that of *either* the initial or final scores. In addition to this tendency to be unreliable is the fact that simple change scores are necessarily dependent on initial scores (Cohen and Cohen, 1975; Green et al., 1975; Mintz et al., 1979). This fact is important when patients have not been randomized to treatment groups. Therefore, there are likely to be important pretreatment differences between two comparison groups, and a simple comparison of raw change scores could reflect not only treatment effects but these group pretreatment differences as well.

Another expected effect when extreme groups are selected for study, e.g., patients high on anxiety or low on self-esteem, is regression to the mean. What this means is that the more an initial set of observations deviates above or below the mean of the population distribution, the more a second set of observations will move in the direction of the mean, even in the absence of any true change (Bordin, 1974a, 1974b). If, for example, one is interested in the effect of crisis intervention on a sample of severely depressed patients and has them complete a depression scale prior to and at the end of therapy, it is predictable that the average for this sample will be less extreme at the second point in time regardless of whether or not the intervention was effective.

These and additional considerations have led to the recommendation of "residual" change scores (Cronbach and Furby, 1970; Fiske et al., 1970; Manning and Dubois, 1962).

> A gain is residualized by expressing the post-test score as a deviation from the post-test-on-pretest regression line. The part of the post-test information that is linearly predictable from the pretest is thus partialled out. (Cronbach and Furby, 1970)

More simply, a residual change score represents the difference between actual outcome and that which could be predicted from initial scores. The residual gain is, therefore, "a statistically adjusted measure that rescales an individual's simple gain score relative to typical gains made by others at the same initial level" (Mintz et al., 1979). Essentially, then, this approach reduces but does not completely eliminate initial group differences. However, the reliability of residual change scores is always greater than that of a comparable raw-gain score (Manning and Dubois, 1962). A closely related method of reducing the effect of initial differences between groups is the analysis of covariance. Valid application of this method of adjustment for initial differences requires that groups be chosen randomly and that measurement techniques be highly reliable. However, the application of analysis of covariance to studies in which initial assignment was nonrandom violates its basic assumptions. A number of methodologists (Bryk and

Weisberg, 1977; Cronbach and Furby, 1970) agree with Lord's conclusion that

> there is simply no logical or statistical procedure that can be counted on to make proper allowances for uncontrolled pre-existing differences between groups. (Lord, 1967)

At present there is no consensus among psychometricians on whether statistical adjustments designed to correct for initial differences among groups are good enough to yield useful inferences about "true change."

Perhaps the most reasonable conclusion from this discussion of various ways to measure the outcome of psychotherapy is that when patients are assigned to treatment groups at random, when initial differences among groups are small, and when the correlations between initial and final scores are low, then one may feel reasonably confident with almost any of the methods. However, these conditions are seldom, if ever, met. So the use of the residual gain score appears to be the most reliable and most frequently recommended method (Cronbach and Furby, 1970; Green et al., 1975; Manning and DuBois, 1962; Mintz et al., 1979).

Inter-Rater Agreement and Reliability

It is frequently necessary when interpreting the results of psychotherapy research to assess the degree to which different judges or therapists are in agreement. When numerical scales are used, inter-rater agreement usually means that exactly the same values have been assigned to the subject. No information is presented about the variability among subjects. In contrast, inter-rater reliability is very much concerned with intersubject variability. In this sense, it is more than agreement. It is agreement with regard to discrimination among subjects (Spitzer and Cohen, 1968). There are, however, situations in which an investigator is working with categorical rather than scaled data, e.g., with diagnostic categories. In such cases, agreement is either present or not; and variability in ratings, central to the estimation of inter-rater reliability, is no longer an issue.

A frequently used method for measuring agreement has been percentage or proportion of agreement (P). Although intuitively reasonable, this method suffers from a number of deficiencies. One is that it includes agreement that can be accounted for by chance alone. The true absolute agreement among raters can be overestimated by an amount related to the number of points on the scale. For example, the larger the number of raters and the fewer the points on the scale, the greater the likelihood that percent agreement will be inflated by chance factors.

Another problem with the use of percent agreement is that it is insensitive to degrees of agreement, i.e., agreement is treated as an all-or-nothing phenomenon with no credit given for partial agreement; in this sense, the percentage underestimates the actual extent of inter-rater agreement

(Mitchell, 1979). A third problem with P is that while it is the most common method used in reporting agreement, it is almost never accompanied by a significance test (Spitzer et al., 1967).

When an investigator is working with categorical rather than scaled data, Cohen's (1960) Kappa (K) provides an indication of the proportion of agreement between two raters over and above chance agreement; and because its sampling characteristics are known, it can be subjected to statistical significance testing. The assumptions for the use of K are that the subjects to be rated are independent, that the judges make their ratings independently, and that the categories to which subjects are assigned are independent, mutually exclusive, and exhaustive of the domain under consideration.

The measure of inter-rater reliability most frequently used for quantitatively scaled data is the intraclass correlation (ICC). There are a number of formulas for computing ICC, all of which use the computational procedure of analysis of variance. In the most general terms it can be interpreted as the proportion of the total variance in judges' ratings which is due to variability among the subjects rated (Spitzer and Cohen, 1968; Tinsley and Weiss, 1975). It thus represents the amount of variability among subjects in relation to the amount of variability among raters. For the usual situation in which a number of raters all rate a number of subjects each, ICC may be described as the component of variance due to individuals divided by the sum of this component plus error variance (Fleiss and Cohen, 1973).

In summary, despite its deficiencies, percent agreement (P) continues to be the most frequently used index of agreement for scaled data. For categorical data, Cohen's (1960) Kappa (K) is the most widely used and the most highly recommended index for inter-rater agreement. The intraclass correlation coefficient is generally regarded as the best available choice for estimating the reliability of judges' ratings of scaled data. However, despite all the advances that have been made in the development of statistical techniques for measuring reliability of judgment, all existing coefficients provide somewhat ambiguous solutions.

Statistical versus Clinical Significance

Statistical measures of significance are often misleading, largely because the word "significant" in its nontechnical meaning connotes "large," "important," or "consequential." There is, therefore, the temptation to consider a difference that is highly significant statistically to be one that is also very large. However, differences found to be highly significant in the statistical sense may have little clinical relevance. The reason is that statistical significance may be achieved if study samples are large, even though the actual effect obtained may be minimal. The significance level says nothing about the relative magnitude of the effect that has been observed. The level at which an investigator is willing to declare findings significant simply reflects the risk he is willing to take that he is reporting a real effect when, in fact, there is none (Spitzer and Cohen, 1968).

In 1969, Cohen developed a measure of effect size (ES) that he called *d* which was designed to avoid arbitrary choices among outcome measures and the scales used for their measurement and to transform the magnitude of differences found to a common scale. Although the terminology used to define ES, or *d*, has varied somewhat (e.g., Cohen, 1969; Plutchik, 1974), the following definition provided by Smith et al. (1980) is probably the most useful when considering the outcome of research in psychotherapy: The effect size is the difference in average score between the experimental and control group divided by some measure of variability (e.g., standard deviation) of the control group. In essence, *d* changes raw scores to standard scores by expressing them in standard deviation units. The advantages of this procedure are that (a) *d* is an unambiguous function of the relative magnitude of the experimental effect and does not depend on the size of the samples on which it was determined, and (b) the results of studies using different types of measures may be directly compared. ES, or *d*, becomes the common unit of measurement (Cohen, 1969).

Statistical Power Analysis

An investigator can make two kinds of interrelated errors when drawing conclusions from his or her data. The investigator can conclude that a difference between two populations exists when in fact it does not or can conclude that a difference does not exist when in fact it does. The first kind of error (Type I) has received much attention and is taken into account by setting typically low statistical criterion levels of probability, for example .05 or .01, for rejecting the null hypothesis (the hypothesis that no difference between groups exists). However, the second kind of error, that of concluding that no difference exists between groups when in fact it does, has been largely neglected in research in psychotherapy. If the investigator is a typical researcher in this area, not only has he or she exerted no prior control over the risk of committing this type of error (Type II), but the magnitude of the risk will be unknown (Spitzer and Cohen 1968).

"The technical term used to describe the probability of obtaining a result which is statistically significant when the phenomenon actually exists is statistical power" (Spitzer and Cohen 1968). In somewhat simpler terms, power refers to the probability of rejecting the null hypothesis when it is in fact false, and a true difference between groups exists. A number of factors enter into the determination of statistical power.

Statistical power analysis may be viewed as the formal study of the complex relations among the following four parameters:

A. The *power* of the test (that is, the probability of correctly rejecting the null hypothesis). Theoretically, this may range from zero to 1.00.

B. The significance criterion that leads to rejecting the null hypothesis. As the criterion level increases, that is, becomes *less* stringent (i.e., goes from .01 to .05), power increases.

C. The sample size *n*. As *n* increases, power increases.

D. The magnitude of the phenomenon in the population, *d*, or effect size (ES). As this increases, power increases.

In conclusion, it is important to note that merely increasing sample size is no panacea for all the problems of psychological research. A large *n* can never replace good planning, reliable and valid measures, optimally efficient experimental designs, random sampling procedures, and all the other factors that have been explored at length earlier in this chapter. Increasing *n* when appropriate can, however, serve to reduce the probability of spurious negative results.

Techniques for Combining Results of Different Studies

The term "combinatory techniques" refers to an important approach that has resulted from the rapid expansion of research dealing with the efficacy of psychotherapy. As this research has grown from a few controlled studies in the 1950's to hundreds of investigations that have used reasonably scientific standards in the 1970's, the complex nature of the results and the inconsistent findings have created many problems of interpretation. Those investigators who have tried to review various segments of the literature have had to develop schemas for deciding, on methodological grounds, which studies to include in their reviews and also how to combine the often conflicting results of large numbers of investigations. The present section will describe two recent approaches for dealing with these problems.

The Box-Score Method. The box-score method is essentially a way of summarizing, evaluating, and comparing the outcome of studies using different modalities or techniques of treatment. Studies that have assessed the effect of a specific treatment modality on a specific outcome variable are examined. Three outcomes are possible: The treatment can result in significantly positive or significantly negative effects or it can have no significant effect in either direction. Studies falling into each of these three categories are simply tallied. If a majority of studies falls into one of the three categories, with fewer falling into the other two, the category containing the majority of studies is assumed to give the best estimate of the true effect of that particular mode of treatment (Light and Smith, 1971).

In 1975, Luborsky et al. examined published studies that paid at least some attention to the main criteria of controlled comparative research. The research quality of each study was evaluated according to 12 criteria, such as the following: Controlled assignment of patients to each group, either by random assignment or by appropriate matching on important variables; the use of real patients; outcome measures related to target goals; the gathering of information about concurrent treatment (e.g. drugs); and adequate sample size (Luborsky et al., 1975).

The authors then graded each study on a scale from A (a well-designed study) to E (deficiencies so serious as to deserve exclusion from the analysis) according to how well they fit the criteria. For each type of comparison made (e.g., individual versus group psychotherapy), a "box-score" was provided, with the number of studies in which the treatments were significantly better or worse. "Tie-scores," the term used for therapies showing no statistical differences, were also used.

Critique of the Box-Score Method. Kazdin and Wilson (1978) present a number of criticisms of the box-score method. Although these criticisms are specific to the method used by Luborsky et al. (1975), they would apply to most reviews that have used this combinative approach or modified versions of it in their data analysis.

First, Kazdin and Wilson (1978) point out that so many of the experiments cited by Luborsky et al. (1975) have flawed designs that the "best" studies are not necessarily much better than the poorest studies. A second criticism of the box-score strategy is that by essentially ignoring their own grading system, Luborsky et al. (1975) often give equal weight to different investigations despite great differences in methodology and outcome criteria. This procedure is a "kind of majority rule whereby two poor experiments are given twice as much weight as a single sound one" (Gardner, 1966).

Third, even though Luborsky et al. (1975) concluded that behavior therapy is "tied" with other psychotherapies in effectiveness, Kazdin and Wilson (1978) point out that behavior therapy was slightly or significantly more effective than the alternative treatments in almost all cases. Fifth, Kazdin and Wilson (1978) criticize the box-score method as providing no rational statistical basis for combining the results of different investigations, regardless of what their ratings are. For example, in Luborsky et al.'s (1975) comparison of behavior therapy and psychotherapy, 13 studies showed "tied" scores, and six showed results in favor of behavior therapy. The authors then concluded that these results indicate that there are no differences in outcome between these two modalities. Such a judgment is obviously arbitrary, and it is likely that an evaluator representing another point of view might come up with an entirely different conclusion.

Finally, Kazdin and Wilson (1978) claim that the box-score approach obscures the real differences between techniques that happen to be given the same global labels. Behavior therapy is not synonymous with systematic desensitization, "cognitive modification," or rational therapy; nor is psychotherapy the same as psychoanalysis, brief psychoanalytically-oriented therapy, dynamic group therapy, or supportive counseling. The box-score strategy tends to reify the convenient labels describing therapeutic endeavors.

Smith et al. (1980) also make some cogent criticisms of this method. In their opinion, its most serious shortcoming is that it ignores considerations of sample size in the studies integrated. Quite simply, large samples are likely to produce more statistically significant findings than small samples. Thus, it is possible that nine small-sample studies could yield results falling just short of the specified level of statistical significance, while a tenth large-sample study showed significant results. Although intuitively it does not seem right, the box-score is still one for the therapy and nine against it. A second deficiency pointed out by these authors is that it discards good descriptive information. For example, "To know that aversive conditioning beats directed imagery in 25 of 30 studies—if, in fact, it does—is not to know whether it wins by a nose or a walkaway" (Smith et al., 1980).

These criticisms of the box-score strategy are cogent and largely appropriate, and they highlight the need for a more defensible way of making judgments about the often conflicting results of large numbers of investigations that deal with the same general problems. Meta-analysis represents Smith et al.'s (1980) attempt to overcome the deficiencies of past techniques.

Meta-Analysis of Outcome Studies. Meta-analysis, the integration of large numbers of research studies through statistical analysis of the data of individual studies, was first described by Glass (1976). It was used by Smith and Glass in 1977 to integrate the results of 375 psychotherapy outcome studies and in a more extended analysis of 475 outcome studies in 1980 (Smith et al., 1980).

For a study to be included in a meta-analysis, it must have at least one therapy treatment group that is compared to an untreated or waiting-list control group or to a different therapy group. Rigor of research design is not a selection criterion but is, rather, one of several characteristics of the individual study to be related to the effect of the treatment in that study.

For each study included in a meta-analysis, information of the following type is obtained: date and form of publication; type of therapy used; duration of therapy; professional affiliation and number of years' experience of the therapist; diagnosis, age, and IQ of patients; source of patients; method of assignment to groups; therapist-patient similarity; type and reactivity or "fake-ability" of outcome measures; patient attrition; internal validity of the research design; and effect size.

As conceived by Smith et al. (1980), the most important feature of an outcome study is the magnitude of the effect of the therapy used. The concept of effect size as an unambiguous common unit of measurement of the relative magnitude of an experimental effect that does not depend on the size of the samples on which it was determined has already been discussed.

It is important to note that an effect size may be calculated on any outcome variable a researcher chooses to measure and that in many cases a study may yield more than one effect size, since effects might be measured on more than one type of outcome variable. Typical outcome measures on which effect sizes are obtained are self-esteem, anxiety, depression, work/school achievement, physiological stress, etc. Mixing different outcomes is also defensible on a number of grounds, including the fact that all outcome measures are more or less related to "well-being," and so are comparable at a general level (Smith and Glass, 1977).

Meta-analysis has its limitations, and various criticisms have been leveled against it. For example, Parloff* has pointed out that the patients represented in the survey were not the typical clientele served by most psychotherapists. Sixty-two percent of the 1,766 reported treatment effects were derived from subjects who either responded to an advertisement or who were directly solicited by the experimenter; furthermore, only three percent were described as "depressed," a diagnosis that accounts for approximately half of all patients seen in the "real" world.

The therapists in the studies surveyed by Smith et al. (1980) are also considered by Parloff to be nonrepresentative of therapists in general inasmuch as the majority were relatively inexperienced. Furthermore, not only were the therapists biased in favor of a particular form of treatment in 88 percent of the 475 studies reviewed, but Parloff quotes the authors as stating that "where the allegiance was in favor of the therapy, the magnitude of effect was greatest. Where there was bias against the therapy, the effect was least" (Smith et al., 1980).

It is important to note that this critique by Parloff is not meant to impugn the significance of what he calls "this elegant survey." Rather, it is meant to show that as a consequence of the research field's dependence on voluntary participation, the body of evidence for the effectiveness of psychotherapy does not seem fully to represent psychotherapy as it is actually offered to the public. It thus appears that although meta-analysis is an important new statistical advance, considerably more research, and particularly more research that adequately represents psychotherapy as it is practiced today, is needed before existing conflicts among facts and interpretations can be resolved.

NEED FOR A NEW PARADIGM

The various methodologic and content issues that have been described imply that psychotherapy research is difficult and unwieldy at best and that it has not provided unequivocal conclusions about the effectiveness of psychotherapy.

*Parloff MB: Psychotherapy evidence and reimbursement decisions: Bambi meets Godzilla. Presented at the annual meeting of the Society for Psychotherapy Research, Aspen, Colorado, June 1981.

The surprising and perhaps disappointing results of the research of the last few decades raise important issues for the future. The most important of these is whether the model of psychotherapy research which is currently considered to be the appropriate paradigm is in fact correct. In much of the current literature, approval is given to the idea of strict control of independent variables and to the absolute necessity of a control group. This is a model that is based on the laboratory research that is typical of certain aspects of psychology such as animal learning, memory, and psychophysiology, which in turn is based on a model of research developed for the physical and biological sciences. In other branches of medicine and in drug research it is known as the controlled clinical trial. One can raise the question of whether this model is appropriate to all forms of psychotherapy research. One criticism concerns the practical problem of applying the experimental model to psychotherapy. For example, Frank (1979) points out that criteria for selection of patient samples are often vague or inadequate; therapies are defined in such a way that large and unrecognized variations in style of application by different therapists occur; measures of outcome are not comparable from one investigation to the next; outcome measures are sometimes trivial; and independent variables are too often demographic measures such as age, sex, and social class, which are, at best, indirectly related to therapeutic outcome.

Frank (1979) has pointed out several other problems with experimental/control group designs which have not been given sufficient attention. Although one of the criticisms of contemporary psychotherapy research is that different therapists do not do the same things, Frank believes that this is not only an impossible criterion to meet but an undesirable one as well. He believes that standard measures of outcome, and manuals on how to do each particular brand of therapy, are largely irrelevant to long-term, open-ended therapies. "To the extent that the spontaneity of the therapists' actions is considered crucial, and the patient's improvement is defined solely by changes in his or her subjective state, it is hard to see how either the therapy or the measures of benefit could ever be standardized" (Frank, 1979). Any therapeutic encounter is necessarily characterized by therapeutic improvisations.

Frank also notes that since therapy occurs in the midst of complex social and family systems, many of the determinants of outcome lie outside the specific interaction between patient and therapist. This implies that causal statements about the relation between therapy modality and outcome cannot be made. Finally, Frank states that the types of symptoms and signs of distress which patients exhibit often shift in idiosyncratic ways during the course of long-term psychotherapy, creating problems for both standard outcome measures and diagnostic classification systems.

Another problem with controlled trials concerns the use of a "placebo" condition. First, few therapists would accept the task of implementing a true placebo condition for more than a few sessions. Second, if the placebo condition were applied for a long time, the patients would probably become disenchanted with their lack of progress and might even feel that they were harmed by the treatment. Third, placebo conditions are, by definition, theoretically inert, and yet are presented to the patients as potentially effective treatment. This practice is an ethically questionable deception and has been criticized as a research tool. Fourth, patients in a placebo condition may postpone seeking treatment elsewhere and thus possibly harm themselves. Finally, if patients suffer deterioration when in a placebo condition, not only does this harm them but it acts to reduce the confidence of the public-at-large in the therapeutic endeavor.

A number of alternatives to the experimental group/control group traditional research design may usefully contribute to research in psychotherapy. Some of these alternatives are (a) the use of special groups, (b) the use of analogue research, and (c) the use of computer simulation. Although future research may show each to have its own drawbacks, these methods provide a new range of possibilities that need to be explored.

The Use of Special Control Groups

This research strategy includes several aspects. One uses component control designs, a second uses alternative treatments, a third uses community controls, and a fourth uses scaled comparison groups.

Component Controls. This approach involves either the omission of an active ingredient of therapy for the control group or the use of *only* one element of therapy for the control group (e.g. relaxation training without biofeedback). Using these procedures, both experimental and control groups have expectations of improvement; Borkovec and Nau (1972) have shown that each treatment component is likely to generate an improvement expectation that is comparable to that generated by the whole treatment package.

Alternative Treatment Controls. Given the fact that many studies have shown that psychotherapy produces better results than doing nothing, it seems reasonable to conclude that each new study is not required to document this point. Instead, and in view of the difficulties of long-term research, therapies should now be compared against each other. In this way every patient is treated for an equivalent period of time, and therapy may continue for long periods.

In addition, research of this type may help deal with one of the limitations of meta-analysis, namely, that in the effort to standardize effect sizes, the actual outcome variables are not standardized so that different therapies are really not comparable. For example, the statement that behavioral therapies have higher effect sizes than gestalt therapies is largely meaningless. Behavioral therapies may be concerned with reducing anxiety as the primary (or only) focus of therapy, while gestalt therapies may be concerned with restructuring personality and reducing defensiveness. A meta-analysis of different therapies will be meaningful only when equivalent outcome measures are used.

Community Controls. In medical research it is often possible to obtain data on the degree to which a disease or condition exists in the community through epidemiological surveys. The same idea can be applied to psychotherapy research. Over the years a number of surveys (Hollingshead and Redlich, 1957; Srole et al., 1962) have tried to determine the extent to which various psychiatric conditions exist in the general population. As an extension of these findings it should be possible to identify and follow people who have a defined illness or diagnosis but who have not sought psychotherapeutic treatment. To the extent that this can be done norms will become available on the natural course of untreated mental illnesses. For example, if a community survey identified five percent of the population as moderately to severely depressed, these identified persons could be reinterviewed each year for several years to determine what happens to the depression over time for those individuals who do not seek formal psychiatric treatment.

Such data can be used as base-rate information for future studies of psychotherapy without requiring that each investigator provide untreated controls of his own. Such community controls can also provide base-rates for long-term as well as short-term therapy. Although it is unlikely that such epidemiological surveys can provide base-rates for all diagnostic entities (e.g., schizophrenia), they can probably provide data on many conditions usually treated by psychotherapy (e.g., anxiety states, phobias, depressions, adjustment reactions, and character disorders). In England, a community survey has established the levels of measured hopelessness in the general population (Greene, 1981).

Scaled Control Groups. Many critics have noted that the concept of an untreated control group is probably an illusion. What it means at most is that an identified potential patient has not sought formal treatment. It certainly does not imply that they have not discussed their problems with family members, friends, teachers, pastors, or others. What this observation implies is that a *zero* level of treatment is unattainable.

A similar situation exists in physics and chemistry. Certain conditions cannot be studied directly because they cannot be obtained in the real world, for example, absolute zero degrees on the Kelvin scale, zero levels of friction, or extremely high temperatures or pressures. Despite these limitations physicists can describe a great many of the properties of these extreme conditions. They do so, in part, by a method of successive approximations and by extrapolation as a result of the use of scaled variables.

The same idea can be used in psychotherapy research. This can be illustrated by a hypothetical extension of a study by Imber et al. (1957). One group of patients (randomly selected) could see their therapists three times a week for one year. Another group could see their therapists once a week for a year. A third group could see their therapists once every two weeks, and a fourth group could see their therapists once a month. If one measures (for example) decreases in level of depression, one might find a gradual decrease in the amount of change as a mathematical function of the frequency of therapeutic contacts. From the curve one could then estimate (extrapolate) the change in depression to be expected if the potential patient did not see the therapist at all.

Use of Analogue Research

Analogue research refers to research that is carried out under more restricted, simplified conditions than are found in the natural clinical settito take the role of patients. Such restricted research designs appear to have certain advantages, for example, to enable a greater degree of control over the selection of "patients" and "therapists" and what they do and say. Other advantages include the opportunity to manipulate variables systematically, to introduce unusual control groups, and to test specific, if limited, hypotheses. These advantages must be considered in the light of the limited generalizability of results to the clinical situation.

A number of important issues need to be considered, however. Perhaps the most important is the concept of an analogue experiment itself. One can argue that all research in psychotherapy represents an analogue of the "real" clinical situation and also represents the result of various restrictions and simplifications. There is little doubt that "real" psychotherapeutic interactions are carried out in a looser, more improvisational style than the experimental protocols would permit. Finally, therapists in practice are undoubtedly older and more experienced than the graduate students, interns, and residents who typically act as therapists in most psychotherapy research. It is probably safe to conclude that there is no sharp line of distinction between analogue research and "real" psychotherapy research.

Computer Simulation

At one time computers were used almost exclusively as high speed automatic calculators. They made it possible to do statistical computations of great complexity in a very brief period, and this use of computers remains an important one. However, over the years many additional functions have been added to the repertoire of the computer. These include such tasks as natural language translation, pattern recognition, medical and psychiatric diagnoses, content analyses of verbal interactions, interactive teaching, and simulation, among others. Although all of these roles of the computer have a place in psychotherapy research, potentially the most important is the computer as a simulator of personality and as a simulator of the techniques of therapy interaction.

Loehlin (1968) has presented details of four computer models of personality. The simplest is called "Aldous" in honor of Aldous Huxley, author of *Brave New World*. Aldous is able to evaluate stimuli (written input to the computer); "feel" anger, fear, or attraction; and report behaviors of attack, withdrawal, or approach. If several emotions are aroused by an event (input), conflict occurs according to certain defined rules. Aldous is able to store the results of interaction in short- or long-term memory so that they may influence, to some degree, the results of new encounters.

Colby has developed a model of the paranoid patient (Colby et al., 1971). In this simulation, the "patient" can have different levels of anger, fear, or mistrust. The responses of the model (PERRY) to statements or questions by the interviewer depend on two factors: (a) current levels of these emotional states, and (b) the connections between the "therapist's" words and special "sensitive" words in PERRY's memory (e.g., related to the delusion or personal references). The level of emotion determines PERRY's sensitivity to symbols that are capable of triggering defenses or evoking his delusions. When the thresholds are high (anger and fear are low), PERRY is capable of relatively "normal" conversation. When anger and fear are high, PERRY will defend himself by a verbal attack or by withdrawal. Emotions, once evoked, subside gradually, even if not aroused again. It has been shown that records of PERRY interacting with a psychiatrist cannot be reliably distinguished by other psychiatrists from records of interactions produced by real paranoid patients.

Development of computer simulation models of the kind described has several important implications. First, since personality and psychotherapy theories are often wordy, ambiguous, and sometimes contain unstated assumptions, the computer model will bring some of these weaknesses to light. Second, the fact that the model's assumptions are made explicit (in the form of explicit programs and subroutines) means that the rules of interaction can be changed in systematic ways to explore the consequences of such changes. Thus, for example, changes in the assumptions of the model created the different versions of Aldous that were tried out. Third, it may theoretically be possible to simulate at least the major features of patients of any diagnostic type and allow these "patients" to interact with "therapists" of any defined school of psychotherapy. The parameters of the interaction can be manipulated easily, and standard output measures can be obtained (e.g., affect, behavior, defenses, etc.). Fourth, the process of interaction can be speeded up as much as one might wish so that a major compression of time can occur. This would enable long-term psychotherapy to be modeled or simulated over a relatively brief real time period. Last, but not least, the computer models will allow students to receive training in technical skills and, in particular, modes of psychotherapy, thus allowing greater consistency of strategies to be developed among practitioners of any given therapy.

CONCLUSIONS

Controlled psychotherapy research is, relatively speaking, still in an early stage of its development. Before the 1960's, clinical research was largely anecdotal or without adequate control or comparison groups. Only in the last two decades or so have the many problems inherent in the conduct of research in psychotherapy been recognized. As more methodological sophistication has come to the field, there has been an increased realization of at least what needs to be done.

Available research data do not adequately reflect the work of clinicians as actually practiced. This is especially true for long-term psychotherapy and psychoanalysis. However, lack of evidence for the efficacy of long-term psychotherapy should not be interpreted as an indication of its lack of effectiveness. A large body of clinical experience and knowledge has been accumulated by practitioners over many decades which must be taken into consideration in the overall evaluation of psychotherapy. The future of psychotherapy research lies in the integration of the already considerable body of experience and knowledge possessed by clinicians with newly developed technological advances and innovative approaches to research.

REFERENCES

Baekeland F, Lundwall L: Dropping out of treatment: a critical review. Psychol Bull 82:738-783, 1975

Bednar RL, Lawlis GF: Empirical research in group psychotherapy, in Handbook of Psychotherapy and Behavior Change. Edited by Bergin AE, Garfield SL. New York, John Wiley & Sons, 1971

Bergin AE, Lambert MJ: The evaluation of therapeutic outcomes, in Handbook of Psychotherapy and Behavior Change: An Empirical Analysis, 2nd ed. Edited by Garfield SL, Bergin AE. New York, John Wiley & Sons, 1978

Bergin AE: The evaluation of therapeutic outcomes, in Handbook of Psychotherapy and Behavior Change. Edited by Bergin AE, Garfield SL. New York, John Wiley & Sons, 1971a

Bergin AE: Some implications of psychotherapy research for therapeutic practice. J Abnorm Psychol 71:235-246, 1971b

Bordin ES: Outcome or process? in Research Strategies in Psychotherapy. Edited by Bordin ES. New York, John Wiley & Sons, 1974a

Bordin ES: Tactics in process studies, in Research Strategies in Psychotherapy. Edited by Bordin ES. New York, John Wiley & Sons, 1974b

Borkovec ID, Nau SD: Credibility of analogue therapy rationales. J Behav Ther and Exper Psychiatry 3:257-260, 1972

Bryk AS, Weisberg HI: Use of the nonequivalent control group design when subjects are growing. Psychol Bull 84:950-962, 1977

Campbell DT, Stanley JC: Experimental and Quasi-Experimental Designs for Research. Chicago, Rand McNally, 1963

Cochrane R, Sobol MP: Myth and methodology in behaviour therapy research, in Theoretical and Empirical Bases of the Behaviour Therapies. Edited by Feldman MP, Broadhurst A. London, John Wiley & Sons, 1976

Cohen J, Cohen P: Applied Multiple Regression/Correlation Analysis for the Behavioral Sciences. Hillsdale, NJ, Lawrence Erbaum Associates, 1975

Cohen J: Statistical Power Analysis for the Behavioral Sciences. New York, Academic Press, 1969

Cohen J: A coefficient of agreement for nominal scales. Educational and Psychological Measurement 20:37-46, 1960

Colby KM, Weber S, Hilf FD: Artificial paranoia. Artificial intelligence 2:1-25, 1971

Cronbach LJ, Furby L: How we should measure "change"—or should we? Psychol Bull 74:68-80, 1970

Cronbach LJ: Designing Evaluations. Stanford, Calif, Stanford Evaluation Consortium, 1978

Cross HJ: The outcome of psychotherapy: a selected analysis of research findings. J Consult Psychol 28:413-417, 1964

Dittman AT: Psychotherapeutic processes, in Annual Review of Psychology. Edited by Farnsworth P, McNemar O, McNemar Q. Palo Alto, Calif, Annual Reviews, 1966

Erwin E: Psychoanalytic therapy: the Eysenck argument. Am Psychol 35:435-443, 1980

Eysenck HJ: The effects of psychotherapy: an evaluation. J Consult Psychol 16:319-324, 1952

Fiske DW, Hunt HF, Luborsky L, et al: Planning of research on effectiveness of psychotherapy. Arch Gen Psychiatry 22:22-32, 1970

Fiske DW: Methodological issues in research on the psychotherapist, in Effective Psychotherapy: A Handbook of Research. Edited by Gurman AS, Razin AM. New York, Pergamon Press, 1977

Fleiss JL, Cohen J: The equivalence of weighted kappa and the intraclass coefficient as measures of reliability. Educational Psychological Measurement 33:613-619, 1973

Frank JD: The present status of outcome studies. J Consult Clin Psychol 47:310-316, 1979

Frank JD: Issues in selection and assignment of patients to groups, in Psychotherapy Research: Selected Readings. Edited by Stollak GE, Guerney BC, Rothberg M. Chicago, Rand McNally, 1966

Gardner RA: On box score methodology as illustrated by three reviews of overtraining reversal effects. Psychol Bull 66:416-418, 1966

Garfield SL: Psychotherapy: a 40-year appraisal. Am Psychol 36:174-183, 1981

Garfield SL: Research problems in clinical diagnosis. J Consult Clin Psychol 46:596-607, 1978

Glass GV: Primary, secondary, and meta-analysis of research. Educational Researcher 10:3-8, 1976

Gottman JM, Markman HJ: Experimental designs in psychotherapy research, in Handbook of Psychotherapy and Behavior Change: An Empirical Analysis, 2nd ed. Edited by Garfield SL, Bergin AE. New York, John Wiley & Sons, 1978

Green BL, Gleser GC, Stone WN, et al: Relationships among diverse measures of psychotherapy outcome. J Consult Clin Psychol 43:689-699, 1975

Greene SM: Levels of measured hopelessness in the general population. Br J Clin Psychol 20:11-14, 1981

Gurman AS, Kniskern DP: Research on marital and family therapy: progress, perspective and prospect, in Handbook of Psychotherapy and Behavior Change: An Empirical Analysis, 2nd ed. Edited by Garfield SL, Bergin AE. New York, John Wiley & Sons, 1978

Hampton P: Placebo treatment techniques in behavior therapy. Behavior Therapy 4:481-482, 1973

Hollingshead AB, Redlich C: Social Class and Mental Illness: A Community Study. New York, John Wiley & Sons, 1958

Horowitz MJ: Stress Response Syndromes. New York, Jason Aronson, 1976

Imber SD, Frank JD, Nash EH, et al: Improvement and amount of therapeutic contact: an alternative to the use of no-treatment controls in psychotherapy, Psychotherapy Research: Selected Readings. Edited by Stollak GE, Guerney BG, Rothberg M. Chicago, Rand McNally, 1957

Karasu TB, Skodol AE: DSM-III: psychodynamic evaluation. Am J Psychiatry 137:607-610, 1980

Karasu TB: The ethics of psychotherapy. Am J Psychiatry 137:1502-1512, 1980

Kazdin AE, Wilson GT: Evaluation of Behavior Therapy: Issues, Evidence, and Research Strategies. Cambridge, Mass, Ballinger, 1978

Kiesler DJ: Some myths of psychotherapy research and the search for a paradigm. Psychol Bull 65:110-136, 1966

Klein DF, Gittelman R, Quitkin F, et al: Diagnosis and Drug Treatment of Psychiatric Disorders: Adults and Children, 2 ed. Baltimore, Williams & Wilkins Co, 1980

Lambert MJ, DeJulio SS, Stein DM: Therapist interpersonal skills: process, outcome, methodological considerations, and recommendations for future research. Psychol Bull 85:467-489, 1978

Lambert MJ, Utic JM: Therapist characteristics and psychotherapy outcome, in The Effects of Psychotherapy, vol 2. Edited by Lambert MJ. New York, Human Sciences Press, 1982

Liberman BL: The maintenance and persistence of change: long-term follow-up of investigations of psychotherapy, in Effective Ingredients of Successful Psychotherapy. Edited by Frank JD, Hoehn-Saric R, Imber SD, et al. New York, Brunner/Mazel, 1978

Light RJ, Smith PV: Accumulating evidence: procedures for resolving contradictions among different research studies. Harvard Educational Review 41:429-471, 1971

Loehlin JC: Computer Models of Personality. New York, Random House, 1968

Lord FM: A paradox in the interpretation of group comparisons. Psychol Bull 68:304-305, 1967

Luborsky L, Singer B, Luborsky L: Comparative studies of psychotherapies: is it true that "everyone has won and all must have prizes"? Arch Gen Psychiatry 32:995-1008, 1975

Malen DH: The outcome problem in psychotherapy research: a historical review. Arch Gen Psychiatry 29:719-729, 1973

Manning WH, DuBois PH: Correlational methods in research on human learning. Percept Mot Skills 15:287-321, 1962

Marks IM: Empiricism is accepted. Int J Psychiatry 7:141-148, 1969

May PRA: Psychotherapy research in schizophrenia—another view of present reality. Schizophr Bull 9:126-132, 1974

Meltzoff J, Kornreich M: Research in Psychotherapy. New York, Atherton Press, 1970

Mintz J, Luborsky L, Christoph P: Measuring the outcomes of psychotherapy: findings of the Penn Psychotherapy Project. J Consult Clin Psychol 47:319-334, 1979

Mitchell SK: Interobserver agreement, reliability, and generalizability of data collected in observational studies. Psychol Bull 86:376-390, 1979

Mosher LR, Keith SJ: Psychosocial treatment: individual, group, family, and community support approaches, in Schizophrenia 1980. Washington, DC, US Government Printing Office, 1980

O'Leary KD, Borkovec TD: Conceptual, methodological, and ethical problems of placebo groups in psychotherapy research. Am Psychol 9:821-830, 1978

Parloff MB, Wolfe B, Hadley S, et al: Assessment of Psychosocial Treatment of Mental Disorders: Current Status and Prospects. National Technical Information Service PB 287 640, 1978

Parloff MB, Dies RR: Group psychotherapy outcome research 1966-1975. Int J Group Psychother 27:281-319, 1977

Paul GL: Strategy of outcome research in psychotherapy, in Prescriptive Psychotherapy. Edited by Goldstein AP, Stein N. New York, Pergamon Press, 1976

Paul GL: Insight versus desensitization in psychotherapy two years after termination. J Consult Psychology 31:333-348, 1967

Plutchik R: Foundations of Experimental Research, 2nd ed. New York, Harper and Row, 1974

Plutchik R: Foundations of Experimental Research. New York, Harper and Row, 1968

Rogers CR, Gendlin ET, Keisler DJ, et al: The Therapeutic Relationship and Its Impact: A Study of Psychotherapy with Schizophrenics. Madison, University of Wisconsin Press, 1967

Rosenthal D, Frank JD: Psychotherapy and the placebo effect. Psychol Bull 53:294-302, 1956

Sloane RB, Staples FR, Cristol AH, et al: Psychotherapy Versus Behavior Therapy. Cambridge, Mass, Harvard University Press, 1975

Smith ML, Glass GV, Miller TI: The Benefits of Psychotherapy. Baltimore, Johns Hopkins University Press, 1980

Smith ML, Glass GV: Meta-analysis of psychotherapy outcome studies. Am Psychol 32:752-760, 1977

Spitzer RL, Cohen J, Fleiss JL, et al: Quantification of agreement in psychiatric diagnosis. Arch Gen Psychiatry 17:83-87, 1967

Spitzer RL, Endicott JE, Robins ES: Research Diagnostic Criteria (RDC) for a Selected Group of Functional Disorders, 3rd ed. Rockville, Md, NIMH Clinical Research Branch Collaborative Program on the Psychobiology of Depression, 1978

Spitzer RL, Cohen J: Common errors in quantitative psychiatric research. Int J Psychiatry 6:109-118, 1968

Spitzer RL, Endicott J: Assessment of outcome by independent clinical evaluators, in Psychotherapy Change Measures, DHEW Publication No (ADM) 74-120. Edited by Waskow IE, Parloff MB. Washington, DC, US Government Printing Office, 1975

Srole L, Langner TS, Michael ST, et al: Mental Health in the Metropolis: The Midtown Manhattan Study, vol 1. New York, McGraw-Hill, 1962

Stotsky BA, Zolik ES: Group psychotherapy with psychotics: 1921-1963—a review. Int J Group Psychotherapy 15: 321-344, 1965

Strupp HH, Bergin AE: Some empirical and conceptual bases for coordinated research in psychotherapy: a critical review of issues, trends, and evidence. Int J Psychiatry 7:18-90, 1969

Strupp HH, Hadley SW: A tripartite model of mental health and therapeutic outcomes with special reference to negative effects in psychotherapy. Am Psychol 32:187-196, 1977

Strupp HH: Psychotherapy research and practice: an overview, in Handbook of Psychotherapy and Behavior Change; An Empirical Analysis, 2nd ed. Edited by Garfield SI, Bergin AE. New York, John Wiley & Sons, 1978

Tinsley HEA, Weiss DJ: Interrater reliability and agreement of subjective judgments. J Counsel Psychology 22:358-376, 1975

Truax CB, Mitchell KM: Research on certain therapist interpersonal skills in relation to process and outcome, in Handbook of Psychotherapy and Behavior Change. New York, John Wiley & Sons, 1971

Vandenbos GR, Pino CD: Research on the outcome of psychotherapy, in Psychotherapy: Practice, Research, Policy. Edited by Vandenbos GR. Beverly Hills, Calif, Sage Publications, 1980

Waskow IE: Selection of a core battery, in Psychotherapy Change Measures, in DHEW Publication No (ADM) 74-120. Edited by Waskow IE, Parloff MB. Washington DC, US Government Printing Office, 1975

Weissman MM: The psychological treatment of depression: evidence for the efficacy of psychotherapy alone, in comparison with, and in combination with pharmacotherapy. Arch Gen Psychiatry 36:1261-1269, 1979

Reprise

Reprise

All human beings share certain universal needs. In essence, these are:

A. Physical: For vitality, skills, and longevity to explore and control the environment.

B. Psychosocial: For interpersonal securities and cultural hegemony.

C. Existential: For emotional security derived from beliefs in metapsychologic or religious systems.

COMMON DYNAMICS OF THERAPY

An integrative analysis indicates that many if not all modes of treatment attempt, covertly or overtly, to meet one or more of these universal needs by one or more of the following parameters of influence:

The Prestige of the Therapist. Whether derived from current personal fame, popular school, or prominent institution, the therapist's reputation is what attracts the patient to therapy, sometimes with great difficulty over long distances. The patient's wishful expectations of cure give a powerful preliminary advantage to the prospective practitioner, whether psychopharmacologist, group therapist, psychoanalyst, or promiser of miracles. As to the latter role, Western psychiatrists, though still endowed with some measure of mystique, are inhibited about taking explicit advantage of the sanctioned myths and practices that aid their colleagues in other cultures.

Rapport. Patients seek help when they suffer from pervasive anxieties, which, though often initially unformulated, eventually are related to real or fantasied threats to one or more of their basic needs. In effect, they seek help when (a) they fear that their physical welfare and bodily integrity are endangered by disease, trauma, or deterioration; (b) their sense of adequacy, emotional security, or need for self-fulfillment is impaired and/or their familial, sexual, or social interrelations appear to be failing; or (c) their cherished convictions (i.e., rationalized or mystically wishful beliefs) are no longer an adequate source of comfort.

Each of the appeals for help exemplified in the above examples, regardless of the seeker's "objective" physical state, social status, or ultimate fate, indicates some anticipation of impending difficulties. The therapist can increase the patient's trust and collaboration by showing competency in all therapeutic roles:

A. As a clinician well trained to diagnose and treat somatic illnesses;

B. As a person whose interest and empathy will show the patient that he or she has found a trustworthy ally in an otherwise unpredictable or hostile world;

C. And less explicitly, as a mentor capable of exploring and resolving psychologic or philosophic dilemmas.

Hippocrates wrote in his *Precepts*:

> Human illnesses are due to excessive indulgences or repressions, . . . disappointments in love or war, sustained tensions, fears and superstitions . . . [i]n the race for fame and fortune. . . . Only where there is love of man is there love of medicine.

Relief. Two principal modes of relief are open: medical and psychosocial. The therapist must be cognizant of the psychologic and behavioral dysfunctions that accompany somatic illnesses, which require accurate diagnoses, consultants as indicated, and specific treatment (Schwab, 1982). Medications, with due precautions as to incompatibilities, overdoses, plasma levels, and addictions, may include the benzodiazepines for tension; a mild flurazepam for insomnia; carefully monitored lithium for manic states; tricyclics, MAO inhibitors, or electroconvulsive therapy for depression; and the phenothiazines, butyrophenones, or other drugs for psychotic behavior. Concurrent environmental therapy may consist of relief from external stresses, which may require day, night, or continuous hospitalization.

Retrospection. With psychosomatic distress partially controlled, the patient, under gentle, empathetic, and skillfully directed questioning, will be more willing to consider the real or imagined circumstances that precipitated current personal or social dysfunctions. In modalities that decry anamnestic inquiries in favor of "emphasis on the here and now," patients' character development may also be inferred from their current behavior— dress, voice, mannerisms, and a multitude of other overt or subtle indications. Confessions of past or current misconduct may be therapeutic not only because of any inherent "cathartic" or "abreactive" effect also but insofar as they are received by a reassuringly sympathetic and helpfully constructive therapist in an atmosphere of trust and expectancy. A truly comprehensive survey of each patient's familial, educational, sexual, social, occupational, marital, aesthetic, and related experiences should reveal not only significant physical and psychological vulnerabilities but also prognostically important talents, skills, and existential potentialities.

Re-education. Regardless of the patient's position on a chair or couch, the number of participants in each session, or duration of therapy, the therapist, through words, gestures, examples, or more subtle modes of communication, explores the patient's motivations, concepts, symbolisms, values, and conduct, and explicitly or implicitly conveys clarifying and evaluative reactions. If the therapy is skillfully conducted, the patient will reconsider whether, even at the price of surrendering formerly cherished covert gratifications, he would secure more substantial and lasting rewards by changing his behavior. If the patient brings to the therapist unacceptable interpersonal demands, these may be analyzed and corrected.

Rehabilitation and Resocialization. In these procedures the patient uses newly acquired perspectives and reorientation to alter his conduct in a more personally and socially acceptable direction, first in individual or group therapeutic sessions and concurrently or eventually outside the treatment environment—thereby demonstrating true operational adaptabilities.

Recapitulation. Finally, as in any other form of re-education, it is often necessary to re-establish faltering rapport, relieve reoccurrences of symptoms, correct previous misunderstandings, reconsider remaining departures from rational conduct, and repeat portions of the process as often as necessary until the patient feels capable of continuing growth on his own. During all these phases the therapist can maintain both optimism and humility in the knowledge that many patients—even those who had been labeled chronically ill—spontaneously achieve viable social adaptations (Bleuler, 1979; Ciompi, 1980; Harding and Brooks, 1980; Huber et al., 1980).

SURVEY OF COROLLARY FORMULATIONS OF THE COMMON DYNAMICS OF PSYCHIATRIC THERAPIES

Representative concepts are cited chronologically but with the order of implicit dynamics rearranged serially to correspond with the basic parameters outlined above:

S. Rosenzweig (1936): The therapist's "good personality" and "acceptable ideology" elicit confidence and catharsis so that, by unspecified nonverbal influences, the patient is helped toward "personality-reintegration."

R. White (1952): An interested, friendly, and permissive therapist induces expressions of feeling, interprets them transferentially, and thus elicits new behavior.

Jerome Frank (1961, 1972): An attractive setting and a "trusting and expectant therapist-patient relationship" lead to sufficient emotional arousal for the patient to accept a "therapeutical ritual" and a compatible "myth" as to his difficulties with which to explore more successful reality experiences despite his previous "demoralization." Frank (1978) adds: "Our psychotherapeutic literature has contained precious little on the redemption value of suffering, acceptance of one's lot in life, filial piety, adherence to tradition, self-restraint and moderation."

Judd Marmor (1962, 1968, 1979; Marmor and Woods, 1980): A good patient-therapist relationship and implicit emotional catharsis and support encourage identification with the therapist, whose suggestions and persuasions, combined with cognitive (re-) learning and operant (re-) conditioning lead to reality testing and adaptations.

R.J. Corsini (1966): The therapeutic factors are acceptance ("cohesion"), interaction, instillation of hope, catharsis, guidance, learning, existential insight, and altruism.

S. Garfield (1971): A sympathetic, nonmoralizing healer establishes an emotional relationship that promotes catharsis and understanding, leading to reorientation of conduct.

E. Fuller Torrey (1972): The socially designated therapist explains "what is wrong" and by various modalities analogous to faith healing fulfills the patient's expectations of treatment.

Hans Strupp (1973a, 1973b): A therapist with "tact, maturity and a firm belief in his ability to help" encourages a cooperative patient's "honest self-scrutiny" through interpretation of unconscious material and by suggestion, persuasion, and personal example manipulates deterrents or rewards so as to improve the patient's behavior in the "here and now."

P.A. Dewald (1976): The therapeutic relationship helps alleviate anxiety through catharsis, abreaction, and exploration of basic drives, thus clarifying defensive, regressive, and other mechanisms, including identification with the therapist, thereby leading to personality changes, which are enhanced by external reinforcements.

Toksoz B. Karasu (1977): The "therapeutic troika" comprises cognitive mastery, affective experiencing, and behavioral modification.

W. Tseng and W. McDermott (1979): A properly qualified "sensitive, empathetic and benevolent" therapist operating in a therapeutic atmosphere (as to "dress, milieu, license," etc.) orients the expectant patient cognitively and emotionally to a healing rationale and then prescribes changes in conduct which the patient variably implements.

L. Wolberg (1979): Therapeutic influences are derived from "the relationship position" (i.e., client-centered, existential, etc.) in which the receptive, empathetic, helpful attitude of the therapist is in itself sufficiently salutory; from "the reward/punishment position" in which maladaptive behaviors are pragmatically "reconditioned"; and/or from the "cognitive position," which requires that repressed early experiences be recalled and "interpreted" before conscious "insight" can produce permanent personality change. Directed communication with a trusted therapist establishes a productive learning relationship in which the patient's difficulties are verbally or manipulatively elucidated so that, despite problems of resistance, transference, and countertransference, compliant insight and operant (re-) conditioning lead to changes in behavior for constant review.

Other authors add various ancillary parameters such as reciprocal inhibition (Wolpe, 1958), Zen meditation (Ben-Ave, 1959), operant reconditioning (Skinner, 1971), cognitive learning (Beck, 1976), social modeling (Bandura, 1977), psychodynamic motivation (Silverman, 1979), crisis mobilization (Speck and Reuveni, 1980), dyadic or group monitoring (Burton, 1980), stress relief (Horowitz et al., 1980), and biodynamic integrations (Masserman, 1955, 1966, 1973, 1974, 1975, 1978, 1980, 1981).

CODA

Ideally, all therapies designed to alleviate somatic dysfunctions, psychosocial maladaptations, or existential anxieties should use every medical, environmental, and psychosocial means to relieve somatic distress; every ethical form of influence to encourage patients to explore modes of conduct which they will ultimately find more satisfactory and profitable; and to assist them in evolving a philosophy of life in which they can find greater measures of well-being, creativity, security, and metapsychologic serenity. However, it would be presumptuous to specify in greater detail how every mode of therapy reviewed in this volume could be exclusively subsumed under one or another of the seven parameters outlined above; there would be too much dovetailing and overlapping rather than precise fits. As discussed in Chapter 1, comprehensive treatment must be exquisitely individualized as to age, physical state, education, intellectual level, familial and economic status, cultural and religious orientations, special talents and potentialities, treatment objectives, and many other factors and contingencies. How each therapist, acting as clinician, social ombudsman, and philosophic mentor, combines elements of various parameters of influence constitutes his or her unique therapeutic craft. Analysis of the interrelated vectors of physical, psychosocial, and metapsychologic influences can then lead to a more comprehensive rationale for, and more specific and effective applications of, various modalities of psychiatric therapy.

REFERENCES

Bandura A: Social Learning Theory. Englewood Cliffs, NJ, Prentice-Hall, 1977

Beck AT: Cognitive Therapy and the Emotional Disorders. New York, International Universities Press, 1976

Ben-Ave A: Zen buddhism, in An American Handbook of Psychiatry. Edited by Arieti S. New York, Basic Books, 1959

Bleuler M: The long-term course of the schizophrenic psychoses. Psychol Med 4:244-259, 1979

Burton A: Monitoring therapy, in Current Psychiatric Therapies, vol 19. Edited by Masserman JH. New York, Grune & Stratton, 1980

Ciompi L: Long-term study of schizophrenics. Schizophr Bull 6:606-618, 1980

Corsini RJ: Roleplaying in Psychotherapy. Chicago, Aldine, 1966

Dewald PA: Psychotherapy: A Dynamic Approach. New York, Basic Books, 1976

Frank JD: Psychotherapy and the Human Predicament. New York, Schocken, 1978

Frank JD (ed): Effective Ingredients of Successful Therapy. New York, Jason Aronson, 1972

Frank JD: Persuasion and Healing. Baltimore, Johns Hopkins Press, 1961

Garfield S: Research in clinical variables, in Handbook of Psychotherapy and Behavior Change. Edited by Bergin AE, Garfield S. New York, John Wiley & Sons, 1971

Harding CM, Brooks GW: Longitudinal assessment of schizophrenics discharged 20 years ago. Psychiatric Journal of the University of Ottawa 5:274-278, 1980

Horowitz MJ, Kelner H, Kaltreider N, et al: Signs and symptoms of post traumatic stress disorder. Arch Gen Psychiatry 37:85-92, 1980

Huber G, Gross G, Schüttler R, et al: Longitudinal studies of schizophrenic patients. Schizophr Bull 6:592-605, 1980

Karasu TB: Psychotherapies: an overview. Am J Psychiatry 134:851, 1977

Marmor J, Woods S: Psychodynamic and Behavior Therapies. New York, Plenum, 1980

Marmor J: Changes in psychoanalytic treatment. J Am Acad Psychoanal 7:34-357, 1979

Marmor J (ed): Modern Psychoanalysis. New York, Basic Books, 1968

Marmor J: Common denominators in psychoanalytic schools, in Science and Psychoanalysis, vol 5. Edited by Masserman JH. New York, Grune & Stratton, 1962

Masserman JH: The behavior therapies, in Current Psychiatric Therapies, vol 20. Edited by Masserman JH. New York, Grune & Stratton, 1981

Masserman JH: Biodynamics, in Comprehensive Textbook of Psychiatry, 3rd ed. Edited by Kaplan HI, Freedman AM, Sadock BJ. Baltimore, Williams & Wilkins Co, 1980

Masserman JH: Threescore and thirteen psychiatric therapies: an integration, in Current Psychiatric Therapies, vol 17. Edited by Masserman JH. New York, Grune & Stratton, 1978

Masserman JH: Myth, mystic and metapsychiatry, in Psychiatry and Mysticism. Edited by Dean SR. Chicago, Nelson-Hall, 1975

Masserman JH: Psychiatric syndromes and modes of therapy, in Serial Handbook of Psychiatry, vol 2. New York, Stratton Intercontinental Medical Book Corp, 1974

Masserman JH: Theory and Therapy in Dynamic Psychiatry. New York, Jason Aronson, 1973

Masserman JH: The biodynamic roots of psychoanalysis, in Frontiers of Psychoanalysis. Edited by Marmor J. New York, Basic Books, 1966

Masserman JH: Practice of Dynamic Psychiatry. Philadelphia, WB Saunders, 1955

Rosenzweig S: Common factors in psychotherapy. Am J Orthopsychiatry. 6:412-415, 1936

Schwab JJ: Psychiatric manifestations of organic diseases, in Current Psychiatric Therapies, vol 21. Edited by Masserman JH. New York, Grune & Stratton, 1982

Silverman HL: The unconscious fantasy as therapeutic agent in psychoanalytic treatment. J Am Acad Psychoanal 2:184-218, 1979

Skinner BF: Beyond Freedom and Dignity. New York, Alfred A Knopf, 1971

Speck RV, Reuveni U: Treating the family in time of crisis, in Current Psychiatric Therapies, vol 19. Edited by Masserman JH. New York, Grune & Stratton, 1980

Strupp HH: Psychotherapy: Clinical Research and Theoretical Issues. New York, Jason Aronson, 1973a

Strupp HH: On the basic ingredients of psychotherapy. J Consult Clin Psychol 41:1-8, 1973b

Torrey EF: The Mind Game. New York, Emerson, 1972

Tseng WS, McDermott WJ: Triaxial family classification. J Am Acad Child Psychiatry 18:22-27, 1979

White RW: Lives in Progress. New York, Dryden, 1952

Wolberg LR: Techniques of Psychotherapy, 3rd ed. New York, Grune & Stratton, 1979

Wolpe J: Psychotherapy by Reciprocal Inhibition. Stanford, Calif, Stanford University Press, 1958

Index